Disease Management

Michael D Randall

MA, PhD
Senior Lecturer in Pharmacology
University of Nottingham Medical School
Nottingham, UK

Karen E Neil

BPharm (Hons), PhD, MRPharmS
Special Lecturer in Clinical Pharmacology
University of Nottingham Medical School
Nottingham, UK

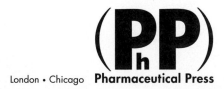

London • Chicago Pharmaceutical Press

Published by the Pharmaceutical Press
Publications division of the Royal Pharmaceutical Society of Great Britain

1 Lambeth High Street, London SE1 7JN, UK
100 South Atkinson Road, Suite 206, Grayslake, IL 60030-7820, USA

 is a trade mark of Pharmaceutical Press

First published 2003

Text design by Barker/Hilsdon, Lyme Regis, Dorset
Typeset by Type Study, Scarborough, North Yorkshire
Printed in Great Britain by The Bath Press, Bath

ISBN 0 85369 523 7

This book is dedicated to our other halves, Clare and Geoff, and to Thomas and Tamsin Randall.

Contents

Preface

OUR AIM IS TO PUT PHARMACOLOGY, which is being learnt or was learnt some time ago, into the context of clinical practice. We believe that this book will be of use to later-year pharmacy students who are encountering clinical pharmacy and pharmacology for the first time, and to pre-registration pharmacists who are putting their training into practice, and will be of general interest to pharmacists in practice. However, the prescribing role of other healthcare professions is likely to expand and we believe that *Disease Management* will also prove a useful resource for introducing and dealing with important issues associated with medicines management.

Disease Management has grown from a new course in clinical pharmacy and pharmacology (Disease and the Goals of Treatment) with which we have been involved at the University of Nottingham Pharmacy School. In that course, we have used a case study-based approach, coupled to summary lectures, to introduce important therapeutic areas. In doing this we have become aware of the value of a disease-based approach to learning. In *Disease Management* we have sought to build on the course by taking common diseases such as diabetes, hypertension, asthma, depression and peptic ulceration, and dealing with the therapeutic issues. The structure we have adopted is to provide a brief outline of the disease characteristics and clinical features. We have generally worked on the basis that diagnosis is beyond the scope of this book but have provided clinical features, particularly in the context of alerting symptoms for referral. These are followed by brief accounts of the pharmacology of the agents used to manage the conditions. Where guidelines exist and are in widespread use, we have incorporated brief summaries. The reader is of course referred to the more detailed guidance available and should also recognise that there are currently a wealth of resources which provide clinical guidance, such as Prodigy, National Service Frameworks (NSFs) and the National Institute of Clinical Excellence (NICE).

We have focused on drug choice and have taken a holistic approach to recognise that a patient may have several related or unrelated conditions. For example, rational drug choice in hypertension should be based on managing the hypertension without affecting other concurrent conditions such as asthma. Similarly, drug interactions represent an important therapeutic challenge and here we have attempted to highlight important examples of interactions and how they may be dealt with. Given the plethora of information on drug interactions we have largely drawn on *Drug Interactions* by Stockley (2002) for information, as this provides an evidence-based approach with considered advice.

The topics of drug choice are intended to enable the reader to appreciate the rationale behind logical prescribing and advice in medicines management. We have also considered the patient rather than the disease and here we have produced some points in which patients should be counselled regarding their disease and their drug treatment.

Our initial concept was to produce a short textbook focused on primary care but we now believe that we have produced an introduction to the management of diseases which are commonly encountered in, but not exclusive to, primary care. As such, we believe that *Disease Management* will provide a useful generalist introduction to medicines management.

Reference

Stockley I H (2002). *Drug Interactions*, 6th edn. London: Pharmaceutical Press.

General reading

In producing this book we have used an extensive range of excellent standard textbooks and reference sources. These are listed here both as acknowledgement and to enable the reader to carry out further reading. More specific references, further reading and resources are provided in each chapter.

General medicine

Haslett C, Chilvers E R, Hunter J A A *et al.* (1999). *Davidson's Principles and Practice of Medicine*, 18th edn. Edinburgh: Churchill Livingstone.

Hope R A, Longmore J M, McManus S K *et al.* (1998). *Oxford Handbook of Clinical Medicine*, 4th edn. Oxford: Oxford University Press.

Kumar P, Clark M (2002). *Clinical Medicine*, 5th edn. Edinburgh: W B Saunders.

Basic and clinical pharmacology

Grahame-Smith D G, Aronson J K (2002). *Oxford Textbook of Clinical Pharmacology and Drug Therapy*, 3rd edn. Oxford: Oxford University Press.

Hardman J G, Limbird L E, Goodman Gilman A (eds) (2001). *Goodman & Gilman's The Pharmacological Basis of Therapeutics*. New York: McGraw-Hill.

Page C, Curtis M, Sutter M *et al.* (2002). *Integrated Pharmacology*, 2nd edn. Edinburgh: Mosby.

Rang H P, Dale M, Ritter J M (1999). *Pharmacology*, 4th edn. Edinburgh: Churchill Livingstone.

Waller D G, Renwick A G, Hillier K (2001). *Medical Pharmacology and Therapeutics*. Edinburgh: W B Saunders.

Clinical pharmacy

Blenkinsopp A, Paxton P (2002). *Symptoms in the Pharmacy*, 4th edn. Oxford: Blackwell Science.

Edwards C, Stillman P (2000). *Minor Illness or Major Disease?* 3rd edn. London: Pharmaceutical Press.

Green R J, Harris N D (2000). *Pathology and Therapeutics for Pharmacists*. London: Pharmaceutical Press.

Harman R J (ed.) (2001). *Handbook of Pharmacy Health Education*, 2nd edn. London: Pharmaceutical Press.

Harman R J (ed.) (1990). *Handbook of Pharmacy Health-Care*. London: Pharmaceutical Press.

Lee A (ed.) (2001). *Adverse Drug Reactions*. London: Pharmaceutical Press.

Lee A, Inch S, Finnigan D (2000). *Therapeutics in Pregnancy and Lactation*. Oxon: Radcliffe Medical Press.

McGhee M (2000). *A Guide to Laboratory Investigations*, 3rd edn. Oxford: Radcliffe Medical Press.

Stockley I H (2002). *Drug Interactions*, 6th edn. London: Pharmaceutical Press.

Walker R, Edwards C (1999). *Clinical Pharmacy and Therapeutics*, 2nd edn. Edinburgh: Churchill Livingstone.

Wills S (1997). *Drugs of Abuse*. London: Pharmaceutical Press.

Dietary supplements and clinical nutrition

Barnes J, Anderson L A, Phillipson J D (2002). *Herbal Medicines*, 2nd edn. London: Pharmaceutical Press.

Kayne S B (2002). *Complementary Therapies for Pharmacists*. London: Pharmaceutical Press.

Mason P (2000). *Nutrition and Dietary Advice in the Pharmacy,* 2nd edn. Oxford: Blackwell Science.

Mason P (2001). *Dietary Supplements,* 2nd edn. London: Pharmaceutical Press.

Morrison G, Hark L (1999). *Medical Nutrition and Disease,* 2nd edn. Blackwell Science.

Online resources

Bandolier is an excellent site with extensive summaries of recent clinical trials and experiments and is at www.jr2.ox.ac.uk/bandolier/ (accessed 4 December 2002).

British National Formulary may be accessed and interacted with at www.BNF.org.uk (accessed 4 December 2002).

Cochrane Collaboration for access to systematic reviews of healthcare interventions at www.cochrane.org/ (accessed 4 December 2002).

Department of Health is at www.doh.gov.uk (accessed 4 December 2002).

Electronic Medicines Compendium, for user-friendly access to summary of product characteristics and patient information leaflets and available at www.emc.vhn.net/ (accessed 4 December 2002).

Medicines Control Agency is at www.open.gov. uk/mca contains the latest information on adverse drug reactions and withdrawal of drugs (accessed 4 December 2002).

Medicines information is available for healthcare professionals at www.ukmi.nhs.uk/ and www.

druginfozone.org, with daily news headlines available by e-mail (accessed 4 December 2002).

NHS centre for reviews and dissemination is a source of searchable databases including systematic reviews (DARE), economic evaluation of healthcare interventions (NHSEED) and assessment of healthcare technology (HTA) at www.nhscrd.york.ac.uk/ (accessed 4 December 2002).

NICE is at www.nice.org.uk, which is the site of the National Institute of Clinical Excellence, providing guidance on prescribing policies (accessed 4 December 2002).

National Patient Safety Agency (www.npsa.org.uk) for information regarding adverse incidents in healthcare and the latest safety alerts (accessed 4 December 2002).

Pharmacy abbreviations: a searchable site of pharmacy abbreviations is available at www.pharma-lexicon. com (accessed 4 December 2002).

Prodigy is at www.prodigy.nhs.uk which is an excellent site, providing comprehensive details of disease management (accessed 4 December 2002).

Public health laboratory service www.phls.co.uk/ for information and evidence-based guidelines relating to infectious disease (accessed 4 December 2002).

SIGN for access to Scottish evidence-based clinical guidelines via www.sign.ac.uk/ (accessed 4 December 2002).

Virtual Hospital www.vh.org is a general medical site with a good dermatology section. American recommendations are not necessarily the same as those in the UK (accessed 4 December 2002).

http://medicine.iupui.edu/flockhart/ provides specialist information on drug interactions and cytochrome P450 (accessed 4 December 2002).

Note to the reader

In producing this book we have attempted to provide a logical background to disease management. Whilst we have summarised some key guidelines, this book is not intended to provide definitive guidance and the reader should of course consult appropriate national and local guidelines. The examples of drug interactions, adverse drug reactions and counselling points are not exhaustive and are included to illustrate common or important examples. Similarly, *Disease Management* is not intended to replace professional experience and the reader is reminded of the need to consult the latest information presented in the latest *British National Formulary,* summary of product characteristics and evidence-based resources for the latest drug information.

The case studies may deliberately contain less than ideal regimens and are intended to illustrate important therapeutic issues. Once again, the reader is reminded of the importance of consulting the *British National Formulary*.

Acknowledgements

In producing *Disease Management* we are grateful to a number of colleagues who have provided comments on our drafts. In particular, we are indebted to Professor Tony Avery, Professor of Primary Health Care at the University of Nottingham Medical School and a general practitioner, who commented on much of the clinical content. We are also extremely grateful to Dr Guy Mansford, a Nottinghamshire general practitioner, and to Mrs Katie Grundy, a community pharmacist, for the much appreciated comments on many of the chapters. We would like to thank Professor Dave Kendall and Dr Ivan Stockley for their encouragement and shared enthusiasm for pharmacology. We should also like to thank Dr Tony Short for introducing us to the value of case study based teaching.

In addition we would like to thank the many colleagues within the University of Nottingham Medical and Pharmacy Schools who have also provided detailed comments and criticisms on individual chapters: Dr Claire Anderson, Reader in Pharmacy Practice; Sandra Beatty, Pharmacist Teacher Practitioner; Dr Sue Chan, Lecturer in Cell Signalling; Dr Vicky Chapman, Lecturer in Pharmacology; Dr Dick Churchill, General Practitioner and Clinical Lecturer in General Practice; Dr Jeff Fry, Reader in Molecular Toxicology; Dr Katie Hewitt, Research Fellow; Dr Roger Knaggs; Professor Charles Marsden, Professor of Neuropharmacology; Dr Rob Mason, Senior Lecturer in Neuroscience; Dr Kishor Patel, Research Registrar; Dr Nick Pierce, Consultant; Dr Nick Shaw, Senior Lecturer; Dr Gary Whitlock. We are also indebted to Dr Anna Cadogan; Anne Lee, Principal Pharmacist, Glasgow Royal Infirmary; Dr Swaran P Singh, Senior Lecturer in Community Psychiatry, St George's Hospital, London; Miss Alison Wallace, Preregistration Pharmacist, Alder Hey Children's Hospital, Liverpool and Mrs Louise Walmsley, Health Visitor, Nottingham, for their most helpful comments and advice. We are indebted to the staff of the Pharmaceutical Press and especially Paul Weller and Tamsin Cousins for their invaluable assistance and advice.

Despite the extensive help that we have received, any of the errors and omissions within *Disease Management* are the sole responsibility of the authors and we would very much appreciate any constructive comments directed to michael.randall@nottingham.ac.uk or k.neil@ntlworld.com.

About the authors

Michael Randall read natural sciences at the University of Cambridge and specialised in Pharmacology. After his first degree, he remained at Cambridge, carrying out research into the vascular actions of the endothelial factors, nitric oxide and the endothelins, and obtained a PhD in cardiovascular pharmacology. He was then a postdoctoral research fellow at the University of Wales College of Medicine, continuing research into vascular pharmacology. In 1993 he was appointed to a lectureship, and subsequently a senior lectureship in pharmacology at the University of Nottingham Medical School, teaching pharmacology to both medical and pharmacy students. He is also on the editorial board of the *British Journal of Pharmacology*.

Karen Neil studied pharmacy at the University of Nottingham, before completing preregistration training based at Broadgreen Hospital in Liverpool. She then returned to Nottingham to develop an interest in pharmacology gained during her final year as an undergraduate. She researched a variety of mechanisms involved in mediating second-messenger cross-talk, with particular interest in pathways associated with beta-adrenoceptors, nitric oxide and phosphodiesterases, and achieved a PhD in molecular pharmacology. The application of pharmacology to clinical pharmacy beckoned and this developed from experience gained as a community pharmacist and researcher investigating adverse drug events and particularly drug interactions. She has been involved in teaching clinical pharmacy to pharmacy undergraduates, using problem-based learning, for a number of years.

Abbreviations

ACE angiotensin-converting enzyme
ADH antidiuretic hormone
ADP adenosine diphosphate
ADR adverse drug reaction
AED antiepileptic drug
AF atrial fibrillation
AIDs acquired immune deficiency syndrome
AIN acute interstitial nephritis
ALP alkaline phosphatase
ALT alanine transaminase
AMP adenosine monophosphate
ANP atrial natriuretic peptide
APTT activated partial thromboblastin time
ARDS adult respiratory distress syndrome
5-ASA 5-aminosalicylate
ASH Action on Smoking and Health
AST aspartate transferase
AT angiotensin
ATP adenine triphosphate
AUC area under the curve
AV atrioventricular
BCG bacille Calmette-Guérin
b.d. bis die (twice daily)
BDP beclometasone dipropionate
BHF British Heart Foundation
BMI body mass index
BNF *British National Formulary*
BP blood pressure
BTS British Thoracic Society
C concentration
CABG coronary artery bypass grafting
CAD coronary artery disease
CAI cholesterol absorption inhibitors
cAMP cyclic adenosine-3'-5'-monophosphate
CAPD continuous ambulatory peritoneal dialysis
CAPP Captopril Prevention Project
CBT cognitive behaviour therapy
CCK cholecystokinin

CDH chronic daily headache
CFC chlorofluorocarbon
cGMP cyclic guanosine-3'-5'-monophosphate
CGRP calcitonin gene-related peptide
CHAOS Cambridge Heart Antioxidant Study
CHD coronary heart disease
CHF chronic heart failure
CK creatine kinase
CL clearance
CNS central nervous system
CO_2 carbon dioxide
CoA coenzyme A
COMA Committee on Medical Aspects of Food and Nutrition Policy
CONSENSUS Cooperative North Scandinavian Enalapril Survival Study
COPD chronic obstructive pulmonary disease
COX cyclooxygenase
CPK creatine phosphokinase
CRF corticotrophin-releasing factor
CRP C-reactive protein
CSM Committee on Safety of Medicines
CTZ chemoreceptor trigger zone
CVA cerebrovascular accident
DCCT Diabetes Control and Complications Trial
DCT distal convoluted tubule
DDT dichlorodiphenyltrichloroethane
DEET diethyltoluamide (diethylmethylbenza-mide)
DEXA dual-energy X-ray absorptiometry
DHA docosahexanoic acid
DHEA dehydroepiandrosterone
DHP dihydropyridine
DIG Digitalis Intervention Group
DMARD disease-modifying antirheumatoid drug
DNA deoxyribonucleic acid
DOH Department of Health (UK)

DSM-IV *Diagnostic and Statistical Manual of Mental Disorders*
DVT deep-vein thrombosis
e.c. enteric-coated
ECG electrocardiogram
ECT electroconvulsive therapy
EEG electroencephalogram
EPA eicosapentaenoic acid
EPO erythropoietin; evening primrose oil
ESR erythrocyte sedimentation rate
ET endothelin
F bioavailability
FBC full blood count
FDA (US) Food and Drug Administration
FEV$_1$ forced expiratory volume in the first second
FVC forced vital capacity
GABA gamma-aminobutyric acid
GAD general anxiety disorder
GFR glomerular filtration rate
GGT gamma-glutamyl transferase
G6PD glucose-6-phosphate dehydrogenase
GI gastrointestinal
GLUT glucose transporters
GORD gastro-oesophageal reflux disease
GP general practitioner
GSK-3 glycogen synthase kinase-3
GTN glyceryl trinitrate
H histamine
Hb haemoglobin
HbA$_{1c}$ glycated haemoglobin
HCT haematocrit
HDL high-density lipoprotein
HIV human immunodeficiency virus
HMG hydroxymethylglutaryl
HOPE Heart Outcomes Prevention Evaluation
HOT Hypertension Optimal Treatment
HPA hypothalamic-pituitary-adrenal axis
5-HT 5-hydroxytryptamine (serotonin)
HRT hormone replacement therapy
IARC International Agency for Research on Cancer
IBS irritable bowel syndrome
IBW ideal body weight
ICD-10 *International Statistical Classification of Diseases and Related Health Problems*, 10th edn
IDDM insulin-dependent diabetes mellitus
Ig immunoglobulin
IHD ischaemic heart disease

i.m. intramuscular
INR international normalised ratio
IONA Impact Of Nicorandil in Angina
IP$_3$ inositol triphosphate
IV intravenous
JVP jugular venous pressure
K$_{ATP}$ ATP-sensitive potassium channels
LDH lactate dehydrogenase
LDL low-density lipoprotein
LFT liver function test
LIFE Losartan Intervention for Endpoint Reduction in Hypertension
LMWH low-molecular-weight heparin
LVH left ventricular hypertrophy
MAOI monoamine oxidase inhibitor
MCA Medicines Control Agency
MCH mean corpuscular haemoglobin
MCV mean corpuscular (cell) volume
MDI metered dose inhaler
MDMA 3,4-methylenedioxymethamfetamine or ecstasy
MI myocardial infarction
MMR measles, mumps and rubella
MODY maturity-onset diabetes of the young
MOH medication overuse headache
MRSA methicillin-resistant *Staphylococcus aureus*
MS multiple sclerosis
NACC National Association for Colitis and Crohn's Disease
NANC non-adrenergic non-cholinergic
NARI noradrenaline (norepinephrine) reuptake inhibitors
NaSSAs noradrenergic and specific serotonergic antidepressants
N&V nausea and vomiting
NHS National Health Service
NICE National Institute of Clinical Excellence
NIDDM non-insulin-dependent diabetes mellitus
NK neurokinin
NMDA *N*-methyl-D-aspartate
NPA National Pharmaceutical Association
NPC National Prescribing Centre
NRT nicotine replacement therapy
NSAIDs non-steroidal anti-inflammatory drugs
NSF National Service Framework
NSP non-starch polysaccharides
OA osteoarthritis

OCD obsessive compulsive disorder
o.d. omni die (daily)
o.m. omni mane (every morning)
o.n. omni nocte (every night)
ORT oral rehydration therapy
OTC over-the-counter
PAF platelet-activating factor
PCV packed cell volume
PDEI phosphodiesterase inhibitor
PE pulmonary embolism
PEF peak expiratory flow
PG prostaglandin
PGRs prandial glucose regulators
PI phosphatidyl inositol
PLA$_2$ phospholipase A$_2$
PMR patient medication record
POM prescription-only medicine
PPAR peroxisome proliferator-activated receptors
PPI proton pump inhibitor
PRISM Platelet Receptor Inhibition in Ischemic Syndrome Management
PROGRESS Perindopril Protection Against Recurrent Stroke Study
p.r.n. pro re nata (when required)
PSA prostate-specific antigen
PTCA percutaneous translumenal coronary angioplasty
PTH parathyroid hormone
PUFA polyunsaturated fatty acids
q.d.s. quater die sumendus (four times a day)
RA rheumatoid arthritis
RAAS renin–angiotensin–aldosterone system
RAS renin–angiotensin system
RBC red blood cell
REIN Ramipril Efficacy In Nephropathy
REM rapid eye movement
RICE rest, ice, compression and elevation
RIMA reversible inhibitor of MAO-A
RPSGB Royal Pharmaceutical Society of Great Britain
4S Scandinavian Simvastatin Survival Study
SACN Scientific Advisory Committee on Nutrition

SAD seasonal affective disorder
SERM selective oestrogen receptor modulator
SIADH syndrome of inappropriate secretion of antidiuretic hormone
SIGN Scottish Intercollegiate Guidelines Network
SJS Stevens–Johnson syndrome
SLE systemic lupus erythematosus
SM smooth muscle
SMAC Standing Medical Advisory Committee
SNRI serotonin–noradrenaline (norepinephrine) reuptake inhibitors
SPC summary of product characteristics
SRM serotonin receptor modulator
SSRI selective serotonin reuptake inhibitor
T$_3$ triiodothyronine
T$_4$ thyroxine
TB tuberculosis
TCA tricyclic antidepressant
TDM therapeutic drug monitoring
t.d.s. ter die sumendus (three times a day)
TEN toxic epidermal necrolysis
TENS transcutaneous electrical stimulation
TFT thyroid function test
THC Δ^9-tetrahydrocannabinol
TIA transient ischaemic attack
TNF-α tumour necrosis factor-α
TPN total parenteral nutrition
tRNA transfer ribonucleic acid
TrT troponin T
TSH thyroid stimulating hormone
Tx thromboxane
U and Es urea and electrolytes
UKPDS UK Prospective Diabetes Study
UT urinary tract
UTI urinary tract infection
UV ultraviolet
V$_d$ volume of distribution
VLDL very-low-density lipoprotein
VSM vascular smooth muscle
VTE venous thromboembolism
WBC white blood cells
WFSBP World Federation of Societies of Biological Psychiatry
WHO World Health Organization

Part A

The patient

1

Signs and symptoms

Symptoms and patient histories in the pharmacy

Role

The pharmacist has a central role in assessing a patient's complaint or condition, with a view to providing information, recommending appropriate treatment or referring patients to their general practitioner (GP). Indeed the pharmacist may be the first health professional consulted by many patients, especially as an appointment is not required.

The consultation

Unlike the hospital doctor or GP, the community pharmacist is unlikely to have the luxury of carrying out a full medical history and may not have access to the patient's medical records. The consultation may well be happening in a busy shop. Hence the pharmacist has to establish the relevant facts, to differentiate between minor complaints and potentially serious conditions and make a judgement or even diagnosis 'on the spot'. First, the patient must be identified, and once this is established the pharmacist might then ask the person to explain what the problem is and this may be followed by more specific questions related to the condition. Throughout the interview, the pharmacist should observe the person (if this is the patient) to determine 'how ill he or she appears' and perhaps to observe for obvious physical signs, which might point to underlying disease such as jaundice in liver disease. The pharmacist should also attempt to make a judgement as to the educational background or medical knowledge of the person, so that the questioning and any subsequent counselling may be appropriately phrased. A patient volunteering specific facts or requesting a specific medicine may reveal medical knowledge or a lack of it.

Establishing the facts

The questioning should be directed towards aiding a diagnosis or making a judgement as to the need for referral or over-the-counter (OTC) treatment. Relevant lines of questioning might be related to (Edwards and Stillman, 2000):

3

- the nature of the symptoms
- the severity of the symptoms
- the duration of the symptoms
- the location of the symptoms
- accompanying symptoms
- provoking factors
- alleviating factors
- social factors (if relevant)
- a drug history, with particular attention to the use of OTC treatments

The drug history may be relevant to the current symptoms or influence the recommendation of OTC medicines or referral. In addition, it is clearly important for the pharmacist to establish if the patient is suffering from a previously diagnosed chronic condition such as diabetes mellitus, asthma, chronic obstructive pulmonary disease (COPD), epilepsy, liver disease, renal disease and cardiovascular disease or receiving long-term treatment, e.g. corticosteroids. It may be that the presenting complaint is associated with this condition or its treatment but this may not be obvious to the patient. Chronic conditions will also influence the use of OTC medicines and the importance of referral. In the case of women of child-bearing age it is important to establish if the patient could be pregnant.

The above may be summarised by the popular mnemonic, WWHAM (Blenkinsopp and Paxton, 2002):

Who is the patient?
What are the symptoms?
How long have the symptoms been present?
Action taken, medicines tried?
Medicines taken for other conditions?

Once the presenting complaint has been established, the pharmacist should use professional skills to select relevant searching questions. For example, a patient may complain of a cough and an opening and open-ended question might be:

'Tell me about the cough'

and, depending on the response, detailed questioning may enable the pharmacist to determine the underlying nature of the complaint (and thus the course of action). For example, the questioning might proceed:

What are the symptoms?

'Is there any sputum?'

'What colour is the sputum?'

'Have you noticed any blood in the sputum?' or ask the patient to describe the sputum.

Indeed, the last question is a more indirect approach than the question 'Have you coughed up any blood?' Using appropriate questions is important as patients may wish to deny to themselves sinister symptoms such as haemoptysis or by contrast they may not appreciate their importance.

How long?

'How long have you had the cough?'

Action taken, medicines tried? Medicines taken for other conditions?

'Are you taking any medicines prescribed by a doctor or bought from a pharmacy?'

This essential question enables the identification of iatrogenic problems such as drug-induced blood dyscrasias in patients prescribed immuno-suppressants or a cough induced by an angiotensin-converting enzyme (ACE) inhibitor. It may also identify problems where a drug has already been prescribed but the treatment has failed. Medicines taken for other conditions should also be considered. A drug history is imperative when OTC medication is recommended, allowing the exclusion of contraindications and avoidance of drug interactions.

Additional relevant questions might be:

'Have you ever smoked?' This is a more searching question than 'Do you smoke?' as the person may have given up yesterday (perhaps in response to the symptom) and the answer would be no! Alcohol consumption is also likely to be under-reported by patients.

'Are you having any difficulty in breathing?'

'Have you noticed a wheezing noise or rattle?'

The outcome

The interview should enable the pharmacist to make a reasonable attempt at identifying the condition and then to decide on the appropriate course of action, whether it is advice, treatment or referral. If the outcome is that the pharmacist believes it to be in the patient's best interests to consult the GP, the importance of this should be emphasised but the pharmacist should not unduly worry the patient. It is, however, important to give an indication of the urgency of referral. For example, a patient presenting with cystitis and with systemic symptoms such as fever should be seen urgently rather than wait for the next available appointment.

Signs and symptoms

In dealing with responding to symptoms the reader is referred to *Minor Illness or Major Disease?* by Edwards and Stillman (2000) and *Symptoms in the Pharmacy* by Blenkinsopp and Paxton (2002), which deal with responding to a range of common symptoms.

Symptoms

A symptom is a perceived change in well-being by the patient that may or may not be associated with significant illness. The patient complains of a symptom and it is different from 'normal'. Several symptoms may present together to suggest a disease or exclude a disease. Indeed, they may appear unrelated, e.g. breathlessness and swollen ankles in chronic heart failure. The following are some examples of symptoms:

- cough
- tiredness
- aches
- chest pains
- breathlessness
- indigestion

Signs

A sign is a clinical change in a person, which may be observed by a clinician and indicates a disease. The following are some common examples of signs:

- changes in skin (colour, markings)
- digital clubbing (fingers clubbed in lung and hepatic diseases)
- heart murmurs
- sounds on listening to the lungs (wheezes (rhonchi), crackles (crepitations))
- dullness to percussion of the thorax (changes in sound on tapping)
- changes to the retina
- enlarged lymph nodes

There is obviously some overlap between signs and symptoms as a patient might notice ankle oedema but not realise that it is a significant sign of heart failure.

Important examples of signs and symptoms

Cough

A cough may be a trivial symptom, reflecting a minor ailment, or may point to a serious underlying disease (Table 1.1).

Chest pains

Once again, chest pains represent an important symptom, which may be due to a minor illness or a serious condition, and some common causes are detailed in Table 1.2.

Given the above presentations and diverse conditions, then questioning should be directed towards establishing:

- the location and nature of the pain and additional symptoms
- what provokes the pain?
- what relieves the pain (including the use of OTC medicines)?
- past medical history
- is the patient's GTN in date?

Breathlessness

Similarly, breathlessness may be due to a whole range of conditions and the possible aetiologies include:

- congenital – cystic fibrosis
- infection – chest infection, tuberculosis
- inflammatory – asthma, anaphylaxis

Table 1.1 Some causes of a cough

Underlying condition	Comments
Coryza (cold) (Chapter 18)	Associated with cold symptoms
Acute bronchitis (Chapter 18)	Often following a cold: there may be production of sputum, with wheezing and a temperature
Tracheitis	A dry, rasping and painful cough which is often associated with a viral infection
Pneumonia (Chapter 18)	Infection of the alveoli which leads to sputum (which may be blood-stained, and is often rusty in appearance), breathlessness, pleuritic chest pains and fever
Chronic bronchitis (Chapter 20)	• COPD • Associated with exacerbations • The 'smoker's cough' may herald the onset of COPD
Asthma (Chapter 20)	• May be associated with wheezing and breathlessness • Often a nocturnal cough and this may be the only symptom in a child
Drug-induced (Chapters 11 and 14)	For example, with angiotensin-converting enzyme (ACE) inhibitors
Anxiety	A long-term 'nervous cough'
Foreign body	Associated with recent inhalation of an object
Tuberculosis (Chapter 30)	Associated with tiredness, malaise, weight loss, fever and haemoptysis
Bronchiectasis	• Dilated bronchioles with persistent infections and mucus • Copious amounts of sputum which may be blood-stained
Congestive heart failure (Chapter 14)	Associated with breathlessness and oedema
Lung cancer	A history of smoking associated with haemoptysis. A change in a 'smoker's cough' is a serious alerting symptom

COPD, chronic obstructive pulmonary disease; ACE, angiotensin-converting enzyme.

- neoplastic – carcinoma
- haematological – secondary to anaemia
- psychogenic – panic attacks
- degenerative – COPD
- cardiac – chronic heart failure, acute left ventricular failure, myocardial infarction
- thromboembolic – pulmonary embolism
- functional – in pregnancy, ascent to altitude, obesity
- iatrogenic – bronchospasm secondary to drug treatment (e.g. beta-blockers, non-steroidal anti-inflammatory drugs (NSAIDs)); chronic pulmonary damage (e.g. amiodarone). See Chapter 5
- traumatic – physical damage to the chest

In all cases, the serious nature of the potential conditions should lead to a referral and the key question is the degree of urgency required.

Pain

In considering pain, the following features should be considered:

Onset and duration

For example, a headache of sudden onset may indicate subarachnoid haemorrhage. Alternatively, chronic joint pain may be due to rheumatoid arthritis.

Site and radiation

Poorly localised pain may indicate visceral pain. For example, chest pain radiating to the left arm or jaw may indicate angina or myocardial infarction. Gallbladder pain may be referred to the back or shoulder tip. The pain of appendicitis tends to originate around the umbilicus and then move to the right iliac fossa with tenderness on the right.

Table 1.2   Some causes of chest pains

Underlying condition	Comments
Musculoskeletal in origin (Chapter 28)	Pain may be worse on moving an arm or follows strenuous or unusual exercise. This is a common explanation and is often the default diagnosis
Respiratory (Chapter 20)	The pain is likely to be associated with breathing and to be due to an underlying respiratory disease, e.g. asthma
Pleuritic pains	This may be due to some form of respiratory disease but, if associated with calf swelling, haemoptysis or risk factors for thromboembolism, may point to pulmonary embolism
Gastric origin: peptic ulceration, reflux oesophagitis (Chapter 7)	Here there may be a relationship to food, either being brought on by a meal (reflux oesophagitis) or relieved by food (peptic ulceration). It should be relieved rapidly by antacids In patients over 45 years of age, if this symptom is of recent onset it raises the suspicion of carcinoma, which should be excluded
Angina (Chapter 13)	Angina has the following characteristics which often allow it to be diagnosed by a history: • A crushing feeling in the chest • Often accompanied by pains down the arm (often left) • Pains may be radiating to the jaw • Stable angina is induced by exercise, emotional stress, cold weather or a meal • Unstable angina may occur at rest • It should be relieved by rest (unless unstable) or glyceryl trinitrate (GTN) • Characteristic ECG changes
Myocardial infarction (Chapter 13)	• This must be differentiated from angina and is characteristically severe chest pains, which are not relieved by rest or GTN • May be accompanied by nausea, breathlessness, pallor, sweating and pains down the arms and/or jaw • Often diagnosed by ECG changes and so-called 'cardiac enzymes' • Some patients may experience a silent myocardial infarction, which does not cause chest pains

ECG, electrocardiogram.

Precipitating and relieving factors

A diagnosis of angina is likely if chest pain is brought on by activity and relieved by rest and/or treatment with nitrates. Conversely, chest pain triggered by food, alcohol or posture may be more suggestive of indigestion. Gallbladder pain may follow a fatty meal. Joint pain relieved by exercise may be indicative of osteoarthritis.

Tenderness

Tenderness may indicate tissue damage or injury. The location of tenderness may identify the cause of pain such as appendicitis, fractures or tumours.

Timing

For example, the joint pain associated with rheumatoid arthritis may be worse in the morning.

Preceding events

Preceding events may indicate trauma or, in the case of chest pain, pain at rest may be more suggestive of a myocardial infarction.

Past medical history

Pain in the left upper quadrant may indicate a recurrence of peptic ulcer disease. A history of alcohol abuse may implicate pancreatitis.

Nature

Colicky, constant, sharp or dull, wakening at night may point to the origin and severity of pain. Radiating pain may be visceral or due to a neck problem, ear or dental disease. Swelling, redness and warmth are indicative of inflammation.

Pattern

Intermittent pain associated with movement may indicate injury. The pain of gallstones may follow a pattern linked to the ingestion of fatty food. Continuous pain tends to be associated with chronic pain such as cancer, back pain or be due to infection.

Severity

Due to the subjective nature of pain, a patient's interpretation of pain as the 'worst ever' indicates increased severity. It often helps to rate it on a scale of one to 10.

Associated features

Symptoms such as vomiting, dyspepsia, altered bowel habit, pyrexia or sudden weight loss may help determine underlying causes of pain such as infection, gastric ulceration, irritable bowel syndrome or cancer. Peripheral pain associated with discoloured skin may indicate peripheral neuropathy. Anxious patients may have a lower pain threshold and the psychological component of pain should not be overlooked.

A 'funny turn'

This symptom encompasses a range of events from dizziness to total loss of consciousness which may involve fitting. As one might imagine, the range of events has a wide number of possible causes, including:

- Cardiovascular events such as a cerebrovascular accident (including a transient ischaemic attack), arrhythmias and postural (orthostatic) hypotension, which is particularly prevalent in the elderly and those taking vasodilators or diuretics. Vasovagal syncope (fainting) may involve bradycardia with vasodilatation as a response to fear, pain, emotion or standing for a prolonged period and result in a faint.
- Neurological causes include epilepsy, cerebrovascular accidents, migraine and infections including meningitis.

- Endocrine causes include postural hypotension due to Addison's disease, thyrotoxicosis and diabetes with hypoglycaemia or hyperglycaemia.
- Psychological causes include panic attacks.
- Iatrogenic causes include postural hypotension in those taking vasodilators or diuretics as mentioned above or confusion with benzodiazepines.

In response to a funny turn, the following questions may help to implicate or exclude certain causes:

- What provokes an attack? e.g. flashing lights in certain forms of epilepsy.
- Were there any prodromal symptoms? e.g. an aura in epilepsy.
- Was there loss of consciousness?
- Was there injury? Tongue biting would be consistent with epilepsy.
- Were there any unusual movements? This might implicate epilepsy.
- Was there incontinence? Incontinence of urine is common in epilepsy.
- What colour did the patient go? Extreme pallor during the episode and flushing after the attack might suggest a cardiac cause.
- How did the patient recover? With neurological causes there may be confusion.
- How long did it last?
- Does the patient have a current illness or is he or she receiving any drugs?

Given the potential seriousness of the above causes of a 'funny turn', it is likely that a referral would be made.

Referral

The pharmacist has a major role in responding to symptoms. Initially, the pharmacist should respond with advice and where necessary counterprescribe for 'minor' conditions which would respond to OTC medicines. Compliance problems with prescribed medicines can often be rectified by the pharmacist. Equally, the pharmacist should be able to recognise potentially serious symptoms and refer patients to their GP, National Health Service (NHS) drop-in centres, or in an emergency to a hospital Accident and Emergency department. Consultation via telephone, publications or online resources with NHS Direct is also a valuable source of referral information, triage and algorithms for patients.

In general, referral should be made for patients with potentially serious symptoms, for persistent symptoms and high-risk patients such as:

- babies
- children
- elderly
- diabetics
- pregnant or breast-feeding mothers
- immunocompromised patients

In addition, many other disease states represent high risk (e.g. ischaemic heart disease, epilepsy, COPD, asthma) and deterioration might warrant referral.

One should also be mindful of patients who frequently request OTC medicines for symptomatic relief, as they may be used to hide symptoms, for example the use of OTC H_2-receptor antagonists in peptic ulceration. Another reason to refer would be due to the failure of OTC medicines to control or relieve a condition or requests for OTC medicines which are not covered by their licence. In addition, the following examples of alerting symptoms should prompt a referral.

Gastrointestinal

Some important gastrointestinal referral points are shown in Table 1.3.

Cardiorespiratory

Some important cardiorespiratory referral points are shown in Table 1.4.

Neurological and psychiatric

Some important neurological and psychiatric referral points are shown in Table 1.5.

Others

Some other important referral points are shown in Table 1.6.

The above list of referrals is intended as a list of common examples which should prompt referral to the patient's GP or urgent referral to hospital. Obviously, if there is any doubt then the patient should be referred and, as emphasised in Chapter 5, the pharmacist should be alert to the possibility of patients presenting with an adverse drug reaction. The list is clearly not exhaustive and local referral protocols may already be established with GPs.

CASE STUDIES

Case studies on coughs
A cough may be a trivial symptom, reflecting a minor ailment, but may be associated with serious underlying disease. The following cases are intended to illustrate the possible causes.

Case 1
A 4-year-old boy with a cough as the presenting symptom was taken to the pharmacist. The pharmacist asked the following questions:

- 'Is it nocturnal?' This may point to asthma.
- 'Is there a family history of asthma?' A family history of asthma and/or atopy may suggest asthma.
- 'Is it productive?' This may point to a bacterial chest infection.
- 'Is it productive of vast quantities of sputum?' Large amounts of sputum which may contain blood may point to bronchiectasis.

continued

CASE STUDIES (continued)

- 'Is it a dry cough?' This may point to a simple upper respiratory tract infection.
- 'Is it associated with wheezing?' This may point to bronchiolitis or asthma.
- 'Is he eating and drinking normally?' This may give an indication as to how ill he is.

It was found that the cough was non-productive and of recent onset and a diagnosis of a viral infection was made. Reassurance was given and paracetamol was recommended for any fever and the mother was advised to take the child to the GP if he was no better after 2 weeks or it became worse in that time.

Case 2
In the course of a morning, a number of 60-year-olds present to their GP with coughs and additional questioning went along the lines of:

- 'Have you ever smoked?'
- 'Is it a dry or productive cough?'
- 'How long have you had it?'

Patient A: A productive cough of recent onset with green sputum.

- This is consistent with bacterial infection and a chest infection was diagnosed.

Patient B: A smoker with a productive cough over many years which is worse in winter and the sputum is grey or sometimes green.

- Smoking is a major risk factor for respiratory diseases and a 'smoker's cough' is an early sign of COPD. His present condition is consistent with COPD with an infection. Haemoptysis (coughing up blood) may occur in other serious conditions such as tumour, which should be excluded. An exacerbation of COPD was diagnosed.

Patient C: Smoker with changes in cough characteristics or persistent dry cough and coughing up blood.

- This may be a presenting symptom of carcinoma and other signs (which may include haemoptysis, digital clubbing, pleural pain, weight loss, signs of metastasis, central nervous system changes including fits) are all ominous symptoms of carcinoma. The suspicion of carcinoma was raised.

Patient D: Non-smoker with productive cough, haemoptysis, weight loss, night sweats and risk factor for tuberculosis (TB) (homeless).

- A productive cough is a major respiratory symptom and night sweats are consistent with TB and also Hodgkin's disease. The suspicion of TB was raised.

Patient E: Cough and breathlessness at mild exertion and lying down in bed at night.

- The suspicion of chronic heart failure was raised.

Patient F: Cough whilst taking an ACE inhibitor for chronic heart failure.

- These might point to inadequate treatment or an ACE inhibitor-induced cough.

Table 1.3 Some important gastrointestinal referral points

Leading feature	Features and comments
Mouth ulcers	• Recurrent and/or failure of OTC therapy • Possible ADR • Associated with agents which may cause neutropenia such as carbimazole, carbamazepine and clozapine (Chapter 5)
Swallowing	• Dysphagia (difficulty in swallowing) • Odynophagia (painful swallowing) which is not simply due to a sore throat
Vomiting (Chapters 8 and 9)	• Haematemesis (vomiting blood) – any and urgent referral if profuse. Bleeding may be profuse or present as 'ground coffee' in appearance (Chapter 7) • Symptoms of dehydration such as decreased output of urine, headache and confusion – care in special groups; taking laxatives or diuretics (advise to omit doses). • Nausea of more than 3–4 days
Dyspepsia/'Indigestion' (Chapter 7)	• Indigestion persisting after 2 weeks of OTC H_2-receptor antagonists • Pain consistent with peptic ulceration • Following use of NSAIDs • Prolonged indigestion, also new or changed symptoms in patients over 45 years of age, or alerting symptoms including anorexia, weight loss, anaemia and upper abdominal masses
Bowel habits (Chapter 9)	• Sustained (>2 weeks) alteration in bowel habits (particularly in those over 45 years old) • Passing blood (frank or melaena, black 'tarry' stools) – this may be due to gastrointestinal bleeding • Severe diarrhoea whilst taking antibiotics, especially clindamycin – antibiotics may lead to colitis • Steatorrhoea – significant if not explained by concomitant orlistat • Pale stools
Weight loss	• Weight loss or wasting which is unexplained
Liver problems (Chapter 10)	• Jaundice

OTC, over-the-counter; ADR, adverse drug reaction; NSAIDs, non-steroidal anti-inflammatory drugs.

References

Blenkinsopp A, Paxton P (2002). *Symptoms in the Pharmacy*, 4th edn. Oxford: Blackwell Science.

Edwards C, Stillman, P (2000). *Minor Illness or Major Disease?* 3rd edn. London: Pharmaceutical Press.

Online resource

www.nhsdirect.nhs.uk is the website of NHS Direct, with advice on how patients should respond to symptoms (accessed 4 December 2002).

Table 1.4   Some important cardiorespiratory referral points

Leading feature	Features and comments
Chest pain (Chapter 13)	• Chest pain at rest or on exertion • Chest pain suggesting a myocardial infarction and which is not relieved by nitrates should prompt emergency hospital referral. Consider administering aspirin (150–300 mg)
Breathlessness	• Any of new onset or deterioration • Including breathlessness at night whilst lying down (Chapter 14) • Breathlessness (often wheezy) with signs of anaphylaxis such as urticaria, angioedema with swollen lips or eyelids, should lead to urgent hospital referral (Chapter 19)
Wheezing	• Any
Cough	• Persistent cough of greater than 2–3 weeks, or with a history of bronchitis or green sputum (Chapter 18) • A change in smoker's cough • Persistent dry nocturnal cough in a child, which may indicate asthma (Chapter 20) • Haemoptysis (coughing up blood) • Cough with ACE inhibitors (Chapters 11 and 14), if the cough is intolerable
Symptoms consistent with anaemia	• Any (Chapter 16) – identify possible cause, including use of NSAIDs and associated gastrointestinal bleeding
Dizziness on standing (postural hypotension)	• Especially in patients taking ACE inhibitors, diuretics, alpha-blockers and antipsychotics
Painful unilateral calf swelling	• Especially if accompanied by breathlessness and/or pleuritic pain, this should lead to urgent referral to hospital (Chapter 15)
Ankle swelling	• Any – new or deterioration
Xanthomata	• Yellowish lipid deposits especially on eyelids (xanthelasmata), cornea and tendons (Chapter 12)
Sore throat	• Persistent sore throat (Chapter 18) • Sore throat with rash, fever, enlarged lymph nodes or infected tonsils (Chapter 18) • Sore throat or rashes, especially in patients taking drugs known to cause neutropenia such as carbimazole, clozapine and carbamazepine (Chapter 5)
Sinusitis	• Sinus pain or discharge which does not resolve after 7 days (Chapter 18)

ACE, angiotensin-converting enzyme; NSAIDs, non-steroidal anti-inflammatory drugs.

Table 1.5   Some important neurological and psychiatric referral points

Leading feature	Features and comments
Headache (Chapter 21)	• Headache which is severe, follows injury, or is accompanied by other alerting signs • Recurrent or persistent migraine not relieved by OTC medicines
Seizures or loss of consciousness (Chapter 22)	• Any, including absences
Signs or behaviour pointing to psychiatric disorders	• Any (Chapters 23–26)
Insomnia	• With repeat requests (> 2 weeks) for OTC sleeping remedies (Chapter 25)

GP, general practitioner; OTC, over-the-counter.

Table 1.6   Some other important referral points

Leading feature	Features and comments
Symptoms suggestive of diabetes mellitus (Chapter 33)	• Including polydipsia (increased drinking), polyuria, recurrent thrush, frequent skin infections, ketone breath
Symptoms suggestive of hyperthyroidism (Chapter 34)	• Including tachycardia, palpitations, fine tremor, warm peripheries, bulging eyes
Symptoms suggestive of hypothyroidism (Chapter 34)	• Including tiredness, weight gain, cold intolerance, dry skin and hair, goitre, puffiness around the eyes
Cushingoid symptoms	• Features include moon face, thinning of the skin, easy bruising and central weight gain • Including patients taking corticosteroids
Problems with urination	• Difficulty in passing urine • Blood in urine • Recurrent thrush or cystitis • Urinary dysfunction suggestive of prostatic hypertrophy
Urogenital problems	• Vaginal bleeding; in pregnancy this should lead to urgent referral • Recurrent infections • Urinary dysfunction, including haematuria (passing blood) and prostate problems • Any renal problems
Somatosensory problems	• Eye problems • Eye infections where OTC treatment is not appropriate or is ineffective • Hearing problems • Otitis media not responding to simple analgesia • Disturbances of balance

Continued

Table 1.6 *Continued*

Leading feature	Features and comments
Dermatological problems (Chapter 32)	• Eczema for the first time • Infected eczema (bacterial infection; eczema herpeticum) • Impetigo • Use of OTC topical steroids for greater than 1 week • Secondary infection of bites • Psoriasis • Rosacea • Acne after 2 months of OTC treatment or risk of scarring • Jaundice • Spider naevi • Changes in moles • Rodent ulcers • Chickenpox in patients taking steroids • Shingles • Rashes: especially following drugs. Non-blanching rashes where there is suspicion of meningitis should lead to immediate hospital referral • Burns larger than a thumbnail in size • Purpura (easy bruising), especially in patients taking drugs associated with thrombocytopenia or taking warfarin
Lumps	Especially in: • Breast • Testicles • Neck • Armpit
Muscloskeletal	• Pain on weight-bearing • Significant pain not relieved by simple analgesia • Any significant trauma at high speed or significant load • Any significant limb or motor dysfunction • Muscle pains with statins and/or fibrates (Chapter 12) • Tendon pain with certain drugs, including quinolones
Drugs	• Overdose of drugs (especially paracetamol) requires urgent referral to hospital, even in the absence of any symptoms
Travel	• Ill after foreign travel

OTC, over-the-counter.

2

Clinical laboratory tests

The following sections are intended as a guide to the most commonly used laboratory tests. Reference values are included as a guide and represent average population values. It should be noted that these values may alter according to the assay procedure, particularly when measuring enzymes, and local values should be sought when interpreting clinical data.

Clinical biochemistry

The monitoring of clinical biochemistry is used alongside clinical symptoms to diagnose disease, regulate drug therapy and identify adverse drug reactions. Biochemical blood tests include:

- urea and electrolytes (U and Es): a standard request may provide sodium, potassium, urea and creatinine levels
- liver function tests (LFTs)
- lipid profiles
- glucose and glycated haemoglobin (HbA_{1c})
- thyroid function tests (TFTs)

Urea and electrolytes

The plasma concentration of urea and the electrolytes sodium, potassium, calcium and magnesium in blood plasma is used to indicate renal function, dehydration and electrolyte disturbances caused by drugs or disease. For example, the retention of electrolytes may indicate impaired renal function or electrolyte loss may occur due to diarrhoea and vomiting, or the overuse of diuretics. See Table 2.1.

Drugs and the monitoring of U and Es

The requirement for electrolyte monitoring is discussed in individual chapters. A summary of some important drug-related electrolyte disturbances is given in Table 2.2.

Renal function tests

Renal function is often predicted from the results obtained from U and E monitoring. The main indicators are urea and creatinine. Urea is a product of protein metabolism and may be raised

Table 2.1 Measurement of blood plasma concentrations of urea and electrolytes and glycated haemoglobin (HbA$_{1c}$)

Biochemical parameter	Reference ranges	Comments
Sodium (Na$^+$)	135–145 mmol/L >155–160 mmol/L confusion and coma <120 mmol/L weakness and confusion	• Sodium controls the volume of extracellular fluid • Sodium is involved in neuronal action potentials and is therefore important for neuronal and muscle function
Potassium (K$^+$)	3.5–5.3 mmol/L >6.5 mmol/L or <2.5 mmol/L are medical emergencies	• Potassium levels determine membrane potential and influence the functioning of excitable tissues such as muscles and neurons • Hypokalaemia increases toxicity with digoxin therapy
Calcium (Ca^{2+})	2.25–2.6 mmol/L >3.50 mmol/L danger of cardiac arrest <1.6 mmol/L tetany (muscle spasm/twitching)	Calcitonin and parathyroid hormones maintain calcium blood plasma levels. As well as its role as a component of bone and teeth, calcium is essential for many metabolic processes, including nerve function, muscle contraction and blood clotting
Magnesium (Mg^{2+})	0.7–1.2 mmol/L	Magnesium is found in bones and is essential for the functioning of nerves and muscles. It is also a cofactor for many enzymes
Creatinine (plasma)	60–120 µmol/L	When calculating creatinine clearance as an indication of renal function, creatinine levels are adjusted according to age, weight and sex (see text)
Creatinine clearance	97–140 mL/min males 85–125 mL/min females	Used to estimate GFR (see text)
Urea	2.0–6.5 mmol/L	See text
Uric acid (Chapter 28)	0.15–0.47 mmol/L	• Elevated by thiazide diuretics • Excess may present as gouty arthritis due to deposits of uric acid crystals in joints
Bicarbonate (HCO$_3^-$)	22–29 mmol/L	• Important for acid–base balance. • Reflects renal and metabolic function
Glucose	3.0–5.0 mmol/L (fasting) <10.0 mmol/L (non-fasting)	Chapter 33
HbA$_{1c}$	4–5% (non-diabetic); in diabetes the aim is to keep it below 7%	• Glycated haemoglobin • Measured to assess the glycaemic control by diabetics during the previous 2 months • Higher levels are accepted during pregnancy and in elderly patients

GFR, glomerular filtration rate.

following high protein intake, renal impairment, tissue damage and/or catabolism. Elevated urea levels alone therefore do not provide an accurate estimation of renal function as required when adjusting doses of drugs excreted renally.

Creatinine is a product of muscle metabolism of creatine and in normal catabolic states is a more reliable parameter than urea. The level of creatinine in the blood however varies with age, sex and weight due to differences in muscle turnover.

Table 2.2   Examples of drugs causing electrolyte disturbances

Electrolyte disturbance	Symptoms	Drugs implicated
Hypokalaemia (reduced potassium)	Hypokalaemia due to fluid loss (consider diuretics, vomiting, diarrhoea); may occur in hepatic failure due to aldosterone release; may lead to neuromuscular disturbances, cramps, muscle weakness, and tetany leading to paralysis and respiratory failure. Arrhythmias may also occur, especially in patients at increased risk, e.g. taking digoxin	Especially thiazide and loop diuretics; beta$_2$-adrenoceptor agonists, corticosteroids, lithium and theophylline
Hyperkalaemia (increased potassium)	Hyperkalaemia may lead to a limp paralysis, arrhythmias and sudden death, but is initially asymptomatic	ACE inhibitors, aldosterone receptor antagonists, analgesics, angiotensin II receptor antagonists, potassium salts (salt substitute, effervescent preparations, e.g. low-sodium cystitis products and potassium citrate mixture), potassium-sparing diuretics and heparin
Hyponatraemia (reduced sodium)	Symptoms of hyponatraemia include orthostatic hypotension, reduced skin turgidity, confusion and ultimately convulsions. Hyponatraemia due to excess water may present as anorexia, heart failure, muscle weakness and oedema	ACE inhibitors, aldosterone inhibitors, analgesics, antidepressants, carbamazepine, loop diuretics, omeprazole, potassium-sparing diuretics, thiazide diuretics, chlorpropamide and tolbutamide
Hypernatraemia (increased sodium)	Hypernatraemia occurs in renal failure, producing symptoms of confusion, drowsiness, lethargy, dry skin, hypotension, muscle twitching, peripheral vasoconstriction and ultimately coma	Corticosteroids, NSAIDs, lithium
Hypomagnesaemia (reduced magnesium)	Hypomagnesaemia increases the risk of arrhythmias	Aminoglycosides, bisphosphonates, immunosuppressants, loop diuretics and thiazide diuretics
Hypercalcaemia (increased calcium)	Symptoms of hypercalcaemia include abdominal pain, anorexia, constipation, fatigue, nausea and vomiting, polyuria with nocturia and thirst. Progression to confusion, delirium, psychosis, gallstones, renal impairment (due to calculi or stones), stupor and coma may occur	Androgens, antacids, calcium salts, fat-soluble vitamins, sex hormones, thiazide diuretics, vitamin A derivatives and vitamin D derivatives
Hypocalcaemia (decreased calcium)	Hypocalcaemia tends to be asymptomatic. Worsening hypocalcaemia may produce paraesthesia of the face, fingers and toes, tetany or prolonged tonic muscle spasms and ultimately convulsions and psychosis	Loop diuretics, bisphosphonates

ACE, angiotensin-converting enzyme; NSAIDs, non-steroidal anti-inflammatory drugs.

A more precise predictor of renal function is therefore calculated as an estimate of the glomerular filtration rate (GFR) calculated from the plasma creatinine levels (Chapter 17) and adjusted for age, weight and sex. The ideal body weight (IBW) should be used if the patient's weight is greater than 20% in excess of IBW. A more accurate GFR may be calculated by comparing the amount of creatinine collected in a 24-h urine sample to the blood plasma measurement. Cockcroft Gault equation:

$$\text{Creatinine clearance (ml/min)} = \frac{1.23 \text{ (males) } 1.04 \text{ (females) } \times (140 - \text{age (years)}) \times \text{weight (kg)}}{\text{serum creatinine (µmol/L)}}$$

The use of drugs in renal impairment may involve the avoidance or reduction of doses, according to the extent to which the kidneys are involved in the elimination of drugs. Individual chapters should be consulted for more detail. Important examples of drugs to be used with caution, often at reduced doses and with regular monitoring, or avoided in renal failure include:

- non-steroidal anti-inflammatory drugs (NSAIDs)
- angiotensin-converting enzyme (ACE) inhibitors
- tetracycline
- metformin
- digoxin
- gold salts
- penicillamine
- ciclosporin
- lithium

Liver function tests

Impaired liver function may be detected from: deranged bilirubin; the enzymes transaminase, alkaline phosphatase and/or gamma-glutamyl transferase; albumin and coagulation factors. The range of biochemical parameters (Table 2.3) reflects the diverse functions of the liver. Diagnosis can broadly be defined as acute or chronic cellular damage and/or cholestasis. For further discussion of liver disease see Chapter 10 and for drug-related liver disease see Chapter 5.

Acute cellular damage

Damage to hepatocytes results in an increased permeability of these cells and a subsequent leaching of hepatic enzymes into the hepatic circulation. Blood plasma levels of the enzymes alanine transaminase (ALT) and aspartate transaminase (AST) are found to be elevated in patients with acute hepatocyte damage. It should be noted that AST is also found in cardiac muscle and skeletal muscle and therefore blood levels may be raised following damage to cardiac cells after myocardial infarction or following non-specific muscle damage.

The damaged liver also fails to clear bilirubin, a breakdown product from the haem component of red blood cells. The unconjugated form of bilirubin, termed free bilirubin, therefore builds up in the blood, causing a yellowing of the skin together with pruritus (Chapter 10).

Chronic cellular damage

Chronic cellular damage, such as alcohol-induced cirrhosis, results in the deposition of fibrous tissue in place of dysfunctional hepatocytes. Transaminase levels are often normal but the decline in function of the damaged liver results in a reduction of components in the blood, which are normally produced by the liver, for example, albumin and clotting factors. These patients therefore suffer from hypoalbuminaemia and an increased prothrombin time or international normalised ratio (INR: Chapter 15) due to reduced clotting ability.

Cholestasis

Cholestasis results from a blockage of the bile duct and therefore substances that would usually be excreted in the bile build up in the liver. These substances, such as conjugated bilirubin and alkaline phosphatase (ALP) are therefore present in increased concentration in blood plasma. The enzyme gamma-glutamyl transferase (GGT) is also elevated but is not a reliable indicator of cholestasis as it may also be induced by drugs such as alcohol and anticonvulsants, thereby increasing levels in the absence of cholestasis. In addition, the presence

Table 2.3   Summary of parameters measured in liver function tests but local values should be checked

Parameter	Reference range (check local ranges)	Comment
Aspartate transaminase (AST)	< 50 IU/L	Elevated in acute hepatocyte damage but considered to be a non-specific parameter as it may also be elevated following myocardial infarction and other muscle damage
Alanine transaminase (ALT)	< 45 IU/L	Elevated following hepatocyte damage and tends to indicate acute damage
Alkaline phosphatase (ALP)	39–117 IU/L	Indicator of cholestasis but non-specific as it is also found in bone, placenta and intestine. Levels are therefore raised in Paget's disease, osteomalacia and the last trimester of pregnancy. Consider also the level of GGT as levels of ALP may be increased in other types of liver disease
Gamma-glutamyl transferase (GGT)	Up to 70 IU/L (males) Up to 40 IU/L (females)	Often used in the diagnosis of cholestasis but may also be elevated in acute or chronic hepatitis, alcoholism and in patients prescribed inducers such as anticonvulsants
Unconjugated (free) bilirubin	5–17 µmol/L (>35 µmol/L produces jaundice)	Increased levels indicate impaired liver function
Prothrombin time	10–14 s	Prolonged when clotting factor synthesis is reduced, e.g. chronic hepatitis and/or malabsorption of vitamins, warfarin treatment
INR	1–1.2	Ratio of prothrombin time compared to a control
Albumin	30–48 g/L	Since albumin is synthesised in the liver, chronic damage results in hypoalbuminaemia. May include a corrected calcium level (2.2–2.6 mmol/L)

INR, international normalised ratio.

of ALP in tissue such as bone, placenta and the intestine limits the reliability of ALP as an indicator of cholestasis. Both ALP and GGT are therefore considered, together with the clinical presentation and history. A drug history is useful in determining alternative causes of raised GGT levels.

Summary of LFT interpretation

In general, LFTs are considered abnormal when a value is more than double the maximum value of the normal reference range.

Acute hepatitis

- large elevations of ALT and AST
- possible slight increases in ALP and GGT
- possible large elevation of bilirubin
- prothrombin time may occasionally be increased
- no change in albumin levels

Chronic cellular damage

- ALP, ALT and AST tend to be normal or only slightly increased.
- GGT levels may show an elevation.

- Albumin levels are low.
- Bilirubin levels may show marginal to large increases.
- Prothrombin time is prolonged.

Cholestasis

- ALP levels show a large increase.
- GGT is usually elevated.
- ALT and AST tend to be only marginally raised or normal.
- Bilirubin levels may show marginal to large increases.
- Albumin levels are normal.
- Prothrombin time may occasionally be increased.

Drugs requiring regular LFTs (see also individual chapters)

The requirement for monitoring LFTs when prescribing is indicated in individual chapters. Examples where monitoring is appropriate include:

- statins
- fibrates
- amiodarone
- isotretinoin
- isoniazid
- methyldopa
- rifampicin
- rosiglitazone, pioglitazone
- sodium valproate
- sulfasalazine

Herbal preparations should also be considered when patients present with signs of hepatic disease. For example, the Committee on Safety of Medicines and Medicines Control Agency have requested the withdrawal of the preparation kava-kava, pending further investigation into its safety.

Lipids

A full screen of lipids (Chapter 12) from patients when fasting includes the measurement of:

- total cholesterol (ideal target <5.2 mmol/L)
- high-density lipoprotein (HDL) cholesterol (ideal >0.9 mmol/L males, >1.2 mmol/L females and >20% of total cholesterol)
- low-density lipoprotein (LDL) cholesterol (<3.35–4.0 mmol/L)
- triglyceride (<1.9 mmol/L)
- ratio of total to HDL cholesterol (<4.5)

Isotretinoin treatment may alter serum lipids and monitoring is recommended 1 month after treatment is initiated and again at the end of treatment (Chapter 5).

Glucose

See Chapter 33.

Thyroid function tests

Thyroid function is determined by comparing clinical features, as discussed in Chapter 34, with biochemical values of thyroid-stimulating hormone (TSH), free thyroxine (T_4), and free triiodothyronin (T_3). Drug treatments requiring regular monitoring of thyroid function include lithium and amiodarone (Chapters 5 and 34).

Summary

Monitoring requirements are also considered within individual chapters. Further information can be found in the SPCs or in the latest *British National Formulary* or direct from the drug manufacturer. It should be noted that requirements for monitoring change according to the clinical presentation of the patient, together with risk factors. For monitoring of drug levels in blood plasma, see Chapter 6.

Haematology

Haematological monitoring is used as a general screening test to aid the diagnosis of inflammatory conditions or drug-related blood dyscrasias, to identify anaemias and to monitor coagulation such as during warfarin therapy. Tests include:

- full blood count (FBC) – standard request provides haemoglobin, white blood cell count (WBC), platelets, mean cell volume (MCV), mean corpuscular haemoglobin (MCH), red blood cells (RBC), haematocrit (HCT) (Table 2.4) and estimates of differentiated types of white blood cells
- erythrocyte sedimentation rate (ESR)
- blood coagulation
- vitamin B_{12} and folate

Full blood count

Table 2.4 summarises some of the main haematological parameters measured. Drugs requiring a regular FBC include immunosuppressants, clozapine and methyldopa.

Monitoring of oral anticoagulants

See Chapter 15.

Zinc protoporphyrin

This test is used to detect porphyria, a genetic abnormality of haem synthesis, in which abnormal concentrations of haem precursors accumulate (Chapter 5).

Immunological tests

These tests generally involve the detection of antibodies that may point to autoimmune disease or may indicate general immune status. The following tests are used:

- Autoantibody or autoimmune screening includes the detection of antibodies to preparations of thyroid cytoplasm, parietal cells, mitochondria, smooth muscle and liver or kidney microsomes.
- Rheumatoid factor – a positive test confirms a diagnosis of rheumatoid arthritis/autoimmune rheumatoid disorders.
- C-reactive protein (CRP) is elevated during infection and/or severe inflammation and may be repeated to monitor the outcome of treatment. CRP is more specific for inflammation, necrosis or infection and changes more rapidly than ESR (Table 2.4, see page 23).
- Thyroid antibodies (Graves disease: see Chapter 34).
- Immunoglobulins: patients presenting with epigastric pain may be tested for the presence of serum immunoglobulin G (IgG) against *Helicobacter pylori* infection (Chapter 7).
- Paul–Bunnell test (infectious mononucleosis or glandular fever) in response to persistent sore throat, lethargy, fever, headache and cervical adenopathy.
- Prostate-specific antigen (PSA): a positive test provides an early indication of prostate cancer even when the patient is asymptomatic. This is, however, a relatively non-specific test, as only a proportion of patients who have a high value have malignancy.

Microbiology

Microbiology tests are performed on samples such as urine, sputum, cerebrospinal fluid, faeces or swabs from the vagina or cervix, nose or eyes. These tests tend to be requested when treatment has failed, or sinister causes are suspected, for example, in symptoms suggestive of meningitis or if there is a risk of sexually transmitted diseases such as *Chlamydia*, gonorrhoea or syphilis.

Reference

Mehta D K (ed.) *British National Formulary*, latest edition. London: British Medical Association and Royal Pharmaceutical Society of Great Britain.

Further reading

Barber N, Wilson A (eds) (1999). *Clinical Pharmacy Survival Guide*. London: Churchill Livingstone.

Harman R J, Mason P (eds) (2002). *Handbook of Pharmacy Health Care*, 2nd edn. London: Pharmaceutical Press.

Hoffbrand A V, Pettit J E, Moss P A H (2001). *Essential Haematology,* 4th edn. Oxford: Blackwell Science.

Lee A (ed.) (2001). *Adverse Drug Reactions.* London: Pharmaceutical Press.

McGhee M (2000). *A Guide to Laboratory Investigations,* 3rd edn. Oxford: Radcliffe Medical Press.

Table 2.4 Monitoring of haematological parameters

Haematological parameter	Reference value(s)	Comments
White blood cells (leucocytes: WBC): Differential:	$4–11 \times 10^9/L$	• Increased levels (leucocytosis) during infection or malignancy
Neutrophils	$2.5–7.5 \times 10^9/L$	• Reduced levels (leucopenia) due to drugs (Chapter 5), viral infections, chronic infections or hypersensitivity reaction
Lymphocytes	$1.5–3.5 \times 10^9/L$	
Monocytes	$0.2–0.8 \times 10^9/L$	
Eosinophils	$0.04–0.4 \times 10^9/L$	• Types of WBC are cell counter estimates
Basophils	$0.01–0.1 \times 10^9/L$	• Patients of Afro-Caribbean origin have a lower normal range
Erythrocyte sedimentation rate (ESR)	0–9 mm/h male 0–20 mm/h female	Elevated with increasing age, during pregnancy, chronic infection, dysproteinaemias, cancer and inflammatory diseases (e.g. giant cell arteritis, rheumatoid arthritis)
Serum ferritin	15–300 µg/L male 15–200 µg/L female	A measure of iron stores
Haemoglobin (Hb) (Chapter 16)	13.5–17.5 g/dL male 11.5–15.5 g/dL female	Symptoms of anaemia appear at levels <9–10 g/dL
Platelets	$140–400 \times 10^9/L$	• Low due to vitamin B_{12}/folate deficiency, infections, drug-induced thrombocytopenia (Chapter 16), bone marrow hypoplasia, uraemia, liver disease and alcohol abuse • Increased following trauma, infection and inflammation or malignancy
Mean cell volume (MCV)	76–95 fl	• Raised in vitamin B_{12} or folate deficiency, excess alcohol consumption or liver disease • Reduced in iron-deficient anaemia or chronic blood loss or thalassaemia • May be normal during acute blood loss or anaemia of chronic disease (e.g. renal anaemia)
Red blood cells (RBC, erythrocytes)	$4.5–6.5 \times 10^{12}/L$ male $3.8–5.8 \times 10^{12}/L$ female	
Haematocrit (HCT) or packed cell volume (PCV)	0.37–0.54 male 0.35–0.47 female	• PCV of anticoagulated blood • The HCT gives a crude indication of red cell volume but the RBC and MCV reveal more specific details
Mean corpuscular haemoglobin (MCH)	27–33 pg	• Consider with other red cell parameters • Raised in vitamin B_{12} or folate deficiency • Lowered due to chronic blood loss, iron deficiency, thalassaemia or megaloblastic anaemia
Vitamin B_{12}	211–911 ng/L	• Deficiency may result in macrocytic anaemia (Chapter 16) • Vitamin B_{12} deficiency may be due to low dietary intake (vegans or Hindu vegetarians)
Folate (serum)	2.9–18 µg/L	• Deficiency may result in macrocytic anaemia (Chapter 16) • Folate deficiency may be due to malabsorption or drug causes (Chapter 16)

3

Lifestyle advice

Healthcare professionals have a vital role to play in health promotion, with a view to both the prevention and treatment of diseases, including ischaemic heart disease, cancer and mental health, as outlined in the Department of Health white paper (1999) *Saving Lives: Our Healthier Nation*. Key issues include:

- encouraging smoking cessation
- reducing alcohol intake. Binge drinking should be avoided, with limits of 3–4 units per day for males and 2–3 units per day for females. The maximum weekly intake should not exceed 14 units for females or 21 units for males
- promoting a healthy diet and increased physical activity. Approximately three exercise sessions of 20 min each per week are recommended
- reducing blood pressure (Chapter 11), plasma cholesterol (Chapter 12) and stress
- promoting safe sex
- improving cancer screening
- preventing skin cancer by education on protection from the sun

- encouraging increased education in basic first aid

Dietary recommendations are made according to the Scientific Advisory Committee on Nutrition (SACN), which replaced the Committee on Medical Aspects of Food and Nutrition Policy (COMA). Healthcare professionals should particularly be aware of specific requirements for different life-stages and disease states.

In the following sections, the role of dietary supplements is discussed and situations for appropriate recommendation of these products are suggested. Dietary supplements include vitamin and mineral preparations, natural oils, enzymes, amino acids and other substances often endogenous to the body but for which a precise role or deficiency state has not been elucidated fully. Herbal products are also described as dietary supplements (Chapter 4).

Recommendations for healthy living

The following summary highlights the main recommendations by the COMA and SACN for the prevention of disease and reduction of disease severity:

- Aim to maintain a body mass index (BMI) of 20–25 kg/m². This is a guide to ideal body weight calculated as weight (kg) divided by height (m) squared. It should be noted that this calculation is only a guide. Limitations occur, for example, a muscular athlete with low body fat may be classed as obese using the BMI. The measurement of percentage body fat should therefore be considered.
- At least five portions of fruit and vegetables should be consumed daily.
- Reduce the intake of saturated fat to provide no more than 10% of energy requirements. Total fat should provide no more than 35% of energy.
- Increase the intake of n-3 polyunsaturated fatty acids (PUFA) e.g. from oily fish.
- Reduce the intake of salt to no more than 6 g/day.
- Reduce the intake of added sugars to provide no more than 10% of energy requirements.

- Complex carbohydrate should provide 50% of energy.
- The intake of non-starch polysaccharides (NSPs), previously described as dietary fibre, should be increased to 18 g/day and consumed from a wide variety of food sources, including cereals.

A useful description for patients is that their plate should contain mainly vegetables, and complex carbohydrates such as potatoes or pasta with the smallest portion being meat (preferably oily fish or white meat such as chicken rather than red or processed meat). The consumption of jacket potatoes and brown rice or pasta can help to increase the intake of NSPs and reduce the saturated fat found in chips or roast potatoes. Advice should be supplemented with written information.

Adverse drug reactions and nutritional status

The effect of adverse drug reactions (ADRs) on nutritional status should not be overlooked (Chapter 5). For example:

- Drugs may increase appetite or cause fluid retention, leading to weight gain.
- The palatability of food may be reduced as a result of taste disturbances, dry mouth or nausea.
- Food absorption may be disrupted by drugs such as colestyramine, requiring the supplementation of fat-soluble vitamins.
- Metabolic effects include altered glucose and lipid profiles that may be problematic in long-term treatment of patients with diabetes mellitus and/or hypercholesterolaemia. Glucocorticoid-induced hyperglycaemia has been known to necessitate increased doses of hypoglycaemic drugs and treatment of non-diabetic patients.

Food–drug interactions

When treating diseases, consideration should be given to the nutritional status and diet of patients to prevent possible food–drug interactions (Table 3.1). As with drug–drug interactions (Chapter 5), food may affect pharmacokinetic parameters such as absorption, metabolism or excretion of drugs. Alternatively, pharmacodynamic interactions may occur due to similar pharmacological targets. The result may be increased toxic effects or treatment failure.

Risk factors applicable to drug–drug interactions also apply to drug–nutrient interactions:

- drugs with a narrow therapeutic window (phenytoin, theophylline, digoxin, lithium and anticoagulants)
- extremes of age
- chronic illness, e.g. requiring enteral or parenteral feeding
- polypharmacy
- malnourished and/or nutritional or metabolic disorders
- restrictive diets such as high-protein or vegan
- the use of high-dose supplements
- increased or decreased BMI during treatment may result in altered drug metabolism

General precautions for avoiding drug interactions with enteral and parenteral feeds

Food–drug interactions may also result from the administration of enteral or parenteral feeds. The following points are intended as a checklist to highlight some important considerations for drug administration to patients prescribed supplemental feeds:

Enteral feeds

- Drug administration should be separated from the enteral feed.
- The feeding tube should be thoroughly washed before and after drug administration.
- Antacids may interact to form an obstructive plug in the oesophagus.
- Phenytoin absorption is reduced by enteral feeds.
- The bioavailability of theophylline and levodopa is reduced by high-protein feeds.

- The vitamin K content of feeds should be checked in patients prescribed anticoagulants as fluctuations in vitamin K intake will alter the efficacy of anticoagulants (Chapter 15).

Parenteral feeds

- Drugs should never be given down intravenous (IV) lines in an attempt to keep the lines clean and free from infection.
- Drugs are not generally added to total parenteral nutrition (TPN) due to altered stability. Occasionally heparin, insulin, H_2-receptor antagonists or corticosteroids are added.
- The vitamin K content should be considered for patients taking warfarin.
- The bioavailability of theophylline and levodopa is reduced by high-protein feeds.

Tobacco smoke

Tobacco smoking has a profound adverse effect on health. Strong evidence links it to the main causes of mortality: cancer, respiratory disorders and heart disease. As many as 90% of lung cancers, 90% of COPD deaths and 25% of deaths due to heart disease are smoking-related. Smoking cessation may therefore be considered to be the most important intervention by health professionals in the treatment and prevention of disease. The powerful addictive nature of nicotine however makes this an extremely difficult task.

Pharmacological activity

Tobacco smoke contains nicotine, carcinogenic tars (polycyclic hydrocarbons) and carbon monoxide, with the main pharmacologically active ingredient being nicotine. Nicotine stimulates subtypes of nicotinic receptors leading to neuronal excitation. These receptors are distributed on neurons in the brain and on autonomic ganglia and neuromuscular synapses (mainly in the heart and lungs) in the periphery. The effects produced by smoking lead to:

Table 3.1 Examples of food–drug interactions

Dietary component(s)	Drug	Comment
Caffeine	Cimetidine	Cimetidine may increase the effects of caffeine
	Oral contraceptive	Possible increased and prolonged effects of caffeine
	Fluconazole, fluvoxamine	Increased effects of caffeine
	Disulfiram	Increased effects of caffeine, such as irritability, insomnia, anxiety, may be deleterious during alcohol withdrawal
	Theophylline	Increased theophylline levels and therefore increased risk of ADRs. Note that both caffeine and theophylline are methylxanthines and may therefore exhibit similar pharmacology
Calcium salts	Calcium channel blockers, captopril, levodopa, levothyroxine	• Calcium carbonate may reduce the absorption of captopril and levothyroxine and doses should be separated by at least 2 h • Calcium carbonate may reduce the bioavailability of levodopa and patients should be monitored for reduced efficacy
Calcium and iron-rich foods	Tetracyclines	Reduced absorption and antibacterial activity due to chelation. Tetracycline should be taken at least half an hour before food and milk
Calcium salts and/or vitamin D	Diuretics, thiazides	Risk of hypercalcaemia and metabolic alkalosis with high doses of calcium salts and/or vitamin D since diuretics reduce the excretion of calcium ions. Monitoring of calcium levels is therefore important (see also Chapter 2)
Co-enzyme Q	Warfarin	Reduced effect of warfarin. Monitor for changes when supplements are initiated or stopped
Evening primrose oil (EPO)	Antiepileptics, phenothiazines, SSRIs, bupropion	• Possible increased risk of seizures. Evidence is poor but monitoring is advised during concurrent use • Some evidence suggests that EPO may improve seizure control in patients with epilepsy • Until more information becomes available, it may be prudent not to recommend EPO for patients with a history of epilepsy or taking drugs known to lower the convulsive threshold
Ferrous sulfate	Levodopa	• Reduced absorption of levodopa • The separation of doses and/or increased dose of levodopa is required

Continued

Table 3.1   *Continued*

Dietary component(s)	Drug	Comment
Ferrous salts	Antacids, levothyroxine, tetracyclines, quinolone antibiotics (ciprofloxacin, levofloxacin, norfloxacin)	• Separate doses as antacids reduce iron absorption • Ferrous sulfate and possibly other ferrous salts may reduce the absorption of thyroid hormones, tetracyclines and quinolone antibiotics. Doses should be separated by at least 2 h
Fibre (NSPs)	Amoxicillin	Reduced absorption and therefore possibly reduced response to amoxicillin with a high-fibre diet
Fish oils	Anticoagulants, aspirin, dipyridamole, clopidogrel	Increased risk of bleeding and additional monitoring when changing the intake of fish oils, particularly supplements, is therefore advised
Folic acid	Anticonvulsants (phenytoin, phenobarbital, primidone), co-trimoxazole, sulfasalazine, oral contraceptives, methotrexate, proguanil	• Folic acid supplementation may be required following long-term treatment with the drugs listed, particularly in women of child-bearing age • High-dose folic acid (5 mg) is required with anticonvulsants or proguanil in pregnancy • The anticonvulsant serum levels may fall, therefore monitoring and possible dose adjustment are recommended • Folic acid may reduce the adverse effects but also the desired effects of methotrexate
Food in general but particularly high-protein	Levodopa	The timing and composition of food may alter the response to levodopa
Food in general	Antifungals (griseofulvin, ketoconazole, itraconazole), phenytoin	• Possible increased dissolution and therefore absorption at acidic pH. Take with or after food. Fatty meals increase the absorption of griseofulvin • Phenytoin absorption may be reduced by food and particularly enteral feeds such as Ensure and also nasogastric feeding
Glucose	Corticosteroids, thiazides	Increased levels of blood glucose (Chapter 33)
Grapefruit juice	Terfenadine, calcium channel blockers (particularly nifedipine, felodipine and nicardipine)	Cytochrome P450 inhibition. Reduced metabolism may increase the drug effects
Ispaghula husk	Lithium	Serum levels of lithium may be reduced. Monitoring with appropriate dose adjustment is recommended
Milk	Alcohol	Reduced absorption of alcohol and therefore reduced blood levels and intoxication effects

Continued

Table 3.1 *Continued*

Dietary component(s)	Drug	Comment
Potassium-containing foods or salt substitute	Potassium-sparing diuretics (amiloride, spironolactone), ACE inhibitors, valsartan and losartan	Risk of hyperkalaemia
Sodium chloride (salt)	Lithium	Reduced lithium levels due to increased excretion of sodium and lithium ions
Sodium chloride (salt)	Diuretics	Sodium chloride opposes the beneficial effects of diuretics by increasing water retention by the kidney
Sodium chloride (low intake)	Amphotericin B	Increased risk of renal toxicity
Tyramine (cheese, yeast extracts, salami, pickled herring, chicken or beef livers, soy sauce, avocado, some beers, lagers and wines)	MAOIs	Avoid. Risk of hypertensive crisis
Vitamin A (retinol)	Isotretinoin	• A condition similar to vitamin A overdose may result from concurrent administration of isotretinoin and vitamin A • Intracranial hypertension ('pseudotumour cerebri') may occur
Vitamin B_6 (pyridoxine)	Levodopa (excluding co-careldopa and co-beneldopa); Anticonvulsants (phenytoin, phenobarbital)	Reduced or abolished efficacy of levodopa and large doses may reduce levels of phenytoin and phenobarbital
Vitamin C	Aspirin, warfarin	• Reduced absorption of vitamin C by aspirin. Particularly relevant if taken in combination to treat the common cold • There is a small risk that large doses of vitamin C could reduce the effects of warfarin
Vitamin D	Antiepileptics	High-dose supplements may be required due to altered vitamin D metabolism
Vitamin E	Warfarin	A small risk of increased anticoagulant effect but monitoring is advised when vitamin E is added
Vitamins, fat-soluble (A, D, E, K)	Colestyramine, orlistat, liquid paraffin	• Supplements should be taken at least 2 h after administration of orlistat, or at bedtime • Supplements may be required for patients prescribed colestyramine and should be administered 1 h before or 4–6 h after colestyramine • Liquid paraffin is not recommended due to adverse effects such as lipoid pneumonia, anal seepage and irritation with prolonged use

Continued

Table 3.1   *Continued*

Dietary component(s)	Drug	Comment
Vitamin K (consider supplements, enteral feeds, beetroot, green vegetables such as spinach, Brussels sprouts, lettuce)	Warfarin	Reduced or abolished effects of warfarin, a vitamin K antagonist
Zinc	Calcium supplements, tetracyclines, quinolone antibiotics (ciprofloxacin, levofloxacin, norfloxacin)	• Calcium salts reduce the absorption of zinc and doses should be separated • Separate doses by at least 2 h as zinc reduces the absorption of these antibiotics. The interaction with doxycycline is minimal

ADRs, adverse drug reactions; SSRIs, selective serotonin reuptake inhibitors; NSPs, non-starch polysaccharides; ACE, angiotensin-converting enzyme; MAOIs, monoamine oxidase inhibitors.

- increased or decreased arousal, as observed on electroencephalogram (EEG)
- autonomic reflexes such as tachycardia, increased cardiac output, increased arterial pressure, reduced gastrointestinal activity and sweating
- the secretion of adrenaline (epinephrine) and noradrenaline (norepinephrine) from the adrenal medulla, which also contributes to the cardiovascular effects
- reduced urinary flow due to the release of antidiuretic hormone
- increased plasma concentration of lipoproteins (increased low-density lipoprotein (LDL) and very-low-density lipoprotein (VLDL)) and therefore risk of atherosclerosis
- increased platelet aggregation and therefore risk of thrombosis
- reduced immunity of lungs, leading to respiratory infections and exacerbation of asthma and COPD
- increased diabetic complications due to adverse effects on microvascular circulation

Carbon monoxide reduces the oxygen-carrying capacity of haemoglobin, contributing further to the adverse cardiovascular effects outlined above. Irritant, carcinogenic and other toxic substances found in cigarette smoke include arsenic, benzene, lead, DDT (dichlorodiphenyltrichloroethane, an insecticide), nitric acid and toluene (methylbenzene). Carcinogenic tars may lead to COPD and cancer of the lungs, upper respiratory tract, oesophagus, pancreas and bladder.

Treatment of nicotine addiction

Patients who smoke more than 10 cigarettes per day may benefit from nicotine replacement, counselling and support. All preparations of nicotine replacement therapy (NRT) have been shown to be effective in smoking cessation, with cessation rates increased by 1.5–2-fold (systematic review by Silagy *et al.*, 2002). The dosage form is selected according to patient preference. Bupropion may also be used but current National Institute of Clinical Excellence (NICE) guidelines do not recommend concurrent use with NRT.

Withdrawal symptoms include:

- dysphoric or depressed mood
- insomnia
- irritability, frustration or anger
- anxiety
- difficulty concentrating
- restlessness
- decreased heart rate
- increased appetite and weight gain

Concurrent disease

Table 3.2 considers the use of NRT and bupropion for patients with concurrent disease. It should also be noted that many preparations are not licensed for patients aged less than 18 years.

Drug interactions and adverse effects

Tobacco smoke

Components of tobacco smoke, thought to be polycyclic hydrocarbons, induce cytochrome P450 enzymes in the liver, thereby increasing the metabolism of some drugs. For example, the dose of theophylline may need to be reduced on cessation of smoking, due to reduced metabolism.

Increased insulin-opposing hormones caused by smoking necessitate greater insulin doses in diabetics who smoke and a reduced dosage on cessation of smoking (Stockley, 2002). Smoking also adds to the cardiovascular risk of these patients. A further increased risk of thromboembolic disease in women taking oral contraceptives occurs if they also smoke.

Nicotine

The use of nicotine patches may also lead to drug interactions. For example, the clearance of nicotine is reduced when combined with cimetidine and possibly ranitidine. This may reduce the requirement for high doses of NRT.

Bupropion

The increased risk of seizures should be considered when coprescribing drugs known to lower the seizure threshold (Table 5.9 and Chapter 22). The long half-life of drugs such as fluoxetine may also increase the risk of interactions following the cessation of treatment. There may also be an increased risk of hypomania or mania in patients coprescribed fluoxetine and bupropion. Evidence of these problems is limited but careful monitoring is recommended if coprescribing is deemed appropriate (Stockley, 2002). Bupropion has also been shown to increase imipramine levels in an interaction at the level of hepatic cytochrome P450 enzyme.

General counselling

For smoking cessation to be successful, patients must make the decision to stop. Health professionals therefore need to recognise the different stages involved in arriving at this decision. This ranges from the patient who has never considered stopping smoking to the patient who is ready to stop. Information leaflets may be given to patients who smoke and encouragement to stop smoking given at every opportunity. A successful attempt to quit is more likely when the patient has actually made the decision and is ready to stop. The patient should be advised to set a date to stop smoking completely and discard all remaining cigarettes. The importance of willpower and the use of NRT to alleviate the symptoms of withdrawal should be stressed.

The following points may help the patient to be successful:

- Explain that chest symptoms such as increased secretions may occur initially due to the withdrawal of nicotine but these should abate within 2–3 weeks.
- Try to avoid situations associated with smoking. For example, take up a hobby in the evening if this is when most cigarettes are smoked.
- Encourage the patient to return with questions or difficulties.
- Avoid excess intake of caffeine as this may worsen the withdrawal effect of nicotine.
- A list of the benefits of smoking cessation may particularly help patients who are long-term smokers. Rapid improvements in taste and sense of smell, circulation and lung function are experienced. After only 5 years, the risk of experiencing a heart attack is reduced to half that of a smoker.
- Money usually spent on cigarettes could be saved in a jar. Other benefits include increased exercise capacity, reduced odour, avoiding premature ageing of the skin and tooth loss.

NRT (patches, gum, inhalator, lozenges, sublingual, nasal spray)

- The nasal spray should not be used when driving due to the risk of sneezing or watery eyes.

Table 3.2 Concurrent disease and prescribing of smoking cessation aids (derived from the *British National Formulary* (BNF))

Disease	Cautions and contraindications	Comments
Cardiovascular disease, including peripheral vascular disease	Nicotine products are contraindicated in severe cardiovascular disease such as: • severe arrhythmias • recent myocardial infarction, TIA or CVA Monitoring is appropriate for other conditions	• These patients should be encouraged to stop smoking due to the adverse effects outlined in the text • Monitoring for signs of deterioration is required. The harmful effects produced by toxic components of smoke are obviously removed but unwanted effects due to nicotine remain. This information may be useful for patients reluctant to stop using NRT
Depression, bipolar disorder	The use of bupropion is contraindicated	Increased risk of precipitating or exacerbating the manic phase
Diabetes mellitus	NRT and bupropion should only be used with caution	• See risk of seizures with bupropion use in diabetes mellitus • The effects of nicotine may mask the signs of hypoglycaemia and increase the risk of damage to the microvascular circulation • Smoking cessation is imperative in these patients due to the increased risk of diabetic complications (Chapter 33) and NRT may be useful in the short term with monitoring
Epilepsy, risk of seizures	Bupropion is contraindicated when there is a risk of seizures as follows: • a history of seizures or eating disorders • a CNS tumour • during acute withdrawal from alcohol or benzodiazepines	Buproprion may be used with caution and close monitoring when benefit exceeds risk in the following situations: • alcohol abuse • history of head trauma • diabetes • concurrent use of stimulants or anorectic drugs, which may lower the seizure threshold
Hyperthyroidism	NRT should only be used with caution	Nicotine may exacerbate symptoms of hyperthyroidism and complicate its management
History of gastritis and peptic ulcer	NRT should be used with caution	Nicotine may worsen gastritis and peptic ulcer disease and patients should be monitored accordingly. Smoking cessation is however particularly important for these patients
Pregnancy and breast-feeding	Both bupropion and NRT are currently contraindicated	Smoking cessation should be strongly encouraged in pregnant women and those with young children
Chronic generalised skin disease	Nicotine patches are contraindicated	NRT patches should not be used on broken skin
Renal and hepatic impairment	NRT and bupropion should be used with caution	• Dose adjustment may be required (BNF appendices 2 and 3) • Avoid bupropion in severe hepatic cirrhosis

TIA, transient ischaemic attack; CVA, cerebrovascular accident; NRT, nicotine replacement therapy; CNS, central nervous system.

- Side effects include nausea, dizziness, headache, cold and influenza-like symptoms, palpitations, dyspepsia, insomnia and vivid dreams (particularly with the 24-h patch). The 24-h patch should be removed if these symptoms are troublesome: a 16-h patch may be more suitable.
- Patches should not be applied to broken skin.
- Patches are not appropriate for occasional smokers.

Bupropion

- Side-effects include dry mouth, gastro-intestinal disturbances, insomnia, tremor, tachycardia and hypertension.
- Blood pressure should be monitored weekly if bupropion is used with NRT. Patients who relapse should be encouraged to self-refer due to the risk of increased blood pressure.
- Bupropion should be used with caution when driving or performing skilled tasks.

Alcohol

Pharmacological activity

The main effects of alcohol result from central nervous system (CNS)-depressant and disinhibition effects with comparable mechanisms to volatile general anaesthetics that are also highly lipid-soluble. Pharmacological changes include increased activity of inhibitory gamma-aminobutyric acid (GABA) transmission similar to the effects of benzodiazepines, and reduced excitatory pathways such as Ca^{2+} entry through voltage-gated Ca^{2+} channels, and reduced N-methyl-D-aspartate (NMDA) receptor function.

Peripheral effects include increased salivation and gastric secretions. Excess consumption of alcohol may damage the gastric mucosa, resulting in chronic gastritis and gastric bleeding. Adrenal steroid hormone production is increased, resulting in a 'pseudo-Cushing's syndrome' and characteristic 'moon face' due to raised plasma cortisol. Diuresis occurs in response to reduced antidiuretic hormone (ADH) secretion. Impotence may follow reduced testicular steroid synthesis and increased deactivation by the liver.

Long-term effects

Chronic alcohol abuse produces liver and brain damage. Increased fat accumulation in the liver (fatty liver) leads to hepatitis, which may progress to irreversible necrosis and fibrosis and oesophageal varices. The latter results from increased pressure in the hepatic portal vein leading to obstruction and subsequent formation of collateral vessels, for example in the oesophagus and stomach. These vessels allow portal blood flow to pass directly to the systemic circulation, bypassing the liver. Thiamin (vitamin B_1) deficiency occurs due to reduced deamination and therefore storage of vitamins by the liver, resulting in chronic neurological damage. Chronic malnutrition occurs since the high calorific content of ethanol prevents the consumption of nutrient-containing foods. Other effects include immunosuppression and a greater risk of cancer of the mouth, larynx and oesophagus.

Protective effects

Moderate consumption of alcohol of 2–3 units per day increases high-density lipoprotein (HDL) and reduces platelet aggregation, thereby reducing the risk of cardiovascular disease.

Drug interactions

Table 3.3 highlights some interactions occurring between prescribed drugs and alcohol. It is important that patients are warned about these interactions as many patients do not consider alcohol to be a drug and therefore rarely enquire as to problems with prescribed medicines.

Alcohol misuse

Treatment of alcohol misuse

Withdrawal from excessive drinking produces symptoms of tremor, insomnia, anxiety and cravings. More severe symptoms include severe agitation, seizures and hallucinations. Alcohol dependence is treated with disulfiram, acamprosate, long-acting benzodiazepines or clomethiazole (inpatient setting only).

Table 3.3   Examples of drug interactions with alcohol

Drug(s)	Consequences	Comments
Antibiotics (erythromycin, doxycycline)	Reduced absorption of erythromycin and doxycycline and possibly increased alcohol levels may occur	There is a popular misconception that all antibiotics interact with alcohol. In fact, very few antibiotics are known to interact with alcohol: see metronidazole
Metronidazole (including vaginal preparations), edible fungi, disulfiram, ketoconazole (oral)	Flushing and fullness of face and neck, tachycardia, breathlessness, giddiness, hypotension, nausea and vomiting. Disulfiram or Antabuse reaction	• Patients should be warned that disulfiram-like reactions could occur if alcohol is taken during treatment with metronidazole • A rare reaction with ketoconazole but patients, particularly heavy drinkers, should be warned
Antidiabetic agents	Risk of hypoglycaemia, particularly if liver glycogen stores are depleted, e.g. following intense exercise	• CNS-depressant effects with hypoglycaemia are particularly hazardous • Facial flushing (a disulfiram-like reaction) occurs with chlorpropamide
Antihypertensives	Reduced efficacy of antihypertensives	• Excess alcohol consumption increases blood pressure • A reduction in alcohol intake may allow the dose of antihypertensives to be reduced • There is also a risk of postural hypotension when antihypertensives (particularly ACE inhibitors and/or diuretics) are initiated
CNS-depressants (antihistamines, analgesics, antidepressants, cough and cold remedies, psychotropics, tranquillisers, travel-sickness tablets)	Additive CNS-depressant effect, resulting in increased drowsiness and reduced alertness	Patients should be warned of an increased risk of accidents when driving or operating machinery
H_2-receptor antagonist (cimetidine, ranitidine and nizatidine)	Blood alcohol levels may be increased in patients taking certain H_2-blockers	It should also be noted that alcohol may worsen dyspepsia
Lithium	Possible risk of impairment of skilled tasks such as driving	Patients should be warned that lithium taken alone or with alcohol may make driving more hazardous
Phenytoin	Reduced phenytoin levels	Alcohol induces hepatic enzymes
Retinoids (acetretin, isotretinoin)	• Increased levels of the teratogenic etretinate may occur in patients taking acetretin • Alcohol may reduce the effects of isotretinoin	The long half-life of acetretin should be considered on cessation of treatment
Verapamil	Blood alcohol levels may be increased and the effects of alcohol prolonged	Patients should be informed, due to the implications for drivers
Warfarin	INR may be increased or decreased. Heavy drinkers may require increased doses	This interaction mainly occurs with liver disease and/or heavy drinking and binge drinking. Moderate consumption appears safe

CNS, central nervous system; ACE, angiotensin-converting enzyme; INR, international normalised ratio.

Patient counselling

Health professionals should be particularly aware of the vicious circle whereby patients drink alcohol for its temporary euphoric and/or sedative effects but the CNS-depressant activity and insomniac effects of alcohol may worsen the original problem. Patients at risk of abusing alcohol include those with depression, anxiety and/or insomnia, chronic illness, social isolation (including the elderly) and following redundancy. The importance of drug interactions should also be considered (Table 3.3).

Other recreational drugs

Cannabis (marijuana, hashish, weed)

The pharmacological effects of cannabis result from Δ^9-tetrahydrocannabinol (THC)-mediated activation of predominantly CNS cannabinoid receptors.

These include:

- CNS-depressant and psychomimetic effects
- impairment of short-term memory
- impaired motor coordination
- catalepsy
- amnesia
- increased appetite

Peripheral effects include tachycardia, dry mouth and vasodilatation, including the scleral and conjunctival vessels of the eyes, and reduced immunity. A reduction in plasma testosterone and sperm count may occur.

Potential beneficial effects and therapeutic targets include:

- bronchodilation
- antiemetic (available as nabilone on prescription for restricted indications)
- analgesia (mechanism includes the activation of cannabinoid receptors in the brain and spinal cord)
- multiple sclerosis (antispastic actions)
- reduced intraocular pressure

Abuse potential and drug interactions

THC produces drowsiness and confusion in overdose with apparent safety in comparison to alcohol, opioids and other drugs, which produce life-threatening respiratory depression and cardiovascular effects. The risk of tolerance and dependence is less than with nicotine, alcohol and opioids, and cannabis is not considered to be addictive. Excess use may however produce withdrawal symptoms such as nausea, confusion, agitation, irritability, tachycardia and sweating. Long-term psychological effects may also occur.

Table 3.4 is included as a guide for health professionals since it is recognised that cannabis use is increasing. It may therefore be necessary to warn patients to avoid cannabis with prescribed medication. This may also be considered a cause of ADRs, requiring sensitive questioning in confidence.

Concurrent disease

The management of concurrent disease in patients abusing drugs represents another challenging area for health professionals. Indeed, the presentation of some diseases may be the first indication that a patient is abusing drugs. Table 3.5 has been included to highlight disease states that may be particularly complicated by drug abuse.

Over-the-counter (OTC) medicines are also prone to misuse. For a detailed discussion and useful suggestions for controlling the problem, the reader is referred to *Drugs of Abuse* (Wills, 1997). Examples of OTC drugs associated with abuse include the following:

- Sedative antihistamines, including those contained in cough medicines, may be used chronically for insomnia, leading to dependence (Chapter 25).
- Laxatives may be misused for weight loss, particularly by female patients and those suffering from anorexia nervosa.
- Patients addicted to opioids may misuse codeine and other opioid-containing preparations, such as kaolin and morphine. The

Table 3.4 Drug interactions with cannabis

Drug	Consequences	Comments
Alcohol	Additive effects. Peak blood alcohol levels reduced and delayed	Additive adverse effects
Chlorpromazine	Increased metabolism of phenothiazines possibly due to enzyme induction by smoke	Increased dose may be required with concurrent cannabis smoking. Dose reduction on cessation of smoking
Anticholinergics (including tricyclic antidepressants, antihistamines and phenothiazines)	Tachycardia due to additive anticholinergic and beta-adrenergic effects. Other anticholinergics are likely to interact similarly	Avoid concurrent use
Theophylline	Cytochrome P450 induction by polycyclic hydrocarbons in smoke. Increased metabolism	Possible increased dose required. Dose reduction on cessation of heavy smoking
SSRIs (fluoxetine)	THC is a potent inhibitor of serotonin uptake	Synergistic effect, including risk of hypomania and mania

SSRIs, selective serotonin reuptake inhibitors; THC, Δ^9-tetrahydrocannabinol.

antihistamine cyclizine is also subject to misuse by these patients and is thought to increase the effects of opioids.

- Sympathomimetics such as ephedrine, pseudoephedrine and phenylpropanolamine are used for their alerting and euphoric effects, for fatigue, improving athletic performance (see banned substances in the *British National Formulary*), for weight loss, to reduce craving for amphetamines and for the manufacture of amphetamines.
- Caffeine-containing products include some analgesics and preparations marketed for increased energy, e.g. Pro Plus. Added to consumption from tea and coffee, patients may become restless, nervous and prone to tachycardia or cardiac arrhythmias. Symptoms of excess caffeine intake may exacerbate or be mistaken for symptoms of anxiety and insomnia (Chapters 24 and 25). Withdrawal effects such as headache and exhaustion then lead to further intake and dependence.

Drug interactions associated with these products

can be found in chapters addressing each disease state. For example, for interactions of OTC medicines with those prescribed for depression, consult Chapter 23.

Patient counselling and the recommendation of food supplements

In general, a balanced diet as indicated above should provide all the necessary nutrients. The following section will consider situations requiring specific advice and a possible requirement for the recommendation of food supplements. The differing demands of various life-stages and nutritional status are considered. The effects of disease on nutritional status are addressed within specific chapters. All recommendations should be evidence-based with consideration given to possible toxicity and drug interactions.

Table 3.5   Adverse effects of drugs of abuse and concurrent disease, compiled from *Drug Interactions* by Stockley (2002) and *Drugs of Abuse* by Wills (1997)

Disease	Abused drug	Effects
Asthma	Inhaled cocaine	Cough, bronchospasm, wheezing, status asthmaticus
	Smoked cannabis, tobacco	As above and bronchitis. Dosages of theophylline may need to be increased
	Overdose of IV opioids	Bronchospasm, respiratory arrest
	Heroin (diamorphine) injected or vaporised	Bronchospasm (this may be an excipient effect)
Epilepsy	Cocaine, amphetamines, alcohol, benzodiazepine withdrawal, some opioids	Epileptics may be prone to convulsant effect
Depression	Ecstasy, alcohol, cannabis	CNS-depressant effects may lead to depression. Also many drug interactions
Renal failure	Opioids, benzodiazepines,	Increased sensitivity to CNS effects
Immunocompromised	Alkyl nitrites, opioids, alcohol, cannabis, smoking, anabolic steroids, ecstasy	Risk of reduced immunity and therefore infection, particularly in immunocompromised patients
Hypertension	Cocaine, amphetamines, anabolic steroids, chronic alcohol consumption	Increased blood pressure. Note increased postural hypotension due to interaction between alcohol and antihypertensive medication
Diabetes	Anabolic steroids	Reduced insulin requirement
	Smoking	Increased insulin requirement
	Alcohol	Risk of hypoglycaemia, particularly if liver glycogen stores are depleted, e.g. following intense exercise. CNS-depressant effect with hypoglycaemia is particularly hazardous
	Cannabis	Slight increase in blood glucose but rare
	Stimulants (amphetamine, ecstasy, cocaine)	Loss of appetite requiring reduced insulin dose. Also overactivity resulting in hypoglycaemia

IV, intravenous; CNS, central nervous system.

Pregnancy

Ideally, the provision of nutritional advice should occur prior to conception, with the aim of correcting the mother's nutritional status before pregnancy. Of particular importance is the supplementation of folic acid 400 µg to all women when planning a pregnancy or likely to become pregnant and continued until the 12th week of pregnancy to help prevent neural tube defects. A review of chronic disease states and

drug treatment is also important. Preconception interventions might include:

- reducing a high caffeine and/or alcohol intake
- the provision of smoking cessation advice
- reducing the intake of artificial sweeteners
- referral for support of drug abuse
- discussions about long-term medication such as for epilepsy, depression or Crohn's disease
- a review of the disease history and/or screening and treatment of current symptoms of

diabetes, hypertension, vomiting, constipation, heartburn and dyspepsia
- a review of general dietary habits and supplementation with 400 µg of folic acid daily
- ideally, oral contraception should be stopped 3 months before a planned pregnancy due to the reduced absorption of micronutrients

General nutritional advice during pregnancy

The following points summarise the main nutritional issues during pregnancy:

- Pregnancy is an opportunity to promote healthy eating. Of particular importance are:
  - folate-rich foods, including fortified bread and breakfast cereals, Brussels sprouts and spinach, in addition to supplementation
  - iron-rich foods, including red meat, breakfast cereals, baked beans and soya beans. These should be eaten with sources of vitamin C such as citrus fruits, to optimise iron absorption
  - calcium-rich foods, such as milk, Cheddar cheese, Edam, yogurt, canned sardines and whitebait
- Avoid *excessive* consumption of vitamin A, found in products such as liver and pâté, as this has been associated with an increased risk of birth defects.
- Alcohol intake should be limited to less than 10 units per week and spread across the week. Excessive intake and dependency (approximately 6 units per day or more) causes fetal alcohol syndrome, including facial abnormalities, CNS defects and growth retardation. Chronic alcohol abuse may also reduce the nutritional status of the mother.
- Artificial sweeteners should not be consumed in excessive quantities.
- Nausea and vomiting may be avoided or reduced by eating frequent nutritious snacks and small meals.
- Avoiding triggers such as spicy food, eating smaller meals and more frequently, eating slowly and the avoidance of eating late may control heartburn. It should be noted that antacid preparations should not be taken at the same time of day as iron supplements.

- To prevent constipation, pregnant women can increase their dietary intake of NSPs, including wholemeal bread, brown pasta, fruit and vegetables, whilst maintaining an adequate fluid intake.
- Patients with hypertension should restrict sodium intake, including intake from soluble preparations such as paracetamol and antacids.
- Due to the risk of *Listeria*, the following foods should be avoided during pregnancy: undercooked meat, pâté, unwashed salad, soft and blue cheese and unpasteurised food. Flu-like symptoms should be reported to exclude *Listeria*.

Appropriate recommendation of supplements

Generally, supplements other than folic acid are not required if the mother has a healthy diet. Herbal supplements should be avoided due to the lack of safety data of use in pregnancy together with the pharmacological activity of these products. Vitamin A supplements, with the exception of the precursor beta-carotene, should be avoided due to the risk of birth defects associated with a high intake of vitamin A.

The following situations indicate appropriate recommendation of supplements during pregnancy:

- All women likely to become pregnant require a supplement of folic acid (see above). Patients prescribed proguanil or antiepileptic drugs such as phenytoin require a higher dose of folic acid (5 mg/day), which is only available on prescription.
- Asian and vegan women and indeed all women with a low intake of vitamin D and/or little exposure to sunlight, particularly during the winter, may benefit from a supplement of 10 µg/day of vitamin D.
- Vegan women may require a supplement of vitamin B_{12} and calcium (with vitamin D for absorption), although the absorption of calcium increases during pregnancy.
- Iron supplements may be required in iron-deficient anaemia and particularly if iron stores were low prior to pregnancy. Vitamin C

intake should be maintained for optimum iron absorption.

- Patients who abuse alcohol require multi-vitamin and mineral supplementation.
- Adolescent mothers have an increased requirement for nutrients required for growth. A diet rich in calcium, iron, zinc and folate is required and supplements may be of benefit.

Lactation

The nutritional requirements of breast-feeding women are also altered. Breast-feeding should be encouraged and women provided with support and reassurance. The following summarises the general advice to be given during lactation:

- the importance of a healthy diet based on current recommendations
- to eat according to appetite in order to meet increased energy requirement
- the importance of a diet high in calcium-rich foods such as dairy products to meet increased calcium requirements (double the normal requirement)
- the requirement for increased fluid intake for establishing and maintaining lactation. For example, fluid intake should be increased according to thirst
- avoid excess alcohol and caffeine-containing drinks, which may affect the baby
- mothers requesting advice about starting formula milk should be referred to their health visitor or midwife
- the importance of good attachment by pushing both the nipple and areola into the baby's mouth
- to report symptoms of redness, swelling and painful breasts for early diagnosis and treatment of mastitis
- dieting should be discouraged during lactation and any weight loss should be gradual
- soya-based formula milk should not be recommended without prior diagnosis of lactose intolerance or cow's-milk sensitivity and only following medical advice

Appropriate recommendation of supplements

Supplements are generally not necessary during lactation unless the diet is poor. It should also be considered that excess intake may be harmful. For example, excess vitamin D could lead to hypercalcaemia in the infant. The following situations may prompt supplementation:

- Vegan diets may be deficient in vitamins D and B_{12} and calcium.
- Asian women may lack vitamin D.

Infants

The following points are intended as a guide to general requirements and advice for mothers of infants from 1 to 5 years of age:

- Unmodified cow's milk should ideally not be given until 1 year, as it may not contain sufficient iron. From 1 to 5 years, half a litre or a pint of full-fat milk per day is recommended. Semiskimmed or skimmed milk is not usually recommended for children aged less than 5 years. Semiskimmed milk may however be suitable for children over 2 years if the diet is adequate.
- Unmodified soya milks are not recommended for children under 5 years as they are considered to be nutritionally inadequate.
- Bottles should not be heated in the microwave oven due to uneven heating.
- Weaning should generally not be started before 6 months of age. Nutritious food such as baby rice, puréed fruit or vegetables is introduced gradually, giving 1–2 teaspoonfuls initially. Food to avoid under the age of 6 months includes eggs, wheat, nuts, sugar, salt and citrus fruit.
- Vitamin drops may be given from 1 month if the mother of a breast-fed baby has a poor diet. They may also be indicated from 6 months to 5 years if sources of vitamins A and D are lacking in the diet. Vitamin D deficiency may also result from low exposure to sunlight.

Children

The following points refer to the general nutritional requirements and advice for children aged over 5 years:

- Height and weight are monitored according to standard reference curves.
- Reducing weight gain while height increases rather than advising weight loss is the method of treating overweight children.
- Frequent and small meals should be encouraged.
- Sweets should be restricted to once or twice a week and not given as a reward, due to the risk of dental caries.
- Important components of the diet are nutrient-dense food such as meat, poultry, fish, milk, cheese, eggs, bread, cereals, fruit and vegetables.
- Diets high in NSPs or dietary fibre are avoided, as they may be too bulky for children. Low-fat diets are also inappropriate as they provide insufficient energy.
- High levels of food additives including colours, preservatives and antioxidants may be associated with hyperactivity.

Adolescence

The following recommendations reflect the dietary needs of teenagers during puberty:

- Vegetarians should be advised to include pulses, soya products and dairy products (unless they are vegans) and to take multivitamin and mineral supplements to avoid nutrient deficiency. Supplements are particularly relevant for vegans.
- Smoking and alcohol consumption are to be discouraged as nutritional requirements, particularly for thiamin, folic acid and vitamin C, are increased.
- Encourage healthy eating as before. Increase the intake of complex carbohydrates according to appetite, to meet increased energy requirements. Avoid a diet high in fat and sugar.
- Emphasise, particularly in females, the importance of weight-bearing exercise for the

prevention of osteoporosis in later life. Calcium supplements may be indicated if the diet is poor.
- Iron-rich foods are important, particularly for females. Supplements may be required in the presence of menorrhagia or vegetarianism.
- Slimming should be avoided due to a risk of calcium, iron, vitamin A, B_6, folate and riboflavin deficiency. Slimming may also trigger anorexia nervosa in this age group. Overweight adolescents should be advised to increase exercise and advised of the importance of a healthy diet.

Elderly

Nutritional care of elderly patients presents a particular challenge to healthcare professionals, due to the many social, pharmacological and age-related factors combining to make eating difficult. These include an age-related loss of taste, loss of interest in food, living alone, reduced mobility and concurrent disease such as COPD. The following points outline the main problems to address:

- The regular monitoring of the BMI (see above) is a useful tool to aid diagnosis of malnutrition and disease states associated with weight loss. Subsequent interventions such as the initiation of drug treatment and/or supplemental feeds can also be monitored.
- Vitamin D deficiency may result from poor diet and low exposure to sunlight.
- Regular drug reviews should consider the effect of drugs on nutritional status and the risk of drug–nutrient interactions. For example, eating may be easier for COPD patients if medication is administered to improve breathing prior to eating. Alternatively, patients prescribed warfarin should avoid changing their intake of vitamin K provided by foods such as avocado and green vegetables (Table 3.1).
- The elderly have reduced energy requirements but their nutrient requirements are unchanged, with the exception of iron for women. A nutrient-dense diet is therefore required.
- It is important to avoid causing anxiety by recommending lots of changes.

- Elderly patients may be referred to Age Concern for advice and support and may be directed to a 'meals on wheels' service.

Appropriate recommendation of supplements

The following situations may warrant dietary supplements for elderly patients:

- multivitamin and mineral supplements for patients unable to eat a healthy diet
- meal replacements such as Build-up and Complan to increase energy, but not for more than 2 weeks as the sole source
- vitamin C supplements if there is a lack of fresh food available and particularly to increase iron absorption
- vitamin D for the housebound
- vitamin B_{12} in malabsorption conditions
- calcium to slow bone loss if the diet lacks calcium and/or the patient is at risk of osteoporosis. Risk factors include a family history, early menopause and regular treatment with corticosteroids (Chapter 28)
- iron supplements may be required if the dietary intake is low and following blood loss, which may be caused by non-steroidal anti-inflammatory drugs (NSAIDs)

Lifestyle advice and the role of the community pharmacist

Lifestyle advice is an important component of the prevention and treatment of disease and a multidisciplinary approach is essential. Community pharmacists have an important role to play in the provision of health promotion as part of the primary care team and are increasingly providing services such as:

- blood pressure monitoring
- glucose testing of the blood and/or urine
- cardiovascular risk assessment
- osteoporosis screening
- cholesterol testing
- smoking cessation advice and the use of NRT
- dietary advice, including the appropriate use of supplements
- patient counselling to avoid drug–food interactions
- advice on weight control according to the measurement of BMI

Practice points

- The provision of lifestyle advice in accordance with the latest evidence is important for all patients with the aim of both preventing and treating disease.
- Medication review should include an assessment of ADRs as a possible cause of poor nutritional status. Conversely, dietary factors should be considered as a possible cause of drug interactions.
- Drugs of abuse should be considered as a cause of both disease and interactions with prescribed medicines.
- Dietary advice specific to the different life-stages is required due to changing nutritional requirements.
- Patients most likely to benefit from vitamin and mineral supplements include those at risk of inadequate intake from the diet such as vegetarians, the elderly and those who smoke and/or misuse alcohol.

CASE STUDIES

Case 1
An elderly patient comes into the pharmacy for her prescription:

Ramipril 5 mg o.d.	furosemide (frusemide) 40 mg o.m.
Digoxin 125 μg o.d.	aspirin 75 mg o.d.
Simvastatin 10 mg o.n.	glyceryl trinitrate spray p.r.n.

A neighbour has advised her that reducing her salt intake would benefit her hypertension. She has heard that you can buy salt substitute and would value your opinion. You notice from your patient medication record that her husband takes lithium tablets.

This case illustrates a range of nutritional issues and highlights the importance of patient education. The main issues are summarised here:

- There is a requirement for reinforcing advice regarding a low-fat diet in view of the patient's hypercholesterolaemia (Chapter 12).
- She is right to reduce the sodium content of her diet in view of her hypertension and diuretic treatment (Chapter 11), but this will impact on her husband's treatment.
- Changing from salt (sodium chloride) to salt substitute (potassium salt) would reduce sodium intake and risk an increase in her husband's serum lithium levels to toxic levels. Patients stabilised on lithium should not alter sodium intake and should maintain an adequate fluid intake. Any change in salt and water intake should be discussed first with their general practitioner (GP), who may then monitor plasma levels of lithium. A lithium treatment card should be given.
- The potassium content of salt substitute interacts with her angiotensin-converting enzyme (ACE) inhibitor (although this may be negated by the loop diuretic), increasing her risk of hyperkalaemia. Since she is also taking digoxin, her urea and electrolytes (Chapter 2) should be monitored regularly and checked prior to a change in sodium and/or potassium intake.

In summary, the patient could reduce her salt intake, for example not use salt at the table, and reduce her consumption of processed food and this may have some effect on her blood pressure. However, more importantly, she should reduce her intake of saturated fat and follow a healthy diet. Her intake of oily fish should be increased.

Case 2
The mother of a 14-year-old boy asks your advice about antibiotics for acne. She comments that her son has been taking the antibiotic for a month with no improvement.
Current treatment: tetracycline 250 mg b.d.

- This case may represent compliance issues and/or a potential food–nutrient interaction. For example, the patient should be asked if he takes the antibiotics regularly and an hour before food? Does he take any mineral supplements or indigestion remedies? The absorption of tetracycline is reduced by milk, dairy products, iron, calcium, magnesium and zinc and this could be a cause of treatment failure.

In this case, compliance problems were identified and corrected with explanation. In addition, the patient had only been taking the treatment for 1 month and was therefore advised to continue if possible as an alternative antibacterial would not be tried unless no improvement was observed

continued

CASE STUDIES (continued)

after 3 months (see also Chapter 32). Tetracycline is usually given at a dose of 500 mg b.d. for the treatment of acne. The dose should therefore be queried. Maximum improvement may take several months. The patient was advised to consult his GP if there was no improvement within another 2 months or if he experienced a worsening of his condition. Compliance problems may be addressed by prescribing minocycline once daily, which does not interact with milk and dairy products, but has cost implications.

Case 3
A 22-year-old female is taking fluoxetine for depression and presents with symptoms of hypomania. What is the course of action?

- Further questioning is required to establish a possible cause prior to dose adjustment and/or stopping her treatment. This example represents a student who was smoking cannabis and consuming excess alcohol. Symptoms were improved following the cessation of cannabis and she was also advised that alcohol may work against her antidepressant treatment (see also Chapter 23). This case highlights the importance of questioning patients about the use of substances such as alcohol and cannabis as they have the potential to interact with conventional medicines.

References

Department of Health (1999). *Saving Lives: Our Healthier Nation*. London: HMSO.

Mehta D K (ed.) *British National Formulary*, latest edition. London: British Medical Association and Royal Pharmaceutical Society of Great Britain.

Silagy C, Lancaster T, Stead L, Mant D, Fowler G (2002). (3) Nicotine replacement therapy for smoking cessation (Cochrane review). *Cochrane Database Systematic Review* issue 3. Oxford: Update Software.

Stockley I H (2002). *Drug Interactions*, 6th edn. London: Pharmaceutical Press.

Wills S (1997). *Drugs of Abuse*. London: Pharmaceutical Press.

Department of Health (2002). *Paper for Information: Key Dietary Recommendations*. Scientific Advisory Committee on Nutrition. London: Department of Health.

Raw M, McNeill A, West R (1998). Smoking cessation guidelines for health professionals. A guide to effective smoking cessation interventions for the health care system. *Thorax* 53: S1–S18.

Useful contacts

Quit line 0800 0022000 is available between 9 a.m. and 9 p.m. for counselling and support for those attempting to stop smoking.

Further reading

Anon (1999). Nicotine replacement therapy. *MeReC Bull* 10: 9–12.

Online resources

www.ace.org.uk. Age Concern provides information and access to local services relating to care of the elderly (accessed 4 December 2002).

www.alcoholics-anonymous.org.uk. Alcoholics Anonymous, for access to local contacts, including groups of recovered and recovering alcoholics who provide support to those committed to controlling their problem (accessed 4 December 2002).

www.ash.org.uk Action on Smoking and Health (ASH) for education and research with the aim of preventing some of the 120 000 deaths from smoking-related diseases in the UK each year (accessed 4 December 2002).

www.doh.gov.uk. The Department of Health site provides a search facility and a useful A–Z index for access to government information, e.g. smoking cessation advice, Standing Medical Advisory Committee (SMAC) reports and health promotion (accessed 4 December 2002).

The Royal Pharmaceutical Society has produced a guide to the provision and auditing of smoking cessation campaigns as part of the 'Ready-to-go-series' available from www.rpsgb.org.uk (accessed 4 December 2002).

4

Herbal medicine and homeopathy

Herbal preparations contain pharmacologically active substances and should therefore be considered as drugs. Plant extracts for these preparations are derived from leaves, buds, roots, flowers, fruit, seed, stems, wood, bark, rhizomes or other plant parts, which may be fragmented or powdered.

Reporting of drug interactions and adverse drug reactions (ADRs) due to herbal drugs remains low due to the perception by the general public that these preparations are natural and therefore 'safe'. They are considered to be 'alternative remedies' and the presence of pharmacological activity comparable with conventional medicines is underestimated. Useful examples include the origin of digoxin from foxgloves and the powerful laxative effect of senna. Professional judgement and pharmacological knowledge are important when considering the suitability of herbal preparations for patients with concurrent disease and taking conventional medicines. This was highlighted by reports of interactions involving St John's wort (Table 4.1), which is thought to exert antidepressant activity by inhibiting serotonin, dopamine and/or noradrenaline (norepinephrine) uptake, although the precise mechanism is not known.

Drug history-taking and responding to symptoms should involve active enquiry about herbal medicines. Any change in clinical outcome should be assessed for possible drug interactions or ADRs thought to result from concurrent use of conventional and herbal drugs. Suspected problems should be reported to the Committee on Safety of Medicines (CSM) using the yellow card system.

Evidence

It is difficult for health professionals to recommend the use of many herbal preparations in the absence of good evidence of safe efficacious use, particularly in combination with conventional medicines. Added to this, an extensive variety of preparations is available, doses and purity may vary. The Code of Ethics for Pharmacists (Royal Pharmaceutical Society of Great Britain) recommends that pharmacists 'should not recommend any [herbal] remedy where they have any reason to doubt its safety or quality.' Herbal preparations should be obtained from reliable sources and licensed products stocked

Table 4.1 Examples of interactions between herbal and conventional medicines for which clinical evidence exists or potential interactions based on *in vivo* or *in vitro* pharmacological activity

Physiological effects	Implicated herbs and interactions with conventional drugs	Comments
Antiplatelet activity	Garlic, arnica, aniseed, angelica, celery, camomile, feverfew, ginkgo biloba, red clover, turmeric and green tea with warfarin or antiplatelet drugs (aspirin, dipyridamole, clopidogrel)	• An isolated report of spontaneous bleeding from the iris in a patient taking low-dose aspirin and ginkgo biloba • It may be sensible for patients prescribed antiplatelet treatment to avoid these herbal preparations • Patients reporting increased bleeding, e.g. bruising, should be asked about their use of herbal preparations • These products should also be avoided or discontinued at least 24–48 h before surgery
Cardioactive activity, e.g. antiarrhythmic, inotropic or calcium channel effects	Cola, coltsfoot, ginger, ginseng (Panax), motherwort, shepherd's purse and wild carrot with antiarrhythmics (amiodarone), digoxin and other cardioactive agents	Patients at increased risk include those with cardiovascular disease and/or taking drugs with cardiovascular activity
Cholinergic activity	Ginkgo leaf with donepezil, rivastigmine or galantamine	Risk of additive effects and therefore increased cholinergic side-effects such as diarrhoea, urinary incontinence and insomnia
Diuresis	Artichoke, burdock, celery, dandelion, elder, java tea, juniper, nettle, shepherd's purse and squill	• Potential to interact with concurrent diuretic and other antihypertensive treatment (Chapter 11) • Particular caution may be required with drugs associated with significant hypotensive effects such as ACE inhibitors, alpha-adrenoceptor antagonists and antipsychotics
Hormone activity	Dong quai (Chinese), vitex berry, hops flower, ginseng root, black cohosh root with tamoxifen	• There is little evidence of a problem but these products demonstrate binding to oestrogen receptors and may therefore oppose the action of tamoxifen and possibly stimulate the growth of oestrogen-sensitive tumours of the breast
	Saw palmetto with antiandrogens (finasteride)	• Saw palmetto has been reported to possess antiandrogen activity and this should be considered when prescribing antiandrogens for prostatic hyperplasia
Hyperglycaemic	Ginseng (Panax), liquorice, rosemary	Increased risk for patients with diabetes mellitus and also concurrent treatment with corticosteroids (Chapters 20 and 33)

Continued

Table 4.1 *Continued*

Physiological effects	Implicated herbs and interactions with conventional drugs	Comments
Hypoglycaemic	Aloe vera, burdock, celery, cornsilk, dandelion, garlic, ginger, ginseng (Panax), ispaghula, juniper, marshmallow, nettle, sage	Increased risk for patients with diabetes and concurrent disease treated with ACE inhibitors (Chapters 11 and 14)
Hypertension and risk of hypokalaemia	Liquorice with antihypertensives	• Effects are due to weak mineralocorticoid properties of glycyrrhizic acid found in liquorice • People with hypertension, CHF or taking drugs with the potential to cause hypokalaemia should avoid large quantities of liquorice
Immunostimulant	Echinacea with immunosuppressants (corticosteroids, azathioprine)	Avoid, as echinacea may be predicted to oppose immunosuppressant effects
Increased levels of digoxin	Ginseng (Siberian) with digoxin	Siberian ginseng contains glycosides related to digoxin
Increased effects	Ginseng with MAOIs (phenelzine)	Increased side-effects such as headache, tremor and psychoactive effects
Increased effects	St John's wort with triptans, SSRIs	The CSM/MCA warn of an increased risk of serotonergic effects
Decreased effects	St John's wort with anticonvulsants, warfarin, digoxin, theophylline, ciclosporin, oral contraceptives	• St John's wort induces cytochrome P450 isoenzymes • Avoid concurrent use • Dose adjustment is not appropriate due to varying doses of St John's wort according to preparation
Laxative effects	Aloes, cascara, ispaghula, rhubarb and senna	• Consider the risk of abuse by patients with anorexia nervosa • Increased risk of dehydration of patients taking drugs such as diuretics (Chapters 11 and 14)
Sedation	Celery, kava, camomile, ginseng, hops, nettle, sage, St John's wort and valerian with opioids, antihistamines, alcohol, antidepressants, benzodiazepines	• Possibility of severe sedation with concurrent use of St John's wort with SSRIs (paroxetine) and other antidepressants • Avoid concomitant use and if possible leave a washout period when stopping St John's wort and starting any SSRI • It may be a sensible precaution to avoid concurrent use of St John's wort with all antidepressants due to the risk of additive pharmacological effects Increased effects of CNS-depressants

Continued

Table 4.1 *Continued*

Physiological effects	Implicated herbs and interactions with conventional drugs	Comments
		• Patients requesting herbal products for insomnia should be advised as for conventional hypnotics (Chapter 25)
		• Valerian root may increase concentrations of the inhibitory neurotransmitter, GABA, in the brain
		• As a precaution, patients should not take herbs such as valerian up to 2 hours before driving or performing other skilled tasks
Sympathomimetic activity	Aniseed, caffeine, arnica, borage, capsicum, echinacea, ephadra, Chinese ginseng (Panax), gentian, valerian, nettle, parsley, passionflower and vervain	• Reduced effect of antihypertensives
Thyroid effects	Kelp with amiodarone, thyroxine, lithium and antithyroid drugs	Iodine content of kelp may alter thyroid function
Urinary effects (increased flow)	Saw palmetto	• Patients at risk include those with concurrent prostatic hyperplasia, incontinence or taking drugs such as diuretics
		• If possible, patients requesting herbs for bladder problems should be asked about symptoms, which may indicate prostatic hyperplasia requiring referral to their general practitioner, including:
		• a sensation of incomplete bladder emptying on urination
		• needing to urinate within 2 h of previous urination
		• frequent urination during the night
		• non-continuous urine flow
		• a weak urinary stream
		• difficulty starting urinating
		• difficulty postponing urination

Derived from *Drug Interactions* by Stockley (2002), *Dietary Supplements* by Mason (2001) and *Herbal Medicines* by Barnes *et al.* (2002).
ACE, angiotensin-converting enzyme; CHF, chronic heart failure; MAOIs, monoamine oxidase inhibitors; SSRIs, selective serotonin reuptake inhibitors; CSM, Committee on Safety of Medicines; MCA, Medicines Control Agency; CNS, central nervous system; GABA, gamma-aminobutyric acid.

whenever possible. It should be noted that unlicensed products will not have been assessed by the Medicines Control Agency (MCA) and licensed products will not have been tested as vigorously as conventional drugs, which undergo controlled clinical trials.

The most important role of health professionals in the use of herbal preparations is to advise patients of potential problems, particularly associated with concurrent use of conventional medicine (Table 4.1) and to help identify adverse effects, which should be reported to the CSM. When available, the evidence of efficacy and safety may be communicated to patients and this information is increasingly available in systematic reviews of current trials, for example Cochrane and Bandolier reviews (see Online resources at the end of this chapter). Health professionals without training in prescribing herbal medicines should refer patients to suitably trained herbalists, who may be located via the National Institute of Medical Herbalists' website provided at the end of the chapter.

Current problems

Current safety issues reported by the MCA and CSM relate to interactions between herbal remedies and conventional medicines, the accidental inclusion of toxic or potent herbal ingredients, contamination with heavy metals or the illegal addition of some prescription-only medicines. Further information is available from the MCA or US Food and Drug Administration (FDA) websites given at the end of the chapter. Examples of recent reports include:

- interactions between conventional drugs and St. John's wort (Table 4.1)
- hepatotoxicity with kava-kava and renal failure with certain Chinese herbs
- the substitution of plantain by digitalis, leading to serious cardiac arrhythmias
- the addition of corticosteroids, warfarin, alprazolam and sildenafil to herbal remedies

Interactions between herbal and conventional medicines

Examples of interactions between herbal and conventional medicines, for which clinical evidence exists are given in Table 4.1. The possibility of drug interactions extrapolated from *in vitro* and *in vivo* pharmacological activity is also considered.

For further information the reader is referred to Stockley's *Drug Interactions* (2002) and *Herbal Medicines* by Barnes *et al.* (2002) and the online resources listed at the end of the chapter.

The risk factors for adverse reactions to herbal medicines are the same as those for conventional medicines, for example, polypharmacy, extremes of ages, impaired renal or hepatic function, history of allergy, use of high doses and chronic use. The source of the product and existence of a product licence should also be considered.

Homeopathy

The main principle of homeopathy is the treatment of 'like with like', as implied by the prefix 'homeo-'. For example, insomnia is treated with an extract from the green coffee bean (*Coffea*). Extremely small quantities of the homeopathic preparation are administered following serial dilution, agitation and formulation. A product is recommended according to the presenting complaint but also the individual, providing a holistic approach.

Nomenclature used to express potency uses centesimal and decimal systems. For the centesimal system, mother tincture is prepared from an extract of the source material, which may be plant, animal, insect, biological or chemical material, in a mixture of alcohol and water. One drop of mother tincture is then added to 99 drops of diluent (20–60% triple-distilled alcohol and water). The resulting solution is shaken vigorously (a process known as succussion) and then serial dilutions are made, indicated by a multiple of 'c' representing the number of successive dilutions of one in 100. For example, a potency of 6c gives a concentration of 10^{-12}. It is the process of serial dilution and claims of increased therapeutic potency (potentisation) with each dilution which many people find difficult to accept.

The decimal system involves the addition of one drop of mother tincture to nine drops of diluent and represented as a multiple of 'x'. The letters M and CM are used to represent greater dilution levels of 1000 and 10 000, respectively. If one compares the two systems for denoting potency, therefore, 6c is equivalent to 12x.

To date, there is no proven scientific or pharmacological theory for the efficacy of homeopathic remedies and evidence of efficacy is limited. However, these remedies continue to be available on the National Health Service (NHS) and many patients choose homeopathy. Healthcare professionals should be alert for a possible delay in consulting advice for serious symptoms (Chapter 1) by patients choosing homeopathy. Advice should only be provided following adequate training. It should be noted that adverse effects involving an exacerbation of symptoms may be reported. Patients should discontinue treatment and consult a homeopath. There are no known interactions with conventional medicines, although steroids are thought to inactivate homeopathic preparations.

The following points of advice may be given to patients taking homeopathic preparations. The active ingredient is placed on the surface of the dosage form and absorbed through the oral mucosa. Inappropriate handling is therefore thought to inactivate the product. Patients should be counselled as follows:

• The product should be kept in its original container.
• Homeopathic medicines should not be handled but transferred to the mouth via the container cap.
• Take at least 30 min before or after food.
• Suck or chew tablet before swallowing.
• Mother tincture should be diluted in a mouthful of water, gargled and then swallowed.

• Highly flavoured or aromatic foods should be avoided, e.g. peppermints.
• Avoid the inhalation of aromatic products containing eucalyptus and camphor, as well as smoking and coffee or tea.
• Stop the treatment when the condition improves.

Homeopathy and pregnancy

Highly diluted homeopathic remedies are considered safe for use during pregnancy but should not delay referral to exclude serious conditions.

Practice points

• Health professionals should enquire routinely about the use of herbal remedies by patients.
• Herbal remedies should be avoided in pregnancy and lactation, due to the absence of safety data.
• The risk of ADRs caused by herbal preparations is increased, as for conventional drugs, with polypharmacy, long-term use, high doses, patients at extremes of age and impaired renal and hepatic function.
• Information relating to the safe and effective use of herbal preparations is increasing rapidly and the latest information can be found online: useful websites are provided at the end of the chapter.

  CASE STUDIES

Case 1
A 25-year-old woman has recently been diagnosed with Crohn's disease. She has been given dietary advice and her symptoms have improved. Her symptoms have however worsened in the last 24 h and she does not understand why. She says she feels very low and is tearful. She has started taking St John's wort. She is also complaining of a sore throat and chest infection. Should she take echinacea? She is very keen on taking herbal remedies, as they are natural. She gives you her prescription:

→

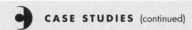

CASE STUDIES (continued)

Venlafaxine 75 mg b.d.
Azathioprine 50 mg t.d.s.
Prednisolone 5 mg e.c. tablets as directed
Mesalazine 400 mg e.c. tablets 2 t.d.s.

Whilst you dispense her medication, she starts to tell you about a party she went to the previous night.

Is it appropriate for this patient to take St John's wort with echinacea? What general advice would you give to this patient about herbal medicines?

There were a number of issues to consider from this case:

- Was she taking a calcium supplement to reduce the risk of osteoporosis due to her prednisolone treatment, particularly in view of malabsorption as a result of her Crohn's disease (Chapter 9)?
- How much alcohol was she consuming? Alcohol is a central nervous system-depressant and may therefore worsen her depression (see venlafaxine) and could also exacerbate her Crohn's disease. The corticosteroid may also contribute to her low mood (Chapter 5).
- St John's wort should not be given with antidepressant therapy. She should be referred back to her general practitioner (GP) if her antidepressant treatment is not effective. Perhaps check first how long she has been taking the venlafaxine, as there may be a delay in efficacy at the start of treatment.
- Hopefully her sore throat is the result of too much singing the night before. However, in view of her immunosuppressant therapy, she should be referred to her GP for a full blood count.
- Echinacea may interfere with immunosuppressive therapy as it is thought to have immuno-stimulant activity.
- It may be wise to advise this patient to avoid herbal medicine in view of her drug treatment.

Case 2
A 21-year-old female asks what you think about kelp tablets for weight loss. Her gym instructor recommended them.

What further questions would you ask?

- It is important to establish if the patient is overweight and to consider her lifestyle and diet (Chapter 3). Her medical history and any current medication should also be considered.
- Further questioning reveals a history of thyroid dysfunction and excessive calorie intake from lager.

Are kelp tablets suitable for this patient?

- No. Kelp tablets contain iodine, which could exacerbate her thyroid problem (Chapter 34). There is also a risk of the presence of toxic heavy metals. Possible mechanisms for the weight-loss effect of kelp tablets include increased thyroid activity and/or laxative effects and are not, therefore, a healthy option for weight loss. General lifestyle factors should be considered and the patient advised that the best way to lose weight is to increase exercise and reduce her calorie intake (Chapter 3). This patient was only marginally overweight and this was corrected by avoiding lager and continuing her exercise routine.

continued

CASE STUDIES (continued)

Case 3

A 56-year-old female informs you that she has been taking a herbal remedy containing ginseng root to relieve her menopausal symptoms. She has found that her symptoms have improved and thought you would like to know so that you could recommend them to other patients. You notice from her computer records that she is currently taking tamoxifen 20 mg/day for breast cancer.

Are you happy for the patient to continue with the herbal remedy?

- No. In view of her tamoxifen treatment and the absence of sufficient safety data, the ginseng root is not recommended since it has been shown to possess oestrogen receptor-binding activity. There is a risk that the herbal preparation could interfere with her tamoxifen treatment. This case illustrates the importance of asking patients about their use of herbal preparations, as the information is not always volunteered.

References

Barnes J, Anderson L A, Phillipson J D (2002). *Herbal Medicines*, 2nd edn. London: Pharmaceutical Press.

Mason P (2001). *Dietary Supplements*, 2nd edn. London: Pharmaceutical Press.

Royal Pharmaceutical Society of Great Britain (2002). *Medicines, Ethics and Practice – A Guide for Pharmacists*, 26th edn. London: Royal Pharmaceutical Society of Great Britain.

Stockley I H (2002). *Drug Interactions*, 6th edn. London: Pharmaceutical Press.

Further reading

Barnes J (2002a). Herbal therapeutics (1) An introduction to herbal medicinal products. *Pharm J* 268: 804–806.

Barnes J (2002b). Herbal therapeutics (2) Depression. *Pharm J* 268: 908–910.

Barnes J (2002c). Herbal therapeutics (3) Cognitive deficiency and dementia. *Pharm J* 269: 160–162.

Barnes J (2002d). Herbal therapeutics (4) Hyperlipidaemia. *Pharm J* 269: 193–195.

Barnes J (2002e). Herbal therapeutics (5) Insomnia. *Pharm J* 269: 219–221.

Barnes J (2002f). Benign prostatic hyperplasia. *Pharm J* 269: 250–252.

Fugh-Berman A (2000). Herb–drug interactions. *Lancet* 355:134–138.

Kayne S B (2002). *Complementary Therapies for Pharmacists*. London: Pharmaceutical Press.

Online resources

http://www.cfsan.fda.gov/~dms/supplmnt.html   For the US Food and Drug Administration, information relating to dietary supplements, including warnings and safety information on the use of herbal preparations (accessed 4 December 2002).

http://www.mca.gov.uk The Medicines Control Agency with policy information for the use and licensing of herbal medicines and the latest safety information. There is also a new online information service to give up-to-date advice on herbal medicines safety (accessed 4 December 2002).

http://www.who.int/medicines/organization/trm/orgtr mmain.shtml. The World Health Organization's policy and strategy on traditional medicine (accessed 4 December 2002).

Royal Pharmaceutical Society of Great Britain (2002) Homeopathy, Useful Information for Pharmacists. Available from the RPSGB at www.rpsgb.org.uk.

www.homeopathy-soh.org. The Society of Homeopaths provides information and maintains a register of qualified homeopaths (accessed 4 December 2002).

www.nimh.org.uk. The National Institute of Medical Herbalists provides information and research relating to herbal medicines and access to suitably trained herbalists (accessed 4 December 2002).

www.trusthomeopathy.org/trust/tru_faq.html. For the British Homeopathic Association, information relating to homeopathy and access to qualified homeopaths (accessed 4 December 2002).

Part B

Treatment

5

Adverse drug reactions and interactions

Adverse drug reactions (ADRs) and drug interactions are related topics. For example, a drug interaction results in a change to the expected treatment outcome and occurs as a result of concurrent exposure to a second drug, food or chemical. The result may be an adverse event but this is not always the case. ADRs may occur during monotherapy and, by definition, are always unwanted effects.

The purpose of this chapter is to explore the nature and mechanisms, when known, resulting in ADRs and interactions. The inclusion of tables listing causative drugs is intended to give examples for familiarisation. Further information for a suspected drug-induced reaction should be sought from the summary of product characteristics (SPCs: see www.emc.vhn.net), manu-

facturers and published reports or the Committee on Safety of Medicines (CSM). The information presented in tables relating to ADRs was largely derived from Lee's *Adverse Drug Reactions* (2001) and the *British National Formulary*. Information relating to drug interactions was mainly derived from *Drug Interactions* by Stockley (2002).

Adverse drug reactions and side-effects

These terms are difficult to distinguish and in practice the two are often used interchangeably. It may be helpful to consider side-effects of a medicine as predictable secondary effects that may be beneficial (e.g. sedation with antihistamines when used as an over-the-counter (OTC) sleep medicine) or undesirable (e.g. sedation with antihistamines used for allergy relief). By contrast, ADRs are side-effects which are always deleterious. So, when considering drug treatment, one must balance both benefits and risks and be vigilant of established and previously unrecognised ADRs.

Recent evidence indicates that the problem of adverse reactions is of enormous proportions (Wiffen *et al.*, 2002). It must be appreciated that many patients may experience ADRs, which may limit the success of treatment and be associated with morbidity and mortality. Drugs most commonly implicated in causing ADRs as reported in hospital studies include:

- non-steroidal anti-inflammatory drugs (NSAIDs)
- antibiotics
- anticoagulants
- digoxin
- diuretics
- hypoglycaemic agents

ADRs are divided into type A (augmented response) and type B (bizarre or idiosyncratic reactions).

Type A: augmented response

This type of undesirable effect can be explained or predicted on the basis of the drug's pharmacology. Type A reactions are often dose-dependent and may often be managed by dose adjustment. If they are anticipated, measures may be taken to ameliorate or prevent the problem; for example, the use of antiemetics in patients receiving chemotherapy, or laxatives with opioid analgesics.

Type B: bizarre or idiosyncratic reactions

These ADRs are unrelated to the known pharmacology of the drug, which makes them less common and unpredictable; they may also be severe. This group of ADRs is often related to genetics or immunology, which means that certain individuals may be at a higher risk than others.

Risk factors for developing ADRs

When considering ADRs there are a number of risk factors which may predispose a patient to adverse responses:

- polypharmacy
- extremes of age
- gender
- concurrent disease
- pharmacokinetic variables, e.g. renal or hepatic function
- pharmaceutical factors, e.g. nature of dosage form or excipients
- race, e.g. glucose-6-phosphate dehydrogenase (G6PD) deficiency (see below) in African, Middle Eastern and South-east Asian populations.

Mechanisms of adverse reactions

The effects of a drug may be enhanced by various pharmacodynamic or pharmacokinetic factors, leading to enhanced side-effects or adverse reactions. Pharmacodynamic factors include those relating to the pharmacological activity of the drug, for example, the induction of bronchoconstriction in patients taking beta-adrenoceptor antagonists.

Pharmacokinetic ADRs result from impaired absorption, distribution, metabolism or excretion. For example, a reduced rate of elimination, often due to impaired renal function, is likely to increase plasma concentrations, leading to augmented effects. These are the most common causes of ADRs and may often be prevented. Impaired renal function is common in the elderly and neonates and this may be measured and drug doses adjusted as appropriate to prevent an ADR. Important examples where serious toxicity may arise as a consequence of renal impairment are:

- digoxin
- lithium
- NSAIDs
- metformin

- angiotensin-converting   enzyme   (ACE) inhibitors
- aminoglycoside antibiotics

Alterations in metabolism and pharmacogenetics

Alterations in drug metabolism may also lead to increased plasma concentrations. Metabolism may be altered at the extremes of age, such that neonates conjugate drugs at a slow rate (see phase II reactions below), while microsomal enzyme activity in the liver by cytochrome P450 isoenzymes decreases variably with age. An example of this is the prolonged half-life of diazepam with age, and hence the increased propensity to side-effects, including oversedation.

Genetic differences in the expression of cytochrome P450 isoenzymes may also contribute to variations in metabolism. Ninety per cent of the population are described as extensive metabolisers; the remaining 10%, however, possess defective isoenzymes of cytochrome P450, which slows down the metabolism of drugs such as debrisoquine, nortriptyline, flecainide, metoclopramide, nortriptyline, clomipramine, paroxetine and venlafaxine. These drugs are metabolised by cytochrome P450 isoenzyme CYP2D6 pathways. CYP2C9 inactivity requires reduced doses of warfarin.

Drug metabolism is described in two phases. Phase I reactions include oxidation, reduction or hydrolysis, resulting in the formation of charged metabolites. Phase II reactions involve coupling reactions such as acetylation or conjugation, which tend to produce an inactive product. For example, glutathione may couple to toxic metabolites of paracetamol. Drug metabolism by acetyation demonstrates genetic variability, with patients being described as slow or fast 'acetylators'.

Clinically, hepatic failure is an important cause of reduced metabolism and is dealt with in Chapter 10.

Hepatic porphyria

Affected individuals lack one of the enzymes for haemoglobin synthesis and there is an accumulation of porphyrin precursors, leading to gastro-intestinal (GI), neurological and behavioural disturbances. Cytochrome P450 inducers including barbiturates, carbamazepine, griseofulvin and oestrogens, tend to provoke an attack by inducing amino laevulinic acid synthase, giving rise to porphyrins.

Glucose-6-phosphate dehydrogenase deficiency in erythrocytes

This is a common example and is especially prevalent in Mediterraneans. G6PD is an enzyme present in erythrocytes (red blood cells), which provides reducing power, thereby maintaining glutathione in the reduced form. This prevents oxidative damage to the cells. The absence of G6PD therefore leads to fragile membranes and haemolysis, resulting in anaemia. Patients with G6PD deficiency are therefore sensitive to the effects of oxidative drugs such as antimalarials, sulphonamides, quinolones, nalidixic acid, nitrofurantoin, sulfasalazine and aspirin (refer to the *British National Formulary*), leading to oxidative damage with haemolysis and anaemia.

Immunological responses

Drugs are foreign molecules and some may induce an immunological response. These reactions may be delayed and tend not to be dose-related, occurring with the smallest doses of drug. They are usually reversible on cessation of the causative agent. Allergic reactions vary from skin rashes to life-threatening angioedema, bronchospasm and hypotension. Patients with a history of allergic disorders such as hayfever, asthma and atopic eczema are at increased risk. Important examples of causative agents are penicillins and streptokinase.

Penicillins couple to proteins, forming immunogens, which may precipitate hypersensitivity reactions. Management includes stopping the drug and treating the patient with antihistamines, adrenaline (epinephrine) and/or parenteral steroids according to severity. In extreme cases potentially life-threatening anaphylactic shock may also occur (Chapter 19). In the case of penicillins, the allergic reaction is a class effect due to the presence of the beta-lactam ring in the drug molecule and approximately 10% of penicillin-allergic patients are also sensitive to cephalosporins. It is therefore appropriate that non-penicillin, non-cephalosporin antibiotics are chosen for patients with a history of penicillin allergy.

Steptokinase carries the risk of anaphylaxis or may be ineffective on second use due to the presence of antibodies produced in response to previous use (Chapter 15).

Withdrawal responses

The withdrawal of certain drugs may lead to predictable symptoms and patients should be counselled appropriately. This type of reaction tends to result from physiological adaptation during the course of treatment. For example, chronic treatment with beta-blockers leads to receptor up-regulation. That is, an increase in the number of beta-adrenoceptors occurs in response to the blockade of existing receptors. Sudden withdrawal of beta-blockade may therefore result in overstimulation of beta-adrenoceptors. In the heart this may predispose to arrhythmias and is associated with increased mortality. Common examples of drugs where abrupt withdrawal may lead to adverse reactions are given below.

Alcohol
Delirium tremens and seizures occur following chronic excessive alcohol intake. Treatment includes short-term chlordiazepoxide or clomethiazole (inpatients only) (*British National Formulary* section 4.10).

Barbiturates
With barbiturates there is a risk of seizures: withdrawal of treatment for epilepsy may take months. A serious withdrawal syndrome includes rebound insomnia, tremor, dizziness, convulsions, delirium and death.

Clonidine
Clonidine may produce a rebound increase in blood pressure. Withdraw gradually to avoid a hypertensive crisis (*British National Formulary* section 2.5.3).

Antidepressants
Selective serotonin reuptake inhibitors (particularly paroxetine), tricyclic antidepressants and monoamine oxidase inhibitors (MAOIs) of 8 weeks' use or more should be withdrawn gradually over at least 4 weeks (up to 6 months after long-term maintenance). Monitor for withdrawal symptoms such as nausea, vomiting, anorexia, headache and panic-anxiety (Chapter 23 and the *British National Formulary* section 4.3).

Benzodiazepines
Withdrawal from benzodiazepines requires a gradual reduction of dose to prevent symptoms of confusion, toxic psychosis, convulsions or those similar to delirium tremens following alcohol withdrawal. These symptoms may take from a few hours to 3 weeks to develop with longer-acting agents. Milder symptoms include insomnia, loss of appetite, anxiety, weight loss, tremor, sweating, tinnitus and disturbances of perception. Patients are transferred to the equivalent dose of diazepam (section 4.1.1 of the *British National Formulary*). The dose is then reduced by increments of approximately one-eighth of the daily dose (or 2–2.5 mg) every fortnight, maintaining the new dose for a longer period if withdrawal symptoms occur. The time taken to withdraw completely from long-term benzodiazepine use can take from 4 weeks to a year or occasionally longer. Specialist counselling may benefit some patients, including education about the risks and benefits of withdrawing from these drugs.

It should be noted that antipsychotics aggravate the symptoms of benzodiazepine withdrawal and should not be used (the *British National Formulary* section 4.1).

Anticonvulsants
See Chapter 22.

Opioids
'Cold turkey' may be experienced after opioid addiction but is rare when opioids are prescribed for pain relief. Debilitating diarrhoea may occur; this may be treated with loperamide.

Baclofen
The CSM warns of serious withdrawal effects. The dose should be reduced gradually over at least 1–2 weeks, or longer if symptoms develop (*British National Formulary* section 10.2.2).

Corticosteroids

Prolonged use of corticosteroids results in the suppression of endogenous production and treatment should therefore be withdrawn gradually according to CSM recommendations (*British National Formulary* section 6.3.2).

The CSM currently recommends gradual withdrawal in patients whose disease is unlikely to relapse and who have:

- recently received repeated courses
- taken a short course within 1 year of stopping long-term therapy
- other possible causes of adrenal suppression
- received more than 40 mg prednisolone (or equivalent) daily
- repeat doses given in the evening
- received more than 3 weeks' treatment

Sympathomimetics

Prolonged use of topical decongestant vasoconstrictors causes tolerance and rebound congestion, probably due in part to down-regulation of alpha-adrenoceptors.

Antipsychotics

Withdraw gradually after long-term therapy and monitor closely for acute withdrawal syndromes or rapid relapse (*British National Formulary* section 4.2.1).

Type A ADRs

In the simplest case, one may predict many common type A ADRs on the basis of the known pharmacology of the drugs. Some common examples are given in Table 5.1.

Gastrointestinal ADRs

ADRs commonly affect the GI tract and may range from nausea or dyspepsia to life-threatening haemorrhage. GI ADRs are summarised in Table 5.2.

Oesophageal disorders

These may be induced by the local effects of drugs such as aspirin, tetracycline, doxycycline and bisphosphonates on the oesophagus, leading to irritation, or by drug-induced relaxation of the gastro-oesophageal sphincter producing reflux (e.g. opioids, calcium channel antagonists, nitrates). Symptoms include dysphagia or odynophagia (difficult or painful swallowing, respectively), heartburn, substernal chest pain or the feeling of something lodged in the throat (Chapter 7). Diagnosis is by endoscopy or contrast radiography. Alternative causes include reflux oesophagitis or, rarely, Crohn's disease or herpes infection of the oesophagus.

Treatment may include cessation of the causative agent, particularly alendronic acid, and the use of proton pump inhibitors (PPIs) for cases of ulceration and/or reflux. Sucralfate may be used for ulceration and chronic gastritis unless patients are seriously ill, particularly those receiving enteral feeding or with a history of delayed gastric emptying. The CSM has warned that these patients are at increased risk of bezoar formation. A bezoar is a mass of material in the stomach, causing gastric obstruction – parenteral or liquid analgesics may be required.

NSAID gastrotoxicity

NSAID-induced gastrotoxicity is discussed in Chapter 7.

Antiplatelet drugs and gastrotoxicity

The adenosine diphosphate (ADP) receptor inhibitor clopidogrel is used as an alternative antiplatelet agent to low-dose aspirin for patients with aspirin sensitivity. Clopidogrel has been shown to exhibit comparable efficacy and fewer adverse GI effects when compared with low-dose aspirin but is not free of GI side-effects and should not be used for patients at risk of GI bleeding (Chapter 13; Harker *et al.*, 1999).

Diarrhoea

Drug-induced diarrhoea is discussed in Chapter 9.

Antibiotic-induced diarrhoea

Most cases resolve on completion of the antibiotic course. Opportunist pathogens such as

Table 5.1 Examples of adverse drug reactions which may be predicted from the pharmacology of the drug class; futher information is given in the relevant chapters

Drug class	Side effect	Pharmacological mechanism	Possible solutions
Beta-blockers	Cold extremities	Antagonism of peripheral $beta_2$-adrenoceptors	• Choose a more cardioselective agent such as atenolol, which has less affinity for $beta_2$-adrenoceptors • Choose a beta-blocker with vasodilator actions, e.g. nebivolol
Beta-blockers	Bradycardia	Antagonism of chronotropic cardiac $beta_1$-adrenoceptors	• Withdraw beta-blockers gradually
Beta-blockers	Bronchospasm	Antagonism of bronchial $beta_2$-adrenoceptors	• All beta-blockers are contra-indicated in asthma and COPD. A cardioselective one may be used with extreme caution under specialist supervision
Alpha-blockers, diuretics, ACE inhibitors	Postural hypotension	Impairment of blood pressure regulation	• Caution on standing • Take first dose of alpha-blocker or ACE inhibitor on retiring to bed
Nitrates	Flushing, headache	Vasodilatation	• Headache relieved by paracetamol • Sublingual tablets may be discarded by spitting them out
Oral anticoagulants	Increased bleeding	Plasma concentration too high or increased bleeding tendency	• Monitoring of INR required and dose adjustment may be required
Opioids	Constipation	Inhibition of lower GI tract motility	• Use a laxative such as lactulose or senna
Tricyclic antidepressants; certain older antihistamines (e.g. promethazine)	Antimuscarinic effects such as dry mouth, blurred vision, constipation and urinary retention	Antagonism of muscarinic receptors	• Consider an SSRI for depression • Choose a newer antihistamine with less muscarinic binding, e.g. loratadine
Sulphonylureas	Hypoglycaemia	Augmented pharmacological effect	• Careful monitoring with dose adjustment • Use short-acting agents

Continued

Table 5.1 *Continued*

Drug class	Side effect	Pharmacological mechanism	Possible solutions
Broad-spectrum antibiotics	Diarrhoea	Alterations of lower GI flora	• Caution: severe diarrhoea should alert one to the risk of pseudomembranous colitis. Otherwise a short course of loperamide may be used with caution
NSAIDs	Gastric damage	Inhibition of the production of cytoprotective prostaglandins	• Use a less irritant NSAID such as ibuprofen • Consider a COX-2 inhibitor • Combine NSAID with misoprostol or a proton pump inhibitor
NSAIDs	Bronchospasm	Inhibition of the production of prostaglandins, favouring the production of leukotrienes	• Avoid in asthma • Leukotriene receptor antagonists as a logical treatment to oppose the effects of NSAID-mediated leukotriene production
Cytotoxic agents	Myelosuppression	Cytotoxic effects on bone marrow	• Prophylactic antibacterial and antifungal agents • Use of transfusions or colony-stimulating factors to increase white blood cell counts

COPD, chronic obstructive pulmonary disease; ACE, angiotensin-converting enzyme; INR, international normalised ratio; GI, gastrointestinal; SSRI, selective serotonin reuptake inhibitor; NSAIDs, non-steroidal anti-inflammatory drugs; COX-2, cyclooxygenase 2.

Clostridium difficile may, however, lead to the rare but potentially fatal pseudomembranous colitis. Symptoms include profuse watery diarrhoea, abdominal pain, fever and bloating with raised plaques covering the colonic mucosa (pseudomembranes). Risk factors include duration of treatment, multiple or repeated antibiotic treatments, severe illness, immunocompromised state, advanced age and prolonged hospital stay. Antimotility drugs may be appropriate for treating mild cases of antibiotic-induced diarrhoea. These drugs should not be used to treat more severe episodes of diarrhoea, particularly when associated with abdominal distension, ulcerative colitis, diverticular disease or pseudomembranous colitis.

Drugs with antimuscarinic activity

Antimuscarinic effects (also know as anticholinergic effects) are caused by the blockade of muscarinic receptors otherwise activated by acetylcholine. These effects may be peripheral or central and may be serious according to underlying disease (such as glaucoma, urinary retention, prostatic hypertrophy or constipation), and the concurrent use of drugs with anticholinergic effects:

• dry mouth
• dry eyes
• blurred vision
• urinary retention or difficulty urinating

Table 5.2 Examples of important adverse drug reactions affecting the alimentary system

Adverse GI effects	Causative drugs	Comments
Taste disturbance	**ACE inhibitors, calcium channel blockers**, etidronate, griseofulvin, isotretinoin, levodopa, losartan, penicillamine, terbinafine	• Usually resolves on cessation of treatment but this may take months
Metallic taste	Allopurinol, gold, lithium, metformin, metronidazole, penicillamine, zopiclone	
Gingival overgrowth	**Dihydropyridine calcium channel blockers**, ciclosporin, phenytoin	• Usually within 3 months of starting treatment. Increased risk if there is poor oral hygiene
Pigmentation of oral mucosa	Tetracyclines	• Rare • Particularly minocycline
Dental coloration	Tetracyclines	• Avoid tetracyclines in children under 12 years of age
Dry mouth (xerostomia)	**Anticholinergic effects, e.g. antihistamines, tricyclic antidepressants, anticholinergics, CNS stimulants, phenothiazines**	• May cause weight loss, candidiasis, dental caries, poor adherence to drug regimens, reduced efficacy of sublingual drug administration (e.g. GTN)
Saliva secretion (ptylism)	**Cholinergic agonists,** e.g. pilocarpine, clozapine	• Risk of choking at night
Stomatitis and mouth ulcers	Aspirin, **barbiturates**, captopril, griseofulvin, isoniazid, nicorandil, **NSAIDs**, proguanil, sulfasalazine	• Usually resolve quickly after drug is stopped. See also Stevens–Johnson syndrome and erythema multiforme
Oesophageal disorders (Chapter 7)	Ascorbic acid, aspirin, **bisphosphonates** (CSM warning), clindamycin, doxycycline, ferrous sulfate, **NSAIDs**, potassium salts, quinidine, tetracycline, theophylline	• Usually occurs within hours to days of taking causative drug • Most cases heal within days or weeks of treatment cessation
Acid reflux or heartburn (Chapter 7)	**Calcium channel blockers, opioids, nitrates and anticholinergics**	• Due to relaxation of the lower oesophageal sphincter
Nausea and vomiting (Chapter 8)	Many: particularly **cytotoxics**, levodopa, **opioids, SSRIs, iron salts**, bromocriptine, digoxin, theophylline, erythromycin and **oestrogens**	• Symptoms may resolve with continued use or occasionally by taking the drug after food • May indicate toxicity of digoxin or theophylline
Gastrotoxicity (Chapter 7)	**NSAIDs, corticosteroids, calcium channel blockers, SSRIs,** clopidogrel	See text. • Increased risk when coprescribing with NSAIDs

Continued

Table 5.2 *Continued*

Adverse GI effects	Causative drugs	Comments
Duodenal ulceration and perforation	**NSAIDs, less often corticosteroids, but more likely if taken with NSAIDs**	• Difficult to diagnose in the early stages, as the inflammation is asymptomatic • May be a cause of 'unexplained bleeding'. Complications include iron-deficiency anaemia due to blood loss, hypoalbuminaemia due to protein loss, ulceration and stricture formation (resulting in postprandial colicky pain) • Associated with alcohol abuse • Diagnosis may follow the detection of iron-deficiency anaemia, usually after long-term treatment, hypoalbuminaemia (associated with peripheral oedema and other signs of fluid retention due to protein loss from damaged intestinal mucosa) or by endoscopy (Morris *et al.*, 1991; Tibble *et al.*, 1999) • Blood loss is not often sufficient for detection in faecal occult blood test
Paralytic ileus and pseudo-obstruction	Acarbose, **calcium channel blockers**, clozapine, **bulk-forming laxatives**, loperamide **opioids, phenothiazines, potassium salts, tricyclic antidepressants**	• Physical obstruction or anticholinergic effects inhibiting smooth-muscle activity, particularly if more than one anticholinergic agent is prescribed
Malabsorption from the duodenum	Colestyramine, colestipol, liquid paraffin, orlistat, metformin	• Supplements of fat-soluble vitamins may be required • Serum vitamin B_{12} may be reduced in patients taking metformin but the clinical significance appears to be small
Diarrhoea (Chapter 9)	Many: commonly **antibiotics**, acarbose, metformin, **bile salts**, colchicine, **cytotoxics**, dipyridamole, gold, **iron salts, laxatives, magnesium-containing antacids, NSAIDs** (mefenamic acid), orlistat, ticlopidine, misoprostol, olsalazine	• Clindamycin-induced diarrhoea may be the result of pseudomembranous colitis. Treatment should be stopped • Severe diarrhoea may lead to treatment cessation of diarrhoea-causing drugs
Colitis	**Amfetamines**, cocaine, digoxin, ergotamine, sumatriptan, methotrexate, methyldopa, methysergide, **NSAIDs, oestrogens, salicylates**	• Presents as sudden onset of severe abdominal pain, nausea, vomiting, diarrhoea and abdominal distension. Tachycardia, pyrexia, leucocytosis (raised white cell count) and bloody stools may be present

Continued

Table 5.2 *Continued*

Adverse GI effects	Causative drugs	Comments
Constipation (Chapter 9)	Many: commonly **anticholinergics, opioids, iron salts,** verapamil, **tricyclic antidepressants, antihistamines,** clozapine, mebeverine, **MAOIs,** peppermint oil, **phenothiazines,** sucralfate, **diuretics**	• Risk factors include polypharmacy, dehydration, immobility, advanced age and low-fibre diet
Dark faeces	**Iron salts, bismuth salts**	Patient counselling is important
Pancreatitis	**Aminosalicylates, ACE inhibitors,** azathioprine, **furosemide (frusemide), H₂-receptor antagonists,** metronidazole, **oestrogens,** propofol, sodium valproate, sulindac, **thiazide diuretics**	• Rare but mild if causative agent is stopped • Risk factors include gallstones, alcohol consumption, hyperlipidaemia, hypercalcaemia • Presents as sudden onset of upper abdominal pain, vomiting, tachycardia, fever, jaundice and rigid tender abdomen. Serum amylase is raised

Text in **bold** represents drug groups or classes.

GI, gastrointestinal; ACE, angiotensin-converting enzyme; CNS, central nervous system; GTN, glyceryl trinitrate; NSAIDs, non-steroidal anti-inflammatory drugs; CSM, Committee on Safety of Medicines; SSRIs, selective serotonin reuptake inhibitors; MAOIs, monoamine oxidase inhibitors.

- tachycardia
- constipation (risk of paralytic ileus)
- reduced sweating and therefore increased risk of heat stroke
- increased intraocular pressure (may exacerbate narrow-angle glaucoma, due to reduced drainage)
- psychosis
- dementia or confusion

The following drugs are associated with anti-muscarinic activity:

- sedating antihistamines (e.g. chlorphenamine)
- antiemetics (e.g. antihistamines, hyoscine)
- antiarrhythmics (disopyramide, propafenone)
- antiparkinson anticholinergics (procyclidine, trihexyphenidyl or orphenadrine)
- antipsychotics (e.g. thioridazine, trifluoperazine, chlorpromazine, clozapine)
- tricyclic antidepressants (e.g. amitriptyline, clomipramine, imipramine, nortriptyline)
- muscle relaxants (e.g. baclofen)
- mydriatic eye drops (e.g. atropine, hyoscine and tropicamide)
- antispasmodics (e.g. hyoscine, atropine, oxybutynin, propantheline, tolterodine)

Patient counselling

- Recommend the use of artificial saliva or sugar-free chewing gum with drugs causing a dry mouth, particularly if sublingual preparations such as glyceryl trinitrate are coprescribed.
- Promote good oral hygiene in patients prescribed drugs causing gingival hypertrophy.
- Drugs with the potential to cause oesophageal disorders, particularly tetracyclines and bisphosphonates, should be taken with plenty of water (at least a tumbler full) and while sitting or standing. Patients taking the bisphosphonate alendronate are advised to stand or sit upright for at least 30 min after taking the tablets, and not to take them at bedtime.
- Patients should be advised to report diarrhoea

resulting from broad-spectrum antibiotics, particularly clindamycin.

Hepatic ADRs (Table 5.3)

Liver function may be altered by drugs to varying degrees ranging from mild, reversible and asymptomatic changes identified by routine liver function tests (LFTs) to severe damage, leading to hepatic failure. Drugs such as paracetamol, salicylates, tetracycline and methotrexate cause dose-dependent type A changes. Unpredictable type B reactions are less common and include those to chlorpromazine and isoniazid.

Risk factors for developing drug-induced hepatic dysfunction:

- pre-existing liver disease
- female sex
- age
- genetic variations in the expression of cytochrome P450 isoenzymes
- concurrent treatment with enzyme inducers (see Drug interactions, below)
- polypharmacy
- concurrent disease – diabetes mellitus predisposes patients to methotrexate toxicity
- nutritional status – fasting patients lack glutathione required in the non-toxic pathway of paracetamol metabolism
- alcohol misuse

Clinical features

Symptoms may present only as fever and a general appearance suggesting the patient is ill (Chapter 10). The liver may be tender and slightly enlarged. A skin rash may suggest a hypersensitivity reaction. Hepatitis presents with anorexia, nausea and vomiting, abdominal discomfort (right upper abdomen), dark urine, pale stools and jaundice. Pruritus may indicate cholestasis, a failure of bile to reach the intestine, possibly due to blockage of the bile duct. Immunological type B reactions may present with rash, fever and eosinophilia. Jaundice without cholestasis may indicate severe injury to the liver.

Diagnosis of drug-related hepatotoxicity is determined by temporal assessment of drug administration (with particular consideration to

drugs given 3 months prior to onset of symptoms), elimination of causes, LFTs (Chapter 2), biopsy and/or measurement of conjugated bilirubin in suspected biliary obstruction.

Paracetamol-induced hepatotoxicity and patient counselling

Paracetamol is the most common cause of drug-induced hepatotoxicity. This is partly due to a lack of awareness of the potential toxicity of paracetamol or its presence in different medicines taken concurrently leading to accidental ingestion of excessive doses (Chapter 27).

Monitoring

The monitoring of liver function is discussed in Chapter 2. It should be noted that elevated LFTs are not always followed by hepatic injury. Generally an increase of two to three times any baseline value would indicate possible drug-induced hepatotoxicity and the need to stop the drug.

Patient counselling

Patients taking drugs known to cause hepatotoxicity should be advised to report symptoms such as nausea, vomiting, abdominal pain, jaundice, dark urine, pale stools, fatigue and generalised pruritus since early diagnosis improves the outcome.

Cardiovascular ADRs (Table 5.4)

Drug-induced cardiovascular disorders are again common and often predictable type A reactions, particularly in patients with pre-existing heart disease. Additional risk factors include undisclosed self-medication with OTC drugs, electrolyte disturbances and impaired renal function.

The prolongation of the QT interval, as revealed by electrocardiogram (ECG), and subsequent risk of life-threatening torsade de pointes arrhythmias have led to the withdrawal of drugs such as cisapride and astemizole, the reversion to prescription-only medicine (POM) status of terfenadine in the UK and the restriction of licensed indications for thioridazine. Sertindole has been restricted to named patients. The CSM advises

Table 5.3 Summary of adverse drug reactions affecting the liver

Liver condition	Causative drugs (common examples)	Comments
Fatty liver (steatosis – intracellular droplets of lipid)	Sodium valproate, tetracycline, **corticosteroids**, methotrexate, alcohol Steatohepatitis – amiodarone	• Acute or chronic (steatohepatitis). Reduced levels of blood glucose and increased levels of blood ammonia • Chronic steatohepatitis may progress to cirrhosis
Acute necrosis (cell, i.e. hepatocyte death)	Allopurinol, aspirin, **NSAIDs**, carbamazepine, cocaine, dantrolene, ecstasy, isoniazid, labetalol, methyldopa, minocycline, **MAOIs**, paracetamol, halophane, sodium valproate, **sulphonamides**, pennyroyal (herbal)	• Generally rare but potentially fatal type B reaction • LFT: increased levels of alkaline phosphatase and alanine aminotransferase • Jaundice and increased prothrombin time if severe
Acute hepatitis (inflammation of hepatocyctes)	**ACE inhibitors, Chinese herbs**, co-trimoxazole, cyproterone, dantrolene, terbinafine, isoniazid, ketoconazole, methyldopa, **MAOIs**, nicotinamide, nifedipine, nitrofurantoin, phenytoin, rifampicin, sulfasalazine, **sulphonamides,** tizanidine, tolcapone, **tricyclic antidepressants**	• Usually self-limiting and reversible but rarely life-threatening. Prothrombin time used to indicate severity • May be cholestatic, due to hepatocellular destruction or a combination of both
Cholestatic hepatitis	Co-amoxiclav, **ACE inhibitors**, erythromycin, azathioprine, carbimazole, chlorpropamide, cimetidine, co-trimoxazole, dextropropoxyphene, flucloxacillin, fusidic acid, gold, ketoconazole, nitrofurantoin, **NSAIDs** (sulindac), penicillamine, **phenothiazines** (chlorpromazine), phenytoin, ranitidine, **sulphonamides, tricyclic antidepressants**	Increased levels of alkaline phosphatase, alanine aminotransferase and conjugated bilirubin
Chronic active hepatitis	Cimetidine, dantrolene, diclofenac, etretinate, isoniazid, minocycline, nitrofurantoin, paracetamol, phenytoin, sulphonamides, **tricyclic antidepressants**	Duration greater than 3 months. Increased levels of serum transaminases. Reduced serum albumin. Usually resolves when the drug is stopped

Continued

Table 5.3 *Continued*

Liver condition	Causative drugs (common examples)	Comments
Fibrosis and cirrhosis	Methotrexate (dose-related), vitamin A	Fibrosis but not cirrhosis is reversible. LFTs not always good predictors but regular monitoring is advisable
Granulomatous hepatitis (overgrowth of granulation tissue due to inflammation)	Carbamazepine, clofibrate, allopurinol, chlorpromazine, gold, hydralazine, methyldopa, nitrofurantoin, penicillin, phenytoin, quinine, **sulphonamides, sulphonylureas**	• Usually a type B immunoallergic reaction • Reversible on cessation of treatment
Chronic cholestasis	Carbamazepine, chlorpromazine, co-amoxiclav, co-trimoxazole, erythromycin, flucloxacillin, phenytoin, prochlorperazine	• Similar presentation to primary biliary cirrhosis • May persist for several years after treatment is withdrawn • Abnormal LFTs and possible jaundice
Cholestasis (failure of bile to reach the intestine)	**Oral contraceptives,** terbinafine, ciclosporin, flucloxacillin, glibenclamide, griseofulvin, tamoxifen, warfarin	• With terbinafine, this usually occurs within the first 2 months of treatment • Increased levels of bilirubin and normal or small increased levels of alanine aminotransferase • If chronic, may cause inflammation, scarring and cirrhosis
Hepatic tumours	**Oral contraceptives,** danazol, anabolic steroids	Rare
Veno-occlusive disease and Budd–Chiari syndrome	**Oral contraceptives, cytotoxics, herbal remedies** (comfrey, heliotropium), azathioprine	Obstruction of the hepatic vein by connective tissue, blood clot or tumour resulting in ascites and cirrhosis

Text in **bold** represents drug groups or classes.
NSAIDs, non-steroidal anti-inflammatory drugs; LFT, liver function test; ACE, angiotensin-converting enzyme.

against the coprescribing of two or more drugs known to prolong the QT interval. Risk factors for developing this ADR include:

- female sex
- family history of coronary heart disease
- smoking
- high stress levels
- substance misuse, particularly alcohol or cocaine
- renal or hepatic impairment or slow metabolisers
- metabolic-type drug interactions (due to increased drug levels)

- electrolyte disturbance such as hypokalaemia or hypomagnesaemia, e.g. with laxatives or diuretics
- high doses, particularly of antipsychotics
- polypharmacy and particularly concurrent diuretic treatment
- bradycardia
- cardiovascular disease: hypertension, congestive heart failure
- a history of QT interval prolongation

For further information and a list of drugs that prolong the QT interval, see Haddad *et al.* (2002) and www.torsades.org.

Table 5.4 Summary of ADRs affecting the cardiovascular system

Cardiovascular disorder	Causative drugs	Comments
Arrhythmias – prolonged QT interval	**Antiarrhythmics**: amiodarone, disopyramide, procainamide, propafenone, quinidine, sotalol **Antihistamines**: astemizole, terfenadine **Antibacterials**: clarithromycin, co-trimoxazole, erythromycin **Antifungals (azoles)**: ketoconazole, itraconazole, miconazole, fluconazole **Antimalarials:** chloroquine, quinine **Antipsychotics:** chlorpromazine, droperidol, haloperidol, pimozide, sertindole, thioridazine **Antidepressants:** tricyclics (amitriptyline and imipramine) **Others:** cisapride, pentamidine, probucol, tacrolimus, terodiline	• Risk of torsade de pointes or sudden death due to ventricular fibrillation • Refer to text for risk factors • Recommended doses for terfenadine should not be exceeded • Terfenadine should be avoided in hepatic impairment, hypokalaemia and pre-existing QT interval prolongation or with grapefruit juice in addition to the risk factors listed above
Atrial fibrillation	Alcohol **Antidepressants** (trazadone, fluoxetine)	Drug causes are rare. Other causes include hypertension, hyperthyroidism, rheumatic heart disease, infection and pneumonia
Bradycardia (less than 60 beats/min)	**Beta-blockers** (including eye drops)**, histamine H$_2$-receptor antagonists,** carbamazepine, clonidine, digoxin, diltiazem, verapamil	• Serious interaction between beta-blockers and verapamil leading to asystole. Risk of bradycardia with beta-blockers and diltiazem (careful monitoring required) • Adjust dose of digoxin to keep the heart rate above 60 beats/min
Cardiac failure (Chapter 14)		
Hypertension (Chapter 11)		
Postural hypotension	**Alpha-blockers, diuretics, ACE inhibitors, antipsychotics, opioids**	• Caution on standing • Take first dose of alpha-blockers and ACE inhibitors on retiring to bed at night
Myocardial ischaemia	Adenosine, **amfetamines, beta-agonists, beta-blockers (withdrawal),** caffeine, ergotamine, nifedipine (short-acting), theophylline, levothyroxine, verapamil	• In patients with hypothyroidism and cardiovascular disease, the initial dose of levothyroxine should be low and increased every 4 weeks
Dyslipidaemia (Chapter 12)		
Peripheral vasoconstriction	**Beta-blockers**	• Choose a more cardioselective agent such as atenolol, which has less affinity for beta$_2$-adrenoceptors • Choose a beta-blocker with vasodilator actions, e.g. nebivolol

Continued

Table 5.4   *Continued*

Cardiovascular disorder	Causative drugs	Comments
Haemorrhagic stroke	**Anticoagulants, thrombolytics and antiplatelet drugs**	• These should be avoided
Thromboembolic disorders (deep vein thrombosis, pulmonary embolism, thromboembolic stroke)	Bromocriptine, danazol, desmopressin, **hypoglycaemic drugs, oral contraceptives, sympathomimetics** (phenylproanolamine), tranexamic acid	• Risk factors: smoking, obesity, hypertension, diabetes, severe varicose veins, trauma, immobility, and family history of deep vein thrombosis or pulmonary embolism

Text in **bold** represents drug groups or classes.
ACE, angiotensin-converting enzyme.

Patient counselling

- Patients prescribed drugs with the potential to prolong the QT interval should be advised to report urgently symptoms of arrhythmia such as dizziness, light-headedness, irregular pulse, palpitations and fainting. Drugs should be stopped immediately and the ECG monitored.
- Patients with pain in the calf or thigh with swelling, redness and warmth and/or breathlessness and chest pain should be referred urgently.

Renal ADRs (Table 5.5)

The kidneys are responsible for the elimination of many drugs and it is, therefore, not surprising that these organs are common targets for drug-induced toxicity, particularly in elderly patients with age-related renal impairment. Drugs commonly implicated include ACE inhibitors, diuretics and NSAIDs, commonly prescribed for the ageing patient with cardiovascular disease and chronic inflammatory conditions such as rheumatoid arthritis. Common mechanisms for drug-induced renal impairment include:

- reduced renal perfusion, e.g. volume depletion during diuretic therapy
- altered glomerular filtration due to altered tone of renal arterioles in the presence of ACE inhibitors or NSAIDs, which inhibit the effects of angiotensin II or prostaglandins respectively

- damage to renal tubules due to inflammatory reactions triggered by many drugs, including NSAIDs

Additional risk factors for renal ADRs include dehydration, cirrhosis or heart failure (due to sodium retention), diabetes, polypharmacy (particularly of nephrotoxic drugs), high doses of the causative agent, hypotension, sepsis and shock.

Clinical features

See Chapter 17.

Patient counselling

- Patients with risk factors for renal disorders as outlined above should report nausea, vomiting and muscle cramps. Urinalysis should be undertaken to check for the presence of protein.
- Patients taking diuretics and/or laxatives are at risk of prerenal failure due to reduced renal perfusion and should therefore report fatigue, postural hypotension and muscle cramps. This is particularly important in elderly patients and those taking additional nephrotoxic drugs. Patients should be referred to their general practitioner (GP) and/or a dose of diuretic omitted when suffering from conditions that may result in dehydration, for example, excess sweating, diarrhoea and/or vomiting.

Table 5.5   Summary of important adverse drug reactions involving the kidney

Renal disorder	Causative drugs	Comments
Prerenal failure	**Diuretics, laxatives**	Due to reduced renal perfusion
Intrarenal failure – changes to GFR	**NSAIDs (particularly if volume-depleted), ACE inhibitors, diuretics**	• Due to effects on mechanisms controlling the tone of renal arterioles • Increased risk in patients with bilateral renal disease • Monitoring essential in at-risk patients
Intrarenal failure – acute interstitial nephritis (AIN)	**NSAIDs**, **beta-lactam antibiotics**, furosemide (frusemide), allopurinol, azathioprine, captopril, cimetidine, co-trimoxazole, erythromycin, isoniazid, methyldopa, minocycline, omeprazole, phenytoin, rifampicin, **thiazides, sulphonamides**	• Hypersensitive, inflammatory reaction leading to damage of renal tubules • Diagnosed by biopsy • Presents as acute renal failure. Dialysis may be required but most patients recover up to several months after causative agent is withdrawn • Intermittent rifampicin therapy should be avoided due to immunological response. Re-exposure to rifampicin should be monitored closely
Intrarenal failure – acute tubular necrosis	Amphotericin, ciclosporin, ciprofloxacin, gentamicin, methotrexate, **radiological contrast agents**, rifampicin	A common, direct toxic effect
Intrarenal failure – glomerulonephritis: membranous, minimal-change, lupus nephritis	Gold, penicillamine, **NSAIDs**, hydralazine (acetylator status important), procainamide	• Bilateral, immunologically mediated damage to glomeruli • Presents as proteinuria, which may progress to oedema and hypoalbuminaemia (nephrotic syndrome)
Postrenal failure	**Chemotherapy,** aciclovir (intravenous), methotrexate, **sulphonamides**	Due to urinary tract obstruction May also follow drug-induced rhabdomyolysis (deposits of muscle cell contents following muscle cell damage)
Chronic renal failure	**Chronic use of NSAIDs, particularly salicylates**	A problem particularly associated with compound analgesic preparations including combinations of paracetamol with salicylates, codeine or caffeine
Nephrogenic diabetes insipidus	Lithium	Does not respond to desmopressin. Serum lithium and creatinine levels should be monitored regularly (Chapters 2 and 6, respectively)
Haemolytic–uraemic syndrome	Ciclosporin, mitomycin C, **oral contraceptives**, metronidazole (in children), quinine	Destruction of red blood cells (haemolysis) leading to obstruction of renal arterioles. Also causes anaemia, thrombocytopenia (reduced platelets) with risk of severe haemorrhage
Discoloration of urine	Rifampicin, co-danthramer, **dopaminergic antiparkinson drugs**	This may be alarming and therefore patients should be warned before beginning treatment

Text in **bold** represents drug groups or classes.
GFR, glomerular filtration rate; NSAIDs, non-steroidal anti-inflammatory drugs; ACE, angiotensin-converting enzyme.

Haematological ADRs (Table 5.6)

Drugs such as cytotoxic agents cause predictable suppression of bone marrow and could therefore be considered type A reactions. Many drugs may however unpredictably affect the bone marrow and blood cell production. With the exception of cytotoxics, drug-induced blood dyscrasias are rare but potentially fatal and therefore health professionals should be aware of drugs known to cause these effects (Table 5.6). Alerting symptoms include sore throat, mouth ulcers, bruising or bleeding, rash, malaise and fever or non-specific illness.

Respiratory ADRs (Table 5.7)

The respiratory system may be the target of chronic and acute ADRs, including anaphylaxis. More common examples include cough due to ACE inhibitors, asthma with beta-blockers and nasal congestion with chronic use of decongestants.

Patient counselling

- Nasal decongestants are likely to cause rebound congestion if used regularly for more than 7 days.
- Patients with a history of bronchospasm, rhinorrhoea, rash or angioedema following an NSAID or indeed any drug treatment should avoid these agents due to the risk of developing a more severe reaction. Some aspirin-sensitive patients may also be sensitive to paracetamol, particularly after long-term use at high doses. Codeine may be recommended for these patients.
- Patients with a history of asthma or chronic obstructive pulmonary disease should have a fast acting beta$_2$-adrenoceptor agonist available due to the risk of developing broncho-constriction when prescribed the antiviral drug zanamivir.
- Symptoms of dyspnoea, cough and chest pain require prompt reporting by patients prescribed amiodarone due to the risk of pulmonary toxicity.
- Women prescribed combined oral contraceptives should seek urgent medical attention if they develop breathlessness and pleuritic pain due to the slightly increased risk of thromboembolic disease leading to pulmonary embolism.

Psychiatric ADRs (Table 5.8)

These are relatively common and consist mainly of type A reactions predictable from pharmacological activity. Some mental health disorders are also precipitated by drug withdrawal (see above).

Risk factors include a history of mental illness, impaired cerebral function (following stroke or injury), alcohol or drug abuse (see Chapter 3), stress and concurrent physical disease. For example, isotretinoin should be used with caution in patients with a history of depression, due to the risk of suicide. Prophylactic use of the antimalarial mefloquine is contraindicated in patients with a history of neuropsychiatric disorders, including depression, or convulsions.

Prior to identifying a drug-induced mental health disorder, it is important to exclude underlying conditions such as Cushing's syndrome, electrolyte imbalance (dehydration), neurological disorder, megaloblastic anaemia, renal dysfunction or thyroid disease. Diagnosis is particularly difficult as a temporal relationship between the start of drug treatment and the development of symptoms is often not predictable. Conversely, drug treatment may also complicate the diagnosis of an underlying mental health problem. Confirmation of drug involvement is therefore best indicated by an improvement of symptoms following the cessation of treatment.

Dementia

Dementia presents with cognitive decline affecting memory, intellect and changes in personality without altered consciousness. Causes include Alzheimer's disease and age-related decline of cognitive function. Drug-induced dementia is difficult to identify and may be further complicated by the cognitive effects of underlying disease, such as depression, insomnia or hypertension, which should be identified and treated.

Table 5.6   A summary of adverse drug reactions involving the haematological system

Haematological disorder	Causative drugs	Comments
Aplastic anaemia (total or partial failure of the bone marrow)	**Antidiabetic** (chlorpropamide, tolbutamide) **Antiepileptics** (carbamazepine, phenytoin, lamotrigine) **Anti-inflammatory** (diclofenac, gold, indometacin, penicillamine, phenylbutazone, piroxicam, sulindac, sulfasalazine) **Antimicrobials** (chloramphenicol, co-trimoxazole, sulphonamides) **Antiplatelets** (ticlopidine) **Antipsychotics** (chlorpromazine) **Antithyroid agents** (carbimazole, propylthiouracil)	• Reduced red cell (anaemia), white cell (leucopenia) and platelet (thrombocytopenia) counts • Often irreversible despite drug withdrawal
Agranulocytosis (profound reduction of granulocytes with neutrophil count less than 0.5×10^9/L)	**Antibiotics** (penicillins, cephalosporins, co-trimoxazole, chloramphenicol, sulphonamides) **Antidepressants** (imipramine, clomipramine, desipramine, mianserin) **Antiepileptics** (carbamazepine, phenytoin) **Anti-inflammatory** (gold, penicillamine, lefunomide, sulfasalazine, NSAIDs) **Antipsychotics** (chlorpromazine, thioridazine, clozapine) **Antithyroid drugs** (carbimazole, propylthiouracil) **Others** – captopril, procainamide, ticlopidine	• Recovery usually 2–3 weeks after drug is withdrawn • Repeat exposure to causative drug not recommended due to sensitisation
Thrombocytopenia (reduced platelets to $<150 \times 10^9$/L)	**Antimicrobials** (chloramphenicol, co-trimoxazole, trimethoprim, penicillins, sulphonamides, rifampicin) **Antiepileptics** (sodium valproate) **Anti-inflammatory** (gold, NSAIDs, penicillamine) **Diuretics** (thiazides, furosemide (frusemide)) **Others** (tolbutamide, digitoxin, methyldopa, heparin (less likely with low-molecular-weight heparin), quinidine)	• May present as easy bleeding, bruising or purpura • Prolonged bleeding time but INR remains normal • Usually occurs 7–10 days after drug started • Avoid future exposure to the causative agent • Aspirin and NSAIDs reduce the effects of remaining platelets and therefore should be avoided during thrombocytopenia

Continued

Table 5.6 *Continued*

Haematological disorder	Causative drugs	Comments
Pure red cell aplasia (total or partial failure of red cell production)	Azathioprine, phenytoin, isoniazid, penicillamine, chlorpropamide, chloramphenicol, erythropoietin	Anaemia with a marked reduction in reticulocytes (immature red cells)
Haemolytic (red cell destruction) anaemia	**Cephalosporins, penicillins, tetracyclines**, insulin, methotrexate, isoniazid, quinidine, quinine, rifampicin, sulphonylureas, methyldopa, levodopa, mefenamic acid, azapropazone, drugs with oxidant effect on cell membrane (particularly in G6PD deficiency, see text)	• The Coombs test is used to distinguish immune mechanisms • Also G6PD deficiency (see text) • Red cells usually return to normal after 2–3 weeks
Megaloblastic (large, abnormal form of precursors to red blood cells) anaemia	Aciclovir, alcohol, **antiepileptics**, methotrexate (dose-dependent), nitrofurantoin, **oral contraceptives**, proguanil, sulfasalazine, trimethoprim (usually due to worsening of pre-existing folate deficiency)	• Impaired DNA synthesis usually due to folate or vitamin B_{12} deficiency • Folic acid supplements to treat patients taking antiepileptics

Text in **bold** represents drug groups or classes.
NSAIDs, non-steroidal anti-inflammatory drugs; G6PD, glucose-6-phosphate dehydrogenase; INR, international normalised ratio.

Indeed, the drug treatment of hypertension has been associated with improved cognitive function. Drugs associated with cognitive impairment should be used with caution in elderly patients as even a small decline in cognitive function may produce important effects such as increasing the risk of falls or accidents when driving. The reader is referred to an excellent review by Gray *et al.* (1999).

Delirium

The symptoms of delirium include altered consciousness and confusion. Patients are profoundly disoriented and may be frightened, bewildered, restless and aggressive. Delirium has an acute onset with intermittent periods without symptoms. The use of anticholinergics to reduce extrapyramidal effects of antipsychotics (Chapter 26) should be avoided. Depending on the number and severity of risk factors, e.g. age, cognitive impairment, drugs and alcohol abuse, delirium may be triggered with even low doses of drug.

Neuroleptic malignant syndrome

This is a rare but severe reaction to antipsychotics. Symptoms include fever, rigidity, altered mental status and autonomic dysfunction (e.g. loss of bladder and bowel control). Reduced central and peripheral dopamine transmission is implicated. Risk factors include dehydration, mood disorder, Parkinson's disease, male genders, high dosage and intramuscular route of administration.

Table 5.7   Summary of adverse drug reactions (ADRs) affecting the respiratory system

Respiratory disorder	Causative drugs	Comments
Nasal congestion	**Antidepressants, antihypertensives** (methyldopa, prazosin, hydralazine, propranolol), **antipsychotics, oral contraceptives**, aspirin, **NSAIDs, chronic use of topical nasal decongestants** (ephedrine, xylometazoline, oxymetazoline)	• Dilatation of nasal vasculature produces tissue oedema • Prolonged use of topical decongestant vasoconstrictors causes tolerance and rebound congestion, probably due in part to down-regulation of alpha-adrenoceptors
Bronchoconstriction (Chapter 20)	**Antibiotics** (e.g. penicillins and cephalosporins), aspirin, **NSAIDs, dipyridamole, beta-blockers** (including eye drops), **ACE inhibitors, anticholinesterases, pharmaceutical excipients** (tartrazine, benzoates, phenylmercuric salts, parabens, benzalkonium chloride and metabisulfite), **general anaesthetics and muscle relaxants Radiological contrast media**	• Particularly in asthma and COPD patients • Allergic reaction to penicillins may also occur with other beta-lactam antibiotics (cephalosporins, carbapenems and monobactams)
Cough	**ACE inhibitors**	• This is a class effect for ACE inhibitors • Angiotensin receptor antagonists may be suitable alternatives
Reflex bronchoconstriction	**Inhaled beta-agonists, corticosteroids**, ipratropium and cromoglicate, zanamivir	Direct irritation of bronchial mucosa
Lung parenchyma – interstitial pneumonitis	Amiodarone, gold, methotrexate, nitrofurantoin, paclitaxel, penicillamine, sulfasalazine	• Generally allergic reactions presenting as cough, breathlessness and wheeze • Early diagnosis and treatment improve recovery • Patients on methotrexate should not receive nitrofurantoin due to synergy of ADR
Lung parenchyma – pulmonary fibrosis	Amiodarone, gold, sulfasalazine, nitrofurantoin, **anticancer agents**	• Direct toxicity causes inflammation and fibrosis leading to significant morbidity and mortality • Dose and duration of treatment important
Pulmonary oedema (adult respiratory distress syndrome, ARDS)	Amphotericin, diamorphine, haloperidol, hydrochlorothiazide, indometacin, methadone, naloxone, protamine, salbutamol IV and terbutaline IV	• Increased pulmonary vascular permeability presenting as cough, breathlessness and frothy sputum • Close monitoring of women receiving IV beta-agonists in premature labour, especially in the presence of fluid overload

Continued

Table 5.7 *Continued*

Respiratory disorder	Causative drugs	Comments
Pulmonary eosinophilia (increased presence of eosinophils)	Nitrofurantoin, **NSAIDs, antibiotics, antineoplastics**	• Symptoms include cough, dyspnoea and fever • Patients improve on cessation of treatment • May be treated with corticosteroids
Respiratory failure (neuromuscular)	**Calcium-channel blockers, beta-blockers, antirheumatics, aminoglycoside and polymyxin antibiotics, opioids and diuretics**	• Impaired respiratory muscle function • Patients at risk include those with pre-existing impaired respiratory muscle function, renal failure and myasthenia gravis • Reversible on cessation of treatment • Opioids depress the rate and depth of respiration due to reduced sensitivity of the respiratory centre in the brain to increased blood CO_2
Pulmonary thromboembolism	**Combined oral contraceptives**	• May present as sudden collapse, pleuritic pain, breathlessness, cyanosis and haemoptysis

Text in **bold** represents drug groups or classes.

For a review of respiratory ADRs see also Bhatia *et al.* (2001).

NSAIDs, non-steroidal anti-inflammatory drugs; ACE, angiotensin-converting enzyme; COPD, chronic obstructive pulmonary disease; IV, intravenous.

Practice points

- The CSM recommends that patients should be informed about the adverse reactions associated with mefloquine and advised to seek medical advice on alternative treatment if symptoms develop. Mefloquine prophylaxis should ideally be started 2–3 weeks before travel in an attempt to identify ADRs.
- Many drugs require dose reduction when treating elderly patients, to prevent adverse effects such as drowsiness, confusion, dementia and delirium. This is particularly required for drugs undergoing hepatic oxidation (phase I, see Drug interactions, below) such as benzodiazepines, tricyclic antidepressants and antipsychotics or those with extensive renal elimination, including lithium, digoxin, histamine H_2-receptor antagonists, morphine and pethidine. It is recommended that renal function is checked every 6 months for patients aged over 70 years to prevent ADRs with these drugs (Gray *et al.*, 1999).
- As with all ADRs, if a drug is suspected of causing dementia or delirium, consider the temporal relationship between introduction of drug and the development of symptoms and consider a trial without the drug.
- Patients prescribed long-term corticosteroids should be advised about the possibility of psychiatric adverse effects, e.g. depression, severe paranoid states and insomnia.
- Patients prescribed the antiparkinson drugs co-careldopa, co-beneldopa and dopamine receptor agonists should be warned of the risk of sudden onset of sleep during the day.

Table 5.8   Summary of adverse drug reactions leading to mental health problems

Psychiatric problem	Causative drugs
Depression (Chapter 23)	**Antimicrobials** (ciprofloxacin, sulphonamides) **Cardiovascular** (lipophilic beta-blockers, alpha-blockers, calcium channel blockers, digoxin, methyldopa, statins) **CNS** (alcohol, amantadine, amfetamine (withdrawal) benzodiazepines, carbamazepine, levodopa, phenothiazines) **Hormones** (corticosteroids, oestrogens, progestogens) **Other:** disulfiram, isotretinoin, mefloquine, metoclopramide, NSAIDs
Psychosis	Amantadine, **amfetamines**, anticholinergics (including sedating antihistamines), **antiepileptics**, bromocriptine, chloroquine, clonidine, digoxin, disulfiram, donepazil, ganciclovir, isoniazid, levodopa, mefloquine, **NSAIDs**, quinidine, **quinolone antibiotics**, zolpidem, **drugs of abuse**
Mania	Baclofen, bromocriptine, chloroquine, **corticosteroids, dopaminergic agents**, isoniazid, levodopa, **antidepressants**
Behavioural toxicity	Lamotrigine, dextromethorphan (children), diphenhydramine, chlorphenamine, vigabatrin
Confusion	**Antiparkinson drugs, barbiturates, beta-blockers, benzodiazepines, cimetidine, corticosteroids, diuretics, histamine H_2-receptor antagonists, hypoglycaemics, MAOIs, NSAIDs, opioids, sedating antihistamines, tricyclic antidepressants**
Dementia or delirium	Many, but commonly **benzodiazepines, corticosteroids, opioids, anticholinergics** and drugs with anticholinergic effects, including **tricyclic antidepressants, antiarrhythmics, antiparkinson agents, conventional antipsychotics**, ipratropium (high doses), oxybutynin, tolterodine and **sedating antihistamines**. Toxic effect of lithium and digoxin (Gray *et al.*, 1999)
Neuroleptic malignant syndrome	**Dopamine antagonists: antipsychotics** (most commonly phenothiazines, butyrophenones)
Sedation	Many, but commonly **antiparkinson drugs, antipsychotics (phenothiazines,** particularly chlorpromazine**), barbiturates, benzodiazepines,** carbamazepine, **opioids, antidepressants** (amitriptyline, trazodone), **sedating antihistamines, alpha-blockers**

Text in **bold** represents drug groups or classes.

CNS, central nervous system; NSAIDs, non-steroidal anti-inflammatory drugs; MAOIs, monoamine oxidase inhibitors.

Neurological ADRs

Neurological disorders encompass disorders of the nervous system, including the brain, spinal cord and all peripheral nerves. This may result from direct toxicity leading to damage of the nerve and/or surrounding myelin sheath or due to predictable pharmacology such as antagonism of dopamine transmission in drug-induced parkinsonism.

Drug-induced movement disorders

Drugs causing movement disorders are listed in Table 5.9. These are often difficult to recognise, particularly in the elderly where misdiagnosis of Parkinson's disease may occur. Drugs may cause more than one type of movement disorder but it is unusual to see more than one type exhibited by a single patient. Symptoms should resolve on cessation of the suspected drug. In the case of

Table 5.9 Summary of adverse drug reactions leading to neurological disorders

Neurological disorder	Causative drugs	Comments
Headache	**Vasodilators** (calcium channel blockers, nitrates and nicorandil), indometacin, **MAOI** interactions (hypertensive crisis), **analgesics** (rebound after daily administration, particularly in combination with caffeine), **triptans** (overuse), ergotamine (withdrawal), **SSRIs**	• Tolerance usually develops during vasodilator treatment and patients should persist with treatment if possible • Medication overuse headache is discussed in Chapter 27
Aseptic meningitis	**NSAIDs, vaccines**, ciprofloxacin, azathioprine, penicillin, isoniazid, co-trimoxazole	• Particularly in patients with systemic lupus erythematosus • Difficult to distinguish clinically from bacterial/viral meningitis, therefore a drug history should be considered in all cases
Benign intracranial hypertension	Amlodipine, **corticosteroids** (including topical), danazol, etretinate, nalidixic acid, nitrofurantoin, **oral contraceptives, tetracyclines,** isotretinoin, vitamin A (high doses and deficiency)	• Symptoms include headache, oedema of the optic nerve head, nausea, vomiting, tinnitus and visual disturbances • Usually resolves on cessation of treatment
Reduction of convulsant threshold and increasing the risk of seizures	Bupropion, **antihistamines** (sedating), **antipsychotics,** baclofen, chloroquine, ciclosporin, **corticosteroids (systemic),** donepezil, isoniazid, lithium, mefloquine, ecstasy (MDMA), **NSAIDs, oral contraceptives, penicillins,** pethidine, **quinolone antibiotics, antidepressants** (TCAs and SSRIs), **stimulants and anorectics,** theophylline, tramadol, **vaccines**. Withdrawal effects: alcohol, baclofen, **barbiturates, benzodiazepines**	• These drugs should be used with caution in people with a history of epilepsy. Coprescribing should be avoided in epilepsy (particularly NSAIDs with quinolones) • Often dose-dependent • An interaction between NSAIDs and quinolones is highlighted by the CSM but the risk is low in the absence of risk factors • Patients with diabetes and/or a history of head trauma and those who abuse alcohol are also at increased risk of seizures
Peripheral neuropathy	Alcohol (nutritional deficiency), amiodarone, dapsone, disulfiram, gold, hydralazine, isoniazid, metronidazole, nitrofurantoin, phenytoin, pyridoxine (vitamin B_6), **quinolones, taxanes,** zidovudine	• Early drug withdrawal improves prognosis • Risk factors include diabetes mellitus, alcoholism, vitamin deficiency (particularly B_1, B_{12}), reduced renal/hepatic function, poor acetylator status (hydralazine, isoniazid)
Guillain–Barré syndrome (disease of peripheral nerves)	Captopril, **corticosteroid**s, gold, hepatitis B vaccine, influenza vaccine, MMR vaccine, oxytocin, penicillamine, streptokinase	• Rare paraesthesia of toes or fingers progresses to upper and lower limb followed by total body weakness

Continued

Table 5.9 *Continued*

Neurological disorder	Causative drugs	Comments
Myasthenia gravis (chronic muscle weakness involving reduced activity of acetylcholine at neuromuscular junctions)	**Corticosteroids** (high-dose), phenytoin, **aminoglycosides, quinolone antibiotics** (ciprofloxacin), **beta-blockers,** lithium, **anticholinergics**	• Avoid in myasthenia gravis
Movement (extrapyramidal) disorders	**Antiemetics** (prochlorperazine, metoclopramide, cinnarazine), **antipsychotics (also following withdrawal), calcium channel blockers** (verapamil, amlodipine, diltiazem), lithium, methyldopa, **antidepressants** (TCAs and SSRIs), valproate	• Apparent lower risk of drug-induced parkinsonism with newer antipsychotics (risperidone, olanzapine, clozapine) • Dose-related • Metoclopramide should be avoided in patents aged under 20 years
Tinnitus	**NSAIDs,** including aspirin	

Text in **bold** represents drug groups or classes.

MAOI, monoamine oxidase inhibitor; SSRIs, selective serotonin reuptake inhibitors; NSAIDs, non-steroidal anti-inflammatory drugs; MDMA, methylenedioxymethamfetamine; CSM, Committee on Safety of Medicines; TCAs, tricyclic antidepressants; MMR, measles, mumps, rubella.

suspected drug-induced Parkinsonism, anti-parkinson drugs should be withheld for at least 3 months. Anticholinergic agents should be used with caution due to the risk of irreversible tardive dyskinesia (Chapter 26).

Patient counselling

Patients should be educated about the risk of medication overuse headache when making repeated purchases of OTC analgesia or requests for repeat prescriptions for treating chronic headache (Chapter 27).

Endocrine ADRs

ADRs may also affect a variety of endocrine control systems such as the thyroid and adrenal glands.

Glucose control

See Chapter 33.

Thyroid dysfunction

See Chapter 34.

Adrenal function

Cushing's syndrome

Cushing's syndrome is caused by prolonged treatment with corticosteroids. Clinical signs include 'moon face', weight gain, excess growth of facial and body hair, raised blood pressure, raised blood glucose levels, osteoporosis, psychiatric symptoms, including depressed mood, and skin thinning.

Adrenal insufficiency

Abrupt withdrawal of corticosteroids following prolonged treatment may lead to headache, dizziness, joint pain, weakness and emotional changes. Abrupt withdrawal from long-term treatment may be more severe and potentially fatal.

Ketoconazole, a potent inhibitor of adrenal glucocorticoid synthesis, may precipitate adrenal insufficiency after only 2 days' treatment. Clinical signs and symptoms include lethargy, anorexia, weight loss, hyponatraemia and hyperkalaemia.

Acute adrenal insufficiency may occur in patient taking rifampicin and with pre-existing hypoadrenalism. The mechanism involved is thought to involve increased glucocorticoid metabolism due to the induction of hepatic cytochrome P450 enzymes by rifampicin.

Hyperprolactinaemia

Prolactin is synthesised and stored in the anterior pituitary gland, being released following childbirth, stimulating milk production by the breast and progesterone production by the corpus luteum in the ovary. Drug-induced hyperprolactinaemia may occur in patients taking drugs that increase serotonin (5-HT) or reduce dopamine effects (e.g. phenothiazines), leading to galactorrhoea (abnormal milk production), amenorrhoea, impotence or infertility. The condition is usually reversible on cessation of treatment.

Syndrome of inappropriate secretion of antidiuretic hormone (SIADH)

Antidiuretic hormone (ADH or vasopressin) is released by the pituitary gland, stimulating the reabsorption of water by the kidney and therefore reducing water loss from the body. Inappropriate secretion of ADH therefore leads to an increase in extracellular fluid. This is the mechanism by which antidepressants lead to hyponatraemia. Symptoms include confusion, weakness, lethargy, weight gain, headache, nausea and vomiting and ultimately convulsions, coma and death (Table 5.10). Monitoring of baseline serum sodium levels is prudent in patients prescribed drugs known to cause SIADH, particularly antipsychotics, carbamazepine and high doses of antidepressants, particularly if coprescribed with other drugs which may cause hyponatraemia (Chapter 2).

Patient counselling

- Patients taking drugs that may interfere with thyroid function should report signs of hypothyroidism or hyperthyroidism (Chapter 34). Particular caution and increased monitoring are required for patients at increased risk of developing cardiac arrhythmias (Table 5.4 and Chapter 14).
- Patients should be advised not to stop abruptly long-term treatment with systemic corticosteroids. A steroid card should be carried (see also Withdrawal responses, above).
- Abrupt withdrawal is often appropriate following short courses of corticosteroids used in the treatment of asthma since treatment is generally less than 3 weeks and not more than 40 mg of prednisolone (or equivalent) daily.
- Patients who develop drug-induced gynaecomastia can be reassured that the condition resolves when treatment is stopped.
- Patients taking drugs known to cause hyponatraemia secondary to SIADH should report weakness, lethargy, headache, nausea and vomiting and confusion.

Genitourinary ADRs (Table 5.11)

Sexual dysfunction is being increasingly recognised as a factor influencing poor compliance with drug treatment and is a cause of considerable distress to patients. Patients should therefore be warned about the possibility of drug-induced sexual dysfunction, particularly due to long-term prescriptions of antihypertensives, antidepressants and antipsychotics, to promote open discussion if problems arise, thereby preventing unnecessary anguish and possible relationship problems. Table 5.11 provides examples of types of sexual dysfunction and the drugs implicated.

Patient counselling

- Patients prescribed drugs given by intracavernosal injection for erectile dysfunction (alprostadil, papaverine, phentolamine) should be warned about the risk of priapism and

Table 5.10   Summary of some adverse drug reactions affecting endocrine systems

Endocrine effects		Causative drugs
Altered glucose control (Chapter 33)		
Thyroid dysfunction (Chapter 34)		
Adrenal function		**Corticosteroids**, ketoconazole (reduced), rifampicin (reduced)
Aldosterone synthesis		Carbenoxolone, lithium, **loop diuretics, oral contraceptives**, spironolactone, **thiazides**
Hypoaldosteronism		**ACE inhibitors (including angiotensin II receptor antagonists), NSAIDs, heparins**
Gonadotrophin release and gonadal function	Ovarian and testicular function	**Corticosteroids** (reduced), danazol (increased free testosterone), ketoconazole (reduced testicular steroidogenesis)
	Gynaecomastia – oestrogenic	Clomifene, digoxin, **oestrogens**, spironolactone
	Gynaecomastia – (due to reduced testosterone)	Alcohol, **alkylating agents**, cyproterone, flutamide, phenytoin, spironolactone, ketoconazole, cimetidine
	Gynaecomastia – other	**Antipsychotics** (chlorpromazine), **calcium channel blockers**, isoniazid, marijuana, methadone, methyldopa, **protease inhibitors**, stavudine, **TCAs**
Hyperprolactinaemia		Methadone, morphine, **antidepressants, antipsychotics, antiulcer drugs** (e.g. cimetidine, ranitidine), **benzodiazepines, oestrogens**, methyldopa, verapamil
SIADH – syndrome of inappropriate secretion of antidiuretic hormone		**Psychotropics**, carbamazepine, **cytotoxics, hypoglycaemics** (chlorpropamide, tolbutamide)

Text in **bold** represents drug groups or classes.
ACE, angiotensin-converting enzyme; NSAIDs, non-steroidal anti-inflammatory drugs; TCAs, tricyclic antidepressants.

advised to seek urgent medical attention should this occur.

Dermatological ADRs (Table 5.12)

Drugs may induce a range of dermatological reactions and these represent a substantial proportion of ADRs, to which the practitioner should be vigilant. Any drug, chemical, herb or pharmaceutical excipient has the potential to cause a dermatological reaction. The mechanisms involved are often unknown but tend to result from an allergic or toxic reaction or exacerbation of a pre-existing inflammatory condition. Allergic reactions such as urticaria may persist for a long time after a drug is stopped or may occasionally fail to develop for up to a week after a drug is withdrawn. The drugs most commonly implicated in adverse skin reactions include penicillins, NSAIDs, phenytoin, gold, chlorpromazine (health workers are advised to avoid direct contact due to sensitisation) and cytotoxic agents.

Identification of the causative agent of a dermatological reaction can be difficult, as rechallenge

Table 5.11   Adverse drug reactions affecting sexual function

Sexual dysfunction	Causative drugs	Comments
Primary infertility	**Cytotoxics (alkylating agents), anabolic steroids**, colchicine, diethylstilbestrol, methotrexate, **NSAIDs** (females), sulfasalazine (males)	May include a toxic effect on the gonads or altered secretion of gonadotrophin hormones by the pituitary gland
Anovulation and amenorrhoea	**Anabolic steroids**, danazol, isoniazid, metoclopramide, cimetidine, **NSAIDs, SSRIs, oestrogens**, risperidone, spironolactone	• May result from drug-induced hyperprolactinaemia • NSAIDs may inhibit ovulation and should preferably be avoided around the time of ovulation in women trying to conceive
Erectile dysfunction (impotence)	**Anabolic steroids, antiandrogens** (finasteride), **anticholinergics, antidepressants, antipsychotics, benzodiazepines, beta-blockers, antiepileptic** (carbamazepine, gabapentin, phenytoin), digoxin, methyldopa, metoclopramide, omeprazole, prazosin, spironolactone, **thiazide diuretics**	• Other factors include smoking, alcohol, diabetes, heart disease, hypertension, peripheral vascular disease, spinal cord injury, psychological • SSRIs may be used to treat premature ejaculation
Priapism (prolonged erection of the penis)	**Anticoagulants**, alprostadil, sildenafil, **antipsychotics (including atypicals)**, hydralazine, nifedipine, papaverine, prazosin, trazodone	Immediate treatment is required to prevent fibrosis or gangrene
Female orgasm dysfunction, libido changes, reduced vaginal lubrication	**Antidepressants, benzodiazepines,** cimetidine, clonidine, **gonadorelin analogues,** methyldopa, **oestrogens**, propranolol, spironolactone, **thiazide diuretics**, trazodone	• Patients prescribed fluoxetine or clomipramine have reported spontaneous orgasm
Reduced libido	Spironolactone, cimetidine, **oral contraceptives**, propranolol, **thiazide diuretics, antidepressants** (particularly SSRIs)	• Libido may be increased rarely by trazadone, moclobemide or levodopa

Text in **bold** represents drug groups or classes.
NSAIDs, non-steroidal anti-inflammatory drugs; SSRIs, selective serotonin reuptake inhibitors.

is not appropriate, with the possible exception of fixed drug eruptions. When making a diagnosis, it is important to consider the information included in SPCs, previous case reports, the pattern of eruption together with consideration of a temporal relationship between drug administration and ADR development. A temporal relationship may be apparent in some cases but in others a reaction may take anything from hours to years to develop. Any serious skin reaction should be reported to the CSM on a yellow card, particularly angioedema, bullous eruption, epidermal necrolysis and generalised exfoliation. In addition, any dermatological reactions suspected to result from new drugs should be reported.

Table 5.12   Summary of adverse drug reactions affecting the skin

Dermatological condition	Causative drugs	Comments
Angioedema and urticaria	Many, including aspirin, **ACE inhibitors,** codeine, imipramine, paracetamol, penicillins, ranitidine, **sulphonamides** and tartrazine	Report cases of angioedema to CSM
Erythroderma and exfoliative dermatitis	**Sulphonamides,** chloroquine, penicillin, phenytoin	Severe and widespread
Erythema multiforme and Stevens–Johnson syndrome (SJS)	**Sulphonamides, barbiturates,** carbamazepine	Causative agents must be identified and withdrawn due to risk of SJS and TEN
Toxic epidermal necrolysis	**Barbiturates,** phenytoin, **penicillins**	Usually 1–3 weeks after exposure (2–8 weeks' phenytoin)
Erythematous (exanthematous) eruptions	**Penicillins, sulphonamides, diuretics,** carbamazepine, **NSAIDs**	Most common drug-induced cutaneous reaction. May occur with any drug often within first 10 days
Acne (acneiform)	**Androgens, corticosteroids, anticonvulsants, oral contraceptives,** lithium	Acneiform eruptions resemble acne vulgaris
Pigmentation	Amiodarone, **oral contraceptives, tetracyclines,** chloroquine, chlorpromazine, phenytoin	Refer to a dermatologist if skin discoloration occurs with prolonged antimalarial treatment
Fixed drug eruption	Phenolphthalein, **sulphonamides, tetracyclines, NSAIDs**	Occurs within 24 h, affecting any part of skin or mucous membranes
Vasculitis	Furosemide (frusemide), allopurinol, methotrexate, minocycline, **NSAIDs**	Immunological reaction. Develops after 7–21 days. Most recover quickly
Pemphigus-like eruptions	Captopril, enalapril, furosemide (frusemide), **penicillins,** penicillamine	Rare
Lichenoid drug eruptions	Lithium, **NSAIDs, beta-blockers,** captopril	Immunological reaction after weeks or months of treatment
Purpura	Aspirin, quinine, **sulphonamides,** penicillin	A full blood count should be measured (Chapter 2)
Psoriasis and psoriasiform eruptions	Lithium, interferon-alfa, terbinafine, chloroquine, **beta-blockers**	Usually occurs within 1–2 months and resolves on discontinuation of drug
Photosensitivity	Amiodarone, **thiazides, tetracyclines, retinoids, sulphonamides,** chlorpropamide, nalidixic acid, **oral contraceptives, phenothiazines**	• Occurs within 5–20 h and may persist for up to 4 months after drug stopped (occasionally years) • Patients taking amiodarone should be advised to avoid sunlight and wear sunblock
Hair loss	**Cytotoxic agents, antithyroid drugs, antidepressants, oral contraceptives** (withdrawal from), tamoxifen, lithium, **antithyroid drugs, antihyperlipidaemics,** tamoxifen, **anticoagulants**	• Growth phase (anagen, by cytotoxics) or resting phase (telogen) of hair follicles affected • Telogen hair loss usually occurs after 2–4 months' treatment

Continued

Table 5.12   *Continued*

Dermatological condition	Causative drugs	Comments
Hair growth	**Androgens**, nifedipine, phenytoin, verapamil, penicillamine, **corticosteroids**	Androgen-mediated hirsutism (often with acne) or hypertrichosis (affecting forehead, cheeks)
Nail disorders	Lithium, **cytotoxics**, captopril, **thiazides, tetracyclines**	• Occurs within a few weeks of treatment • Usually reversible

Text in **bold** represents drug groups or classes.

ACE, angiotensin-converting enzyme; CSM, Committee on Safety of Medicines; NSAIDs, non-steroidal anti-inflammatory drugs; TEN, toxic epidermal necrolysis.

Potentially serious skin reactions

Angioedema and urticaria

The prefix 'angio-' indicates blood or lymph vessels. The term 'angioedema' therefore describes a reaction in which increased vascular permeability results in oedema of the deep dermis, subcutaneous tissue or submucosal regions. The tongue, lips, eyelids, genitalia or upper respiratory tract may be affected, with the risk of airway obstruction and severe life-threatening respiratory distress. Urgent referral and treatment with adrenaline, corticosteroids and antihistamines is required (Chapter 19).

Urticaria (hives or nettle rash) is an acute or chronic allergic reaction with a genetic predisposition and may occur within 36 h of exposure. Individual lesions tend to resolve within 24 h. Reaction occurs within minutes of rechallenge. Urticaria affecting the tongue and lips may result in angioedema.

Erythroderma (exfoliative dermatitis)

Erythroderma is literally a 'reddening of the skin', comprising a widespread erythematous rash with abnormal flaking and thickening of the skin. Erythroderma may develop from psoriasis or following exanthematous eruptions. Systemic symptoms of fever, lymphadenopathy and anorexia may be present. Complications occur due to hypothermia, fluid loss and infection.

Stevens–Johnson syndrome (SJS)

This is a severe form of erythema multiforme (see below) characterised by bullae formation (large blisters containing serous fluid) involving the eyes, genitalia, oral mucosa and skin. Systemic symptoms include arthralgia, myalgia, fever and malaise. Treatment includes systemic corticosteroids, fluid replacement and antibiotics. SJS can develop into potentially fatal toxic epidermal necrolysis (TEN).

Toxic epidermal necrolysis

TEN is a rare reaction, but which carries a high mortality rate. Epithelial necrosis affects all areas of skin with severe involvement of mucous membranes. A prodromal period that may not be differentiated from an upper respiratory tract infection, may last for 2–3 days. The affected skin may detach in large sheets, resulting in dehydration, systemic infection (septicaemia) or damage to other organ systems and death. TEN continues even after the causative drug has been removed.

SJS and TEN have been reported in patients, particularly children, taking lamotrigine and this was associated with a CSM warning in 1997. Increased risk factors include initial dosing higher than recommended, more rapid dose escalation than recommended and concomitant valproate. Patients should be advised to report rash or influenza-like symptoms associated with hypersensitivity urgently. Most rashes occur within 8 weeks of starting lamotrigine.

Associated systemic lupus erythematosus (SLE)

SLE describes a chronic inflammatory disease of connective tissue, which affects the skin and various internal organs. Patients with SLE have a predisposition to TEN.

Less serious skin reactions

Erythematous (exanthematous) eruptions

This reaction usually occurs in the first 10 days of treatment, for example following the administration of ampicillin or amoxicillin to patients with infectious mononucleosis or less commonly, lymphatic leukaemia. The causative drug should be stopped to prevent progression to exfoliative dermatitis.

Pigmentation

Pigmentation may develop following lichenoid or fixed drug eruptions. Patients taking antimalarials for prolonged periods (greater than 3–4 months) are prone to grey-blue/black discoloration of the shins. Referral should be made for eye examination as irreversible retinal damage may occur.

Fixed drug eruptions

Fixed drug eruptions may affect any part of the skin or mucous membranes, usually within 24 h of drug administration. The term 'fixed' is used as the eruptions always occur at the same site.

Vasculitis

Vasculitis means 'inflammation of the blood vessels'. This may be systemic or cutaneous (raised purpuric lesions on the legs of varying size). Occasionally high-dose corticosteroids and immunosuppressants are required.

Pemphigus-like eruptions

These comprise scattered, large, firm and sometimes haemorrhagic bullae (blisters) with an erythematous base displaying similarities to those occurring as a result of the autoimmune disorders idiopathic pemphigus and bullous pemphigoid.

Lichenoid drug eruptions

Lichen describes round, hard lesions occurring close together. Lichenoid drug eruptions are dermatological reactions resembling lichen. If this is extensive, progression to exfoliative dermatitis may occur.

Purpura

So called because of its purple appearance, purpura results from bleeding of small capillaries into the skin. Thrombocytopenia or platelet dysfunction or alternatively immunological damage of small capillaries producing a change in vascular permeability may cause this.

Psoriasis and psoriasiform eruptions

The appearance of erythematous plaques with large dry silvery scales similar to those of psoriasis may be drug-induced. Alternatively, certain drugs may cause a worsening of pre-existing psoriasis, e.g. beta-blockers.

Photosensitivity

Photosensitivity represents a dose-related reaction whereby the photosensitising agent in or on the skin reacts to ultraviolet or visible light. It is a common phenomenon, presenting as sunburn, and is confined to areas exposed to light. It occurs within 5–20 h of drug administration and may persist for months to years after the causative agent is withdrawn. Photoallergic reactions may be delayed by at least a week and have an eczematous appearance.

Patients taking drugs known to cause photosensitivity should be advised to avoid direct sunlight, particularly between 12 and 2 p.m., and to wear protective clothing in the summer months and abroad. The use of sun cream with a high protection factor is recommended during sun exposure.

Erythema multiforme

Erythema multiforme describes a reddening of the skin due to vasodilatation that may be triggered by infection or, less commonly, by drugs. Lesions can resemble those of urticaria but do not last as long, are more purple in colour and often involve the mucous membranes and palms. Diagnosis and cessation of the suspected drug are imperative due to the risk of developing SJS or TEN.

Treatment

Minor skin reactions are treated with oral antihistamines and/or topical steroids. Hydrocortisone 1% is available OTC for up to 7 days' treatment but normally should not be used on the face or anogenital region or applied to broken skin. Conditions affecting these areas require referral to the GP since the use of hydrocortisone treatment is outside the OTC licence.

Patient counselling

- Educate patients to avoid direct sunlight and sun beds, wear protective clothing and use high-protection factor sunscreen during and for a few months after receiving photosensitising drugs.
- Patients should be aware of previous allergic reactions to drugs and encouraged to report them to health professionals. The distinction between traditional side-effects and allergy should be made to avoid confusion.

Musculoskeletal ADRs (Table 5.13)

Drugs may adversely affect muscles, bone and connective tissues in a number of ways, from fluid retention in muscle producing mild aches and pains, to debilitating osteoporosis or life-threatening rhabdomyolysis. It is important to be aware of drugs causing musculoskeletal pathology as early recognition and cessation of the drug can prevent unnecessary suffering and uncertainty, whilst improving the outcome for patients.

Rhabdomyolysis

An example of the importance of early diagnosis of an ADR is the failure to recognise drug-induced myopathy, resulting in the progression to rhabdomyolysis. Risk factors include renal impairment, acute serious illness, infections, major trauma and hypoxia. In addition, coprescribing two or more of the following drugs increases the risk of a patient developing rhabdomyolysis:

- fibrates
- statins (cerivastatin was withdrawn in 2001 due to myopathy)
- ciclosporin
- erythromycin
- danazol
- itraconazole
- ketoconazole

- nefazodone
- nicotinic acid

Patient counselling

- Patients taking statins and/or fibrates should report muscle weakness, pain or tenderness.
- To prevent drug-induced osteoporosis, patients prescribed long-term steroid courses should be advised to stop smoking, limit alcohol consumption, take regular weight-bearing exercise and ensure an adequate calcium and vitamin D intake.
- The CSM advises patients to stop taking quinolone antibiotics at the first sign of tendon damage such as pain or inflammation. The affected limb should be rested until tendon symptoms have resolved.
- Young patients prescribed minocycline for greater than 6 months should report symptoms such as arthralgia, fever, rash and pleuritic pain which may indicate SLE.

Monitoring for ADRs

- ECG monitoring should be considered for patients taking tricyclic antidepressants, droperidol, thioridazine and other drugs which prolong the QT interval and particularly in the presence of additional risk factors such as coronary heart disease. Consider also regular monitoring of potassium levels and the avoidance, if possible, of drugs known to cause hypokalaemia, such as high-dose beta$_2$-adrenoceptor agonists or diuretics (see Chapter 2).
- Patients prescribed treatment long-term should be monitored regularly for adverse effects. For example, patients taking minocycline for longer than 6 months should be monitored for hepatotoxicity, pigmentation and SLE.
- Consider drugs for which regular blood tests are recommended. Common tests include LFTs, full blood counts, renal function or thyroid function tests (Chapter 2). Monitoring of renal and hepatic function is particularly important for elderly patients taking prescribed drugs.

Table 5.13   Summary of adverse drug reactions affecting muscloskeletal tissue

Musculoskeletal pathology	Causative drugs	Comments
Myalgia (muscle pain), cramps or myopathy	Amiodarone, carbimazole, ciclosporin, cimetidine, colchicine, **corticosteroids** (withdrawal), danazol, **diuretics, fibrates**, nicotinic acid, **opioids**, penicillamine, quinine, chloroquine, **quinolones, statins,** zidovudine	• Myalgia presents as muscle pain, tenderness and/or muscle weakness • Increased serum creatine phosphokinase (CPK) is an indicator of muscle damage (10 × normal level may indicate myopathy)
Metabolic bone disease: osteoporosis (loss of bony tissue)	**Corticosteroids,** heparin, **thyroid hormones**	• Lowest-effective dose of corticosteroids should be used • Consider vitamin D supplement for housebound and frail elderly
Metabolic bone disease: osteomalacia (rickets, abnormal bone softening)	**Aluminium salts** (including prolonged ingestion of antacids), **barbiturates, bisphosphonates** (overdose), phenytoin, long-term total parenteral nutrition	• A lack or defective metabolism of vitamin D • Poor diet and lack of sunlight are contributing factors
Arthralgia (joint pain without swelling)	**Calcium channel blockers,** carbimazole, isoniazid, procainamide, quinidine, **quinolone antibiotics,** rubella vaccine, BCG	• May accompany any drug-induced skin eruption • Severe joint pain with swelling is a component of 'serum sickness' (e.g. penicillin)
Arthralgia: acute gout	**Low-dose salicylates, diuretics,** ciclosporin	Caused by the arthritis (includes inflammation and swelling) of acute gout
Arthropathy (erosion of articular cartilage)	Quinolone antibiotics	• Restricted indications in children, growing adolescents and avoidance in pregnancy • Usually reversible on cessation of treatment
Tendinopathy (particularly Achilles tendon)	**Quinolone antibiotics** (ofloxacin)	• More common in people over 50 years of age • Increased risk if renal impairment and/or corticosteroid treatment
Retroperitoneal fibrosis (development of fibrous tissue behind peritoneum)	Aspirin, **beta-blockers,** bromocriptine, codeine, ergotamine, haloperidol, methysergide	• Symptoms include persistent pain in the loin and groin, oliguria, pain on micturition, myalgia and oedema • Symptoms improve on withdrawal of treatment

Continued

Reporting of suspected ADRs

Doctors, dentists, coroners, pharmacists and nurses may submit yellow cards to the CSM for all suspected ADRs produced by new (black triangle) drugs and serious ADRs for all other drugs. For further information see: http://www.mca.gov.uk/ aboutagency/regframework/csm/csmhome.htm.

Table 5.13 *Continued*

Musculoskeletal pathology	Causative drugs	Comments
Systemic lupus erythematosus (SLE: autoimmune disease of the connective tissue)	Hydralazine, procainamide. **beta-blockers**, carbamazepine, chlorpromazine, disopyramide, isoniazid, methyldopa, nitrofurantoin, penicillamine, phenytoin, quinidine, sulfasalazine, **sulphonamides**, **tetracyclines** (minocycline, particularly young patients), **thiazides**, thiouracil	• Symptoms include arthralgias, myalgias, malaise, fever, pleurisy and pericarditis • Symptoms improve within days or weeks of cessation of suspected drug • Usually occurs after several months or years of continued therapy • Presentation of drug-induced SLE differs from SLE • Leucopenia, thrombocytopenia, anaemia, elevated ESR and antinuclear antibodies may be present (Chapter 2) • Increased risk in slow acetylators

Text in **bold** represents drug groups or classes.
BCG, bacillus Calmette-Guérin; ESR, erythrocyte sedimentation rate.

Practice points

- Health professionals should always consider the adverse effects of drugs, including OTC and herbal supplements when making a diagnosis. Early identification of ADRs may improve the outcome for the patient and prevent unnecessary treatment and intervention.
- Always check the medication history when presented with a rash. Consider drugs stopped recently.
- Take care to identify drug allergies as reintroduction may be more severe. Drug allergies should be recorded prominently on all patient medication records.
- Only prescribe a drug when there is a good indication.
- NSAID-induced gastric damage is a major ADR. To reduce the risk:

  – Only one NSAID should be prescribed at any one time.
  – A less toxic agent such as ibuprofen should be used first-line.
  – The lowest effective dose is recommended.
  – The maximum daily dose should not be exceeded.
  – Patients at risk should be prescribed prophylaxis (Chapter 7).
  – Long-term repeat prescriptions should be reviewed.
  – Patients should be counselled to report warning symptoms (see above).

- Ideally, NSAIDs should be avoided in patients with coronary heart disease and particularly congestive heart failure and hypertension, due to an increase in fluid retention. If essential, the lowest effective dose should be prescribed and drugs with a long elimination half-life avoided.
- The greatest bone loss induced by corticosteroid therapy occurs during the first 6–12 months. Early preventive steps are therefore important. Patients taking prednisolone 7.5 mg or more daily for 3 months or more, particularly aged over 65 years, should be assessed for prophylaxis with hormone replacement therapy, bisphosphonate or calcitriol as appropriate (Chapter 28).
- Always use the lowest effective dose of all drugs.
- Gradually withdraw drugs associated with withdrawal symptoms.
- Increased monitoring and education of patients to improve the recognition and reporting of suspected ADRs are important issues for preventing ADRs (Avery *et al.*, 2002).

CASE STUDIES

Case 1
A man returning from 6 months in India reports a scaly rash on his knees and elbows.
   What is the most likely cause of this rash?

• Possibly drug-induced psoriasis if the patient took chloroquine for malaria prophylaxis.

Case 2
A man prescribed a prolonged course (more than 14 days) of co-amoxiclav for a persistent chest infection reports vomiting, general malaise and pruritus.
   What is the likely cause of his symptoms?

• Clavulanic acid-induced cholestatic hepatitis should be suspected.

Case 3
A woman requested that her GP give her a prescription for antibiotics to treat cystitis. On further questioning the symptoms include polyuria, loin pain and blood-stained urine. There is no pain on urination and no clouding or offensive smell. The only medication the lady takes are painkillers she buys from the supermarket for headaches.

• These symptoms may point to analgesic nephropathy as cystitis normally presents with a burning pain on urination and/or clouding and an offensive smell. Cystitis is more common, but in view of the symptoms, together with the use of painkillers, further investigation is required. Antibiotics may not be appropriate.

Case 4
A middle-aged man requests aspirin tablets to treat pain.
   What further questions should be asked?

• Has he taken it before?
• This real but hard-to-believe case turned out to be a request for analgesia to treat stomach pain. On further questioning about the nature of the pain, the patient reported a past history of peptic ulcer disease, which he thought had returned.

Case 5
A 65-year-old woman presents with a chesty cough of 2–3 weeks' duration. She takes ibuprofen and methotrexate.

• This case includes a possible interaction between ibuprofen and methotrexate leading to reduced clearance of methotrexate with an increased risk of methotrexate toxicity. The combination of methotrexate and ibuprofen is, however, often used without problems but patients should be closely monitored. Signs of infection may indicate a methotrexate-induced blood dyscrasia. In this example, a full blood count is required. The cough may also suggest pulmonary toxicity with methotrexate.

Case 6
A 41-year-old woman has been taking imipramine since the birth of her baby, now 2 years old. She has been troubled with a persistent sore throat and has white spots on the back of her tongue and is feeling tired and run-down.

→

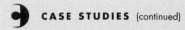

- On checking the SPC for imipramine, you are alerted to the possibility of agranulocytosis and order a full blood count to be carried out. This is a sensible precaution.

Case 7
A 44-year-old woman prescribed nifedipine for Raynaud's phenomenon reports palpitations. She has been drinking grapefruit juice recently.

- This case illustrates a possible interaction between nifedipine and grapefruit juice. The mechanism is thought to involve inhibition of cytochrome P450 isoenzymes by components of grapefruit juice and therefore increased levels of nifedipine.

Drug interactions

Drug interactions may simply be thought of as the actions of one drug being enhanced or inhibited by the presence or actions of another drug or exogenous substance. These may be adverse or beneficial. In addition to recognising the potential for prescribed medicines to interact, one must always bear in mind the potential for OTC medicines, foods and the constituents of herbal remedies to interact with them.

The potential for drug interactions is increased by polypharmacy in the elderly due to reduced renal and hepatic function and by the use of drugs with a narrow therapeutic window such as digoxin, warfarin and lithium. It is, however, difficult to quantify the true incidence of clinically significant drug interactions due to underreporting. This may result from a failure to recognise a drug interaction, fear of litigation or the patient stopping a drug with the familiar report of 'they didn't suit'. Although the reported incidence of coprescribing of serious drug combinations is low, these combinations continue to be prescribed (Chen *et al.*, 2002b).

Approximately 400 drug combinations may be regarded as hazardous or contraindicated, with more than three times this number leading to interactions requiring close monitoring or dosage adjustments. Add to this the interactions leading to unpleasant effects such as drowsiness and those leading to a reduced therapeutic effect, and the number of drug interactions likely to be experienced is staggering. The prescriber can be reassured by the fact that many drug interactions do not result in serious outcomes, although the impact on the patient's quality of life should not be underestimated.

In practice, drug interactions are continually being identified by automated systems and databases and it is often difficult to differentiate between clinically significant and trivial interactions. Furthermore, limitations of these alerts were highlighted in a recent study of interventions by community pharmacists with preliminary findings presented at the British Pharmaceutical Conference (Chen *et al.*, 2002a). Drug interaction alerts produced by dispensary computers were found to omit some important drug interactions when compared with a database containing drug interactions from a standard reference, *Drug Interactions* by Stockley (2002). Also of interest was a questionnaire study seeking the views of GPs; this revealed that 22% of responders admitted to overriding drug interaction alerts frequently or very frequently (Magnus *et al.*, 2002).

The reader is directed to *Drug Interactions* by Stockley for evidence-based information presented in a user-friendly reference with a concise summary of reported drug interactions. In the following chapters an attempt is made to highlight common, serious and clinically significant drug interactions relevant to each section. The latest information should be obtained from the medical literature, SPCs and the latest version of *Drug Interactions* by Stockley.

Mechanisms of drug interactions

The following is a summary of Chapter 1 from *Drug Interactions* by Stockley (2002).

The mechanisms involved in drug interactions are summarised below to provide the understanding required for the prediction and interpretation of these drug-related problems. The following may alert the prescriber to potential problems:

- drugs with a narrow therapeutic window: anticoagulants, anticonvulsants, digoxin, lithium, theophylline and cytotoxic agents
- enzyme inducers and inhibitors
- drugs with similar pharmacology
- elderly patients and children

Pharmacokinetic interactions

Pharmacokinetic interactions are those involving the absorption, distribution, metabolism and/or excretion of drugs.

Absorption

Absorption reactions are often difficult to predict due to the possible combination of several mechanisms. The effect may be a change in either the rate of drug absorption or a change in the total amount of drug absorbed. For drugs with multiple dosing, a change in the rate of absorption may not be important if the total drug absorbed remains unchanged. However, for single-dose regimens, changes in the rate of absorption may be of increased importance.

Examples are given below.

Altered gastric pH

The passive absorption of drugs occurs best with the uncharged form, which is governed by the pK_a value of the drug. Therefore, rises in pH (in the presence of antacids and acid suppressors) may influence the absorption of other drugs. An example of this is ketoconazole, whose absorption is reduced at increased pH with antacids and ulcer-healing drugs. The importance of other interactions resulting from changes in gastric pH is uncertain due to the involvement of additional mechanisms affecting absorption. It is therefore advisable to separate in time the administration of drugs such as antacids, H_2-receptor antagonists and PPIs from other drugs (Chapter 7).

Binding of drugs

The chelation of tetracyclines with di- and trivalent metallic ions such as calcium, iron and aluminium leads to a reduced antibiotic effect. Easy rectification of this is achieved by separating the doses by approximately 2–3 h. Colestyramine reduces the absorption of digoxin, warfarin and levothyroxine due to the binding ability intended for bile salts (Chapters 10 and 12). Concurrent drugs should be taken 1 h before or 4–6 h after colestyramine.

Altered gastric motility

Since the majority of drugs are absorbed in the upper part of the duodenum, a change in gastric emptying affects the rate of absorption of co-prescribed drugs. For example, anticholinerigic drugs and opioids decrease GI motility, reducing gastric emptying, which may delay absorption. By contrast, metoclopramide accelerates gastric emptying, and has the opposite effect. This latter interaction is used to enhance the rate of onset of action of paracetamol in some compound antimigraine preparations.

Malabsorption syndrome

The malabsorption of a number of drugs occurs when taken with neomycin.

Distribution

Protein-binding interactions

Drugs may be dissolved in plasma or bound to plasma proteins, mainly albumin. Equilibrium exists between the bound and free pharmacologically active molecules. Protein-binding interactions occur due to competition for binding sites, resulting in an increased proportion of free drug. The clinical importance of these interactions is debatable due to the consequent metabolism and excretion of the free molecules and a dose adjustment is not usually required. Highly bound drugs with a low volume of distribution are considered the most important participants in this type of interaction.

Metabolism

Drug metabolism occurs in serum, kidneys, skin and intestines but predominantly in the presence of microsomal enzymes found in liver cells. The end result is a less lipid-soluble compound, which is easier to excrete. In the liver, metabolism results from two phases (see Mechanisms of adverse reactions, above).

The most important mechanism resulting in altered drug metabolism is by the induction or inhibition of a family of related isoenzymes, cytochrome P450. Because the cytochrome P450 family comprises a range of isoenzymes, there is added complexity as some forms will be affected by specific inhibitors or inducers and others will not. Even with a detailed understanding of the particular isoenzymes and drug effects, it is difficult to predict interactions at this level, as the metabolism of a drug may involve several enzymes. However, a clear appreciation of the different mechanisms and principal drugs involved is important in medicines management.

Enzyme inhibition

Some drugs inhibit cytochrome P450 enzymes, resulting in reduced metabolism of other drugs. These are dose-dependent and interactions generally develop within 2–3 days with an increase in plasma concentrations and pharmacological effects of the affected drug. Important example of drugs that may inhibit the various isoenzymes include:

- cimetidine
- ciprofloxacin
- erythromycin
- clarithromycin
- metronidazole
- allopurinol
- dextropropoxyphene
- disulfiram
- fluoxetine
- ketoconazole
- fluconazole
- itraconazole
- grapefruit juice
- verapamil
- omeprazole

Enzyme induction

This forms an extremely common mechanism for drug interactions and leads to increased metabolism of the affected drug, reducing plasma concentrations. The result may be failure of treatment and an important example of this occurs with oral contraceptives. An increased dose may be required due to the increased metabolism of a coprescribed drug. For example, the polycyclic hydrocarbons contained in tobacco and cannabis smoke induce enzymes, resulting in increased clearance of theophylline, and an increased dose may be required. This also includes people exposed to high levels of passive smoke but does not include nicotine replacement therapy. Any effects of smoke on phenytoin and warfarin do not appear to be clinically significant.

Additionally, autoinduction occurs, whereby a drug enhances its own metabolism, so that the doses need to be built up. Important examples of this include barbiturates and carbamazepine. Enzyme induction involves an increase in the amount of microsomal enzymes and cytochrome P450 levels in liver cells. Such interactions take from days to 2–3 weeks to develop and also to reverse when a drug is stopped. Good monitoring is essential, particularly as any change in dose may need to be corrected on cessation of the enzyme inducer to prevent overdose.

Agents associated with induction include:

- barbiturates
- rifampicin
- omeprazole
- phenytoin
- ethanol
- carbamazepine
- St John's wort
- tobacco and cannabis smoke (polycyclic hydrocarbons)

Changes in liver blood flow

First-pass metabolism by the liver following transport from the GI tract via the hepatic portal vein is particularly important for highly lipid-soluble drugs such as propranolol. Drugs that alter blood flow through the liver may therefore change the activity of these drugs. For example, cimetidine increases the availability of propranolol by reducing hepatic blood flow.

Excretion

Urinary pH
This is a mechanism of limited clinical importance since mainly inactive compound is excreted in urine following metabolism in the liver.

Competition for renal tubular excretion (methotrexate and NSAIDs)
Changes in active excretion from renal tubules result from competition between drugs using these active transport systems. An example of this interaction is the risk of methotrexate toxicity developing in patients coprescribed salicylates or some NSAIDs. Another important example of this interaction occurs between digoxin and verapamil, resulting in reduced elimination of digoxin, requiring a dose reduction.

Influence of renal blood flow (lithium and COX inhibitors)
Renal blood flow is partly regulated by vasodilator prostanoids. A reduction in synthesis of these prostanoids by COX inhibitors may reduce the excretion of lithium, resulting in increased and possibly toxic levels.

Biliary excretion and enterohepatic shunt (oral contraceptive and antibiotics)
This explains a possible mechanism whereby antibiotics (penicillins or tetracyclines) may reduce levels of oral contraceptives. Drugs excreted in the bile may subsequently undergo metabolism by gut flora to the parent compound, which is then reabsorbed. A reduction in gut flora in the presence of some antibiotics may therefore lead to more rapid loss of drugs undergoing this transformation from the body.

Pharmacodynamic interactions

They occur when different drugs have similar pharmacological targets. They may occur at the level of the same receptor, transduction systems or target responses. This may result in either augmented action or antagonism. Some important examples are listed in Table 5.14.

Practice points

- The key point is clearly vigilance to any changes in a patient's condition which may point to an ADR or interaction.
- Become familiar with clinically significant interactions.
- Warfarin, lithium, theophylline and digoxin therapy should always alert practitioners to be vigilant for ADRs or interactions.
- The change to a patient's therapy which involves a drug known to influence metabolism should prompt a review of all concurrent drugs, whether prescribed, OTC or herbal remedies.
- Consider the pharmacology of drugs when prescribing to allow for the prediction of pharmacodynamic reactions. Avoid using drugs with similar pharmacology.
- It is good practice to be familiar with common interactions as current computer systems have been found to be lacking in the management of drug interactions.

Conclusions

The management of ADRs and drug interactions remains central to the prevention of drug-related problems. Key issues include the implementation of updated computer warning systems to support health professionals in interpreting the ever-increasing number of potential drug interactions, together with the avoidance of polypharmacy, particularly in elderly patients.

Table 5.14   Examples of pharmacodynamic interactions

Interacting drugs	Consequences	Explanation
Beta-adrenoceptor agonists and beta-blockers	Antagonism	These agents will oppose each other
Adrenaline (epinephrine) and beta-blockers	Antagonism	• Adrenaline used in anaphylaxis treatment will be opposed by beta-blockers • Risk of hypertensive crisis (especially with non-selective beta-blockers) as the vasoconstrictor activity of adrenaline via alpha-adrenoceptors will no longer be opposed by $beta_2$-adrenoceptor-mediated vasodilatation
Beta-blockers and verapamil	Addition of actions	The combined negative inotropic and chronotropic effects may lead to asystole
Nitrates and sildenafil	Potentiation, leading to severe hypotension	Nitrates act via cGMP, whose metabolism is prevented by the phosphodiesterase inhibitor, sildenafil
Antihypertensives and antihypertensives	Potentiation, leading to a severe hypotension or used clinically for more effective blood pressure control	Summation of actions (see Chapter 11)
Antihypertensives and oral sympathomimetic decongestants	Opposing actions	Avoid sympathomimetics in hypertension, particularly if poorly controlled
SSRIs and 5-HT$_1$ agonists	Serotonin syndrome (Chapter 23)	SSRIs will prevent the breakdown of endogenous 5-HT, leading to overstimulation of serotonergic system
Betahistine and antihistamines	Antagonism	Betahistine is a histaminergic agent whose actions will be opposed by antihistamines
Warfarin and vitamin K	Antagonism	Warfarin is a vitamin K antagonist
Hypoglycaemic drugs and corticosteroids	Antagonism	Corticosteroids have a diabetogenic effect
Alcohol and sedative agents (including sedative antihistamines)	Potentiation	Potentiation
Potassium-sparing diuretics, ACE inhibitors and potassium	Potentiation, leading to hyperkalaemia	All cause potassium retention
Levodopa activity and some antipsychotic and antiemetic drugs	Antagonism	Some antipsychotic drugs may induce parkinsonism
Drugs which cause QT prolongation (Table 5.4)	Potentiation	Risk of torsade de pointes, arrhythmia and potentially fatal ventricular fibrillation
Drugs with antimuscarinic side-effects (e.g. tricyclic antidepressants; certain older antihistamines, e.g. promethazine, see above)	Enhanced antimuscarinic side-effects	Side-effects include blurred vision, urinary retention, dry mouth and possibly cardiac effects

cGMP, cyclic guanosine monophosphate; SSRIs, selective serotonin reuptake inhibitors; ACE, angiotensin-converting enzyme.

CASE STUDIES

Case 1

A man has been taking timolol tablets long-term for the treatment of hypertension. A colleague prescribed an adrenaline injection for emergency treatment of peanut allergy over the last few years. The patient has administered a single dose in the last year without apparent problems.

- In this case, the blockade of beta-adrenoceptors will render the adrenaline less effective but could lead to unopposed alpha-adrenoceptor vasoconstriction. A number of alternative agents are available, and the timolol should be changed.

Case 2

A 22-year-old woman requests some medicine for a dry cough. The counter assistant asks the pharmacist if it is appropriate to sell a product containing dextromethorphan to this lady. Her records indicate she is taking paroxetine.

- This is a rare but potentially serious drug interaction, due to the risk of the patient developing a serotonin-like syndrome (Chapter 23). Symptoms include tremor, confusion, tachycardia, hypertension and abnormal movements. It would therefore not be appropriate to recommend this product with paroxetine.

Acknowledgement

The information in this chapter was largely derived from *Adverse Drug Reactions* (Lee, 2001) and *Stockley's Drug Interactions* (Stockley, 2002) and we are most grateful to Anne Lee and Dr Ivan Stockley for their advice.

References

Avery A J, Sheikh A, Hurwitz B *et al.* (2002). Safer medicines management in primary care. *Br J Gen Pract* 52 (suppl): S17–S22.

Chen Y F, Neil K E, Avery A J *et al.* (2002a). Prescriptions with potentially hazardous/contraindicated drug combinations presented to community pharmacies. *Int J Pharm Pract* 10 (suppl): R29.

Chen Y F, Avery A J, Neil K *et al.* (2002b). Incidence and possible causes of prescribing potentially hazardous/contraindicated drug combinations in general practice. *Drug Safety*: in press.

Gray S L, Lai K V, Larson E B (1999). Drug-induced cognition disorders in the elderly: incidence, prevention and management. *Drug Safety* 21: 101–122.

Haddad P M, Anderson I M (2002). Antipsychotic-related QTc prolongation, torsade de pointes and sudden death. *Drugs* 62: 1649–1671.

Harker L A, Boissel J P, Pilgrim A J *et al.* (1999). Comparative safety and tolerability of clopidogrel and aspirin. Results from CAPRIE. *Drug Safety* 21: 325–335.

Lee A (ed.) (2001). *Adverse Drug Reactions*. London: Pharmaceutical Press.

Magnus D, Rodgers S, Avery A J (2002). GPs' views on computerized drug interaction alerts: questionnaire survey. *J Clin Pharm Ther* 27: 377–382.

Mehta D K (ed.) *British National Formulary*, latest edition. London: British Medical Association and Royal Pharmaceutical Society of Great Britain.

Morris A J, Madhok R, Sturrock R D *et al.* (1991). Enteroscopic diagnosis of small bowel ulceration in patients receiving non-steroidal anti-inflammatory drugs. *Lancet* 337: 520.

Stockley I H (2002). *Drug Interactions*, 6th edn. London: Pharmaceutical Press.

Tibble J, Smale S, Bjarnason I (1999). Adverse effects of drugs on the small bowel. *Adverse Drug React Bull* 198: 755–758.

Wiffen P, Gill M, Edwards J *et al.* (2002). Adverse drug reactions in hospital patients. A systematic review of the prospective and retrospective studies. *Bandolier Extra* June 2002: 1–15 at www.ebandolier.com

Further reading

Bhatia P, O'Reilly J F, Li-Kam-Wa E (2001). Adverse reactions and the respiratory system. *Prim Care Respir J* 10: 39–43.

Dean T (2000). Withdrawing drugs not the solution. *Prescriber* 11: 11.

Merlo J, Liedholm H, Lindblad U, *et al.* (2001). Prescriptions with potential drug interactions dispensed at Swedish pharmacies in January 1999: cross sectional study. *BMJ* 323: 427–428.

Sipilä J, Klaukka T, Martikainen J *et al.* (1995). Occurrence of potentially harmful drug combinations among Finnish primary care patients. *Int Pharm J* 9: 104–107.

Stockley I H (2000). Interaction warnings. *Prescriber* 11: 120.

6

Clinical pharmacokinetics and therapeutic drug monitoring

Basic principles

The processes of absorption, distribution, metabolism and excretion determine the concentration of a drug in the plasma. These processes are therefore considered when calculating drug dosages with the aim of producing an optimum concentration to elicit a clinical response whilst avoiding toxicity, i.e. within the therapeutic range or window. In clinical practice, the most important application of this is therapeutic drug monitoring (TDM) and this tends to be used for drugs with a narrow therapeutic window. Important examples where this is applied are lithium, phenytoin, theophylline, gentamicin and digoxin.

Absorption

Not all dosage forms result in complete absorption of the drug into the blood stream. The absorption of oral preparations may be reduced by a number of factors. These include the acidic conditions of the stomach, the activity of digestive enzymes, the proportion absorbed, interaction with other drugs in the gastrointestinal tract and metabolising enzymes in the liver and, to a lesser extent, in the gastrointestinal tract. The latter process is described as first-pass or presystemic metabolism occurring prior to entry into the systemic circulation. Drugs which exhibit extensive first-pass metabolism include propranolol, morphine, nifedipine, verapamil, some statins and aspirin.

The concentration of drug in the blood may therefore be much lower than would be predicted on the basis of the oral dose administered.

Pharmacokinetic equations take account of variability in drug absorption by adjusting for bioavailability (F). In Figure 6.1 the area under the curve (AUC) for the graph of plasma concentration against time is directly proportional to the total amount of drug entering the blood. The value of F can therefore be determined from the

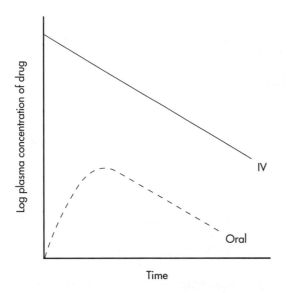

Figure 6.1 Log concentration–time plot comparing the plasma profiles of a drug administered via the intravenous (IV) route and the oral route. This demonstrates the reduced area under the curve for a drug which has reduced oral bioavailability.

AUC following oral administration compared with the AUC from intravenous dosing:

$$F = \frac{\text{AUC oral}}{\text{AUC IV}}$$

Distribution

The volume of distribution (V_d, in L or L/kg) describes the apparent distribution of drugs in the body. By definition, V_d represents the volume of plasma in which the total amount of drug in the body would need to be dissolved in order to reflect the concentration of drug achieved in plasma. Thus:

$$V_d = \frac{\text{Amount in body}}{\text{Concentration}} = \frac{\text{Dose}}{\substack{\text{Concentration} \\ \text{at time zero}}}$$

The importance of V_d is that it gives information regarding distribution; a very large V_d might suggest that the drug is avidly bound to tissues. Indeed, for widely distributed drugs (e.g. digoxin), the V_d may exceed the total volume of

fluid in the body. A small volume of distribution may reflect low tissue binding or fat solubility, or extensive plasma protein binding.

A single-compartment model is used to describe the complete distribution of drug in the plasma. More commonly, drugs enter the plasma and then undergo redistribution to other extravascular sites. This is described as a two-compartment model, and gives rise to two phases in the logarithmic concentration–time plot (Figure 6.2).

In practice, drugs described by the two-compartment model, such as digoxin and theophylline, are sampled for TDM after the distribution phase is complete and one-compartment kinetics are then applied.

Metabolism and excretion

The clearance (CL) of a drug from the body is the theoretical volume of plasma which is cleared of the drug per unit time, and combines the metabolism (e.g. hepatic) and excretion (usually renal) of drug from the body. It is expressed in volume per time, e.g. litres per hour.

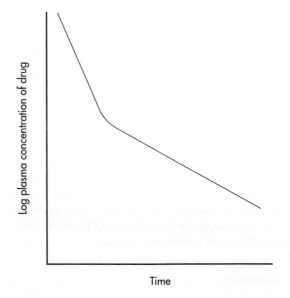

Figure 6.2 Log concentration–time plot for a drug which undergoes extensive elimination and exhibits a two-compartment model.

Generally:

Total clearance = renal clearance + hepatic clearance (+ any other routes)

Knowledge of the relative contributions of the different routes of elimination may influence drug choice. For example, in renal impairment, a drug which is largely eliminated via the liver may be preferred over an alternative which is renally eliminated.

First-order kinetics

Many drugs display first-order kinetics, whereby the rate of elimination of drug from the body is proportional to the drug concentration. The relationship is exponential and, when distribution is rapid compared to elimination, is described by:

$$C_t = C_0 e^{-kt}$$

where C_t is the concentration at time t, C_0 is the concentration at time 0 and k is the rate constant for elimination for a first-order kinetic process:

$$\frac{dC}{dt} = -k[C]$$

In turn, k is given by:

$$k = \frac{CL}{V_d} \text{ and so } CL = k \times V_d$$

Hence

$$C_t = C_0 \exp -\frac{CL}{V_d} \times t$$

As half-life will be the time at which C_t is half C_0 then:

$$\ln 0.5 = -CL/V_d \times t$$

and also

$$t_{1/2} = \frac{0.693 \times V_d}{CL} \text{ or } \frac{0.693}{k}$$

In summary, the half-life of a drug is calculated from its clearance and the apparent volume of distribution. The frequency of administration of a drug is estimated from the half-life. Interacting drugs that alter clearance from the body due to effects on metabolism and/or excretion may lead

to drug toxicity or treatment failure, particularly for drugs with a narrow therapeutic window (Figure 6.3).

Dosage regimens

Drugs are generally given by the oral route for convenience. In normal regimens the mean plasma concentration takes about 5 half-lives (Table 6.1) to reach equilibrium or plateau (the steady-state concentration, C_{ss}) where the amount of drug administered equals that eliminated.

Once this is achieved, the repeated dosing will lead to predictable peaks (C_{ss} max) and troughs (C_{ss} min) with a time-averaged C_{ss}.

In terms of designing dosage intervals for regimens, the drug's half-life is obviously important for determining the longevity. The interval is intended to maintain adequate plasma levels but limit the extremes between peaks and troughs. In terms of therapy, once-daily administration is the

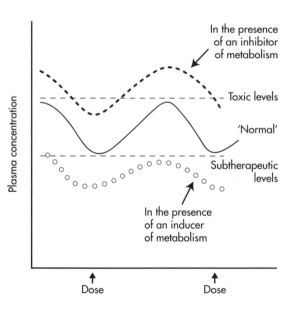

Figure 6.3 The effects of a hypothetical inhibitor and a hypothetical inducer of metabolism on a drug with a narrow therapeutic window. Under 'normal' circumstances the plasma levels are within the therapeutic window on repeat dosing. However, the inhibitor of metabolism leads to toxic concentrations and the inducer to subtherapeutic concentrations.

Table 6.1 Demonstration that steady state is reached after approximately 5 half-lives

Dose	Amount present in the body after one $t_{1/2}$ from dose	Percentage of C_{ss}
First	50%	50%
Second	50% + 25%	75%
Third	50% + 37.5%	87.5%
Fourth	50% + 43.8%	93.8%
Fifth	50% + 46.9%	96.9%

$t_{1/2}$, half-life; C_{ss}, steady-state concentration.

ideal for compliance but other regimens in use tend to be every 12 h (b.d.), 8 h (t.d.s.) or 6 h (q.d.s.). In order to achieve once-daily administration and also limit substantial fluctuations between peaks and troughs, some drugs are formulated as slow-release preparations, where their rate of absorption is reduced and so becomes rate-limiting.

In dealing with infusions or multiple-dosing regimens, the following relationships may be applied (see Hardman *et al.*, 2001).

1. Infusion rate or dose rate:

$$\text{IV infusion rate} = \text{CL} \times C_{ss}$$

Hence for oral dosing dose =

$$\frac{\text{CL} \times C_{ss} \times \tau}{F} \text{ thus } C_{ss} = \frac{F \times \text{dose}/\tau}{\text{CL}}$$

2. Peak-and-trough levels

Maximum plasma concentration

$$\text{(peak level) } (C_{ss}\max) = \frac{F \times \text{dose}}{V_d(1 - e^{-k\tau})}$$

Minimum plasma concentration

$$\text{(trough level) } (C_{ss}\min) = \frac{F \times \text{dose} \times e^{-k\tau}}{V_d(1 - e^{-k\tau})}$$

where F = bioavailability; V_d = volume of distribution; CL = clearance; C_{ss} = steady-state concentration; C_{max} = maximum concentration; t = time; k = rate constant; and τ = dose interval.

Loading doses

In order to produce rapid therapeutic effects, a loading dose (or priming infusion) may be used

to take the plasma concentration up to approximately the steady state (C_{ss}). As it takes approximately 5 half-lives to reach C_{ss} then for drugs with long half-lives, it may take many days or weeks to reach steady state. Therefore, a drug with a long half-life may require a loading dose to reach an efficacious plasma concentration more quickly. For example, loading doses are required when prescribing digoxin ($t_{1/2}$ = 40 h) or amiodarone ($t_{1/2}$ of several weeks) for the treatment of cardiac arrhythmias. Loading doses are also required when an immediate effect is required, for example in using lidocaine (lignocaine: $t_{1/2}$ = 1 h) to treat ventricular arrhythmias.

Determination of the loading dose is simple: all one has to do is calculate the dose required to give the desired concentration in the appropriate volume of distribution:

$$\text{Loading dose} = \frac{\text{required plasma concentration} \times V_d}{F}$$

$$\text{Loading dose} = \frac{C \times V_d}{F}$$

As the loading dose is intended to distribute the drug in the body, then impaired elimination does not influence the dose required.

Maintenance dose

Once C_{ss} is reached or a loading dose is used, then a maintenance dose must be chosen. The maintenance dose must simply equal the elimination and this is the mathematical product of clearance and concentration at steady state, or, put another way:

$$\text{Dose} = \frac{\text{CL} \times C_{ss}}{F}$$

As the maintenance dose is dependent on the rate of elimination, then alterations in elimination through interactions, age and renal or hepatic impairment mean that regimens may need to be altered in terms of either dose or dosage interval.

Saturation kinetics

Saturation or zero-order kinetics describes the kinetics of drugs such as phenytoin and ethanol with metabolic pathways that become saturated as the dose increases, even at therapeutic doses. Metabolism of these drugs consists of two phases: an initial rapid phase followed by saturation with a maximal rate and is no longer proportional to concentration. This results in an unpredictable relationship between the dose and plasma concentration. That is, a small increase in dose may result in a disproportional increase in plasma levels. A practical example of this occurs with ethanol, as after about 2–4 units of ethanol the metabolic enzymes become saturated and the disproportional rise in ethanol concentrations leads to intoxication.

TDM of these drugs uses an application of the Michaelis–Menten enzyme model and parameters such as V_{max} and $K_{M,}$ the maximum rate of metabolism and the concentration giving the half-maximal rate respectively. The V_{max} is ideally calculated using individual patient data since this is most likely to change.

Drugs requiring TDM

Many factors may affect the blood plasma level of a drug by altering the absorption, distribution or metabolism and excretion of drugs and should therefore be considered. These include lean body weight, age, sex, race, hepatic and renal function, concurrent disease states such as thyroid disease or chronic heart failure. Interacting drugs may also alter the dosing requirement due to altered elimination.

The following sections will consider the pharmacokinetics and requirements for TDM of commonly used drugs with a narrow therapeutic index. Clinical monitoring for signs of toxicity or undertreatment may be sufficient in some cases, such as digoxin. However, drugs such as lithium require regular monitoring to ensure concentrations are appropriate for the drug to remain efficacious, whilst avoiding potentially fatal toxicity. Another reason to carry out TDM for a drug is where the desired response is not easy to quantify, for example with antiepileptic drugs where seizures may be infrequent but it is important to know that the drugs used are within the therapeutic range.

Therapeutic drug monitoring

The dose change required to produce a desired level in blood plasma may be readily predicted when drugs exhibit first-order kinetics. That is, a change in dose gives a proportional change in blood level. Despite the clearcut mathematical basis for pharmacokinetics, drug treatments are complicated by other factors, including changes in renal function, hepatic function, age-related changes, concurrent disease and medication. These may lead to alterations in drug levels compared to those expected on a theoretical basis.

Digoxin (Chapter 14)

The appropriateness of digoxin dosing is generally monitored according to clinical response, with the patient maintaining a heart rate of 60 beats/min or greater. Digoxin levels are not monitored routinely during maintenance treatment, unless toxicity or subtherapeutic levels are suspected, although the manufacturers recommend that levels are monitored regularly for elderly patients. Potassium levels should be monitored regularly in patients at risk of hypokalaemia, such as those prescribed diuretics. This is due to the increased sensitivity of the heart to the effects of digoxin in hypokalaemia.

It is useful to consider the pharmacokinetics of digoxin, particularly when predicting doses for patients with impaired renal function, as elimination is principally by the renal route. In patients with chronic heart failure (CHF) the effect of reduced hepatic metabolism is also important to the clearance of digoxin. Additional factors to be considered include drug interactions and thyroid disease.

Theophylline (Chapter 20)

Theophylline has a relatively narrow therapeutic index and consequently toxic side-effects frequently occur with small changes in plasma concentrations. These range from nausea and vomiting, palpitations and arrhythmias to convulsions when plasma concentrations exceed 30 mg/L. Patients should be advised to report nausea and vomiting as an indicator of toxicity. Theophylline is principally metabolised via hepatic cytochrome P450-dependent enzymes. The half-life for theophylline is decreased in smokers, and by the presence of enzyme-inducing drugs (e.g. alcohol, phenytoin, carbamazepine; Chapter 5) but increased in hepatic impairment (including CHF with hepatomegaly) and by enzyme inhibitors (e.g. cimetidine, erythromycin, oral contraceptives). Accordingly, the dose should be increased for smokers and decreased for patients with CHF, liver impairment or severe chronic obstructive pulmonary disease.

Lithium (Chapter 23)

Outside its narrow therapeutic window, lithium is nephrotoxic and may result in convulsions and ultimately coma. Regular monitoring of lithium levels and adherence to a diet with minimum changes in water and salt intake are therefore important. Increased monitoring may be required during periods of dehydration such as in extreme heat, excessive sweating or diarrhoea and vomiting.

Lithium concentrations will also be influenced by renal function, drug interactions and sodium levels.

Carbamazepine (Chapters 22 and 27)

Carbamazepine induces its own metabolism (autoinduction) and this leads to an increase

in clearance and therefore shorter half-life as therapy continues, hence the dose is built up. The dose of carbamazepine may require adjustment when drugs such as phenytoin, which induce hepatic cytochrome P450 enzymes, or enzyme inhibitors such as diltiazem, verapamil, cimetidine, some selective serotonin reuptake inhibitors or erythromycin are initiated or stopped (Chapter 22).

Summary of TDM (Table 6.2)

TDM may then be used to alter dosage regimens, such that:

$$\text{New maintenance dose} = \frac{\text{Target } C_{ss}}{\text{Measured } C_{ss}} \times \text{current dose}$$

Practice points

- Renal function, hepatic function, concurrent disease, age, sex and interacting drugs are all factors to be considered when applying pharmacokinetic models.
- When calculating blood levels of drugs, the following are considered before adjusting the drug dose: drug interactions, time of sampling, compliance, age, body weight, concurrent disease, renal and hepatic function, malabsorption and assay accuracy.
- Advise patients who are prescribed drugs such as lithium, digoxin or theophylline with a narrow therapeutic index to report signs of toxicity.
- Careful consideration of the time of the previous dose compared with the time to reach steady state will ensure accurate interpretation of blood plasma levels.
- The same brand of theophylline and lithium preparations should always be used due to changes in bioavailability between preparations.

Table 6.2 Summary of information on drugs requiring therapeutic drug monitoring (TDM)

Drugs requiring TDM	Optimum plasma concentration	Signs of toxicity	Comments
Digoxin	0.5–2.0 µg/L (0.64–2.56 nmol/L) Increased signs of toxicity > 2.56 nmol/L Toxic >3.84 nmol/L	Diarrhoea, vomiting, abdominal pain, visual disturbances, drowsiness, confusion, arrhythmias	• Regular monitoring not always necessary (see text) • Sampling ≥ 6 h postdose to allow for distribution to occur • Toxicity is potentiated by hypokalaemia and will occur at lower concentrations
Lithium prophylaxis	Acute mania (0.6–1.0 mmol/L) Prophylaxis (0.4–0.8 mmol/L) Elderly patients (0.4–0.7 mmol/L) Toxicity in the elderly occurs at levels > 1 mmol/L	• Blurred vision, polyuria, polydipsia, anorexia, nausea, vomiting, diarrhoea, abdominal pain, muscle weakness, lethargy, drowsiness, tremor, confusion, ataxia, renal impairment (> 1.5 mmol/L) • Serious toxicity occurs at levels of >2–3 mmol/L, resulting in disorientation, convulsions, coma and possibly death	• Blood sampling 12 h after evening dose and 4–7 days after initiation of treatment, following dose adjustment or switching between products • Monitor every 3 months once stabilised
Phenytoin	10–20 mg/L (40–80 µmol/L)	Nystagmus, blurred vision, ataxia, drowsiness, (>30 mg/L) Dysarthria, lethargy and coma (>40 mg/L)	• Sample 1–2 weeks after a dosage change • Marked patient variability for toxic levels. For example, the absence of toxicity has been reported at levels >50 mg/L
Carbamazepine	4–12 mg/L (16–50 µmol/L)	Nystagmus, diplopia, drowsiness, ataxia (>9–12 mg/L)	• Blood sample 2–4 weeks after initiation of therapy or 3–4 days after dose change • Trough level is measured due to variable absorption

Continued

Table 6.2 *Continued*

Drugs requiring TDM	Optimum plasma concentration	Signs of toxicity	Comments
Theophylline	10–20 mg/L (55–110 (μmol/L)	Nausea, vomiting, cardiac arrhythmias, seizures (>30 mg/L).	• Bioavailability differs between brands and they should not be changed • Fast metabolisers, e.g. smokers and children, are more suited to products with a slower rate of absorption (Theo-Dur or Uniphyllin) or three times per day dosing with others (Phyllocontin)

Example of drugs requiring TDM with recommended values from individual summary of product characteristics, the *British National Formulary*, or from the *Oxford Textbook of Clinical Pharmacology and Drug Therapy* by Graham-Smith and Aronson (2002), but local laboratory values should be checked.

References

Grahame-Smith D G, Aronson J K (2002). *Oxford Textbook of Clinical Pharmacology and Drug Therapy*, 3rd edn. Oxford: Oxford University Press.

Hardman J G, Limbird L E, Goodman Gilman A (eds) (2001). *Goodman and Gilman's: The Pharmacological Basis of Therapeutics*. New York: McGraw-Hill.

Mehta D K (ed.) *British National Formulary*, latest edition. London: British Medical Association and Royal Pharmaceutical Society of Great Britain.

Further reading

Barber N, Willson A (1999). *Clinical Pharmacy Survival Guide*. Edinburgh: Churchill Livingstone.

Birkett D J (1998). *Pharmacokinetics Made Easy*. Sydney: McGraw-Hill.

Part C

Gastrointestinal diseases

7

Dyspepsia and peptic ulcer disease

Dyspepsia describes upper gastrointestinal symptoms including heartburn, acidity, nausea, discomfort and wind, and may be referred to as 'indigestion' by the patient.

Disease characteristics

The major problem is one of acidity, in the form of increased acid secretion, reflux of corrosive gastric contents or gastric damage. Clinically, upper gastrointestinal problems encompass simple to serious diseases:

- gastro-oesophageal reflux disease (GORD) is reflux of gastric contents into the oesophagus, which leads to erosion (reflux oesophagitis). Contact oesophagitis also occurs and is induced by contact with certain drugs (Chapter 5)
- gastritis – inflammation of the stomach
- peptic ulceration – gastric and duodenal
- drug-induced peptic damage (largely non-steroidal anti-inflammatory drugs (NSAIDs) and oral steroids)
- Zollinger–Ellison syndrome – a rare gastrin-secreting tumour of D-cells of the pancreas

A patient presenting with symptoms of dyspepsia ('indigestion'), which may include upper abdominal or epigastric pain, requires differential diagnosis from cardiac problems (see Chapter 1). In the context of primary care, there may be alerting clinical features which may suggest more serious underlying pathology, such as carcinoma, which must be excluded and these include:

- aged over 45 years (some authorities say over 55 years)
- weight loss
- anaemia
- dysphagia (difficulty in swallowing)
- haematemesis (vomiting blood)
- melaena (tarry stools)
- upper abdominal masses
- persistent symptoms with repeat requests for over-the-counter (OTC) remedies
- onset of new symptoms

Gastro-oesophageal reflux disease

As the name implies, this is due to the reflux of gastric contents into the oesophagus, causing erosion, which leads to pain, experienced as 'heartburn', although sometimes there may be back or shoulder pain. There may occasionally be wheezing and a cough or an exacerbation of asthma. This condition must be distinguished from oesophageal carcinoma, although dysphagia is also a leading feature. GORD may be caused or exacerbated by an increase in abdominal pressure (due to overeating, obesity or pregnancy) or due to incompetence of the gastro-oesophageal sphincter caused by hiatus hernia or drugs (for example, nitrates, antimuscarinic agents, theophylline, opioids and calcium channel blockers). Reflux oesophagitis may lead to Barrett's oesophagus, a premalignant condition.

Contact oesophagitis

This is caused by local damage due to drugs (see Chapter 5).

Peptic ulceration

Peptic ulceration includes both gastric and duodenal ulceration and is characterised by erosion of the inner lining, which may perforate as a serious complication or erode a major blood vessel, causing haematemesis (vomiting of blood). The leading clinical features of peptic ulceration include:

- epigastric pain, which may be precisely located by the patient by pointing
- hunger pain, which is relieved by eating
- night pain, which is relieved by food, milk or antacids
- waterbrash, which is the appearance of saliva in the mouth
- nausea and, less frequently, vomiting

It may also present as anaemia (Chapter 16) due to chronic blood loss or as melaena (tarry stools) due to bleeding.

It is now well established that infection with the Gram-negative bacterium *Helicobacter pylori* is the cause of up to 95% of cases in duodenal ulceration, and 70–80% of gastric ulceration. The infection leads to chronic inflammation and gastric damage leading to ulceration. There is no evidence that emotional stress or eating spicy foods leads to peptic ulceration.

The other leading cause of ulceration is the use of NSAIDs and, to a much lesser extent, oral steroids, generally with concomitant NSAID therapy. The explanation for the ulcerogenic effect of NSAIDs is that prostanoids synthesised in the stomach are cytoprotective by inhibiting acid release and stimulating the production and release of protective mucus and bicarbonate (Figure 7.1 and Table 7.1). These cytoprotective prostanoids are produced by the constitutive cyclooxygenase (COX-1), which is inhibited by NSAIDs and thus alters the balance in favour of

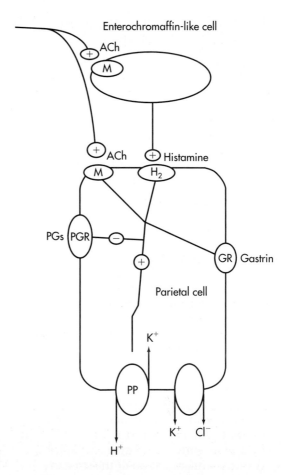

Figure 7.1 A schematic diagram of the parietal cell and the regulation of acid release. M indicates the muscarinic receptor; H$_2$ the histamine H$_2$-receptor; PGs are prostanoids; PGR is a prostanoid receptor; GR is the gastrin receptor; PP the proton pump; + indicates stimulation and − inhibition. This figure is based on diagrams in Rang *et al.* (1999) and Hardman *et al.* (2001).

increased acid activity, predisposing towards gastric damage. This important adverse drug reaction has led to the development of selective COX-2 inhibitors ('coxibs': celecoxib and rofecoxib; etodolac and meloxicam), which inhibit COX-2, associated with inflammation, but leave COX-1 largely unaffected. Despite this, coxibs still appear to cause some gastric damage and their early promise may not be fully realised.

Goals of treatment

Depending on the conditions, the general goals are symptomatic relief or cure. Symptomatic relief may involve lifestyle changes, avoidance of causative drugs, suppression of acid release or activity and mucosal protection. Cure may involve suppression of acid release to allow natural healing and, if appropriate, eradication of *H. pylori* infection. This latter goal is also aimed at reducing the possibility of developing gastric carcinomas, as *H. pylori* is regarded as a carcinogen.

Pharmacological basis of management

Control of acid secretion

In order to understand the mechanisms of drug action, the control of acid secretion must be considered. Figure 7.1 and Table 7.1 show that the release of protons via the proton pump is regulated physiologically.

Antacids

As the name implies, antacids are antiacid. A variety of preparations are available and raise pH:
    Sodium bicarbonate:

$$HCO_3^- + H^+ \rightarrow CO_2 + H_2O$$

with the 'belching' of CO_2, which makes it less suitable in patients who have flatulence.

Magnesium hydroxide ($Mg(OH)_2$) and aluminium hydroxide ($Al(OH)_3$) are also used:

$$Al(OH)_3 + 3HCl \rightarrow AlCl_3 + 3H_2O$$

$$Mg(OH)_2 + 2HCl \rightarrow MgCl_2 + 2H_2O$$

To complicate matters, aluminium compounds are constipating and magnesium salts are laxative, and so they are often used in combination to negate these effects. The use of calcium salts (including ingestion of milk) may in fact stimulate gastrin release and so increase acid secretion, leading to an exacerbation of ulceration.

Antacids provide rapid relief of dyspepsia, removing the symptoms, but they do not lead to a cure. Liquid preparations have a faster onset of action.

Alginates

These are mucopolysaccharides and may be combined with antacids (e.g. Gaviscon). The alginic acid, when combined with saliva, forms a viscous foam which floats on the gastric contents, forming a raft that protects the oesophagus during reflux.

Table 7.1 Regulation of gastric acid production

Increase acid release	Reduce acid release
Histamine via H_2-receptors	Prostaglandins E_2 and I_2 (which are also cytoprotective via mucus and bicarbonate release). Their production is inhibited by NSAIDs
Gastrin Acetylcholine via M_3-receptors and histamine release	

NSAIDs, non-steroidal anti-inflammatory drugs.

H$_2$-receptor antagonists

e.g. Cimetidine, famotidine, ranitidine

These are competitive antagonists at the histamine H$_2$-receptor and inhibit histamine-induced gastric acid secretion. Accordingly, they provide symptomatic relief and in the long-term promote ulcer healing, but if *H. pylori* infection has not been eliminated, then relapse on discontinuation is common. They are most active against basal, as opposed to stimulus-evoked, acid release and are most effective given at night. Ranitidine and famotidine have fewer interactions than cimetidine. Low doses are available OTC for short-term relief of dyspepsia (less than 2 weeks) and higher doses are prescription-only medicine (POM).

Proton pump inhibitors (PPIs)

Lansoprazole, omeprazole (esomeprazole as its S-isomer), pantoprazole, rabeprazole

These are a relatively new class of drugs which are widely used and act via irreversible inhibition of the proton pump (H$^+$/K$^+$-ATPase) and hence suppress proton secretion. This leads to a greater than 90% inhibition of acid secretion which is long-lasting (24 h). The PPIs are converted to active drugs at acid pH, which means that their actions are largely confined to the gastric mucosa, leading to selectivity.

Prostaglandin analogues

Misoprostol

This a stable prostaglandin analogue E$_1$, which inhibits the release of acid and is also cytoprotective by stimulating the release of mucus and bicarbonate.

Bismuth chelate

Bismuth chelate kills *H. pylori*, coats the ulcer, absorbs pepsin, increases prostaglandin production and increases bicarbonate secretion, thereby bringing about ulcer healing.

Prokinetic drugs

Domperidone, metoclopramide

These agents facilitate the movement of gastric contents from the stomach to the duodenum.

Domperidone closes the gastro-oesophageal sphincter and promotes gastric emptying, and this is of benefit in reflux oesophagitis. Metoclopramide acts locally to increase gastric motility and promote emptying. Both agents will provide symptomatic relief of 'bloating'. The prokinetic agent cisapride was withdrawn due to problems associated with cardiac QT prolongation.

Choice of drugs

This is related to the disease and goals of treatment, as occasional heartburn may be effectively relieved by simple antacids or low-dose H$_2$-receptor antagonists, with the antacids having immediate effects. In more serious disease, the first issue is to establish the nature of the complaint as the diagnosis will determine the most appropriate treatment. In the meantime symptomatic relief with antacids, alginates or H$_2$-receptor antagonists is appropriate. Diagnosis may involve breath (^{13}C-urea) tests, serological tests for antibodies for *H. pylori* (these may give false-positive results as they indicate past and not necessarily current infection) or stool antigen testing for *H. pylori* infection and possibly gastroscopy and barium contrast radiology.

The urea breath test involves administering a tablet containing isotope (^{13}C)-labelled urea, as *H. pylori* possesses urease activity which leads to the production of labelled ^{13}CO$_2$ in the presence of infection. The ^{13}CO$_2$ readily and rapidly passes across the stomach wall and is absorbed into the blood stream and appears in the breath, where it may be detected by mass spectroscopy indicating infection. Prior to the breath test or gastroscopy, H$_2$-receptor antagonists, PPIs and antibiotics should be withheld for periods defined by local guidelines to prevent the symptoms being masked.

Gastro-oesophageal reflux disease

The initial approach is lifestyle changes such as reducing overeating, weight reduction if appropriate, reducing the intake of fatty foods and chocolate (which may lubricate the gastro-oesophageal sphincter), smoking cessation, reducing alcohol intake and avoiding tight clothes. If lifestyle changes are inadequate, antacids and then antacids plus alginates will provide rapid relief but limited healing. H_2-receptor antagonists may be used to provide relief in mild to moderate disease but are much less effective than PPIs. If symptoms persist then PPIs are the most effective agents; they remove symptoms and allow healing. They may initially be used for 4–8 weeks, after which a lower maintenance dose should be tried. Prokinetic drugs may also be used, especially when the symptoms include post-prandial bloating, nausea and belching.

Non-*H. pylori* dyspepsia

In the absence of proven *H. pylori* infection, the logical approach to dyspepsia, due to gastritis or ulceration, is a stepped approach, stepping up or down as appropriate:

Step 1: antacid or alginate and antacid
Step 2: H_2-receptor antagonist
Step 3: PPI

At the time of writing, PPIs are the most effective agents and current National Institute of Clinical Excellence (NICE) guidelines (2000) indicate that the cheapest PPI should be used and, once healing has been achieved, the treatment should be stepped down or the lowest possible dose of PPI used.

H. pylori infection

In patients who are infected with *H. pylori* and in patients with duodenal ulceration who are assumed to be infected, eradication is the logical course. This may be achieved by a number of different regimens which involve antibiotics and antisecretory agents ('triple therapy'), and these are associated with 90% eradication rates. Typically, triple therapy involves a PPI (or sometimes ranitidine or ranitidine bismuth citrate) plus two antibacterial agents from clarithromycin, metronidazole and amoxicillin for 1 week. There is significant resistance to metronidazole: patients who have recently received this for other conditions may be harbouring resistant organisms and so this agent should be avoided. Eradication is confirmed by a urea breath test; serology is inappropriate as antibodies to *H. pylori* may persist in the plasma. Following eradication, PPIs may be required for 4–8 weeks after triple therapy to promote further healing, especially if the ulcer was associated with bleeding or NSAID usage.

NSAID-induced ulceration

After *H. pylori* infection, NSAID use is the next commonest cause of ulceration. Gastric damage due to NSAIDs is highest in older patients and is more associated with certain NSAIDs, such as azapropazone, aspirin, naproxen and piroxicam, while ibuprofen, etodolac and nabumentone appear to cause fewer gastric side-effects. It should be recognised that low-dose aspirin (75 mg) for antiplatelet therapy is also associated with a significant incidence of gastric side-effects.

For NSAID-induced damage the initial approach is to stop the NSAID if this is possible and switch to paracetamol for pain relief if this is required. Healing may be brought about by using either an H_2-receptor antagonist, as a cheap first-choice drug, or a PPI.

If the patient must continue with the NSAID or is initially identified as being at a high risk (over 65 years, previous ulcer, concomitant oral steroids, concomitant anticoagulants) then prophylaxis is required, for which omeprazole, lansoprazole and misoprostol are currently licensed. According to Yeomans *et al.* (1998), ranitidine is less effective than omeprazole at preventing and healing NSAID-induced ulceration. Furthermore, cimetidine has been shown to be ineffective at preventing NSAID-induced ulceration (Roth *et al.*, 1987). Misoprostol carries the compliance problem of being required 2–4 times daily and often causes diarrhoea but is available in combination with either naproxen or diclofenac.

The use of selective COX-2 inhibitors (coxibs, etodolac and meloxicam) is controversial. Guidance from NICE (2001) recommends that they are not routinely used in osteoarthritis and rheumatoid arthritis but are reserved for patients at risk of gastrointestinal damage. These patients were identified as those over 65 years of age, those taking additional drugs which may cause gastrointestinal damage or bleeding (e.g. warfarin, selective serotonin reuptake inhibitors), and patients requiring maximum, long-term doses of

NSAIDs. In patients with a history of ulceration or gastrointestinal bleeding it was recommended that selective COX-2 inhibitors should be used, if at all, with great care.

Other considerations

Other considerations concerning drug choice are detailed in Table 7.2.

Significant drug interactions

Cimetidine inhibits cytochrome P450 and therefore the metabolism of other drugs, resulting in important drug interactions. Similarly, omeprazole and lansoprazole also inhibit some isoforms of hepatic cytochrome P450. Additionally, by altering gastric pH, many drugs used in dyspepsia may alter the absorption of other drugs and their

Table 7.2 Considerations of drug choice for dyspepsia in concurrent conditions

Condition	Implications for treatment
Heart failure	Patients should avoid antacids with a high sodium content, especially if they are also receiving diuretics
Prophylaxis of myocardial infarction and stroke with antiplatelet drugs	Low-dose aspirin is associated with gastric bleeding. Clopidogrel is an antiplatelet drug which is used as an alternative to low-dose aspirin. Although it is used when aspirin is contraindicated, there is evidence that by inhibiting platelet aggregation it may also cause gastric bleeding and should not necessarily be regarded as a safe alternative to aspirin in this respect. Indeed, low-dose aspirin with a PPI for prophylaxis would be preferred
Women of child-bearing age	This is a contraindication for misoprostol, a prostaglandin agonist which may cause uterine contractions and subsequent abortion. If misoprostol must be used then effective contraceptive measures should be taken.
Pregnancy	This is associated with an increase in GORD due to increases in intra-abdominal pressure. Alginates are the first-line drugs with efficacy and are safe. If alginates fail, then ranitidine or cimetidine is indicated if essential
Breast-feeding	Antacids, ranitidine or nizatidine are preferred. The BNF should be consulted: some of the other agents are not recommended by their manufacturers until their safety is established
Renal impairment	Patients should avoid antacids with a high sodium content
Liver disease	Most agents require dose reductions; the BNF should be consulted. Ranitidine is often used for gastroprotection
Parkinson's disease	Avoid metoclopramide and domperidone due to extrapyramidal effects (although domperidone is recommended for levodopa-induced nausea). Metoclopramide may antagonise levodopa.
Depression	SSRIs may impair blood clotting, leading to excess bleeding. Accordingly, they should be used with care in patients with gastric damage or with drugs which also impair clotting

PPI, proton pump inhibitor; GORD, gastro-oesophageal reflux disease; BNF, *British National Formulary*; SSRIs, selective serotonin reuptake inhibitors.

administration should be separated. Examples of some important interactions of drugs used in dyspepsia and the management of peptic ulceration are detailed in Table 7.3.

Over-the-counter considerations

OTC antacids and low doses of H_2-receptor antagonists have an important role in the symptomatic

Table 7.3 Examples of some important interactions of drugs used for upper gastrointestinal disease

Interacting drugs	Consequences	Comments
Cimetidine with warfarin, phenytoin, theophylline, carbamazepine, tricyclic antidepressants, diltiazem and nifedipine. Antiarrhythmics (including amiodarone, flecainide, lidocaine (lignocaine), and quinidine) and erythromycin	Cimetidine has been shown to increase the plasma concentration of a number of different drugs, leading to clinically significant interactions	• Monitoring the effects is appropriate and dose reductions may be required for the drug affected • With carbamazepine there are transient increases in the first few days • Generally speaking, these interactions are confined to cimetidine. Other H_2-receptor antagonists do not interact in this way, and so they should be regarded as safe alternatives
Cimetidine or ranitidine with ketoconazole and itraconazole	Reduced absorption of the imidazoles	• Separate dosing by 2–3 h • Fluconazole appears unaffected
Antacids with ACE inhibitors, chlorpromazine, ciprofloxacin, digoxin, ketoconazole, itraconazole, H_2-receptor antagonists, iron, rifampicin and tetracyclines	Antacids may reduce the absorption of these drugs	Their administration should be separated by 1–3 h and in the case of ciprofloxacin by 2–6 h
Sodium-containing antacids with lithium	Sodium may decrease lithium levels	Magnesium or aluminium salts would be appropriate
Omeprazole with benzodiazepines, ciclosporin, digoxin, phenytoin and warfarin	Evidence points to omeprazole having, on occasion, increased the concentration of these drugs	• Omeprazole may inhibit isoforms of cytochrome P450 • Monitoring is appropriate, especially when starting or finishing treatment
Omeprazole with macrolides	Clarithromycin increases the plasma concentration of omeprazole, which may be beneficial. Erythromycin may reduce the effects of omeprazole	
Lansoprazole with amoxicillin; clarithromycin with metronidazole	Glossitis, stomatitis and black tongue coloration have been reported	Monitoring is appropriate
Metronidazole with alcohol	Disulfiram reaction	Alcohol should be avoided with metronidazole

ACE, angiotensin-converting enzyme.

relief of dyspepsia but their use is limited to 2 weeks, after which time referral should be made if symptoms persist.

Counselling

In patients with dyspepsia general counselling should be directed at lifestyle advice. Altering the diet to avoid large meals, fatty foods, hot spicy food, reducing alcohol consumption and smoking cessation should reduce provoking factors. Patients with GORD may (or may not) benefit from raising the head of the bed. Patients taking NSAIDs and other drugs such as doxy-cycline, tetracycline and bisphosphonates, which may cause contact oesophagitis, should be advised to take their medicine while standing or sitting with a glass of water; NSAIDs may be best taken after food but the effectiveness of this is debatable.

Patients taking NSAIDs should be instructed to tell their general practitioner (GP) and pharma-cist that they are taking these agents, even if purchased OTC. Of course they should be avoided if possible in patients with dyspepsia or with a risk of peptic ulceration.

Patients should be advised to report alerting symptoms such as:

- unexplained weight loss
- vomiting blood (with a ground-coffee appearance)
- melaena – black tarry stools which contain blood
- dysphagia (difficulty in swallowing)

Antacids

- These will cause immediate relief but normal doses are unlikely to lead to ulcer healing.
- These are most effective when taken 1 h after food. If they are taken earlier they may be emptied from the stomach.
- Magnesium salts alone may cause diarrhoea.
- Aluminium salts alone may cause constipation.
- Calcium salts will actually stimulate acid release.
- Their administration should be separated in time from a range of other drugs.

Alginates

- These should be taken after food and when retiring to bed.

H$_2$-receptor antagonists

- When used OTC for occasional dyspepsia, H$_2$-receptor antagonists should not be used for more than 2 weeks without consulting the GP.
- They should be taken regularly for prevention and not just for symptomatic relief.
- For ulceration, they are most effective when taken at night; a daily dose taken at night is effective at ulcer healing.
- Their actions may be suppressed by food, which stimulates acid secretion.
- Cimetidine may inhibit the metabolism of warfarin, phenytoin and theophylline and it may increase their plasma concentrations.
- Cimetidine may occasionally cause impotence and gynaecomastia in males due to antiandro-genic actions.

Proton pump inhibitors

- PPIs should be taken regularly for prevention and not just for symptomatic relief.
- They may cause diarrhoea (sometimes secondary to *Campylobacter* infection).

Misoprostol

- Diarrhoea is a common side-effect.
- Misoprostol should not be taken by women of child-bearing age who may be pregnant or become pregnant.

Bismuth chelate

- This may blacken stools and tongue.
- Bismuth chelate should be taken on an empty stomach, avoiding milk and antacids as they prevent the drug coating the ulcer.

Triple therapy for *H. pylori* eradication

- Eradication of the bacteria causing an ulcer is the most effective treatment to prevent a relapse.

- The course should be completed for eradication.
- The course is associated with a high incidence of side-effects, including diarrhoea.

- Is the patient allergic to any antibiotics?
- Avoid alcohol with metronidazole, as there is a risk of a disulfiram-type reaction.

Practice points

- Frequent requests for OTC remedies for dyspepsia should prompt referral.
- Peptic ulceration is largely due to *H. pylori* infection (which should be eradicated).
- NSAID-induced peptic damage is a very important adverse drug reaction. Patients should be asked about their use of OTC NSAIDs and it should be recognised that low-dose aspirin may cause ulceration.
- COX-2 inhibitors may cause gastric damage and should not be used in active ulceration.
- Drugs which alter gastric pH may alter the absorption of other drugs. Cimetidine inhibits hepatic cytochrome P450, with a range of important interactions.
- If PPIs are used, the cheapest agent should be chosen.

 CASE STUDIES

Case 1
A 64-year-old woman who has recently been prescribed rofecoxib (12.5 mg/day) for osteoarthritis complains to her community pharmacist that she has recently developed stomach pains.

1. Explain the likely cause of her new complaint.

- COX-2 inhibitors may cause gastric bleeding. Despite being COX-2-selective, they may inhibit COX-1, which is responsible for the production of cytoprotective prostaglandins in the stomach, altering the balance in favour of gastric damage.

2. How would you respond?

- The patient should discuss the dyspepsia with her GP.

3. What steps may be taken to overcome this new problem?

- Withdrawal of the coxib seems logical, and paracetamol may be used as a substitute. Acid suppression may be required for healing. Alternatively, if the coxib is essential, then a PPI or misoprostol could be added for prophylaxis.

Case 2
A 25-year-old man has developed 'indigestion' and his GP has prescribed cimetidine (400 mg b.d.). He does not smoke, rarely uses NSAIDs and consumes fewer than 21 units of alcohol per week. The GP decides to carry out a ^{13}C-urea breath test before starting the cimetidine.

continued

◗ **CASE STUDIES** (continued)

1. What is the purpose of this test?

• To test for urease in the stomach, which indicates the presence of *H. pylori*.

The ^{13}C-urea breath test proves positive.

2. What is the likely cause of the patient's gastric symptoms?

• Peptic ulceration due to *H. pylori*.

Several weeks later the patient visits his GP for the results of the test and receives the following prescription:

Lansoprazole 30 mg b.d.
Clarithromycin 500 mg b.d.
Metronidazole 400 mg b.d.
For 7 days

3. What is the purpose of this new prescription?

• acid suppression to relieve symptoms and allow healing
• eradication of *H. pylori*.

How should you counsel the patient?

• lifestyle advice regarding food and avoidance of NSAIDs
• to complete the course
• the tablets should be taken together in the morning and evening to aid compliance
• to avoid alcohol, as there is an interaction with metronidazole
• to take the metronidazole with food and plenty of water

As the patient leaves the pharmacy, he asks you whether he should continue to take the cimetidine as well.

5. What advice should you give him?

• He should not take cimetidine as he already has acid suppression. In addition, cimetidine interacts with metronidazole and clarithromycin, increasing their plasma concentrations, but this interaction is probably not significant.

References

Hardman J G, Limbird L E, Goodman Gilman A (eds) (2001). *Goodman & Gilman's The Pharmacological Basis of Therapeutics*. New York: McGraw-Hill.

Mehta D K (ed.) *British National Formulary*, latest edition. London: British Medical Association and Royal Pharmaceutical Society of Great Britain.

NICE Technology appraisal no. 7 (2000). Guidance on the use of proton pump inhibitors (PPIs) in the treatment of dyspepsia. London: NICE (via www.nice.org.uk).

NICE Technology appraisal no. 27 (2001). Guidance on the use of use of cyclo-oxygenase (COX) II selective inhibitors, celecoxib, rofecoxib, meloxicam and etodolac for osteoarthritis and rheumatoid arthritis. London: NICE (via www.nice.org.uk).

Rang H P, Dale M, Ritter J M (1999). *Pharmacology*, 4th edn. Edinburgh: Churchill Livingstone.

Roth S H, Bennett R E, Mitchell C S *et al.* (1987). Cimetidine therapy in nonsteroid antiinflammatory drug gastropathy. Double-blind long-term evaluation. *Arch Intern Med* 147: 1798–1801.

Yeomans N D, Tulassay Z, Juhasz L *et al.* (1998). A comparison of omeprazole with ranitidine for ulcers associated with nonsteroidal antiinflammatory drugs. *N Engl J Med* 338: 719–726.

8

Nausea and vomiting

Clinical characteristics

Nausea (the desire to vomit) and vomiting are common occurrences and may reflect simple disease, for example following exposure to bacterial toxins, they may be associated with motion as occurs in travel sickness, or may reflect more serious underlying pathology. Causes of nausea and vomiting include:

- alcohol (the most common)
- viral and bacterial gastrointestinal infections
- motion sickness
- drugs (such as anticancer drugs, digoxin, erythromycin, levodopa, opioids, selective serotonin reuptake inhibitors (SSRIs), non-steroidal anti-inflammatory drugs (NSAIDs), theophylline, iron salts)
- peptic ulceration
- renal failure with uraemia
- myocardial infarction
- pregnancy
- migraine
- vestibular disorders including Ménière's disease.
- head trauma

Given the range of causative factors, there are several mechanisms of nausea, including local irritation of the stomach involving visceral afferent fibres, the central effects of toxins on the chemoreceptor trigger zone (CTZ) and the conflict between visual and balance information, which is thought to occur in motion sickness. The vomiting pathway is under common, central control leading to a highly coordinated physiological response, involving respiratory, salivary and gastric control, resulting in the expulsion of gastric contents. As shown in Figure 8.1, vomiting is under the control of the vomiting centre, which receives a direct input from visceral afferent nerves and is also regulated by the CTZ. The CTZ is, in turn, sensitive to circulating drugs and toxins, and receives input from the vestibular nuclei, which is linked to the labyrinth of the inner ear. The centres involved in vomiting and their receptors are summarised in Table 8.1.

In the context of gastrointestinal infections, the vomit response may be appropriate for removal of the infective agents, whilst drug-induced nausea may lead to a lack of compliance and failure of treatment. Prolonged vomiting may lead to electrolyte disturbances (including hyponatraemia, hypokalaemia and alkalosis) and dehydration.

123

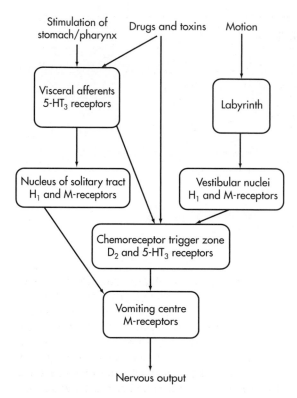

Figure 8.1   A schematic diagram of the stimulation and regulation of vomiting. This figure is based on diagrams in Rang *et al.* (1999) and Page *et al.* (2002).

Pharmacological basis of management

When vomiting is undesirable then removal of any precipitating factors is the first approach and antiemetic agents may be appropriate. Antiemetic drugs encompass a range of different drug classes, with different sites of action. The site of action determines the circumstances in which an agent is effective.

Histamine H$_1$-receptor antagonists

Cinnarizine, cyclizine, meclozine, promethazine (a phenothiazine)
These older, sedative antihistamines also have appreciable antimuscarinic activity, which contributes towards their use as antiemetics. This is shown by the fact that the 'old antihistamine',

chlorphenamine, which lacks antimuscarinic activity is not antiemetic. They act on the vestibular nuclei and are effective in motion sickness.

Antimuscarinic agents

Hyoscine (but also including other groups such as antihistamines and prochlorperazine)
Antimuscarinic agents act in both the vomiting centre and the vestibular apparatus, making them highly effective in motion sickness. They will also reduce gastrointestinal motility. However, substantial antimuscarinic side-effects limit their usefulness.

Histamine analogues

Betahistine
This is a histamine H$_1$-receptor partial agonist and H$_3$-receptor antagonist which has been suggested to increase blood flow to the inner ear and/or decrease endolymph pressure. It is used in vertigo and Ménière's disease.

Dopamine receptor antagonists

Domperidone, metoclopramide, phenothiazines such as prochlorperazine
These act in the CTZ but some may have unwanted central nervous system (CNS) effects (less so with domperidone), which may include extrapyramidal effects and drug-induced parkinsonism. Metoclopramide may also act at 5-HT$_3$-receptors when used at high doses. The prokinetic effects of domperidone and metoclopramide may increase gastric emptying, reducing any feelings of fullness and nausea. They are effective against anticancer drug-induced emesis.

5-hydroxytryptamine (5-HT) receptor antagonists

e.g. Ondansetron (also metoclopramide)
These block 5-HT, acting at 5-HT$_3$-receptors in the gut and CNS, and are particularly effective against anticancer drugs, which may cause the release of 5-HT in the gastrointestinal tract, and also in postoperative nausea and vomiting.

Table 8.1 Summary of the different stimuli, pathways and receptors in vomiting

Stimuli	Site	Receptors
Toxins, irritation, drugs and mechanical	Visceral afferent nerves in the gastrointestinal tract and pharynx	$5\text{-}HT_3$ Dopamine D_2
Toxins and drugs	Chemoreceptor trigger zone	$5\text{-}HT_3$ Dopamine D_2 Opioid
Motion	Labyrinth and vestibular nuclei	Histamine H_1 Muscarinic
Inputs from visceral afferents, vestibular apparatus, chemoreceptor trigger zone	Vomiting centre	Muscarinic Histamine H_1 $5\text{-}HT_3$

Steroids

Dexamethasone

The mechanism of antiemetic actions of steroids is unknown.

Nabilone

This is a cannabinoid receptor agonist whose effects may be mediated via opioid receptors in the CTZ.

Choice of drugs

The initial approach is to remove, if possible, any stimuli which may provoke nausea and vomiting. In the case of infection or alcohol intoxication then vomiting may be considered an appropriate response to eliminate the noxious agents. Not all antiemetics are effective for all conditions, for example $5\text{-}HT_3$ and dopamine-receptor antagonists are ineffective in motion sickness. Some logical drug choices are summarised in Table 8.2.

Other considerations

In addition to selecting the most appropriate antiemetic to suit a specific cause other considerations are as follows.

- Asthma and peptic ulceration are relative contraindications to using betahistine, which

is a histamine analogue and may worsen these conditions through the stimulation of histamine H_1- and H_2-receptors respectively.
- Antimuscarinic side-effects such as blurred vision, urinary retention and constipation of the antihistamines (and of course the antimuscarinic drugs) may be unacceptable, especially if a patient already has, for example, problems of micturition or constipation. Closed-angle glaucoma is a contraindication to using hyoscine. They should also be avoided if there is a risk of dementia in the elderly.
- Sedation may be a desired or undesired side-effect of the antihistamines and hyoscine, which would preclude driving. Of the antihistamines, cinnarizine is the least sedating.
- Extrapyramidal effects may occur with phenothiazines (including prochlorperazine), cinnarizine and metoclopramide. These agents may uncover or worsen existing Parkinson's disease. These effects are far less common with domperidone, which does not extensively penetrate the blood–brain barrier. The phenothiazines will antagonise and reduce the effects of levodopa in patients being treated for Parkinson's disease.
- Young children represent a particular group at risk from vomiting and may require referral at an early stage to prevent dehydration. Projectile vomiting in the first 2 months of life may be caused by pyloric stenosis and requires investigation. Motion sickness is common in

Table 8.2 Some drug choices in nausea and vomiting

Condition	Drug choice	Comment
Motion sickness	Antimuscarinic agents/antiemetic antihistamines	Hyoscine is the most effective but its use is limited by the antimuscarinic side-effects
Vestibular disorders	Prochlorperazine or cinnarizine for acute attacks of vertigo. Betahistine is indicated for prophylaxis of Ménière's disease	Prolonged use of cinnarizine in Ménière's disease may render it less effective. Diuretics have been used but evidence supporting their effectiveness is absent
Anticancer drugs	5-HT$_3$ receptor antagonists, domperidone, metoclopramide, nabilone and dexamethasone	The effects of 5-HT$_3$ receptor antagonists are enhanced by high doses of dexamethasone. The benzodiazepine lorazepam is also used; it may induce a degree of amnesia, reducing the anticipatory nausea associated with subsequent treatment
Use of 5-HT-related drugs such as triptans and SSRIs	5-HT$_3$ receptor antagonists	5-HT$_3$ receptor antagonists will oppose the serotonergic effects of triptans and SSRIs which are associated with transient nausea
Migraine	Metoclopramide, domperidone, prochlorperazine and buclizine	The prokinetic effects of metoclopramide and domperidone may enhance the rate of onset of concomitant analgesics. They should also be taken as early as possible in an attack before gastrointestinal motility is reduced
Radiotherapy	5-HT$_3$ receptor antagonists and dopamine receptor antagonists are used	
Postoperative nausea and vomiting (due to surgical procedures and the use of opioids)	5-HT$_3$ receptor antagonists, phenothiazines and cyclizine	
Myocardial infarction	Cyclizine, prochlorperazine or metoclopramide	Cyclizine should only be used if left ventricular function is satisfactory
Head trauma	Dexamethasone	
Renal failure with uraemia	Dopamine receptor antagonists	
Peptic ulceration	Treat the ulcer (see Chapter 7) with proton pump inhibitors or H$_2$-receptor antagonists	
Pregnancy	Antihistamine or a phenothiazine; promethazine is widely used	Vomiting in pregnancy which is potentially life-threatening requires rehydration and may need short-term drug treatment under expert supervision

Continued

Table 8.2 *Continued*

Condition	Drug choice	Comment
Levodopa-induced nausea in Parkinson's disease	Domperidone	Domperidone does not extensively penetrate the blood–brain barrier and so will not reduce the effectiveness of levodopa in Parkinson's disease

SSRIs, selective serotonin reuptake inhibitors.

children and the following over-the-counter (OTC) availabilities should be noted:

Promethazine hydrochloride 2 years and over
Meclozine 2 years and over
Hyoscine 4 years and over
Cinnarizine 5 years and over

- Promethazine hydrochloride (Phenergan) is available as a syrup and has the advantage of convenient administration to a toddler but may be misused for sedation in children.
- Timing and duration of antiemetics for motion sickness: in choosing an antihistamine for motion sickness the timings shown in Table 8.3 may be helpful.
- Severe vomiting may preclude effective oral administration and transdermal, intramuscular or rectal administration may be preferred.
- Patients receiving diuretics and who are vomiting are at particular risk of dehydration and should be advised to seek advice at an early stage, which may include withholding the diuretic, the use of oral rehydration therapy and the prescription of appropriate antiemetic drugs.

Important interactions

The interactions with antiemetics are reasonably logical. As indicated above, the dopamine receptor antagonists, except domperidone, may antagonise levodopa in Parkinson's disease. The antihistamines which are antiemetic are all sedating and so will synergise with other CNS-depressants. In addition, their antimuscarinic actions (and those of hyoscine) will be enhanced

by other drugs with pronounced muscarinic binding (e.g. tricyclic antidepressants). The combination of betahistine with antihistamines is not appropriate as the former is a histamine analogue.

Counselling

If the patient is taking other drugs for unrelated conditions, then attention should be paid to ensure that measures are taken to overcome the problems of a missed or vomited dose.

Travel sickness

- Any medication should be taken before the journey (promethazine may be taken the night before).
- Measures that may reduce travel sickness include looking out of the car window at the horizon, sitting in the front seat and not reading books. The driver may also help by driving smoothly.
- Patients taking antimotion-sickness preparations should be informed of their sedating properties and duration of action. This may be important as a patient may take an antiemetic for a sea crossing or a flight and may wish to drive on arrival at the destination.

Hyoscine

- This may cause drowsiness, dry mouth, blurred vision and constipation.
- The effects of patches may persist for up to 24 h after removal.

Table 8.3   Dosage timings for drugs used in motion sickness

Antiemetic	Time of dose before travel	Dosage interval
Promethazine hydrochloride	Night before travel and also on the morning of travel if required	6–8 h as required
Meclozine	1 h	24 h
Hyoscine	30 min	6 h
Cinnarizine	2 h	8 h

Information in this table was derived from Goodyer (2001), *Symptoms in the Pharmacy* by Blenkinsopp and Paxton (2002) and the *British National Formulary.*

- Avoid alcohol whilst taking hyoscine.
- Patients should wash their hands after handling patches.

Antihistamines

- Some antihistamines are associated with antimuscarinic side-effects.
- Patients taking sedating antihistamines or prochlorperazine should be advised that their ability to drive or operate machinery may be impaired. The sedation will be enhanced by alcohol.

Ondansetron

- Zofran melts should be placed on the tongue and allowed to disperse before swallowing.

Nabilone

- Patients should be warned of the possible adverse effects such as euphoria, hallucinations and difficulties in concentrating.

Herbal remedies

Ginger is advocated in the prevention of nausea and vomiting in a range of conditions including pregnancy, motion sickness and chemotherapy. There is evidence to support its use with effects significantly better than placebo (Ernst and Pittler, 2000; Vutyavanich *et al.*, 2001).

Over-the-counter considerations

OTC antiemetics play a major role in the management of motion sickness. The pharmacist should be mindful of potential misuse, such as using them for sedation.

Practice points

- Antiemetics should only be used when they are essential.
- Antiemetics have different sites of action. Each class is only effective against certain forms of nausea and vomiting.

References

Blenkinsopp A, Paxton P (2002). *Symptoms in the Pharmacy*, 4th edn. Oxford: Blackwell Sciences.

Ernst E, Pittler M H (2000). Efficacy of ginger for nausea and vomiting: a systematic review of randomized clinical trials. *Br J Anaesth* 84: 367–371.

Goodyer L (2001). Health problems associated with air and sea transport. *Pharm J* 267: 464–469.

Mehta D K (ed.) *British National Formulary*, latest edition. London: British Medical Association and Royal Pharmaceutical Society of Great Britain.

Page C, Curtis M, Sutter M *et al.* (2002). *Integrated Pharmacology,* 2nd edn. Edinburgh: Mosby.

Rang H P, Dale M, Ritter J M (1999). *Pharmacology*, 4th edn. Edinburgh: Churchill Livingstone.

Vutyavanich T, Kraisarin T, Ruangsri R A (2001). Ginger for nausea and vomitting in pregnancy: randomized, double-masked, placebo-controlled trial. *Obstet Gynecol* 97: 577–582.

Further reading

Veysey M, McNair A (2001). Drug treatment of nausea and vomiting. *Prescriber* 12: 41–50.

9

Lower gastrointestinal problems

Diarrhoea

Diarrhoea is characterised by the passing of soft or watery stools at an increased frequency (more than three times a day). It is a common and debilitating condition, and in extreme circumstances can be life-threatening, with some 5 million deaths worldwide due to dehydration. Prolonged diarrhoea, altered bowel habits or the passing of blood should all warrant referral (Chapter 1). Diarrhoea may be acute, for example due to infection, or chronic, for example associated with other gastrointestinal pathologies.

Causes

Acute diarrhoea is often due to bacterial or viral infections. In this regard, rotaviruses cause damage to small-bowel villi and adhesive enterotoxigenic bacteria (such as cholera, *Escherichia coli*, *Yersinia enterocolitica*) adhere to the brush border, and increase epithelial cyclic adenosine monophosphate (cAMP) levels, leading to Cl^- and Na^+ secretion, which are followed by water secretion from the lower gastrointestinal tract. Other agents such as *Shigella* release cytotoxins, causing ulceration of the mucosa. Additional pathogens which may cause diarrhoea include amoebae and *Giardia*.

Other causes of diarrhoea include the following:

- Broad-spectrum antibiotics may alter the natural gut flora, leading to superinfection. An important example of this is pseudomembranous colitis, which is a rare but serious complication of treatment with broad-spectrum antibiotics, especially clindamycin. It involves the growth of *Clostridium difficile* which may lead to colitis, with the possibility of toxic megacolon and perforation of the bowel.

- Proton pump inhibitors may suppress acid secretion sufficiently to cause achlorhydria (an absence of hydrochloric acid), which may allow infection, for example by *Campylobacter*.
- Orlistat, an antiobesity drug, inhibits pancreatic lipases to prevent the breakdown of fat and this may lead to steatorrhoea (fatty diarrhoea), which may be part of its therapeutic action by ensuring that the patient avoids fatty food.
- Misoprostol activates prostanoid receptors in the intestines, increasing cAMP, which may lead to a secretory diarrhoea.

Other drug-induced causes include non-steroidal anti-inflammatory drugs (NSAIDs), magnesium salts, withdrawal in opioid dependence, digoxin toxicity, acarbose, metformin and iron salts.

Chronic diarrhoea may be associated with:

- irritable bowel syndrome (IBS): see later
- ulcerative colitis: see later
- Crohn's disease: see later

Pharmacological basis of management

The first step in the management of acute diarrhoea where a simple cause such as an adverse drug reaction can be identified is to remove the cause, and the condition may resolve. The patient should continue normal feeding with simple foods such as boiled rice, and infants should continue with breast or formula milk feeds. The first active measure is oral rehydration therapy (ORT).

Oral rehydration therapy

The major adverse effect of diarrhoea is dehydration with electrolyte disturbances (which may increase the risk of adverse drug reactions with drugs such as diuretics and digoxin), and rehydration is an important goal. This may be achieved by ORT using an approved and specific mixture of electrolytes and glucose. ORT should be considered for all patients. Soft drinks do not substitute for ORT as they do not have the correct composition. The ORT must be made up to the correct osmolality, as a hyperosmotic mixture may promote further water loss from the gastrointestinal tract. The presence of glucose in ORT is to allow sodium to be cotransported with glucose by a specific transporter on the epithelial cells and this will be followed by water, leading to rehydration.

Antibiotics

Many simple gastrointestinal infections, especially in children, are viral and antibiotics are of no value. If a bacterial causative organism is identified by stool cultures then an appropriate antibiotic can be used. In the case of traveller's diarrhoea (associated with foreign travel and ingestion of contaminated food or water), ciprofloxacin is often effective and is sometimes provided to travellers to take at the start of an attack of diarrhoea. In the case of pseudomembranous colitis, metronidazole and vancomycin are indicated. Giardiasis and amoebic dysentery may be treated with metronidazole, *Salmonella* species with ciprofloxacin and cholera with tetracycline.

Antimotility agents

Opioids (codeine and loperamide) and antimuscarinic agents
These agents provide symptomatic relief by reducing the motility of the lower gastrointestinal tract, allowing reabsorption of fluid and reducing the passage of watery stools. The relief allows bowel control and prevents diarrhoea from interfering with daily activities. They should be used in addition to ORT. The use of antimotility agents does not alter the time course of the diarrhoea; indeed, diarrhoea may serve to eliminate the causative organisms from the body. Antimotility agents should not be used in children or in adults with severe inflammatory bowel disease where they may cause obstruction leading to megacolon.

Opioids reduce tone and peristaltic movements of gastrointestinal muscle by presynaptic inhibition of acetylcholine release from the parasympathetic nerves and this is mediated via μ-opioid receptors. Loperamide is an opioid which is widely used and its efficient enterohepatic cycling means that it is largely retained in the gastrointestinal tract, which limits its systemic action. Furthermore, it does not penetrate the blood–brain barrier, and therefore does not have central opioid effects. Codeine and morphine (in kaolin and morphine mixture) are also available but their use is limited by the potential for central opioid effects. Kaolin may also absorb water and interfere with rehydration or increase the risk of obstruction with opioids.

Atropine is present in co-phenotrope and will reduce peristalsis through inhibition of muscarinic receptors on the gastrointestinal muscle. Its use is limited by the obvious widespread antimuscarinic effects.

Counselling

Patients taking diuretics are at increased risk of dehydration and electrolyte disturbances and may be advised to consult their general practitioner (GP) or omit doses. In patients with diarrhoea it is worth enquiring about drug use and asking about the use of laxatives.

Oral rehydration therapy

- This should be made up with the correct amount of freshly boiled and cooled water.
- The amount required depends on the number of watery stools passed.
- Once reconstituted, ORT may be stored refrigerated for 24 h.

Antibiotics

- Many cases of diarrhoea are viral and so antibiotics are unlikely to be effective.
- Patients who are taking antibiotics (especially clindamycin) and then develop diarrhoea which is severe or bloody should consult their GP immediately.

Opioids

- These are effective at symptomatic relief but will not shorten the course of the diarrhoea.

Constipation

Once again, this is a condition with a range of causes and is defined as altered bowel habits with reduced frequency (e.g. fewer than three motions per week) and the passing of hardened faeces. In the simplest case, constipation may reflect a diet lacking adequate roughage. Other causes may be psychological, due to painful defecation associated with haemorrhoids or anal fissure, due to IBS, postoperatively (secondary to immobility, dehydration or constipating drugs), with ageing, due to serious bowel pathology such as carcinoma of the bowel, secondary fluid restriction in renal failure (Chapter 17) or induced by drug treatment. Drugs which may cause constipation include:

- opioids – when used as analgesics, antitussives or antidiarrhoeal agents
- tricyclic antidepressants
- antimuscarinic agents – including phenothiazines and older antihistamines
- aluminium salts – as antacids and also when used as phosphate binders in renal failure
- iron
- diuretics
- calcium channel blockers
- lithium

The explanation for the constipating effects of opioids is straightforward and is explained by the presynaptic inhibition of the parasympathetic nerves responsible for gastrointestinal motility which underlies their use as antidiarrhoeal agents, as discussed above. The constipating action of antimuscarinic agents, including tricyclic antidepressants, is through postsynaptic inhibition of parasympathetic activity, as mentioned above. Diuretics may cause constipation secondary to dehydration and calcium channel blockers may cause direct relaxation of the gastrointestinal smooth muscle.

In the absence of an obvious cause, constipation, especially in older patients, should warrant referral due to the possibility of carcinoma of the bowel.

Management

The best approach to constipation is a balanced diet with non-starch polysaccharides (NSPs) and fluid or adding bulking agents (e.g. methylcellulose, ispaghula husk) to the diet.

Otherwise laxatives may be indicated.

Osmotic laxatives

Lactulose, magnesium salts

Lactulose is a disaccharide of galactose and fructose and enters the colon unchanged, where it is converted by bacteria to lactic and acetic acid which osmotically raise the fluid volume. This increase in fluid volume leads to larger and softer stools.

Magnesium salts also have an osmotic effect, resulting in a laxative action; this also occurs when magnesium is used as an antacid. Magnesium salts release cholecystokinin which increases gastrointestinal motility.

Stimulant laxatives

Dantron, senna extracts

These provide rapid relief of symptoms. Senna extracts enter the colon and are metabolised to anthracene derivatives which stimulate gastrointestinal activity by irritation. Dantron and sodium picosulfate are also irritants which stimulate lower gastrointestinal activity. Dantron is a carcinogen in animal tests and its use is limited to the elderly and terminally ill patients.

Counselling

- Patients should not expect to pass a motion every day – once every 3 days is within the normal range; it is changes in bowel habits which are significant.
- A diet rich in NSPs and with plenty of water is likely to prevent constipation.
- Lactulose will take 2 days to have an effect.
- Stimulant laxatives given orally take approximately 8–12 h for an effect; when given as suppositories their action is more rapid.

Irritable bowel syndrome

This is a common, long-standing bowel disorder (present for at least 12 weeks within 1 year) with pain, bloating (both of which may be relieved by defecation) and episodes of diarrhoea and/or constipation. Diagnosis is based on the Rome II criteria (see Drossman *et al.*, 1999). The cause of IBS is poorly understood but may have a psychological basis and be associated with depression and stress. It is not thought to be associated with altered gastrointestinal motility but there may be a change in sensitivity of visceral nerves; there is also the concept of a 'brain–gut' interaction. Detailed guidance on IBS and its management has been produced by the British Society of Gastroenterology (Jones *et al.*, 2000).

Pharmacological management

For constipating symptoms

Currently IBS is managed by adding NSPs (such as ispaghula) to the diet when constipation is a leading feature. In this respect, bran fibre is avoided as its fermentation may exacerbate any distension. Lactulose is also used for persistent symptoms.

For bloating and pain

Antispasmodic agents such as antimuscarinic agents and mebeverine are used for the relief of the pain and distension as required. Mebeverine is the most widely used agent and is appropriate for disease with pain and bloating. It causes direct relaxation of gastrointestinal smooth muscle and this is thought to be due to phosphodiesterase inhibition. Dicycloverine is an antimuscarinic agent and inhibits parasympathetic activity, so reducing smooth-muscle tone in the lower gastrointestinal tract. Peppermint oil is also widely used but there is no evidence to support its effectiveness.

Tricyclic antidepressants, such as amitriptyline, are used at low doses and may be effective through their constipating antimuscarinic effects and possible analgesic effects. They may potentially improve depression (although as the dose is low this may be unlikely) and alter visceral nerve activity. The British Society of Gastroenterology guidelines point to tricyclic antidepressants as being the most effective drugs in the management of IBS.

For diarrhoeal symptoms

Any diarrhoea may be managed by loperamide as required.

New treatments

There is some evidence that 5-HT$_3$ receptor antagonists such as alosetron (which is not available in the UK) may reduce the symptoms of IBS in non-constipated subjects, possibly via central actions (Camilleri *et al.*, 2001; Mayer *et al.*, 2002). Also under investigation are the 5-HT$_1$ agonist buspirone, 5-HT$_4$ agonists, selective serotonin reuptake inhibitors, clonidine and neurokinin antagonists.

Counselling

- Patients should be reminded of the importance of a healthy diet which is low in fat but with plenty of fruit (Chapter 3).
- Exclusion of agents which exacerbate the condition may help. Avoidance of excessive caffeine and lactose in milk may help.
- Mebeverine should be taken 20 min before meals.
- If a tricyclic antidepressant is used, it should be pointed out that it is being used for its benefits in IBS as opposed to antidepressant actions (which require higher doses).

Ispaghula

- Ispaghula husk (Fybogel) should be taken with water and not at bedtime.
- Maintain adequate fluid intake.
- Flatulence and abdominal bloating may be worse on starting the treatment. The dose may be reduced to once daily for a few days if necessary.

Inflammatory bowel disease

This condition encompasses both ulcerative colitis and Crohn's disease, distinct inflammatory conditions which represent a high degree of morbidity and run relapsing and remitting courses. In both cases the causes are unclear and possibilities include genetics, microbial and environmental aetiologies, perhaps with an altered or inappropriate immune response to antigens in the gastrointestinal tract.

Clinical features of ulcerative colitis and Crohn's disease

These may include:

- diarrhoea
- faecal incontinence
- rectal bleeding, bloody diarrhoea
- passing of mucus
- cramping pains
- weight loss
- in Crohn's disease there may also be mouth ulcers and anal skin tags
- in Crohn's disease there may be malabsorption, leading to deficiencies of folate, vitamin B$_{12}$ and iron associated with megaloblastic and iron-deficiency anaemia respectively. Blood loss in ulcerative colitis may also lead to iron-deficiency anaemia (Chapter 16)
- inflammatory bowel disease may also occasionally be associated with arthritis, iritis, uveitis and an increased risk of thrombo-embolism

Ulcerative colitis

Ulcerative colitis is characterised by inflammation which involves the rectum and spreads to the colon. In ulcerative colitis the inflammation tends to be superficial, affecting the mucosa.

Crohn's disease

Crohn's disease may affect any part of the gastrointestinal tract but mostly the ileum and/or colon are involved. The features of Crohn's disease and any associated deficiencies reflect the region of the gastrointestinal tract affected. In Crohn's disease T-lymphocytes are activated, leading to transmural inflammation, and the extensive involvement may lead to the formation of fistulae.

Pharmacological basis of management

Drugs used in inflammatory bowel disease are intended to suppress or prevent the inflammatory response.

5-aminosalicylates

Balsalazide, mesalazine, olsalazine, and sulfasalazine

5-aminosalicylates yield 5-aminosalicylic acid (5-ASA), which is the mainstay of therapy for ulcerative colitis, especially in milder disease. Although widely used in Crohn's disease, their effectiveness in maintenance therapy is less clear and a meta-analysis which examined the prophylactic use of mesalazine concluded that it was less effective at maintaining remission but was most effective in postsurgical patients (Camma *et al.*, 1997). Sulfasalazine (5-ASA joined to sulfapyridine), olsalazine (two joined molecules of 5-ASA) and balsalazide (a prodrug) are metabolised in the colon by gut flora to 5-ASA, while mesalazine undergoes pH-sensitive cleavages of its enteric coat to yield 5-ASA. The liberated 5-ASA is thought to act via the inhibition of leukotriene and prostanoid formation, scavenging free radicals and decreasing neutrophil chemotaxis.

Sulfapyridine, derived from sulfasalazine, is a sulphonamide and is unsuitable for patients who are intolerant to sulphonamide: it leads to side-effects which include reversible male infertility. Alternative agents such as mesalazine do not affect fertility. The sulfasalazine-derived sulphonamide is a risk factor for megaloblastic anaemia due to its antifolate properties. The release of 5-ASA renders all of these agents unsuitable for patients who cannot tolerate salicylates, for example patients with asthma who are sensitive to aspirin. They may also cause interstitial nephritis and should be avoided in renal impairment.

The *British National Formulary* recommends that, for patients taking sulfasalazine, a full blood count and a liver function test should be carried out every month for 3 months at the start of treatment.

Significant interactions of 5-aminosalicylates are summarised in Table 9.1.

Corticosteroids

Corticosteroids are used in order to induce a remission in ulcerative colitis and Crohn's disease, especially in more severe disease. Steroid-induced side-effects limit their long-term use for maintenance therapy. Oral prednisolone is widely used and more recently enteric-coated budesonide has been developed: this has poor absorption and extensive first-pass metabolism,

Table 9.1   Some important drug interactions of 5-aminosalicylates

Drugs	Consequences	Comments
Mesalazine, olsalazine or sulfasalazine with azathioprine	5-aminosalicylates may reduce the clearance of azathioprine with enhanced side-effects such as bone marrow suppression	Their concurrent use should be monitored and the dose of azathioprine may need to be reduced
Sulfasalazine with antibiotics	Ampicillin and rifampicin have been shown to eradicate gut bacteria and reduce the release of 5-ASA from sulfasalazine	The effectiveness of sulfasalazine may be reduced by concurrent antibiotics. Metronidazole does not appear to interact with sulfasalazine
Sulfasalazine with digoxin	The plasma levels of digoxin may be reduced	The levels or effectiveness of digoxin should be monitored

5-ASA, 5-aminosalicylic acid.

both of which will limit its systemic side-effects. Oral budesonide is intended for Crohn's disease affecting ileal and ascending colonic regions. Enemas (prednisolone, budesonide and hydrocortisone) are used in more distal or rectal inflammation. The beneficial effects of corticosteroids are via their well-established anti-inflammatory and immunosuppressive actions.

Immunosuppressants

Azathioprine, ciclosporin, methotrexate
The role of immunosuppressants in inflammatory bowel disease is less clear but may have a role in refractory disease and for steroid sparing. In this regard both azathioprine and intravenous ciclosporin are used for inducing remissions. If ciclosporin is given in addition to steroids, there is an increased risk of *Pneumocystis carinii* and prophylactic co-trimoxazole is used. Methotrexate is also effective in Crohn's disease but not in ulcerative colitis.

Infliximab

This is a monoclonal antibody which neutralises the proinflammatory cytokine, tumour necrosis factor-α (TNF-α), which is implicated in the pathology of Crohn's disease, possibly via leucocyte recruitment. The ACCENT I trial (ACCENT I Study Group, 2002) has indicated that patients who show an initial response to a single dose of infliximab are likely to benefit from repeated doses of this agent, leading to remission and discontinuation of corticosteroids. Infliximab has been identified as a risk factor for developing tuberculosis.

National Institute of Clinical Excellence (NICE) guidelines released in 2002 recommend that infliximab can be used by experienced gastroenterologists for patients with severe Crohn's disease which is refractory to immunosuppressants and corticosteroids, where the disease is not fistulating and when surgery is not possible.

Antibacterial agents

Metronidazole and ciprofloxacin (for up to 3 months) may provide some benefit in Crohn's

disease and metronidazole is used in ulcerative colitis. The rationale for their use is that they may eradicate any causative organisms or alter the natural gut flora and so change the local environment.

Loperamide

This may be of some use in diarrhoea associated with mild inflammatory bowel disease but should be used with caution in more severe disease due to the risk of toxic megacolon.

Colestryramine

Colestryramine binds bile salts and may reduce diarrhoea due to malabsorption of bile salts in Crohn's disease.

Fish oils

Fish oils may be of benefit in addition to standard treatments in ulcerative colitis and Crohn's disease, possibly by interfering with leukotriene synthesis.

Nutritional therapy

In Crohn's disease it is well established that parental nutrition allows the gastrointestinal tract to recover ('bowel rest') and results in patients entering remission without the need for steroids. Similarly, elemental feeding with simple, predigested foods is also effective in the management of Crohn's disease.

Probiotics

A small-scale trial has reported that nonpathogenic *E. coli* (Nissle 1917) was equally effective as mesalazine in maintaining a long-term remission in patients with ulcerative colitis (Rembacken *et al.*, 1999). The *E. coli* was given after eradication of endogenous *E. coli* with gentamicin. The authors' explanations for the beneficial effects of *E. coli* were that they may have blocked the binding of adhesive bacteria, produced toxins against pathogenic bacteria or altered the local environment.

Vitamins and minerals

As inflammatory bowel disease may be associated with malabsorption of iron, folate and vitamin B_{12}, leading to anaemia it may be necessary to give appropriate oral or parenteral supplements of these nutrients. Patients taking corticosteroids are at risk of osteoporosis and may benefit from calcium supplementation.

Counselling

- The National Association for Colitis and Crohn's Disease (NACC) provides patient information and support. It produces a 'Can't Wait' card, which is recognised by many shops and is intended to help patients gain access to a toilet in an emergency.
- Smoking makes Crohn's disease (but not ulcerative colitis) worse.
- Inflammatory bowel disease may be exacerbated by NSAIDs.
- Inflammatory bowel disease may be exacerbated by alcohol.
- The effectiveness of dietary modifications is less clear but patients may identify by trial and error which foods exacerbate their condition. Wheat and dairy products may be implicated.
- Patients taking aminosalicylates should report any sore throats, fevers, easy bruising or bleeding due to the risk of blood dyscrasia.
- Aminosalicylates are associated with side-effects which include rashes, headaches and diarrhoea.

- Sulfasalazine may colour urine orange and discolour soft contact lenses.
- Mesalazine and balsalazide tablets should be swallowed whole.
- Patients should be maintained on the same brand of enteric-coated mesalazine.

Practice points

- Changes in bowel habits, including rectal bleeding, should lead to referral to the GP.
- ORT plays a major role in the treatment of diarrhoea.
- Antidiarrhoeal agents provide symptomatic relief but do not alter the course of the diarrhoea.
- Diarrhoea is an important side-effect of antibiotic treatment, and if severe (especially with clindamycin) should lead to prompt referral.
- Constipation is best managed by a healthy diet, adequate fluid intake and exercise.
- Patients receiving chronic opioid treatment should receive a laxative.
- Be vigilant of laxative abuse in eating disorders.
- IBS is poorly defined and is managed according to its leading symptoms.
- Ulcerative colitis and Crohn's disease are distinct relapsing and remitting diseases with high morbidity.
- 5-Aminosalicylates are associated with blood dyscrasias.

 CASE STUDY

A husband requests senna tablets for his wife who has just been discharged from hospital. Suggest further questions you may need to ask prior to making a sale.

- The cause of her admission should be established. Constipation may result from a long stay in hospital with inevitable reduction in physical activity. Dehydration and poor diet and opioid analgesia may also be factors leading to constipation in the convalescing patient. It may appear strange that no laxatives were prescribed at discharge. This patient had received bowel surgery for an obstruction. The constipation could possibly be due to a new obstruction and senna could cause severe abdominal pain if given to this patient. Referral should be made to the GP in the first instance.

References

ACCENT I Study Group (2002). Maintenance infliximab for Crohn's disease: the ACCENT I randomised trial. *Lancet* 359: 1541–1549.

Camilleri M, Chey W Y, Mayer E A *et al.* (2001). A randomized controlled trial of the serotonin type 3 receptor antagonist alosteron in women with diarrhea-predominant irritable bowel syndrome. *Arch Intern Med* 161: 1733–1740.

Camma C, Giunta M, Rosselli M *et al.* (1997). Mesalamine in the maintenance treatment of Crohn's disease: a meta-analysis adjusted for confounding variables. *Gastroenterology* 113: 1465–1473.

Drossman D A, Corazziari E, Talley N J *et al.* (1999). Rome II: a multinational consensus document on functional gastrointestinal disorders. *Gut* 45 (suppl II): 1–81.

Jones J, Boorman J, Cann P *et al.* (2000). British Society of Gastroenterology guidelines for the management of the irritable bowel syndrome. *Gut* 47 (suppl. II): ii1–ii19.

Mayer E A, Berman S, Derbyshire S W G *et al.* (2002). The effect of the 5-HT$_3$ receptor antagonist, alosteron, on brain responses to visceral stimulation in irritable bowel syndrome patients. *Aliment Pharmacol Ther* 16: 1357–1366.

Mehta D K (ed.) *British National Formulary*, latest edition. London: British Medical Association and Royal Pharmaceutical Society of Great Britain.

NICE Technology appraisal no. 40 (2002). Guidance on the use of infliximab for Crohn's disease. London: National Institute of Clinical Excellence (via www.nice.org.uk).

Rembacken B J, Snelling AM, Hawkey P M *et al.* (1999). Non-pathogenic *Escherichia coli* versus mesalazine for the treatment of ulcerative colitis: a randomised trial. *Lancet* 354: 635–639.

Further reading

Camilleri M (2001). Management of irritable bowel syndrome. *Gastroenterology* 120: 652–668.

Farrell R J, Peppercorn M A (2002). Ulcerative colitis. *Lancet* 359: 331–340.

Forbes A (2002). Crohn's disease – the role of nutritional therapy. *Aliment Pharmacol Ther* 16 (suppl. 4): 48–52.

Ghosh S, Shand A, Fergusson A (2000). Ulcerative colitis. *BMJ* 320: 1119–1123.

Jones J, Spiller R (2001). IBS: current approaches to management. *Prescriber* 12: 93–102.

Meeman J (2001). IBD: a guide to ulcerative colitis and Crohn's disease. *Prescriber* 12: 43–59.

Rampton D S (1999). Management of Crohn's disease. *BMJ* 319: 1480–1485.

Scribano M L, Prantera C (2002). Medical treatment of active Crohn's disease. *Aliment Pharmacol Ther* 16 (suppl. 4): 35–39.

Shanahan F (2002). Crohn's disease. *Lancet* 359: 62–69.

Online resource

www.nacc.org.uk is the website of The National Association for Colitis and Crohn's Disease (NACC), which provides patient information and support (accessed 4 December 2002).

10

The liver patient

Hepatic impairment may result from infection (for example, hepatitis), may be drug-induced (see Chapter 5) or associated with chronic alcohol abuse. Liver disease may be acute or chronic and ranges from hepatic impairment through to liver failure. Liver disease may have the following clinical features:

- jaundice – impaired excretion of bilirubin into the bile by the liver leads to hyperbilirubinaemia, resulting in yellow colouration of the skin and sclera of the eyes
- hypoproteinaemia – the ability of the liver to synthesise proteins, including clotting factors, is impaired and leads to a reduction in plasma proteins
- decreased clotting – this occurs as a consequence of impaired synthesis of clotting factors, and may lead to easy bruising and bleeding
- ascites – this is the accumulation of fluid in the peritoneal cavity and in part is due to oedema secondary to hypoproteinaemia and sodium retention caused by secondary hyperaldosteronism, and also portal hypertension

- spider naevi – this is a sign of chronic liver failure and may be an early sign of alcoholic liver disease
- pruritus – hyperbilirubinaemia of jaundice leads to itching
- nausea
- digital clubbing – this may be a non-specific sign in chronic liver failure and its cause is unknown. There may also be white nails due to hypoalbuminaemia
- portal hypertension – this is associated with chronic liver failure due to liver fibrosis altering the haemodynamics and may result in bleeding oesophageal varices
- gynaecomastia – breast development, possibly due to reduced metabolism of oestrogens
- hypoglycaemia – reduced glucose output from the liver's glycogen stores
- encephalopathy – this is associated with both acute and chronic liver failure leading to neuropsychiatric symptoms including changes in personality, disorientation, confusion and drowsiness. The causes of encephalopathy are not fully established but nitrogenous products and false neurotransmitters are believed to

contribute. The gut flora are believed to produce many nitrogenous products, including ammonia, which are normally cleared by the liver. In liver failure these toxins are not adequately cleared and may exert neurological effects

The effects of hepatic impairment

As the liver represents a major site of drug metabolism and elimination, hepatic impairment has significant implications for drugs which are extensively cleared by the liver. On the basis of liver function tests (Chapter 2) it is difficult to predict systematically how a patient will handle various drugs. Appendix 2 of the *British National Formulary* deals with prescribing issues associated with hepatic impairment and details which drugs are affected and how to alter or choose drug treatment. Measures include avoiding certain drugs, selecting alternative drugs which are not extensively eliminated by the liver and reducing doses.

In addition to the role of the liver in drug elimination, its other metabolic activities will be disrupted. In particular, the liver synthesises a number of clotting factors and so their synthesis will be reduced, leading to an increased bleeding tendency. This will have important implications for the use of the oral anticoagulant warfarin, which is also metabolised by the liver. In patients with hepatic impairment receiving warfarin their international normalised ratio or INR (which may be elevated prior to treatment) should be closely monitored and the dose altered accordingly. Hypoproteinaemia will also reduce the plasma protein binding of certain drugs, increasing their free plasma concentration.

Pharmacological management of liver failure

Ascites

In addition to paracentesis (draining off the fluid), patients should have a sodium-restricted diet to limit sodium retention and fluid accumulation. Given the role of aldosterone in secondary hyperaldosteronism, the aldosterone receptor antagonist and potassium-sparing diuretic spironolactone is also used. However, spironolactone may cause gynaecomastia and in liver patients who already have gynaecomastia an alternative potassium-sparing diuretic such as amiloride should be used. Additional diuresis may be provided by loop diuretics. Fluid-retaining drugs such as corticosteroids and non-steroidal anti-inflammatory drugs (NSAIDs) should be avoided. A complication of ascites is spontaneous bacterial peritonitis, for which antimicrobial agents may be used.

Hepatic encephalopathy

To limit the production of nitrogenous products, protein in the diet may be restricted. To limit the production of these toxins, gut flora are eradicated with antibacterial agents such as neomycin or metronidazole. The osmotic laxative lactulose (Chapter 9) is also routinely used in high doses and its beneficial effects may be via regular clearing of the bowel of toxins and/or alterations in the environment for the gut flora.

Sensitivity to centrally acting drugs

Patients with liver disease are especially sensitive to centrally acting drugs such as benzodiazepines, antipsychotic agents and opioids. These drugs should be used with great care, as there is a risk of precipitating a coma.

Hyperbilirubinaemia

Increased levels of bilirubin in the plasma give rise to jaundice and associated pruritus. In order to enhance the removal of bilirubin from the body, colestyramine is used as a bile-binding agent (Chapter 12). Colestyramine binds bile in the intestines and so prevents the reabsorption of excreted bile and leads to enhanced overall excretion. This should limit the jaundice and associated symptoms. However, as discussed in Chapter

12, the binding nature of colestryramine gives rise to a range of interactions with other drugs and those affected should be given at different times.

Pruritus

As commented above, colestyramine reduces bilirubin levels and limits pruritus. Other measures to limit pruritus are the use of menthol in aqueous cream for its local cooling effect and oral antihistamines for patients with mild liver disease. Sedating antihistamines are used with caution especially at night if itching is preventing the patient from sleeping. Non-sedating antihistamines can also be of benefit. The 5-HT_3 receptor antagonist ondansetron has been shown to have a small beneficial effect in managing pruritus associated with jaundice (Muller *et al.*, 1998).

Gastric bleeding

An increased bleeding tendency means that gastric bleeding is more common in liver impairment and to this end antisecretory agents such as ranitidine may be prescribed to reduce the production of gastric acid.

Bleeding oesophageal varices

The bleeding from oesophageal varices is a medical emergency. To limit bleeding, vasopressin is infused and causes vasoconstriction. Octreotide, a somatostatin analogue, is also widely used (unlicensed indication) and is thought to cause vasoconstriction. A beta-blocker may be used in prophylaxis against bleeding varices and this may be secondary to lowering portal pressure.

Impaired clotting

The impaired clotting, secondary to the impaired synthesis of clotting factors, may be managed by parenteral vitamin K. The patient should of course avoid drugs which may inhibit clotting (anticoagulants, antiplatelet drugs) or cause bleeding (NSAIDs).

Hypoglycaemia

This may require intravenous glucose to correct hypoglycaemia.

Considerations in alcoholic liver disease

In addition to caution with the use of drugs when there is liver impairment, patients with alcohol dependence may receive drugs to control their addiction (such as disulfiram, acamprosate) and seizures associated with withdrawal reactions (benzodiazepines, principally chlordiazepoxide, and alternatively clomethiazole). Alcoholism is also associated with deficiencies of thiamin (vitamin B_1) and this may lead to Wernicke's encephalopathy with drowsiness, disorientation, nystagmus and ataxia. To prevent this, alcoholic patients are given vitamin B complex.

Over-the-counter considerations

Obviously greater caution should be exercised when using drugs in liver impairment and failure. Other considerations are the salt content in over-the-counter (OTC) preparations (e.g. antacids, effervescent preparation) if the patient is on a salt-restricted diet. The increased bleeding tendency also means that patients are at increased risk of gastric bleeding with aspirin and ibuprofen. NSAIDs may also lead to fluid retention. These increased risks mean that low-dose paracetamol is a safer alternative for pain relief.

Counselling

• Colestyramine should be mixed with water or a drink and can be used in cooking.
• Colestyramine can interfere with the absorption of other drugs. Therefore, other drugs should be taken at least 1 h before or 4–6 h after the colestyramine.

Practice points

- Liver function should always be taken into consideration when using drugs.
- Blood clotting is impaired in liver failure with increased bleeding tendencies and the actions of warfarin will be potentiated.
- Jaundice may be managed by colestyramine, ascites with spironolactone, and encephalopathy by neomycin and lactulose.

References

Mehta D K (ed.) *British National Formulary*, latest edition. London: British Medical Association and Royal Pharmaceutical Society of Great Britain.

Muller C, Pongratz S, Pidlich J *et al.* (1998). Treatment of pruritus in chronic liver disease with the 5-hydroxy-tryptamine receptor type 3 antagonist ondansetron: a randomized, placebo-controlled, double-blind cross-over trial. *Eur J Gastroenterol Hepatol* 10: 865–870.

Part D

Cardiovascular diseases

11

Hypertension

Disease characteristics

The cause of essential hypertension is not known but may be multifactorial. Indeed, rather than a disease in its own right, one may view hypertension as blood pressure (BP) which is associated with significant cardiovascular risk. The cut-off point between normal and hypertension is arbitrary, and is now generally regarded as a sustained diastolic BP of greater than 90 mmHg or systolic BP of greater than 140 mmHg.

Over the years alterations in many cardiovascular control mechanisms (nitric oxide, endothelins, renin–angiotensin system and sympathetic nervous system) have been proposed as causing essential hypertension but no convincing evidence exists to support a 'universal cause'. Far less commonly, however, hypertension (<10%) may be secondary to another condition: renal disease, renovascular disease, Conn's syndrome (primary hyperaldosteronism), polycythaemia, Cushing's syndrome, hyperthyroidism, phaeochromocytoma and pregnancy, and these should be excluded. Drugs which may cause hypertension include:

- oral contraceptives
- sympathomimetics
- corticosteroids
- non-steroidal anti-inflammatory drugs (NSAIDs)
- ketoconazole
- moclobemide
- erythropoietin
- ciclosporin
- venlafaxine

Clinical features

Hypertension is almost always asymptomatic and is often detected by routine measurement. The main complications are due to end-organ

147

damage, principally left ventricular hypertrophy, ischaemic heart disease, renal failure, retinopathy and peripheral vascular disease. Ultimately hypertension is a major risk factor for stroke (especially), myocardial infarction and the development of chronic heart failure, hence the need to treat this condition effectively.

Goals of treatment

The clear goal is a reduction in BP and, when this involves drug treatment, this should be with as few side-effects as possible. The British Hypertension Society target is a systolic BP of less than 140 mmHg and a diastolic BP of less than 85 mmHg (80 mmHg in diabetics), while the Hypertention Optimal Treatment (HOT) trial (HOT study group, 1998) indicated that there is little benefit from lowering BP further.

As a consequence of treatment the following are ideal goals:

- reduction in cardiovascular damage
- preservation of renal function
- limitation or reversal of left ventricular hypertrophy
- prevention of coronary artery disease and chronic heart failure
- reduction in mortality due to stroke and myocardial infarctions

Pharmacological basis of management

Diuretics

Thiazides and related agents (e.g. bendroflumethiazide, indapamide, metolazone)

Diuretics are first-line drugs in the management of hypertension and cause a reduction in circulating volume, thus reducing preload and afterload, and hence cardiac work. In addition, they may have direct vascular effects leading to vasodilatation, which further reduces preload and/or afterload.

Thiazides act in the distal convoluted tubule to inhibit Na^+/Cl^- reabsorption, leading to

diuresis. Loop diuretics, which are occasionally used when thiazides (except metolazone) are likely to be ineffective in renal impairment, act via inhibition of the $Na^+/K^+/Cl^-$ transporter in the thick ascending limb of the loop of Henle.

It should be noted that, with bendroflumethiazide, the most widely used agent, there is no benefit from increasing the dose above the optimum of 2.5 mg, as there is little additional antihypertensive effect and side-effects are substantially increased.

Beta-blockers

e.g. Acebutolol, atenolol, bisoprolol, metoprolol, nadolol, pindolol, propranolol

Beta-blockers may also be viewed as first-line drugs and have been widely used over many years. Despite this, their precise antihypertensive effect is unclear but is thought to involve a reduction in sympathetic drive to the heart, reducing cardiac output, and a reduction in sympathetically evoked renin release from the kidneys.

Angiotensin-converting enzyme inhibitors (ACE inhibitors)

e.g. Captopril, enalapril, lisinopril, perindopril, ramipril

Angiotensin-converting enzyme (ACE) inhibitors are now recognised as having an important role in hypertension but are no more effective than other agents (CAPP study group, 1999). By inhibiting the ACE, they lead to reductions in angiotensin II, which in turn leads to:

- reductions in arterial and venous vasoconstriction (reduced total peripheral resistance)
- reduced aldosterone production, which leads to reductions in salt and water retention, hence reduced circulating volume (reduced cardiac output)

Clinical use

ACE inhibitors may cause pronounced first-dose hypotension and are best given initially on retiring at night. A low starting dose should be used and titrated up to the maximum effective and tolerated dose.

The renin–angiotensin system is activated in renovascular disease (atheroma of the renal artery) in order to maintain renal perfusion and filtration. Hence ACE inhibitors may cause deterioration of renal function in pre-existing renal disease and these patients should be identified by measuring plasma creatinine and should not receive an ACE inhibitor.

A build-up of bradykinin, usually broken down by ACE, may produce a troublesome dry cough in some patients (10%) treated with ACE inhibitors.

Angiotensin II receptor antagonists

e.g. Candesartan, irbesartan, losartan, valsartan

This new class of drugs blocks the action of angiotensin II at the angiotensin (AT_1) receptor. Hence these agents have similar consequences as ACE inhibitors but do not give rise to a cough. The Lifestyle Intervention for Endpoint Reduction in Hypertension (LIFE) trial (2002) reported that losartan was more effective than atenolol at reducing mortality in hypertensive patients, largely through a reduction in the incidence of stroke. In diabetic patients with hypertension, the effects of losartan were even more impressive at reducing overall mortality, cardiovascular mortality and the development of heart failure. In both classes of hypertensive patients, losartan was also more effective than atenolol at reversing left ventricular hypertrophy.

Calcium channel blockers

e.g. Diltiazem, felodipine, nifedipine, verapamil

There are three main classes of calcium channel blockers: (1) verapamil; (2) dihydropyridines (DHPs) – nifedipine, nicardipine, amlodipine, lacidipine, nisoldipine – and (3) diltiazem. Verapamil exerts most of its effects on the heart compared with DHP effects, which are greater on arteriole smooth muscle. The activity of diltiazem

is between class 1 and 2. Worldwide, calcium channel blockers are currently the most widely used antihypertensives and they act principally to inhibit voltage-operated calcium channels on vascular smooth muscle, leading to vasodilatation and a reduction in BP.

Alpha-blockers

e.g. Doxazosin, prazosin

These should generally be regarded as agents of last choice, being added to therapy that has not achieved target BP. They are competitive receptor antagonists, inhibiting sympathetic activation of alpha$_1$-adrenoceptors on vascular smooth muscle, leading to vasodilatation and a drop in BP. Because of this non-selective action, they lead to widespread side-effects, making them poorly tolerated. They may, however, be useful for diabetics or patients with a lipid disorder (when diuretics or beta-blockers are sometimes avoided) or in older men with prostatic symptoms.

Centrally acting agents

e.g. Clonidine, methyldopa, moxonidine

These agents are occasionally used, for example, methyldopa in pregnancy or when other treatments have failed. Their action is on central vasomotor centres and they lead to a decrease in sympathetic output, causing a fall in BP. The interference with the sympathetic nervous system leads to widespread side-effects. In the case of clonidine and moxonidine (an imidazoline receptor agonist), they should not be withdrawn suddenly, as there is a risk of a hypertensive crisis. For withdrawal, if moxonidine is used concurrently with a beta-blocker, then the beta-blocker should be withdrawn slowly, several days before the centrally acting agent.

The beneficial pharmacological targets of cardiovascular drugs are listed in Table 11.1. Consideration of the distribution in the body of the sites of action for these drugs also explains some of the unwanted but predictable type A adverse drug reactions (Table 11.1).

Table 11.1 Examples of principal type A adverse reactions of drugs used in hypertension

Drug	Pharmacological activity	Unwanted clinical effects
Thiazides	Act on the Na^+/Cl^- transporter of the renal distal convoluted tubule to cause diuresis and reduce circulating volume. May also have vasodilator actions	• Postural hypotension • Adversely alter lipid profile • May induce diabetes
Beta-blockers Hydrophilic (atenolol, acebutolol)	Myocardium: sympathetic drive mediated by beta₁-adrenoceptors SM: bronchoconstriction Reduce lacrimation Peripheral vascular SM: constriction Lipids Liver and pancreas	Bradycardia, cardiac failure, conduction disorders Bronchoconstriction Dry eyes Raynaud's phenomenon, impotence Adversely affect lipid profile: increase LDL and decrease HDL Decrease glycogenolysis, and decrease secretion of insulin
Sotalol (hydrophilic)	As above plus prolongation of QT interval	No longer licensed for hypertension
Lipophilic (propranolol, timolol, metoprolol, labetolol)	As above plus CNS effects	Lethargy, depression, nightmares
Calcium channel blockers	Vascular SM: arteriolar relaxation (mainly dihydropyridines) CNS	Headache, facial flushing, peripheral oedema (ankles), postural hypotension, gum hyperplasia Depression, extrapyramidal symptoms
(1) Verapamil	SM: GI tract Sinus or AV nodes: negative inotrope Myocardium	Constipation Bradycardia or heart block Reduced cardiac output
(2) Dihydropyridines	Reflex sympathomimetic stimulation	Tachycardia or palpitations
(3) Diltiazem	Sinus or AV nodes: negative inotrope SM: GI tract	Bradycardia or heart block Constipation
Alpha₁-blockers (prazosin, doxazosin, indoramin)	Vascular SM: relaxation SM: bronchodilation SM: GI tract constriction SM: GI sphincter relaxation Bladder sphincter relaxation Seminal tract relaxation Liver: reduced glycogenolysis CNS	Impotence, nasal congestion, postural hypotension, tachycardia, oedema Beneficial in concurrent asthma Diarrhoea Vomiting Urinary frequency, incontinence Failure of ejaculation Weight gain (indoramin) Drowsiness, vertigo, headache, lack of energy, extrapyramidal (indoramin)
Centrally acting (e.g. methyldopa)	Inhibition of sympathetic drive to SM CNS	• See alpha- and beta-blockers above • Safe in asthma and heart failure See alpha- and beta-blockers above

SM, smooth muscle; LDL, low-density lipoprotein; HDL, high-density lipoprotein; CNS, central nervous system; GI, gastrointestinal; AV, atrioventricular.

Choice of drugs

For patients with moderate hypertension, life-style and dietary changes (see General counselling, below) should be tried before drug treatment. If these do not bring about a satisfactory reduction in BP, the British Hypertension Society guidelines (Ramsay *et al.*, 1999) suggest that drug treatment should be initiated in the following circumstances.

Younger patients (<60 years old)

Treat if diastolic BP is greater than 100 mmHg, or is between 90 and 99 mmHg if there is evidence of end-organ damage, diabetes mellitus or the patient has a high cardiovascular risk ($\geq$15% over 10 years). Also treat if systolic BP is greater than 160 mmHg, irrespective of the diastolic BP.

Elderly patients (>60 years)

Treat if their diastolic BP is greater than 90 mmHg or their systolic BP is greater than 160 mmHg. However, it should be appreciated that this may encompass a large proportion of the elderly population.

Generally, a thiazide or beta-blocker is the drug of first choice. Indeed, a conclusion from the Captopril Prevention Project (CAPP) trial was that diuretics or beta-blockers should be considered as the mainstay of treatment in hypertension. It should also be noted that, in terms of BP-lowering, each class of drugs should be viewed as equally effective. Recent meta-analyses of hypertension trials have drawn the following conclusions (He and Whelton, 2000):

- There is no evidence that ACE inhibitors are superior to beta-blockers or diuretics in the prevention of cardiovascular disease. (Despite this conclusion, and as commented above, the LIFE trial reported that the AT_1-receptor antagonist losartan was more effective than atenolol at reducing mortality.)
- ACE inhibitors are especially effective in the prevention of heart failure and nephropathy in diabetics.
- Calcium channel blockers are more effective than beta-blockers or diuretics at preventing stroke but may be associated with a higher incidence of coronary artery disease and heart failure.

In drug selection, compelling indications and contraindications are detailed in Table 11.2.

In addition, ethnicity may be considered, as Afro-Caribbean patients respond best to thiazides and calcium channel blockers, while beta-blockers and ACE inhibitors are less effective.

Combination therapy

In the majority of cases the target BP is not reached with the drug of first use and two agents are usually tried in combination. Typically this involves using a thiazide and a beta-blocker. The British Hypertension Society has also specified other logical combinations:

- thiazide with an ACE inhibitor (if an ACE inhibitor is added to thiazide treatment then the thiazide should be stopped for a few days before the ACE inhibitor to prevent severe hypotension. Alternatively, the thiazide should be given in the morning and the ACE inhibitor before retiring to bed at night). The ACE inhibitor will oppose hypokalaemia due to the thiazide
- thiazide with an alpha-blocker
- beta-blocker with a calcium channel blocker, *but not verapamil* as there is a serious risk of asystole
- beta-blocker with an alpha-blocker
- ACE inhibitor with a calcium channel blocker
- ACE inhibitor with an alpha-blocker

The 'AB/CD rules' have been developed in Cambridge (Dickerson *et al.*, 1999), and aim to rationalise the rotation of drugs by using agents with complementary actions. In this case, younger patients are assumed to have high renin levels and are treated with either an ACE inhibitor (A) or a beta-blocker (B) (to suppress the renin–angiotensin system), which may then be combined with either a calcium channel blocker (C) or a diuretic (D). Older patients are initially treated with either C or D, to which A or B may then be added. In this latter case, the use of C or D may provoke activation of the renin–angiotensin system, which would then be suppressed by A or B if they were added.

Table 11.2 Compelling indications and contraindications for antihypertensives

Condition	Drug indicated	Drugs contraindicated or used with caution
Ischaemic heart disease	Beta-blockers; diltiazem verapamil, long acting DHPs	Short-acting dihydropyridines – associated with increased mortality
Heart failure	ACE inhibitors and AT_1-antagonists; diuretics; beta-blockers with caution (see Chapter 14)	Diltiazem and verapamil – due to negative inotropic effects
Left ventricular hypertrophy (LVH)	The AT_1-antagonist, losartan, has been shown to be particularly effective at reversing LVH (LIFE trial)	
Diabetes mellitus	ACE inhibitors – they are renally and vasoprotective in diabetes (HOPE trial). The AT_1-antagonist, losartan, reduces mortality more than atenolol in diabetic patients with hypertension (LIFE trial). Atenolol may be beneficial (UKPDS and CAPP trials). Centrally acting agents and calcium channel blockers are also suitable	Thiazides and beta-blockers may cause hyperglycaemia. Thiazides may adversely affect the lipid profile. Beta-blockers may also mask signs of hypoglycaemia (e.g. tachycardia; Chapter 33)
Elderly	Thiazides	
Chronic obstructive pulmonary disease and asthma	Centrally acting agents are safe	Beta-blockers are contra-indicated – although in the absence of an alternative, $beta_1$-antagonists may be used with extreme caution
History of stroke	Perindopril and indapamide reduce the risk of stroke in both hypertensive and normotensive patients (PROGRESS trial); this may apply to any ACE inhibitor plus a thiazide	
Renal impairment		Thiazides less effective. Dose reduction of hydrophilic beta-blockers (atenolol, celiprolol, nadolol) may be necessary. Caution with ACE inhibitors. ACE inhibitors and AT_1-antagonists should not be used in renovascular disease
Prostatic hypertrophy	Alpha-blocker	Diuretics
Pregnancy	Methyldopa; beta-blockers (third trimester)	Consider all other agents
Gout	Centrally acting agents safe	Thiazides
Migraine	Beta-blocker; clonidine	
Resistant hypertension	Alpha-blocker; minoxidil, hydralazine, sodium nitroprusside	
Depression		Side-effect of beta-blockers, calcium channel blockers, clonidine and methyldopa
Parkinsonism		Indoramin has extrapyramidal side-effects

ACE, angiotensin-converting enzyme; AT_1, angiotensin receptor; LIFE, Losartan Intervention for Endpoint Reduction in Hypertension; HOPE, Heart Outcomes Prevention Evaluation; UKPDS, UK Prospective Diabetes Study; CAPP, Captopril Prevention Project; PROGRESS, Perindopril Protection Against Recurrent Stroke Study.

Resistance

A proportion of patients are resistant to conventional antihypertensive treatment (even after several combined therapies) and there is some evidence that this may be related to hyperaldosteronism. Accordingly, the aldosterone receptor antagonist spironolactone (1 mg/kg) may be added to therapy.

Concurrent illnesses

Hypertension is a major risk factor for cardiovascular disease and so the patient may have other related conditions. Hyperlipidaemia is common in the population at risk of hypertension and should be managed, usually with a statin (see Chapter 12). Guidelines point to using a statin in patients with a 30% or greater 10-year risk of coronary artery disease and who have a plasma cholesterol of 5 mmol/L or greater. Patients with plasma cholesterol of 5 mmol/L or greater who already have evidence of coronary artery disease should also be treated. The goal of treatment is either a 30% reduction in cholesterol levels or low-density lipoprotein to below 3 mmol/L. Despite these guidelines, a large-scale trial of atorvastatin in hypertensive patients with 'normal' cholesterol levels was stopped in late 2002 due to a significant reduction in cardiovascular events in treated patients. Recent evidence from small-scale studies has also suggested that statins may themselves cause modest reductions in BP and, when used in combination with antihypertensives, may augment the regression of left ventricular hypertrophy, an effect which is independent of lipid lowering (Glorioso *et al.*, 1999; Borghi *et al.*, 2000; Su *et al.*, 2000). The concurrent use of a statin would have no bearing on the choice of antihypertensive regimen.

Diabetes mellitus often coexists with hypertension and, as indicated above, may be a compelling reason to use an ACE inhibitor. Hence, all patients presenting with hypertension should have their blood glucose determined.

Heart failure is often a consequence of untreated hypertension and, as reviewed in Chapter 14, may well be treated with an ACE inhibitor, diuretic, beta-blocker or spironolactone, all of which are also indicated for hypertension. In the case of a beta-blocker, a very low dose would be introduced in heart failure initially under the supervision of an appropriately experienced clinician.

Drug interactions

Given the diversity of drugs used in the treatment of hypertension there are a range of drug interactions. Some important interactions of antihypertensive drugs are summarised in Table 11.3.

General counselling

In talking to patients the first obvious aim would be to reduce their overall cardiovascular risk, which may involve weight reduction, reducing fat and salt intake, increasing fruit and oily fish in the diet, increasing exercise and stopping smoking. A recent study has reported that a sustained weight loss of 4.5 kg was associated with an 8–9 mmHg drop in diastolic and systolic BP (Stevens *et al.*, 2001). Particular attention should be paid to alcohol consumption, as excessive alcohol intake is closely associated with hypertension. In many patients the initial treatment will involve lifestyle changes to see whether these bring about a reduction in BP. During this process the patient's BP should be measured on several occasions to determine whether hypertension is established and to exclude 'white-coat' hypertension.

Failure of lifestyle changes alone would then indicate drug treatment. In talking to patients about drug treatment it should be stressed that the purpose is to lower their BP and this should reduce their risk of having a heart attack, stroke or kidney problems. Although hypertension has no symptoms and the drugs may have side-effects, it is important to take the drugs; however, if they find the side-effects intolerable they may find changing their drug is beneficial.

Diuretics

- Diuretics (or 'water tablets') will cause an increase in urine flow, which may subside after a couple of weeks.

Table 11.3 Summary of important interactions within drugs used in hypertension

Interacting drugs	Consequences	Comments
Beta-blockers with beta-agonists	Pharmacological antagonism	Bronchoconstriction may occur due to inhibition of bronchial beta$_2$-adrenoceptors
Alpha-antagonists with calcium channel blockers or beta-blockers	Hypotension	Additive effects require close monitoring and counselling
Calcium channel blockers with beta-blockers	Some combinations are safe (e.g. felodipine and beta-blockers). Bradycardia and heart block with verapamil and beta-blockers (avoid combination or monitor closely); diltiazem, nifedipine and nicardipine with beta-blockers are usually safe but should be monitored	Additive negative inotropic effects. Increased plasma levels of beta-blockers metabolised by the liver
ACE inhibitors with NSAIDs	Risk of renal impairment	Both associated with renal toxicity
Grapefruit juice with nifedipine (and possibly nicardipine, amlodipine)	Increased effects of calcium channel blockers	Inhibition of cytochrome P450 therefore reduced metabolism
Alcohol with antihypertensives	• Chronic: increase in blood pressure • Acute: postural hypotension and dizziness	• Evidence of reduced blood pressure when moderate-heavy drinkers taking antihypertensives reduce alcohol intake • Acutely, alcohol causes vasodilatation

ACE, angiotensin-converting enzyme; NSAIDs, non-steroidal anti-inflammatory drugs.

- It is best to take the diuretic in the morning to limit sleep disturbance. A dose may be taken later in the day to avoid the need for urination interfering with social engagements during the day.
- Diuretic use in the elderly is associated with increased incidence of falls.
- Diuretics may cause impotence and this should be discussed with the patient.

Beta-blockers

- Male patients may experience impotence.
- Report any additional breathlessness (due to worsening of symptoms or blockade of bronchial beta$_2$-adrenoceptors); cold extremities or peripheral weakness may reflect blockade of vasodilator beta$_2$-adrenoceptors.

- Do not stop taking the tablets suddenly (as this may increase the risk of myocardial infarction). Beta-blockers should be withdrawn gradually over at least a week.

ACE inhibitors

- Patients may experience pronounced first-dose hypotension which may be worse if the patient is also taking diuretics; it is best to take the ACE inhibitor on retiring to bed at night. Discuss any cough with their general practitioner. Patients should be encouraged to persist with the ACE inhibitor, as this is an effective treatment. Recent preliminary evidence suggests that iron supplements *may* be effective against the cough.
- Consult a pharmacist before purchasing other

medicines or supplements. For example, avoid the use of potassium salts (salt substitute, effervescent preparations, cystitis treatments) and use NSAIDs with caution.

- If patients experience any lip, facial or tongue swelling (angioedema), they should stop taking the ACE inhibitor and seek immediate medical advice.

Calcium channel blockers

- Calcium channel blockers may cause flushing, constipation and ankle swelling. Gentle exercise or elevation of the foot may reduce ankle swelling. These side-effects should improve after a few weeks. If the side-effects become troublesome, patients should discuss this with their general practitioner.
- Avoid grapefruit juice if taking a DHP.

Alpha-blockers

- Patients should be alert to first-dose hypotension.
- Patients may also experience urinary incontinence.
- Take care when driving, because of possible drowsiness.

Centrally acting drugs

- Take care when driving, because of possible drowsiness.
- Do not stop taking the tablets suddenly (particularly clonidine).

Monitoring

Home and pharmacy blood pressure measurements

Automated devices are available for home monitoring by the patient. These devices measure BP on different principles from auscultation with a sphygmomanometer. Indeed, some devices measure at the wrist rather than the brachial artery and very few of these are accurate. Hence they may give differing absolute values and only a few of the devices have been validated: further

details may be obtained from the British Hypertension Society. The machine should be calibrated annually. Other sources of inaccuracy in home measuring may be poor technique such as cuff placing and inadequate resting before measurement.

'White-coat' hypertension is a well-recognised clinical phenomenon, whereby the patient's BP is significantly higher when recorded by a doctor and this is thought to be induced by anxiety. In a proportion of cases, 'white-coat' hypertension is so pronounced that patients who are normotensive under normal conditions may be classed and treated as hypertensive on the basis of measurements made by a doctor. However, 'white-coat' hypertension may be eliminated by nurses or patients themselves measuring BP. Similarly, the British Hypertension Society (O'Brien *et al.*, 2000) has produced guidelines regarding the use of ambulatory BP monitoring, which also overcomes the problems of 'white-coat' hypertension.

Prior to treatment

The following may be assessed:

- an electrocardiogram (ECG) to test for left ventricular hypertrophy, as up to a third of hypertensives have left ventricular hypertrophy. There may also be the need for an echocardiogram
- electrolytes – especially potassium, as a reduced level may reflect hyperaldosteronism. This is particularly important when initiating diuretics and ACE inhibitors
- plasma lipids and glucose. These may be adversely affected by beta-blockers and diuretics
- renal function; plasma creatinine. This will influence drug choice as thiazides, except metolazone, are ineffective in moderate renal failure and ACE inhibitors may make renal impairment worse. Dose reduction with close monitoring is required if glomerular filtration rate (GFR) is less than 50 mL/min
- urinalysis, as protein and/or blood might indicate renal damage
- full blood count
- liver function test, with mean corpuscular

volume to assess for excess alcohol consumption
- thyroid function test

During treatment

- measurement of BP
- monitor renal function and proteinuria (annually)
- monitor electrolytes, especially potassium, with diuretics and ACE inhibitors

Over-the-counter considerations

Most patients should be considered for low-dose aspirin therapy as this has been shown to reduce the incidence of myocardial infarction in hypertensive patients. Although NSAIDs should not generally be used with ACE inhibitors or thiazides, low-dose aspirin (75 mg) appears safe. Indeed, the HOT trial indicated that low-dose aspirin reduced cardiovascular events but not stroke. The British Hypertension Society recommends that low-dose aspirin is used in primary prevention in hypertensives over 50 years old who have controlled BP (<150/90 mmHg), with end-organ damage, diabetes or a 15% or greater risk of coronary artery disease over 10 years. Even low-dose aspirin is associated with gastric damage and bleeding, to which the patient should be alerted. Ibuprofen may oppose the beneficial effects of aspirin (Chapter 13).

There is some evidence that fish oil supplementation may cause a modest reduction in BP, although this has not been universally reported. None the less, fish oil supplementation appears a sensible approach to reducing overall cardiovascular risk and is advocated by the American Heart Association (Kris-Etherton *et al.*, 2002).

Some considerations of over-the-counter medicines and their use in hypertension are detailed in Table 11.4.

Alternative remedies

Consideration should be given to herbal preparations and supplements with sympathomimetic activity (Chapter 4). Diuretic effects of herbal preparations may also increase side-effects in combination with antihypertensives.

Table 11.4   Summary of the use of over-the-counter (OTC) medicines in hypertension

OTC medicine	Effects	Comments
Low-dose aspirin	Reduces risk of myocardial infarction and stroke	Need to select high-risk patients due to the risk of gastric damage associated with even low doses. Proton pump inhibitor may be used for prophylaxis
Aspirin or ibuprofen	May reduce effects of captopril Aspirin (300 mg) may reduce the effects of enalapril	Caution: blood pressure should be monitored Paracetamol is a safe alternative analgesic
Antacids	Interaction with ACE inhibitors to reduce their absorption	Separate doses
Cimetidine	May increase plasma concentrations of diltiazem and nifedipine	Ranitidine may used as an alternative
Systemic sympathomimetic decongestants	Weak pressor effects	Use topical agents (if not swallowed), steam or saline drops

ACE, angiotensin-converting enzyme.

Future developments

The currently available drug treatments for hypertension are extensive and, in the absence of a single identifiable cause, future directions are limited. Having said that, the selective endothelin receptor antagonists bosentan and darusentan are currently under trial. This class of agents is targeted against the endothelin family of peptides, which are very potent endothelium-derived vasoconstrictors.

Practice points

- The British Hypertension Society guidelines are set out in *BMJ* 319: 630–635.
- The majority of patients do not have their BP adequately controlled by the first drug used.
- Patients should be warned about first-dose hypotension with ACE inhibitors and alpha-blockers (extra caution in combination with diuretics) due to the risk of falls.
- Monitor patients for hypertension secondary to drug treatment, e.g. NSAIDs, oral contraceptives, sympathomimetics, corticosteroids, ketoconazole, moclobemide, venlafaxine and ciclosporin.
- In treatment failure consider over-the-counter drugs, alcohol consumption and compliance.
- The aim of antihypertensive treatment is to reduce cardiovascular risk, reduce/limit end-organ damage, especially kidneys, left ventricular hypertrophy, and reduce the risk of heart failure.
- Aim for BP control without unacceptable side-effects, as hypertension is generally asymptomatic.
- Always enquire about side-effects, particularly impotence.

 ### CASE STUDY

Mr AH was found by his general practitioner during a routine check-up to have a BP of 180/100 mmHg. Mr AH is 44 years old, smokes 20 cigarettes per day, drinks 'several pints each night', has a body mass index of 28 but is otherwise healthy. His father died of 'heart trouble' in his 50s.

1. What would be the first steps in the management of Mr AH?

- 180/100 mmHg is moderate hypertension; there is a need to confirm that this is sustained on several occasions (typically, three readings over 2 months). There is also a need to exclude 'white-coat' hypertension. In the meantime this is not a medical emergency. It is important to get the patient to 'own' the problem and to change his risks, rather than simply leave it as a problem to be solved with tablets. Reduce alcohol intake (a risk factor for essential hypertension), reduce body mass index to <25 (risk factor), cease smoking (whilst not a risk factor for hypertension, smoking greatly enhances the cardiovascular risk from hypertension; smoking is a major risk factor for ischaemic heart disease) and increase exercise.

Two months later Mr AH's BP was 170/98 mmHg.

2. Suggest clinical tests which might be carried out.

- if not carried out at the initial appointment, physical examination: retina for vascular damage, auscultation of heart (and kidneys for renal bruits?)

continued

CASE STUDY (continued)

- ECG to test for left ventricular hypertrophy (up to a third of hypertensives have left ventricular hypertrophy)
- echocardiogram to determine his ejection fraction
- electrolytes – especially potassium (a reduced level may reflect hyperaldosteronism; Conn's syndrome)
- plasma lipids, cholesterol, glucose
- renal function – plasma creatinine (this may influence drug choice; thiazides, except metolazone, are ineffective in moderate renal failure)
- urine – protein/blood may indicate renal damage
- the above would be the ideal, but monitoring may be poor in the community, which may lead to increased hospitalisation, e.g. hypokalaemia

3. What active treatment is he likely to receive?

- He would be started as below on thiazides as a first pharmacological step.

Following 2 months of treatment with 2.5 mg bendroflumethiazide tablets o.m. his BP is now 166/96 mmHg.

4. Why was the bendroflumethiazide o.m.?

- The diuresis would interfere with sleep if taken at night.

5. Given the poor response to bendroflumethiazide, should the dose be increased to 5 mg?

- With thiazides, increasing the dose has no additional benefit and increases the side-effects. Also, thiazides become ineffective in moderate renal failure – this could of course be the explanation for the failure of the thiazide, and so it may be worth measuring creatinine levels.

6. Draw up a plan with the various steps to continue the patient's management.

- Step 1: thiazides as a first pharmacological step. Cheap and effective. Potassium supplements are not normally needed but plasma potassium should be checked after 3–4 weeks.
- Step 2: add a beta-blocker if not contraindicated (e.g. asthma, chronic obstructive pulmonary disease; even cardioselective beta$_1$-adrenoceptor antagonists should be avoided).
- Step 3: add an ACE inhibitor (in place of a beta-blocker) to thiazide but discontinue thiazide for a few days before to prevent a dangerous drop in BP. Replace with an AT$_1$-receptor antagonist if cough is intolerable. *Or* a calcium channel blocker, but there has been some concern over the long-term safety of short-acting nifedipine – it is best to use long-acting versions, e.g. Adalat LA.
- Step 4: consider alpha-blockers, vasodilators or centrally acting agents.
- Generally, thiazides and/or beta-blockers should be regarded as the therapy of choice.

7. What special counselling is appropriate for Mr AH if he receives either atenolol (50 mg/day) or lisinopril (2.5 mg/day) in place of bendroflumethiazide?

- Atenolol: he may experience fatigue, breathlessness and cold extremities. Do not stop taking abruptly, because of receptor up-regulation.
- Lisinopril: dry cough. Take the first dose at night due to the risk of first-dose hypotension. If postural hypotension persists, this should be reported to the doctor.

→

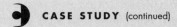

CASE STUDY (continued)

8. What would you make of a prescription for bendroflumethiazide (2.5 mg o.m.) and lisinopril (2.5 mg/day)?

- This should be discussed with the prescriber, as an ACE inhibitor on top of thiazide may cause a dangerous drop in BP. The *British National Formulary* suggests withdrawal of the thiazide temporarily before adding the ACE inhibitor. Alternatively, the ACE inhibitor could be taken at night with the thiazide taken in the morning, so that if hypotension occurs, it will be at night.

9. What are the goals of treatment for Mr AH?

- Target BP of systolic <140 mmHg and diastolic <85 mmHg. Lowering diastolic BP by 5 mmHg reduces the risk of ischaemic heart disease by 21%.
- Reduce cardiovascular risk (both stroke and myocardial infarction).
- Reduce/limit end-organ damage, especially the kidneys.
- Reduce the risk of heart failure.
- BP control without unacceptable side-effects, as hypertension is generally asymptomatic.

References

Borghi C, Prandin M G, Costa F V *et al*. (2000). Use of statins and blood pressure control in treated hypertensive patients with hypercholesterolaemia. *J Cardiovasc Pharmacol* 35: 549–555.

CAPP study group (1999). Effect of angiotensin-converting-enzyme inhibition compared with conventional therapy on cardiovascular morbidity and mortality in hypertension: the Captopril Prevention Project (CAPPP) randomised trial. *Lancet* 353: 611–616.

Dickerson J E C, Hingorani A D, Ashby M J *et al*. (1999). Optimisation of antihypertensive treatment by crossover rotation of four major classes. *Lancet* 353: 2008–2013.

Glorioso N, Troffa C, Filigheddu F *et al*. (1999). Effect of the HMG-CoA reductase inhibitors on blood pressure in patients with essential hypertension and primary hypercholesterolaemia. *Hypertension* 34: 1281–1286.

He J, Whelton P K (2000). Selection of initial antihypertensive therapy. *Lancet* 356: 1942–1943.

HOT study group (1998). Effects of intensive blood-pressure lowering and low-dose aspirin in patients with hypertension: principal results of the Hypertension Optimal Treatment (HOT) randomised trial. *Lancet* 351: 1755–1762.

Kris-Etherton P M, Harris W S, Appel L J (2002). Fish consumption, fish oil, omega-3 fatty acids and cardiovascular disease. *Circulation* 106: 2747–2757.

LIFE (Losartan Intervention for Endpoint Reduction in Hypertension) study investigators (2002). Cardiovascular morbidity and mortality in the Losartan Intervention for Endpoint reduction in hypertension study (LIFE): a randomised trial against atenolol. *Lancet* 359: 995–1003.

Mehta D K (ed.) *British National Formulary*, latest edition. London: British Medical Association and Royal Pharmaceutical Society of Great Britain.

O'Brien E, Coats A, Owens P *et al*. (2000). Use and interpretation of ambulatory blood pressure monitoring: recommendations of the British Hypertension Society. *BMJ* 320: 1128–1134.

Ramsay L E, Williams B, Johnston G D *et al*. (1999). British Hypertension Society guidelines for hypertension management 1999: summary. *BMJ* 319: 630–635.

Stevens V J, Obarzanek E, Cook N R *et al*. (2001). Long-term weight loss and changes in blood pressure: results of the trials of hypertension prevention, phase II. *Ann Intern Med* 134: 1–11.

Su S F, Hsiao C L, Chu C W *et al*. (2000). Effects of pravastatin on left ventricular mass in patients with hyperlipidaemia and essential hypertension. *Am J Cardiol* 86: 514–518.

Further reading

Brown M J (2001). Matching the right drug to the right patient in essential hypertension. *Heart* 86: 113–120.

HOPE (Heart Outcomes Prevention Evaluation) study investigators (2000). Effects of an angiotensin-converting-enzyme inhibitor, ramipril, on cardio-vascular events in high-risk patients. *N Engl J Med* 342: 145–153.

LIFE (Losartan Intervention for Endpoint Reduction in Hypertension) study investigators (2002). Cardio-vascular morbidity and mortality in patients with diabetes in the Losartan Intervention for Endpoint reduction in hypertension study (LIFE): a randomised trial against atenolol. *Lancet* 359: 1004–1010.

McInnes G (2001). Explaining hypertension and its risks to patients. *Prescriber* 12: 19–26.

PROGRESS Collaborative Group (2001). Randomised trial of a perindopril-based blood pressure-lowering regimen among 6105 individuals with previous stroke or transient ischaemic attack. *Lancet* 358: 1033–1041.

Online resources

www.bhf.org.uk is the website of the British Heart Foundation, providing patient information (accessed 4 December 2002).

www.bpassoc.org.uk is the website of the Blood Pressure Association, providing patient information (accessed 4 December 2002).

www.hyp.ac.uk/bhs is the website of the British Hypertension Society, providing professional guidance, including the validation of BP-measuring devices (accessed 4 December 2002).

12

Hyperlipidaemia

Disease characteristics

Hyperlipidaemia represents hypercholesterol-aemia and/or hypertriglyceridaemia and is a major risk factor for atherosclerotic plaque formation on the inner surface of arteries, leading to ischaemic heart disease (IHD), cerebrovascular and peripheral vascular diseases. The cause may be genetic (primary or familial hypercholesterol-aemia) or secondary to disease such as liver disease, renal failure, hypothyroidism or poorly controlled diabetes mellitus, or may be induced by drugs including:

- beta-blockers
- corticosteroids
- thiazides
- anabolic steroids
- retinoids
- oral contraceptives containing levonorgestrel

A number of modifiable risk factors may contribute towards or exacerbate this condition:

- hypertension
- smoking
- obesity
- high-fat diet
- excess alcohol consumption
- hyperglycaemia
- reduced physical activity
- infection?

and should be considered in relation to the lipid profile.

Hypercholesterolaemia

Hypercholesterolaemia is a major risk factor for atherosclerosis and is generally defined as a total plasma cholesterol greater than 6.5 mmol/L,

161

although a desirable level is less than 5.2 mmol/L. It should be recognised that 25–30% of the middle-aged population is hypercholesterolaemic.

The transport of lipids and cholesterol through the blood is carried out by one of four main classes of lipoprotein: high-density lipoprotein (HDL), low-density lipoprotein (LDL), very-low-density lipoprotein (VLDL) and chylomicrons. These lipoproteins, each with a different role, comprise a central core of hydrophobic lipid, encased in phospholipid, cholesterol and apolipoproteins. Classification is determined by differences in density, size and proportion of core lipid.

Lipoproteins

- HDL ('good cholesterol') takes up cholesterol from cell breakdown.
- LDL ('bad cholesterol') is cholesterol rich, and is taken up by the liver and tissues, which is mediated by an LDL receptor. LDL provides cholesterol for cell membranes, steroid synthesis and the production of bile acids.
- VLDL transports cholesterol and triglycerides to muscle and adipose tissue, and becomes LDL with its full complement of cholesterol.
- Chylomicrons transport triglycerides and cholesterol from the gastrointestinal tract to the liver. Free fatty acids are released to tissues and cholesterol is stored, oxidised to bile salts or released to VLDL, LDL and HDL.

Atherogenesis

Especially important in atherosclerosis is a high LDL component or low levels of HDL. Indeed, the ratio of LDL to HDL is of clinical importance (ideally <3). In relation to LDL, blood vessels have LDL receptors for cellular uptake. When injury occurs, monocytes and macrophages are activated and generate free radicals, which oxidise LDL, which in turn destroys the LDL receptor and modified LDL is taken up by macrophages. These macrophages form foam cells which collect below the endothelium, leading to fatty streaks. Platelets, macrophages and endothelial cells release inflammatory mediators and growth factors leading to proliferation of vascular smooth muscle, with vascular changes. In familial hypercholesterolaemia, the LDL receptor is defective and thus LDL is cleared less rapidly and therefore accumulates in the plasma.

In addition, the LDL component lipoprotein (a) inhibits the binding of plasminogen to endothelial receptors (responsible for plasminogen acting as a substrate for plasminogen activator). Accordingly, less plasmin is generated, so acting against fibrinolysis.

In contrast to the above, HDL binds cholesterol and removes it from local sites, taking it to the liver. Hence HDL is viewed as 'good cholesterol'.

Atherosclerosis is an inflammatory disease and there is currently some suggestion, which is not universally accepted, that atherosclerosis may be encouraged by chronic infection with *Chlamydia pneumoniae*. This is based on evidence that antibodies to *C. pneumoniae* are present in plasma of patients with myocardial infarction (MI) and its DNA has been identified in atherosclerotic plaques. It is believed that macrophages transport *C. pneumoniae* from the lungs to the vascular smooth muscle with local infection leading to damage and inflammation.

Hypertriglyceridaemia

This is elevated plasma triglyceride levels, which may or may not coexist with hypercholesterolaemia. Elevated levels of triglycerides are often associated with other conditions such as obesity, diabetes mellitus, high doses of thiazides (transiently) and high alcohol intake. Its association with atherosclerosis is less strong compared to that for hypercholesterolaemia, but at very high levels it is associated with pancreatitis.

Clinical features

The patient may have few obvious symptoms and hyperlipidaemia may only become apparent after determination of plasma lipid levels. In severe hyperlipidaemia there may be physical signs such as xanthomata, which are yellowish lipid deposits especially on the eyelids, cornea and tendons.

Coronary artery disease presenting as angina or MI is a secondary manifestation of hyperlipidaemia. It is currently believed that immediately after a heart attack plasma cholesterol levels fall for the next 3 months and that the plasma cholesterol level is not a reliable indicator during this period. This view is somewhat controversial, but National Institute of Clinical Excellence (NICE) guidelines (2001) point to an assessment of plasma cholesterol 12 weeks after a heart attack in patients who are not already receiving a statin.

Hyperlipidaemia may be associated with diabetes mellitus, renal failure and hypothyroidism, and so blood glucose levels and renal and thyroid functions should be determined to exclude possible contributions from these conditions.

Goals of treatment

The primary objective of treating hyperlipidaemia is to bring about reductions of plasma cholesterol (improving the HDL to LDL ratio) and/or reducing triglyceride levels. The target for cholesterol lowering is either to less than 5 mmol/L total cholesterol or less than 3 mmol/L for LDL. This should lead to a reduction in risk of MI and stroke. The ideal goal would be regression of atherosclerotic lesions. If diet and lifestyle modification fail, the following pharmacological interventions may be considered in addition.

Pharmacological basis of management

HMG-CoA reductase inhibitors or 'statins'

Atorvastatin, fluvastatin, pravastatin, simvastatin

The statins inhibit the hepatic enzyme, hydroxymethylglutaryl coenzyme A reductase (HMG-CoA reductase), which catalyses the first committed step of cholesterol synthesis in the liver:

Statins are hepatoselective with extensive first-pass metabolism, which is advantageous as the liver is the main site of cholesterol synthesis, with extrahepatic sites synthesising essential cholesterol.

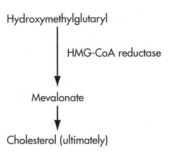

Figure 12.1 Cholesterol synthesis in the liver. HMG-CoA reductase, hydroxymethylglutaryl coenzyme A.

Bile acid-binding resins

e.g. Colestyramine

These agents bind bile salts in the intestines, preventing both their reabsorption and cycling. This interruption in bile cycling leads to incorporation of endogenous cholesterol to form bile salts and there is an increase in the number of LDL receptors, which favours the cellular uptake of cholesterol.

Colestyramine is generally used in addition to other agents and can cause a modest fall in plasma cholesterol, which may lead to a reduction in coronary artery disease. However, the binding nature of these agents will reduce the absorption of fat-soluble vitamins (A, D, E and especially K) and other drugs (including warfarin, digoxin, thiazides, thyroxine and paracetamol), which should not be given at the same time of day. Changes in the absorption of vitamin K may lead to increased effects of warfarin.

Fibrates

Bezafibrate, clofibrate, gemofibrozil

Fibrates are activators of α-peroxisome proliferator-activated receptors (PPAR-α) and lead to alterations in lipoprotein metabolism. This results in the stimulation of peripheral lipoprotein lipases, which promotes the breakdown of VLDL (with small reductions in LDL and increases in HDL) and also leads to reductions in triglycerides. The increased biliary excretion of cholesterol predisposes the patient to gallstones, particularly with clofibrate. Fibrates are therefore contraindicated in gallbladder disease. Their use is associated with a reduction in cardiovascular events but not overall mortality (VA-HIT Trial Study Group, 1999).

Nicotinic acid (niacin)

Vitamin B_3 or its derivatives inhibit hepatic triglyceride production and VLDL secretion. This results in a reduction in LDL and increase in HDL. Nicotinic acid is rarely used due to troublesome adverse effects such as headache and flushing (due to prostaglandin production, which may be reduced by taking aspirin half an hour before the dose), palpitations, pruritus, hyperglycaemia and gout.

Fish oils

Fish oils rich in omega-3 fatty acids (eicosapentaenoic acid and docosahexaenoic acid) are used for hypertriglyceridaemia, although they do increase levels of LDL.

The low incidence of coronary artery disease in Eskimos is attributed to their high dietary intake of omega-3 fatty acids in oily fish. A fish-rich diet following MI has been demonstrated to reduce mortality and reinfarction significantly. The consumption of at least two portions of oily fish per week or supplementation with fish oils is recommended by the American Heart Association (Kris-Etherton *et al.*, 2002). Fish oils should be used with caution in diabetes, haemorrhagic disorders, anticoagulant treatment and aspirin-sensitive asthma.

Antioxidants

Vitamin E is an antioxidant and oxidation of LDL is important in atherosclerosis. The Cambridge Heart Antioxidant Study (CHAOS) (Stephens *et al.*, 1996), in which patients with angiographic coronary atherosclerosis were given 400–800 IU vitamin E, found that this treatment reduced the risk of non-fatal MI but mortality was not affected. However, the GISSI Study Group (1999) found that fish oils but not vitamin E reduced cardiovascular risk in patients who had previously had MI. Furthermore, in patients with a high risk of death from cardiovascular disease (diabetes mellitus, ischaemic heart disease, hypertension or arterial disease), the Heart Protection Study Collaborative Group (2002b) found that supplementation with beta-carotene, vitamin C or vitamin E did not reduce mortality.

Sitostanol

This is a functional food that is added to certain brands of margarine and prevents the absorption of cholesterol. Additions of sitostanol to the diet reduce LDL by 10–15% and may be helpful as an addition to dietary restrictions or statin therapy.

Hormone replacement therapy

The apparent protective effect of oestrogen in premenopausal women has, for a long time, implicated a role for hormone replacement therapy (HRT) in the prevention of IHD in postmenopausal women. One of the effects of oestrogen was thought to be in reducing plasma cholesterol levels. There is now, however, increasing evidence that HRT may not be protective in secondary prevention (Heart and Estrogen/progestin Replacement Study (HERS), 1998) and so the role of HRT in the prevention of IHD is uncertain. Furthermore, a recent large-scale trial involving HRT was stopped in 2002 when there was an increase in both heart attacks and strokes in patients receiving HRT.

Ispaghula

Supplementation with non-starch polysaccharides (NSPs) reduces the absorption of bile acids and therefore leads to a reduction in LDL. It has no effect on triglyceride levels and is used to treat patients with mild to moderate hypercholesterolaemia who have not responded to dietary changes alone. Contraindications include intestinal obstruction, faecal impaction and colonic atony.

Choice of drugs

The number of patients who may potentially benefit from treatment with a lipid-lowering drug is enormous. Hence there is a need to identify those patients who would benefit most. Detailed guidelines produced by the British Hyperlipidaemia Association, in conjunction with the British Cardiac Society, British Hypertension Society and British Diabetic Association, are detailed in Wood *et al.* (1998).

The first group to target are those who have IHD manifest as either angina or previous MI, especially those who have a plasma cholesterol of greater than 4.8–5.2 mmol/L. The next group to target are those who have a greater than 30% risk of a cardiovascular event in the next 10 years through other risk factors (such as hypertension, diabetes mellitus) and whose plasma cholesterol is greater than 5 mmol/L. Risk prediction in primary prevention may readily be determined by referring to appropriate tables, which are now available in the *British National Formulary*. The Heart Protection Study Collaborative Group (2002a) found that treatment of patients at high risk of death from cardiovascular disease (diabetes mellitus, IHD, hypertension or arterial disease) with simvastatin reduced cardiovascular events by a quarter to a third. This effect was irrespective of cholesterol levels and was additive with other protective drugs such as angiotensin-converting enzyme (ACE) inhibitors, beta-blockers and aspirin.

Hypercholesterolaemia

In hypercholesterolaemia, once dietary changes have been tried, statins would be the drugs of choice. Statins are of benefit in types IIa and IIb hyperlipoproteinaemia (elevated LDL and LDL/VLDL respectively). They cause a reduction in plasma cholesterol, while the reduction in hepatic cholesterol synthesis leads to an up-regulation of hepatic LDL receptors, promoting LDL uptake. However, with the exception of atorvastatin, they are less effective in homozygous familial hypercholesterolaemia, a very rare condition where the LDL receptor is lacking.

The 4S trial (Pedersen *et al.*, 1994) (Scandinavian Simvastatin Survival Study) reported that simvastatin, in patients who had previously had an MI or had angina, caused a 35% reduction in LDL (increased HDL) and over 5 years this was associated with a 30% reduction in mortality and a 42% reduction in deaths due to coronary artery disease. The WOSCOPS trial (Shepherd *et al.*, 1995) also confirmed the effectiveness of pravastatin in primary prevention, with a 20% reduction in cholesterol and a 28% reduction in mortality from coronary artery disease in patients with hypercholesterolaemia. Statins also reduce the progression of carotid artery disease and so reduce the risk of stroke. The Heart Protection Study Collaborative Group (2002a) has reported substantial benefits of simvastatin in high-risk patients, with marked reductions in events and mortality, and the protection was related to the level of risk rather than plasma lipid level. The PROSPER study (Shepherd *et al.*, 2002) has also demonstrated that pravastatin is effective at reducing mortality from coronary artery disease in elderly patients (70–84 years) with a history of or risk factors for cardiovascular disease.

The beneficial effects of statins may be due to regression of atherosclerosis, as there is some evidence that not only do they slow down atherosclerosis but they may also cause regression with lipid depletion, leading to stabilisation of lesions. A small-scale study has also indicated that fluvastatin, as a consequence of lipid lowering and direct effects on platelets, may reduce platelet activation (Osamah *et al.*, 1997).

In severe disease it may be necessary to add a fibrate, although this increases the risk of myopathy.

Hypertriglyceridaemia

As a first step, care should be taken in patients with hypertriglyceridaemia to exclude and modify causes such as excess alcohol intake, obesity and diet. Treatment of hypertriglyceridaemia is less compelling but fibrates would be the agents of choice. In this respect bezafibrate has been shown to lower triglycerides and raise HDL in patients with IHD and this was accompanied by a trend in the reduction of fatal and non-fatal MI (BIP Study Group, 2000). Gemfibrozil was also shown to lower triglycerides and raise HDL in secondary prevention and reduced cardiovascular events although not overall mortality (VA-HIT Trial Study Group, 1999). Statins may also cause a modest reduction in plasma triglycerides and may be considered first-choice agents in combined hyperlipidaemia, although only atorvastatin and simvastatin are licensed for this indication. Fish oils are also effective in hypertriglyceridaemia. Anion-exchange resins may aggravate hypertriglyceridaemia.

Homocysteinaemia

This condition is also associated with atherosclerosis and is a genetic impairment of vitamins B_6 and B_{12} and folic acid metabolism, which leads to an increase in plasma levels of homocysteine. This induces oxidative stress, which predisposes towards atherosclerosis and thrombogenesis. Folic acid is thought to reduce plasma homocysteine levels and reduce the progression of atherosclerosis.

Concurrent illnesses

Clinically significant hyperlipidaemia that necessitates treatment is likely to occur in the older patient population where a range of other illnesses may coexist. Of specific importance to atherosclerosis are diabetes mellitus and hypertension, both of which should be treated in concert with lipid lowering. Some considerations of drug prescribing in concurrent conditions are summarised in Table 12.1.

Drug interactions

When considering drug choice within the lipid-lowering agents, interactions should be considered (Table 12.2).

In addition to within-group interactions, anti-hyperlipidaemic drugs show a range of interactions and some important examples are summarised in Table 12.3.

General counselling

In a patient with hyperlipidaemia the counselling should first be directed at lifestyle advice to attempt to reduce plasma cholesterol and other risk factors for atherosclerosis. In relation to hyperlipidaemia it may be worth talking in terms of the blood containing too much of a fatty substance which, over time, can lead to the patient having a heart attack or stroke. The good news is that, by altering diet, with or without taking drugs, the risk of having a heart attack or stroke is reduced. The patient would be advised to reduce the intake of fatty foods, especially dairy products, and perhaps to consider a Mediterranean diet with plenty of oily fish, fruit and vegetables. Dietary changes alone may cause a modest reduction in plasma cholesterol but this is limited, as only 25–30% of cholesterol is derived from the diet. The importance of smoking cessation should be emphasised. Weight reduction, increased physical activity and reduction of excessive alcohol consumption would all be beneficial.

Patients with suspected familial hypercholesterolaemia should be advised that other members of their family should be screened and counselled.

Specific counselling is detailed below.

Statins

- Statins should be taken at night (this offsets a nocturnal increase in cholesterol synthesis), except atorvastatin (which has a prolonged half-life).
- They may cause myopathy (rarely leading to rhabdomyolysis) and so patients should immediately report any unexplained muscle pains, tenderness or weakness to their general practitioner (GP).
- Patients may expect to suffer from headaches, nausea and gastrointestinal pain. These side-effects should improve as treatment continues.
- Statins exhibit a number of interactions. Some statins may enhance plasma levels of warfarin (Chapter 15), and so patients should be advised to inform other healthcare professionals that they are receiving this drug. The international normalised ratio (INR) should ideally be checked before and 5 days after treatment with an interacting drug.
- It is important to continue with the recommended dietary and lifestyle changes.

Table 12.1   Effects of concurrent conditions on drug choice in hyperlipidaemia

Conditions	Effects on drug choice	Comments
Liver disease	A reason to avoid statins and severe disease would be a reason to avoid fibrates	Anion-exchange resins are contraindicated in complete biliary obstruction as they are ineffective
Cholecystectomy	Clofibrate causes gallstones	Clofibrate should only be used in patients who have already had their gallbladder removed
Hypertension	It is well established that thiazides alter lipid profile, by raising cholesterol and triglycerides. Statins may themselves lower blood pressure, when used with antihypertensive drugs	Whether the increase in cholesterol with thiazides is sustained is unclear, but this adverse reaction may have a bearing on the treatment of borderline cases of hyperlipidaemia
Recent heart attack	The PRISM trial (PRISM Investigators, 2002) has indicated that patients who are taking a statin prior to an MI are at increased risk of further cardiac events for the following week if the statin is abruptly withdrawn at the time of the initial event	This effect appeared to be independent of the effects of the statins on plasma lipids and may be due to the loss of other beneficial effects. This suggests that statin therapy should not be abruptly withdrawn in these patients
Renal impairment	May necessitate dose reductions (consult BNF)	The risk of rhabdomyolysis is increased in those with renal impairment (CSM). Modified-release bezafibrate is not appropriate in renal impairment
Diabetes mellitus	Fibrates improve glucose tolerance with an additive effect in combination with hypoglycaemic agents	A reduction in the dose of hypoglycaemic agent may be necessary, particularly with clofibrate. Nicotinic acid should be used with caution
Gout	Nicotinic acid should be used with caution in gout	
Dementia	A recent report (Jick et al., 2000) has also claimed that statins, in the absence or presence of hyperlipidaemia, reduce the risk of dementia and this may also have a bearing on its selection	
Hypothyroidism	Increased risk of rhabdomyolysis with statins and fibrates (CSM)	
Pregnancy	Statins, nicotinic acid and fibrates are contraindicated in pregnancy and breast-feeding	With statins, adequate contraception should be used during treatment and for 1 month after stopping
Postmenopausal osteoporosis	Statins may reduce bone turnover (Rejnmark et al., 2002)	
Peptic ulcer	Nicotinic acid should be used with caution	

PRISM, Platelet Receptor Inhibition in Ischemic Syndrome Management; MI, myocardial infarction; BNF, *British National Formulary*; CSM, Committee on Safety of Medicines.

Table 12.2 Summary of interactions within drugs used in hyperlipidaemia

Interaction	Consequences	Comments
Fibrates and statins	This beneficially results in additional lipid lowering but increases the risk of myopathy	The adverse interaction appears rare but the agents should be used with caution. The interaction is substantial with cerivastatin and gemfibrozil; cerivastatin has now been withdrawn
Colestyramine with fluvastatin/pravastatin	Increased lipid-lowering effect but reduced bioavailability of the statins	Colestyramine binds these statins and so giving the statins several hours afterwards improves bioavailability

Fibrates

- Fibrates may cause myopathy (rarely leading to rhabdomyolysis) and so patients should immediately report any muscle pains to their GP.
- Side-effects include rash, urticaria, weight gain, impotence and headache.

Anion-exchange resins

- Take other drugs or supplements 1 h before or 4–6 h after colestyramine.
- The powder may be used in sauces or added to fruit juice.
- The dose should be increased gradually and then taken regularly.
- Constipation is a common side-effect. Nausea and vomiting, diarrhoea, flatulence and abdominal discomfort may occur but should improve after the first few months of treatment.

Fish oils

- These are best taken with food.
- They may cause occasional nausea and belching.
- Fish oils contain vitamins A and D. Avoid additional supplements containing these vitamins that are stored by the body.

Ispaghula

See Chapter 9.

Monitoring

Liver function

Liver function tests should be carried out before treatment with statins and within 3 months of initiating treatment. Liver function should then be monitored on a fairly regular (6-month to yearly) basis. A sustained rise in transaminase levels of three times the upper limit of the reference range would necessitate discontinuation of treatment.

Monitoring advice for patients prescribed fenofibrate indicates that liver function tests should be repeated every 3 months for the first year. Liver function tests are also recommended before initiating long-term treatment with gemfibrozil.

Creatine kinase

A patient reporting muscle pains should have creatine kinase levels measured. A 10-fold elevation would be consistent with myopathy and treatment would be discontinued.

Over-the-counter considerations

In a patient with IHD or at a high risk from it, it would be sensible to consider low-dose aspirin as an antiplatelet drug and/or referral for a cholesterol test. Some pharmacists offer 'healthy heart checks', including blood pressure and cholesterol

Table 12.3   Summary of interactions with drugs used in hyperlipidaemia

Interacting drugs	Consequences	Comments
Warfarin with fibrates or statins	Fibrates and some statins (Chapter 15) may increase the anticoagulant effect of warfarin	INR should be monitored
Warfarin with fish oils	Fish oils may have anticoagulant effects	Additional monitoring of clotting seems appropriate
Statins or fibrates with ciclosporin	Increased levels of ciclosporin and increased risk of rhabdomyolysis with statins, particularly simvastatin, and fibrates	Pravastatin does not appear to interact adversely with ciclosporin
Statins with itraconazole	Itraconazole increases the levels of simvastatin with an increased risk of rhabdomyolysis	
Pravastatin with orlistat	Possible increase in levels of pravastatin	

INR, international normalised ratio.

measurement, medical history taking and body mass index calculations to estimate the patients' risk of heart disease whilst providing lifestyle advice before coronary artery disease becomes symptomatic. High-risk patients should be advised to wear support hosiery during long flights to reduce the risk of thromboembolism (Chapter 15). These can be purchased over the counter.

Requests for supplements should be considered in relation to prescribed treatment. For example, patients taking warfarin should be advised to have their INR checked if they wish to take fish oils, co-enzyme Q10 or vitamin E supplements. Vitamin K should be avoided. Ideally, general diet and lifestyle advice should be given to all patients requesting food supplements (Chapters 3 and 4).

Garlic supplements have been claimed to reduce plasma cholesterol; however, the evidence for this is weak and any effect is thought to be modest (Neil *et al.*, 1996). It is possible that warfarin effects will be potentiated, particularly if patients consume large quantities of garlic.

Antioxidants

As commented above, the role of antioxidants in hyperlipidaemia is unclear. Furthermore, a recent report has indicated that the antioxidants vitamins E and C, beta-carotene and selenium, when used in combination, reduce the beneficial effects of simvastatin plus niacin in patients with low HDL (Cheung *et al.*, 2001). This interaction should be borne in mind when considering the use of antioxidants.

Recent developments

Cholesterol absorption inhibitors (CAIs), such as ezetimibe, are now available. These agents, which may be used alone or in addition to a statin or fibrate, inhibit the absorption of exogenous and biliary cholesterol in the gastrointestinal tract, bringing about a reduction in total cholesterol and LDL. These agents may be ideal as an addition to statin therapy, instead of increasing the dose of statin which may be associated with side-effects.

Practice points

- Monitoring of cholesterol should be carried out in those at increased risk of heart disease.
- Lifestyle and dietary measures should be tried first and continued alongside pharmacological intervention if ineffective alone. The maintenance of dietary measures may need emphasising to the patient.
- Statins have been shown to be effective in both primary and secondary prevention.
- Fibrates are effective in mixed hyperlipidaemia and hypertriglyceridaemia.
- The Heart Protection Study Collaborative Group (2002a) suggests that simvastatin substantially reduces the risk of MI and stroke. This protection relates to patients' overall risk rather than their lipid profile.
- Statins should be taken at night (except atorvastatin) and liver function tests performed.
- Low-dose aspirin should be considered for all patients at risk of IHD.
- Health professionals should be alert to reports of muscle pain, tenderness or weakness reported by patients taking lipid-lowering drugs.

 CASE STUDY

A 58-year-old woman presents you with a prescription for simvastatin (10 mg daily o.n.). She is also taking atenolol (50 mg daily) having suffered a heart attack last year.

1. Are you happy to dispense the simvastatin? Justify your decision.

- Yes – there is no interaction with atenolol.

2. How would you counsel this patient?

- Take the simvastatin at night.
- Report any muscle pain or weakness immediately: rhabdomyolysis is a rare but important side-effect.
- She may also initially expect headache, nausea and gastrointestinal pain.
- Discuss cardiovascular risks – give up smoking if appropriate; low-fat diet; moderate exercise; weight reduction if appropriate?
- Was she taking low-dose aspirin? If not, might this be appropriate?
- It is important that she continues to take the statin long term.

3. Why is the simvastatin to be taken at night?

- Simvastatin is taken at night, when cholesterol synthesis is greatest.

4. The patient would like to know what this new prescription is for; explain in lay terms why she has this new addition.

- The new medicine is to lower the amount of a fatty substance in her blood called cholesterol which is known to cause heart trouble. Lowering the cholesterol should reduce her chances of another heart attack.

A year later, whilst being maintained on simvastatin (20 mg daily o.n.), she presents with a prescription for erythromycin (250 mg q.d.s.) for sinusitis (she is allergic to penicillin).

→

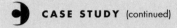 **CASE STUDY** (continued)

4. How would you respond?

• The *British National Formulary* indicates that there is an increased risk of myopathy when simvastatin is used with erythromycin. For the sake of caution the prescriber should be contacted and it might be suggested that a non-penicillin/non-cephalosporin antibacterial such as doxycycline is used as an alternative.

References

BIP Study Group (2000). Secondary prevention by raising HDL cholesterol and reducing triglycerides in patients with coronary artery disease: the bezafibrate infarction prevention (BIP) study. *Circulation* 102: 21–27.

Cheung M C, Zhao X-Q, Chait A *et al.* (2001). Antioxidant supplements block the responses of HDL to simvastatin-niacin therapy in patients with coronary artery disease and low HDL. *Atheroscl Thromb Vasc Biol* 21: 320–1326.

GISSI Study Group (1999). Dietary supplementation with n-3 polyunsaturated fatty acids and vitamin E after myocardial infarction: results of the GISSI-Prevenzione trial. *Lancet* 354: 447–455.

Heart Protection Study Collaborative Group (2002a). MRC/BHF Heart Protection Study of cholesterol lowering with simvastatin in 20 536 high-risk individuals: randomised placebo-controlled trial. *Lancet* 360: 7–22.

Heart Protection Study Collaborative Group (2002b). MRC/BHF Heart Protection Study of antioxidant vitamin supplementation in 20 536 high-risk individuals: randomised placebo-controlled trial. *Lancet* 360: 23–33.

HERS (1998). Randomized trial of oestrogen plus progestin for secondary prevention of coronary heart disease in postmenopausal women. Heart and Estrogen/progestin Replacement Study (HERS) research group. *JAMA* 280: 605–613.

Jick H, Zornberg G L, Jick S S *et al.* (2000). Statins and the risk of dementia. *Lancet* 356: 1627–1631.

Kris-Etherton P M, Harris W S, Appel L J (2002). Fish consumption, fish oil, omega-3 fatty acids and cardiovascular disease. *Circulation* 106: 2747–2757.

Mehta D K (ed.) *British National Formulary*, latest edition. London: British Medical Association and Royal Pharmaceutical Society of Great Britain.

Neil H A W, Silagy C A, Lancaster T *et al.* (1996). Garlic powder in the treatment of moderate hyperlipidaemia: A controlled trial and meta-analysis. *J R Coll Phys Lond* 30: 329–334.

NICE (2001). Prophylaxis for patients who have experienced a myocardial infarction. London: National Institute for Clinical Excellence (via www.nice.org.uk).

Osamah H, Mira R, Sorina S *et al.* (1997). Reduced platelet aggregation after fluvastatin is associated with altered platelet lipid composition and drug binding to the platelets. *Br J Clin Pharmacol* 44: 77–83.

Pedersen T R, Kjekshus J, Berg K *et al.* (1994). Randomized trial of cholesterol-lowering in 4444 patients with coronary-heart-disease – the Scandinavian Simvastatin Survival Study (4S). *Lancet* 344: 1383–1389.

PRISM Investigators (2002). Withdrawal of statins increases event rates in patients with acute coronary syndromes. *Circulation* 105: 1446–1452.

Shepherd J, Cobbe S M, Ford I *et al.* (1995). Prevention of coronary-heart disease with pravastatin in men with hypercholesterolaemia. *N Engl J Med* 333: 1301–1307.

Shepherd J, Blauw G J, Murphy M B *et al.* (2002). Pravastatin in elderly individuals at risk of vascular disease (PROSPER): a randomised controlled trial. *Lancet* 360: 1623–1630.

Stephens N G, Parsons A, Schofield P M *et al.* (1996). Randomised controlled trial of vitamin E in patients with coronary disease: Cambridge Heart Antioxidant Study (CHAOS). *Lancet* 347: 781–786.

VA-HIT Trial Study Group (1999). Gemfibrozil for the secondary prevention of coronary heart disease in men with low levels of high-density lipoprotein cholesterol. *N Engl J Med* 341: 410–418.

Wood D, Durrington P, McInnes G *et al.* (1998). Joint recommendations on prevention of coronary heart disease in clinical practice. *Heart* 80 (suppl. 2): S1–S29.

Further reading

Berger J, Moller D E (2002). The mechanisms of action of PPARs. *Annu Rev Med* 53: 409–435.

Borghi C, Prandin M G, Costa F V *et al.* (2000). Use of statins and blood pressure control in treated hypertensive patients with hypercholesterolemia. *J Cardiovasc Pharmacol* 35: 549–555.

Rejnmark L, Buus N H, Vestergaard P *et al.* (2002). Statins decrease bone turnover in postmenopausal women: a cross-sectional study. *Eur J Clin Invest* 32: 581–589.

Online resources

www.bhaonline.org.uk is the website of the British Hyperlipidaemia Association providing professional information (accessed 4 December 2002).

www.bhf.org.uk is the website of the British Heart Foundation, providing patient information (accessed 4 December 2002).

13

Ischaemic heart disease

Disease characteristics

Ischaemic heart disease (IHD), which is also referred to as coronary artery disease (CAD) or coronary heart disease (CHD), is the biggest killer in the western world and so represents a crucial area for both prevention and treatment. IHD may manifest as either angina or myocardial infarction (MI) and is an important cause of chronic heart failure (Chapter 14). In both cases, IHD is generally associated with atherosclerosis within the coronary artery, leading to impaired blood flow or thromboembolic occlusion. In angina the reductions in coronary blood flow mean that perfusion does not match demand, leading to ischaemia, which provokes the symptoms. In MI, there is often thromboembolic occlusion of the coronary artery, which may lead to acute left ventricular failure and/or arrhythmias, which are the leading cause of early mortality.

Risk factors for IHD include:

- male gender

- family history
- smoking*
- diabetes mellitus*
- hypercholesterolaemia*
- hypertension*
- sedentary lifestyle*
- obesity*

*modifiable

Angina pectoris

Angina may be divided into two groups, stable and unstable angina. Stable angina reflects atherosclerotic disease, which limits the heart's ability to respond to increased demand and is characterised by symptoms which appear on exertion but are relieved by rest. By contrast, unstable angina is generally due to plaque rupture and the formation of a non-occlusive thromboembolism, or, less commonly, vasospasm (Prinzmetal angina), both of which give rise to symptoms at rest.

The Department of Health has produced the National Service Framework (NSF) for Coronary Heart Disease and within this has stated recommendations for the prevention and management of stable angina. This NSF may be accessed via www.doh.gov.uk/nsf/.

The characteristic feature of angina is a crushing chest pain, which may radiate to the arm and jaw. Of course, chest pain may reflect a number of other causes (Chapter 1):

- myocardial infarction
- dyspepsia
- musculoskeletal pain
- pulmonary embolism

A diagnosis may be made on the basis of history and, in the case of stable angina, its provocation by exercise or eating a meal. The pain should be relieved by glyceryl trinitrate (GTN) and in stable angina is relieved by rest. An electrocardiogram (ECG) during an attack would confirm a diagnosis by showing ST-segment depression. Angina may also be secondary to increased cardiac work in anaemia (Chapter 16) and hyperthyroidism (Chapter 34), which should be excluded.

Goals of treatment of angina

Angina is a manifestation of IHD and the principal goal of treatment is the reduction of cardiovascular risk. In relation to the management of angina the specific goals are to:

- reduce symptoms
- improve exercise capacity
- reduce the risk of a heart attack
- stabilise or cause regression of atherosclerotic lesions

Management of angina

In the first instance, attention should be paid to reducing cardiovascular risk by smoking cessation, weight loss and dietary changes (Chapters 3, 11 and 12). Treatment options include percutaneous transluminal coronary angioplasty (PTCA) to open the occlusion and may include placing a stent. This often produces relief but is associated with a high rate of restenosis (reocclusion) as the physical damage caused promotes proliferation of the vascular smooth muscle. Alternatively, coronary artery bypass grafting (CABG) is a surgical option in which the diseased artery is bypassed by a saphenous vein or internal mammary artery. CABG has been proven to offer longer-term relief of symptoms but is associated with a degree of operative mortality.

Pharmacological basis of the management of angina

Drug treatment is aimed at reducing cardiac work or improving coronary blood flow. The first group of agents to consider is the nitrates.

Nitrates

GTN, isosorbide mononitrate

Nitrates cause vasodilatation via the release of nitric oxide, which gives rise to an increase in cyclic guanosine monophosphate (cGMP). In the context of angina, their beneficial effect is largely via venodilatation, leading to a decrease in preload and a reduction in cardiac work, while they may also cause coronary vasodilatation to improve coronary flow.

GTN is widely used for rapid symptomatic relief of an attack or may be given before exercise which may provoke an attack. GTN may be given by a spray under the tongue or as a sublingual tablet. Isosorbide mononitrate tablets may be given orally with the aim of giving longer-term nitrate treatment.

Beta-blockers

These are dealt with in detail in Chapter 11. In the context of angina they should be considered as first-choice drugs for prevention, with their negative inotropic and chronotropic effects reducing cardiac work and preventing symptoms. Because coronary flow only occurs during diastole, then by slowing the heart the diastolic period will be increased, as will be the time for coronary blood flow. They also have antiarrhythmic effects and reduce the risk of MI.

Calcium channel blockers

e.g. Amlodipine, diltiazem, felodipine, nifedipine, verapamil

Once again, these are dealt with in detail in Chapter 11. The calcium channel blockers give rise to vasodilatation and improve coronary blood flow, so preventing symptoms. In addition, verapamil, and to a lesser extent diltiazem, also have myocardial-depressant and bradycardic actions, so reducing cardiac work. Verapamil also exerts class IV antiarrhythmic activity.

Angiotensin-converting enzyme inhibitors

Angiotensin-converting enzyme (ACE) inhibitors are dealt with in detail in Chapters 11 and 14. In addition, the Heart Outcome Prevention Evaluation (HOPE) trial (Yusuf *et al.*, 2000) indicated that ramipril reduced mortality in patients with IHD and it may therefore be worth considering the addition of ramipril (or presumably any ACE inhibitor) to a patient with IHD.

Potassium channel activators

Nicorandil

Nicorandil is a recent addition and is a combined nitric oxide donor and activator of adenosine triphosphate (ATP)-sensitive potassium channels. The release of nitric oxide leads to an elevation in cGMP levels and the independent activation of ATP-sensitive potassium channels leads to vascular smooth-muscle hyperpolarisation with coronary artery vasodilatation and improved coronary flow. The vasodilator actions of nicorandil contribute towards its side-effects of flushing and reflex tachycardia.

Choice of drugs

All patients with angina are at a high risk of having an MI and so all patients should be considered for antiplatelet treatment with low-dose aspirin or clopidogrel. Low-dose aspirin is now well established as playing a major role in the primary and secondary prevention of MI. Aspirin inhibits irreversibly both platelet and endothelial cyclooxygenases (COX). The endothelial cells may regenerate

the COX but the platelets lack nuclei and cannot, hence endothelial production of prostacyclin may be resumed shortly afterwards, whilst the production of thromboxane is impaired until a new cohort of platelets are produced. This leads to a state which opposes platelet aggregation. Other non-steroidal anti-inflammatory drugs (NSAIDs) may cause a reversible inhibition of COX, leading to transient antiplatelet actions and so are not suitable for primary or secondary prevention. A small-scale study has in fact suggested that ibuprofen administered before aspirin may inhibit the actions of aspirin, presumably by protecting the COX against aspirin (Catella-Lawson *et al.*, 2001). The significance of this potential interaction remains to be established, but it may be sensible to avoid ibuprofen with aspirin.

Clopidogrel is an equally effective alternative antiplatelet drug for patients intolerant of aspirin. Clopidogrel inhibits adenosine diphosphate (ADP)-induced expression of platelet glycoprotein IIb/IIIa, which is involved in aggregation by cross linking fibrin.

Attention should be paid to blood pressure (to obtain a target of 140/85 mmHg; Chapter 11) and hypercholesterolaemia (to a target total cholesterol level of less than 5 mmol/L, low-density lipoprotein (LDL) below 3 mmol/L, or a 30% reduction, whichever is greater; Chapter 12).

For symptomatic relief or occasional treatment, a GTN spray or sublingual tablets would be appropriate. In terms of continuous, preventive treatment:

- First choice: beta-blockers should be used for more pronounced stable and unstable angina (but not Prinzmetal angina). Oral long-acting nitrates may be added.
- Second choice: if a beta-blocker is ineffective or contraindicated, then verapamil (or diltiazem) would be used or, failing that, a long-acting dihydropyridine. Calcium channel blockers are particularity effective at reversing vasospasm and are first choice drugs for Prinzmetal angina.
- In refractory disease: a beta-blocker may be used with dihydropyridine calcium channel blockers *but not with verapamil* as there is a severe risk of asystole; diltiazem and beta-blockers may be

used with caution. Nicorandil may also be added to therapy. If two agents fail to control the disease then surgical treatment may be required.

Although the role of nicorandil in therapy has been uncertain, the large-scale Impact Of Nicorandil in Angina (IONA) clinical trial (IONA Study Group, 2002) has found that in stable angina nicorandil, in addition to standard therapy, reduced the incidence of cardiovascular events. This indicated that nicorandil afforded cardioprotection and it was proposed that by activating cardiac mitochondrial K_{ATP}-channels it was able to mimic ischaemic cardiac preconditioning, the natural phenomenon whereby short periods of ischaemia protect the heart. This points to nicorandil as being of particular benefit in IHD.

Some compelling indications and contraindications are indicated in Table 13.1.

In addition, patients with unstable angina are likely to be maintained on a low-molecular-weight heparin.

Drug interactions

Within antianginal drugs, the major within-group interaction is between beta-blockers and verapamil, as in combination they may cause asystole. All of the agents, by acting as vasodilators, may lead to hypotension, with the possibility of a fall in the elderly.

General counselling

Counselling should be directed towards a reduction in cardiovascular risk, with smoking cessation, weight reduction, increased exercise, reduced alcohol intake and dietary changes to reduce the intake of saturated fats and increase oily fish in the diet or supplementation with fish oils. When explaining the disease to patients, one approach might be to tell them that their heart muscle is not getting enough blood to do the job that it used to, and that the pains they experience are similar to muscle cramp.

Table 13.1   Other considerations in the choice of antianginal agents

Condition	Drug choice	Comments
Heart failure	• Beta-blocker can be used with caution (Chapter 14) • Verapamil is contraindicated	
Arrhythmias	May be a reason to use a beta-blocker or verapamil	Both agents are antiarrhythmic
Chronic obstructive pulmonary disease and asthma	Contraindication for beta-blockers	Beta-blockers may lead to bronchospasm
Migraine	Beta-blocker	Beta-blockers are effective in migraine prophylaxis
Diabetes mellitus	May be a reason to avoid beta-blockers	Beta-blockers may reduce the warning signs of hypoglycaemia
Hyperthyroidism	An indication for a beta-blocker	For reduction of cardiac effects in hyperthyroidism
Glaucoma	• Closed-angle glaucoma is a contraindication for nitrates • Chronic simple glaucoma is an indication for a beta-blocker	In glaucoma, beta-blocker eye drops are absorbed and should not be used in addition to an oral beta-blocker

Nitrates

- GTN sprays or sublingual tablets should be used before an event likely to provoke an attack.
- The patient should be counselled on how to use a GTN spray and supervised in its use.
- GTN sprays or sublingual tablets may cause pronounced hypotension and are best taken whilst sitting.
- If a patient feels faint after GTN tablets then the tablet should be spat out or swallowed; the patient could also bend over and place the head between the knees.
- GTN tablets have a short shelf-life of 8 weeks and should be discarded after this time.
- When taking isosorbide mononitrate or dinitrate, then there is a substantial risk of nitrate tolerance. This may be reduced by having a nitrate-free period, usually at night when symptoms are less. Patients may be advised to take their twice-daily nitrate tablets 8 h apart, at say 8 a.m. and at 4 p.m., to give a nitrate-free period. GTN patches should also be removed for several hours each day, perhaps at night.
- If GTN does not relieve an episode of chest pain, then medical help should be sought immediately.
- Drugs which cause a dry mouth may reduce the effects of sublingual GTN (Table 5.2).

Beta-blockers

- See Chapter 11.
- Great emphasis should be made to ensure that patients do not suddenly stop taking the beta-blocker, as this is likely to lead to a worsening of symptoms and may increase their chances of having an MI.

Calcium channel blockers

- See Chapter 11.

Nicorandil

- Nicorandil may affect driving or operating machinery.
- Side-effects are related to vasodilatation and may include headache.

Myocardial infarction

MI is often due to the formation of a thrombus at the site of rupture of an atherosclerotic plaque, leading to cardiac ischaemia and damage, with early deaths due to arrhythmias and late deaths due to damage to the myocardium, which may result in heart failure. The necrotic muscle may rupture, leading to rupture of the ventricles (giving rise to tamponade) or pulmonary oedema if papillary muscles rupture and there is severe mitral regurgitation. Rupture of the septum leads to shunting, which requires surgery.

In full-thickness infarctions, the infarct may undergo thinning and stretch, causing ventricular dilatation and hypertrophy, which may lead to the development of heart failure at a later date.

Symptoms of MI

- prolonged cardiac pain – chest, throat, arms, epigastrum or back
- breathlessness
- collapse
- anxiety
- nausea/vomiting

Signs of MI

- pallor/sweating/tachycardia (due to sympathetic activation)
- vomiting/bradycardia (vagal)
- signs of impaired cardiac function
- hypotension, oliguria, cold extremities
- narrow pulse pressure
- lung crepitations
- some (especially elderly) patients have a 'silent MI' with no signs or symptoms

Differential diagnosis

- dyspepsia
- angina (which is relieved by GTN)
- musculoskeletal pains
- panic attacks
- pulmonary embolism

Diagnosis

The diagnosis is based on ECG changes (including ST-segment elevation) and increases in cardiac enzymes released by infarcted tissue. These are creatine kinase (CK), troponin T (TrT), aspartate aminotransferase (AST) and lactate dehydrogenase (LDH).

Management

The initial management of MI is beyond the scope of this book. However, a brief summary is given in Table 13.2.

For patients who survive the initial MI the outlook can be good, with on average 80% being alive after 1 year, although the outlook is influenced by the initial presentation and development of heart failure. Therefore, in primary care the central issues are secondary prevention and prevention of long-term complications such as heart failure. All patients should be counselled with respect to lifestyle changes:

- weight reduction
- dietary advice – including increased intake of oily fish
- smoking cessation
- appropriate exercise

Secondary prevention

In terms of drug treatment for secondary prevention in patients who have already had an MI there are a number of considerations and the following is, in part, based on the National Institute of Clinical Excellence (NICE) guidelines issued in 2001:

- Antiplatelet therapy with low-dose aspirin (75–150 mg) is established as substantially reducing reinfarction. In patients who are intolerant to aspirin due to asthma, then clopidogrel is indicated, and it is equally effective. Low-dose aspirin is associated with gastric damage, and prophylaxis with a proton pump inhibitor may be required (Chapter 7).

- Beta-blockade: all patients should be considered for a beta-blocker to limit cardiac work and reduce the risk of rupture, to manage stable angina and hypertension and as an antiarrhythmic. Beta-blockers are contraindicated in bradyarrhythmias. Long-term beta-blockade is well established at reducing reinfarction. If the patient has heart failure, then the beta-blocker may be introduced (after an ACE inhibitor) at a low dose and under expert supervision and would be contraindicated in severe heart failure.
- ACE inhibitors: all patients with heart failure should receive an ACE inhibitor. NICE guidelines (2001) point to an ACE inhibitor also being considered for patients without heart failure after they have been considered for a beta-blocker.
- Calcium channel blockers: these should only be considered for patients who are intolerant to beta-blockers or ACE inhibitors and for the relief of angina and/or hypertension, as there is no evidence that they reduce mortality. Diltiazem or verapamil should be used with caution because of their cardiodepressant actions.
- Statins: these should be considered for all patients. Currently plasma cholesterol should be measured within 24 h of the MI as it is believed that cholesterol falls for the first 3 months afterwards. Statins are believed to be equally effective as beta-blockers and antiplatelet drugs in secondary prevention.
- Diuretics: patients with symptomatic heart failure benefit from loop diuretics or thiazides. Patients in moderate to severe failure benefit from the addition of spironolactone.
- Antiarrhythmics: there is no evidence that long-term treatment with these agents confers any benefit in the patient post-MI, but they may be needed in some patients.
- Anticoagulants: these drugs do not appear to have a long-term role in most patients and do not appear to confer any additional benefit to aspirin, except in patients with atrial fibrillation. Fiore *et al.* (2002) have reported that the addition of warfarin to low-dose aspirin does not confer further benefit in the secondary prevention of MI.

Table 13.2   Management of a MI

Treatment	Comments
Immediate	
Soluble or chewable aspirin (150–300 mg)	This may be given as a first-aid measure as an antiplatelet treatment to reduce further thrombus formation
Oxygen	To reduce hypoxia
Nitrates	To reduce ischaemia, but they have no bearing on mortality
Morphine or diamorphine IV with antiemetics (cyclizine (but only if left ventricular function is satisfactory), prochlorperazine or metoclopramide)	• Morphine for relief of dyspnoea; also causes venodilatation to reduce preload and induces a degree of calm • An antiemetic to reduce nausea associated with opioids
Thrombolytic agent (e.g. alteplase, streptokinase, reteplase)	• Should be given to dissolve the clot as soon as possible (ideally within 90 min) and certainly within the first 12 h, unless contraindicated (including recent surgery, peptic ulceration, current menstruation, pregnancy, recent stroke, history of haemorrhagic stroke) • Streptokinase can be given up to 4 days following an initial dose but thereafter it should not be given for at least 12 months, if at all • Streptokinase may be ineffective in patients who have recently had a streptococcal sore throat, due to the production of antibodies • Streptokinase may cause an allergic reaction • Certain thrombolytic agents are now licensed for use before admission
Subsequent acute treatments	
Beta-blocker	• IV atenolol or metoprolol given early reduces arrhythmias and improves survival • Improves myocardial perfusion and reduces infarct size • Reduces chance of cardiac rupture • If beta-blockade is contraindicated and in the absence of heart failure then verapamil might be used
ACE inhibitors	• The European Society of Cardiology recommends the use of an ACE inhibitor within the first 24 h if there is evidence of heart failure emerging
Anticoagulants	• Heparin given for 7–10 days post-MI after thrombolysis may prevent reinfarction
Nitrates	• If systolic blood pressure >100 mmHg they may be given in the first 24 h to reduce cardiac work
Antiarrhythmics	• Despite arrhythmias complicating post-MI, antiarrhythmics may increase mortality • Antiarrhythmics may be proarrhythmic on the ischaemic myocardium • Beta-blockade is likely to have been initiated • Lidocaine (lignocaine) is indicated for ventricular ectopics but is less widely used now
Insulin	• NICE guidelines (2001) recommend that diabetics should receive intensive insulin therapy from admission for 3 months as this reduces mortality

IV, intravenous; ACE, angiotensin-converting enzyme; NICE, National Institute of Clinical Excellence.

Additional considerations

There is a high incidence of depression following an MI. In terms of drug treatment this may present a question of drug choice as tricyclic antidepressants have been associated with increased mortality in patients post-MI, especially if class I antiarrhythmics are also used. Currently, selective serotonin reuptake inhibitors are considered more suitable.

A history of IHD may affect other treatments, which are detailed in Table 13.3.

Specific counselling

All of the counselling for specific drugs or classes is detailed in other sections:

- beta-blockers (Chapters 11 and 14)
- ACE inhibitors (Chapters 11 and 14)
- statins (Chapter 12)

The only additional consideration is to advise patients who have received streptokinase to carry a card to alert medical staff who may treat them at a subsequent MI that they have previously received this agent.

Practice points

- An NSF sets out recommendations for the management and prevention of IHD.
- NICE guidance should be consulted for secondary prevention.
- For secondary prevention after an MI, patients are often prescribed a beta-blocker, an ACE inhibitor, a statin and an antiplatelet drug.

Table 13.3   Examples of conditions which may be affected by a previous myocardial infarction (MI)

Condition	Problems	Comments
Migraine	• 5-HT$_{1D}$ agonists (triptans) are contraindicated in patients with IHD • Ergotamine is contraindicated in IHD	The triptans may cause coronary artery spasm (Chapter 21)
Nicotine addiction	Nicotine replacement products should be avoided immediately post-MI	
Depression	Tricyclic antidepressants are contraindicated after recent MI and used with caution in cardiac disease	SSRIs appear to be more appropriate (Chapter 23)
Hypothyroidism	Levothyroxine	May cause anginal symptoms; monitor and reduce dosage in IHD (Chapter 34)
Impotence	Sildenafil	Risk of severe interactions with nitrates, as sildenafil inhibits phosphodiesterases and prevents the breakdown of cGMP. It is contraindicated after recent MI.

IHD, ischaemic heart disease; SSRIS, selective serotonin reuptake inhibitors; cGMP, cyclic guanosine monophosphate.

CASE STUDY

Mr PS (56 years) has recently suffered an MI and is on a cardiac ward. He was initially treated with streptokinase (1.5 million units IV), diamorphine (5 mg IV), cyclizine (50 mg IV) and atenolol (10 mg IV; then 50 mg b.d. for 2 days). On discharge he is now written up for:

Aspirin 75 mg daily
Atenolol 50 mg daily

1. Explain the use of all of the above drugs.

- streptokinase – to destroy the clot, leading to reperfusion
- diamorphine – pain relief (pain can be severe in MI), and may induce some euphoria
- cyclizine – H_1-receptor antagonist used as an antiemetic to prevent diamorphine-induced emesis
- atenolol – an antiarrhythmic, reduces infarct size and reduces cardiac work (risk of cardiac rupture). It improves survival
- aspirin – antiplatelet drug

2. What considerations were made before streptokinase was administered?

- Had the patient had an MI? This would be confirmed by an ECG.
- Was the MI recent, within the last 12 h? Streptokinase is only of real benefit in the first 12 h.
- Had the patient had any evidence of recent surgery, recent haemorrhagic stroke, active gastric ulceration or previous treatment with streptokinase? All of these are contraindications.

His lipid biochemistry has revealed a total cholesterol level of 7.1 mmol/L (ideal <5.2 mmol/L), triglycerides of 1.9 mmol/L (ideal < 1.9 mmol/L) and HDL of 0.9 mmol/L (ideal > 0.9 mmol/L).

3. What advice would you give concerning the management of this patient?

- Hypercholesterolaemia – there is a need to reduce total cholesterol and LDL. Statins should be given to MI patients. Statins are proven to reduce cardiovascular risk and may cause regression of coronary artery disease.
- Simvastatin (20 mg o.n.) should be prescribed.
- Statins reduce total cholesterol and decrease LDL.
- Statins (except atorvastatin) are taken at night to offset the nocturnal increase in cholesterol synthesis.
- Liver function tests should be carried out before and 1–3 months after starting the statin.
- All post-MI patients should be discharged on an ACE inhibitor if appropriate.

4. How would you counsel the patient with regard to treatment with streptokinase and simvastatin?

- Streptokinase: the patient should carry a streptokinase card. Further treatment with this agent may be ineffective or provoke an anaphylactic reaction due to the antibodies raised.
- Simvastatin: this should be taken at night; the patient should stick to the recommended diet; and report muscle pains straight away as they may indicate rhabdomyolysis. Ten per cent of patients have gastrointestinal disturbances.

On presentation of a repeat prescription to his community pharmacist, Mr PS complains of indigestion-type discomfort.

continued

CASE STUDY (continued)

5. What do you advise?

• Refer to the GP – the discomfort may be due to cardiac symptoms or gastric irritation due to aspirin.

Several years later Mr PS is experiencing chest pains and is prescribed GTN sublingual tablets (500 µg p.r.n.).

6. How would you counsel Mr PS?

• Take the GTN when symptoms develop or before provoking event.
• Sit down whilst taking the GTN.
• Place the tablet under the tongue.
• Spit it out or swallow the tablet if the patient feels faint.
• Keep in the original container and discard after 8 weeks.
• Any headache may be managed with paracetamol.

The above treatment is only partially successful and Mr PS is now prescribed verapamil (80 mg t.d.s.).

7. Are you happy to dispense the new prescription?

• No – we do not know whether he is still taking atenolol. There is a risk of a serious interaction of beta-blockers and verapamil, and the cardiac depression could cause asystole.

References

Catella-Lawson F, Reilly M P, Kapoor S C *et al.* (2001). Cyclooxygenase inhibitors and the antiplatelet effects of aspirin. *N Engl J Med* 345: 1809–1817.

Fiore L D, Ezekowitz M D, Brophy M T *et al.* (2002). Department of Veterans Affairs Cooperative Studies Program clinical trial comparing combined warfarin and aspirin with aspirin alone in survivors of acute myocardial infarction – primary results of the CHAMP study. *Circulation* 105: 557–563.

IONA Study Group (2002). Effect of nicorandil on coronary events in patients with stable angina: the Impact Of Nicorandil in Angina (IONA) randomised trial. *Lancet* 359: 1269–1275.

NICE (2001). NICE guidance on prophylaxis for patients who have experienced a myocardial infarction. London: National Institute for Clinical Excellence (via www.nice.org.uk).

Yusuf S, Sleight P, Pogue J *et al.* (2000). Effects of an angiotensin converting-enzyme inhibitor, ramipril, on cardiovascular events in high-risk patients. The Heart Outcomes Prevention Evaluation Study Investigators. *N Engl J Med* 342: 145–153.

Further reading

ACE Inhibitor Myocardial Infarction Collaborative Group (1998). Indications for ACE inhibitors in the early treatment of acute myocardial infarction. *Circulation* 97: 2202–2212.

Cohen H W, Gibson G, Alderman M H (2000). Excess risk of myocardial infarction in patients treated with antidepressant medications: association with use of tricyclic agents. *Am J Med* 108: 2–8.

de Bono D P, Hopkins A (1994). The management of acute myocardial infarction: guidelines and audit standards. *J R Coll Phys Lond* 28: 312–317.

ISIS-2 (Second International Study of Infarct Survival) Collaborative Group (1988). Randomised trial of intravenous streptokinase, oral aspirin, both, or neither among 17 187 cases of suspected acute myo-cardial infarction: ISIS-2. *Lancet* ii: 349–360.

McGlynn S, Reid F, McAnaw J *et al.* (2000). Coronary heart disease. *Pharm J* 265: 194–205.

Roose S P (2000). Considerations for the use of anti-depressants in patients with cardiovascular disease. *Am Heart J* 140 (suppl. S): 584–588.

Saltissi S, Mushahwar S (1995). Myocardial infarction: prophylaxis after infarction. *Prescribers J* 35: 149–158.

Scandinavian Simvastatin Survival Study Group (1994). Randomised trial of cholesterol lowering in 4444 patients with coronary heart disease: the Scandinavian Simvastatin Survival Study (4S). *Lancet* 344: 1383–1389.

Online resources

www.bhf.org.uk is the website of the British Heart Foundation, providing patient information (accessed 4 December 2002).

www.doh.gov.uk/nsf/ is the website of the Department of Health and contains the NSF for Coronary Heart Disease (accessed 4 December 2002).

14

Heart failure

Disease characteristics

In simple terms, heart failure may be viewed as a failure of the heart as a pump to meet the circulatory needs and this may be either acute (for example following a heart attack or volume loading) or chronic. The underlying cause is failure of the heart muscle, sustained arrhythmias (such as atrial fibrillation) or failure of the heart valves (through infection or ageing-related changes).

The leading causes (70%) of chronic heart failure (CHF) are ischaemic heart disease and hypertension. In the case of hypertension, the increased afterload leads in time to hypertrophy. The cardiac enlargement thus increases the work of the heart and lessens the ejection fraction. Indeed, a compelling reason to treat hypertension is to reduce the likelihood of developing CHF. Heart failure associated with ischaemic heart disease results from reduced blood flow, leading to impaired cardiac muscle function, with a reduction in pump performance. Cardiomyopathies due to alcohol abuse, infection and drug treatment (e.g. anthracycline anticancer drugs) may also cause CHF. Other causes of heart failure are pregnancy, anaemia, thyrotoxicosis, excessive infusion of intravenous (IV) fluids and fluid-retaining drugs (e.g. non-steroidal anti-inflammatory drugs (NSAIDs), glucocorticoids, mineralocorticoids) and these should be excluded.

Underlying pathology

The key change, to which therapy is ideally targeted, is inappropriate neurohormonal adaptation. As a pathophysiological adaptation, in an attempt to compensate for circulatory failure, there is activation of the sympathetic nervous system and the renin–angiotensin–aldosterone

185

system (RAAS), with increased release of anti-diuretic hormone (ADH), although there is also a release of atrial natriuretic peptide (ANP) from the dilated heart. While these activations may seem logical to restore circulatory function, the increased sympathetic and RAAS activities increase arterial vascular resistance (afterload) and venous return (preload), thus increasing the workload of the heart. The increased sympathetic activity will also attempt to increase the force of cardiac contraction but will predispose towards arrhythmias. The attendant increase in circulating volume, evoked principally by the RAAS, will similarly increase preload and afterload on the heart. Consequent to the increased resistance there is impaired renal function, with additional salt and water retention with further activation of RAAS. Hence a vicious cycle develops which further impairs the pump activity of the heart. A consequence of these changes is oedema (congestion) at different sites in the body and the term 'congestive heart failure' is also widely used (Figure 14.1).

The neurohormonal activation also leads to myocyte dysfunction, with increased aldosterone activity leading to fibrosis and stiffening of the cardiac muscle, further impairing pump activity.

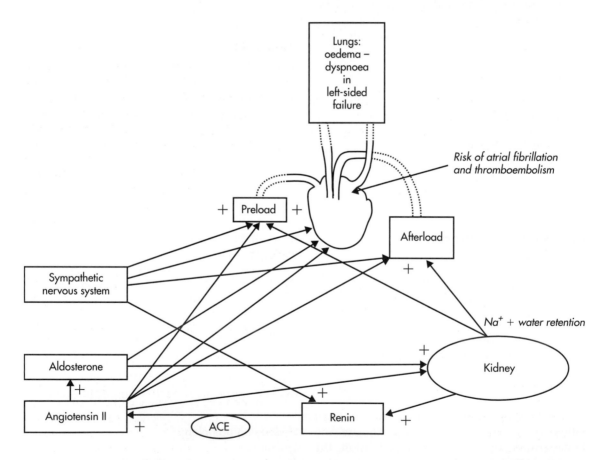

Figure 14.1   Schematic diagram of the principal pathophysiological changes and interactions in chronic heart failure. Activation of the renin–angiotensin systems leads to increased levels of angiotensin II (via angiotensin-converting enzyme (ACE)) which activates (+) the release of aldosterone, promotes sodium retention, causes arterial and venous vasoconstriction and causes cardiac remodelling. The sympathetic nervous system also stimulates renin release and causes both arterial and venous vasoconstriction. Aldosterone promotes sodium retention and is associated with cardiac fibrosis. Sodium and water retention increase the circulating volume, with increases in preload and afterload.

Classification

Left-sided failure

- This is the most common form of heart failure, and is often secondary to hypertension.
- Left ventricular (systolic) function is impaired, with poor output leading to increased left atrial and pulmonary venous pressures with pulmonary congestion and oedema.

Right-sided failure

- Right-sided failure is often due to chronic lung disease (cor pulmonale).
- Right ventricular output falls, leading to increased venous pressure, with peripheral oedema.

Biventricular failure

- Both main chambers are affected as left and right ventricular failure often coincide. Diseases such as ischaemic heart disease may have affected both ventricles.
- Often, left ventricular failure leads to pulmonary congestion, which in turn impairs right ventricular function, causing failure on the right side as well.

Clinical features

As one might predict from a failure of the heart to meet circulatory needs, cardiovascular-related features are:

- reduced ejection fraction (<45%), as identified on an echocardiogram. This leads to impaired exercise tolerance
- hypotension, leading to tiredness and possibly dizziness
- reduced urine flow
- cold peripheries
- breathlessness
- oedema

With associated, non-specific symptoms:

- fatigue, listlessness
- poor exercise tolerance (determines grade)
- weight loss or even gain due to oedema

Left ventricular failure

The key feature is pulmonary oedema, which leads to dyspnoea with a sensation of drowning. There is often marked orthopnoea, as lying down leads to further venous congestion, which is relieved on sitting up or standing. This is particularly pronounced in bed and patients often describe having to go to the window 'to get air'. Using pillows to prop the patient up may relieve orthopnoea in bed and the number of pillows used may be a guide to the severity of this symptom. The pulmonary congestion may also lead to a cough, with sputum which may or may not be frothy and contain blood.

Right ventricular failure

The leading feature of right ventricular failure is raised venous pressure, which leads to peripheral oedema (typically in the ankles on standing, and which may shift to the sacral regions whilst lying down). The raised venous pressure will also manifest as raised jugular venous pressure (JVP, which is raised if greater than 4 cm from the clavicular line). The increased venous pressure may also lead to hepatomegaly (enlarged liver), with abdominal discomfort.

Atrial fibrillation

A major and common consequence of cardiac failure is a build-up of back-pressure in the heart, as there is impaired ejection. This often leads to dilatation of the left atria and the physical distension of the muscle causes disturbances in atrial electrical activity, resulting in atrial fibrillation. This does not greatly impair cardiac function; however, the consequent stasis of blood in the left atria increases the likelihood of thrombi forming. These may dislodge and travel to the cerebral circulation, giving rise to thromboembolic occlusion, resulting in transient ischaemic attacks or stroke.

The key feature of a patient with atrial fibrillation is an irregularly irregular pulse. Atrial fibrillation is readily identified on an electrocardiogram (ECG) as the absence of P waves and irregular QRS complexes.

Goals of treatment

The main goal of treatment is to improve the quality of life by relieving symptoms and if possible to reverse or modify the disease processes. The Department of Health has produced the National Service Framework (NSF) for Coronary Heart Disease and within this has stated recommendations for the prevention and management of heart failure. This NSF may be accessed via www.doh.gov.uk/nsf/.

The simplest approach is to treat any underlying causes, such as valvular disease or ischaemic heart disease or atrial fibrillation. In both cases this may involve cardiac surgery.

The principles of medical management using drugs are to (Greene and Harris, 2000):

- reduce cardiac workload – using diuretics and vasodilators
- increase cardiac output – using positive inotropic agents
- counteract maladaptation – antagonising the neurohormonal adaptation

If atrial fibrillation is present, additional aims are to control ventricular rate and to prevent thrombus formation, reducing the likelihood of a transient ischaemic attack.

Pharmacological basis of management (Table 14.1)

Angiotensin-converting enzyme inhibitors

e.g. Captopril, enalapril, lisinopril, perindopril, ramipril

Angiotensin-converting enzyme (ACE) inhibitors are now recognised as first-line therapy in CHF and may be given to asymptomatic patients. They are proven to both reduce symptoms and improve prognosis (Cooperative North Scandinavian Enalapril Survival Study (CONSENSUS) trial: Swedeberg, 1987). By inhibiting the ACE, they lead to reductions in the neurohormonal adaptation due to angiotensin II and aldosterone, with the following consequences:

- reduction in arterial and venous vasoconstriction (reduced after- and preload)

- reduction in salt and water retention, hence reduced circulating volume
- indirect positive inotropic effect
- prevention and reversal of cardiac remodelling due to RAAS

Clinical use

By the nature of their action, ACE inhibitors may cause severe hypotension (in about 2% of patients) and are best given initially on retiring at night. A low starting dose should be used and titrated up to the maximum tolerated dose. In certain patients at high risk, including those with a systolic blood pressure less than 90 mmHg, treatment should be initiated in hospital under supervision. There should be close monitoring of creatinine, urea and electrolyte levels before and after each dosage change.

The renin–angiotensin system is activated in renovascular disease in order to maintain renal perfusion and filtration. Hence ACE inhibitors may cause deterioration of renal function in pre-existing renal disease and these patients should be identified by measurement of plasma creatinine and should receive ACE inhibitors with great caution.

Angiotensin II receptor antagonists

e.g. Candesartan, irbesartan, losartan, valsartan

This new class of drugs blocks the action of angiotensin II at the AT_1 receptor, which will also reduce the stimulation of aldosterone release. Hence AT_1 receptor antagonists act in a similar manner to ACE inhibitors but do not give rise to a cough. These agents are not currently licensed for heart failure but the ELITE II trial (Pitt *et al.*, 2000) reported that losartan was equally effective at reducing mortality in elderly patients with heart failure as captopril, but it was also better tolerated. Similarly preliminary results from a recent trial (Val-HeFt: Cohn and Tognoni, 2001) have indicated that valsartan improves the quality of life in patients with heart failure. AT_1 receptor antagonists may also be used in conjunction with ACE inhibitors.

Table 14.1   Summary of principal effects of drugs used in heart failure

Drug	Pharmacological targets	Mechanism	Effects
ACE inhibitors	Renin–angiotensin system (RAS)	Inhibition of ACE	• Decreased arterial and venous vasoconstriction • Decreased blood volume • Decreased compensatory effects of RAS
Loop diuretics	Kidney: loop of Henle	Inhibition of $Na^+/K^+/2Cl^-$ transporter in loop of Henle	• Na^+ excretion • Decreased blood volume • Decreased plasma K^+
Thiazide diuretics	Kidney: distal convoluted tubule	Inhibition of Na^+/Cl^- reabsorption	• Na^+ excretion • Decreased blood volume • Decreased plasma K^+
Potassium-sparing diuretics (amiloride)	Kidney: aldosterone-responsive segment of distal tubule	Decreased Na^+ permeability due to blockade of Na^+ channels	• Weak diuretic effect (increased Na^+ excretion) with decreased K^+ excretion
Potassium-sparing diuretics (spironolactone)	Kidney: as above	Aldosterone receptor antagonist	• Weak diuretic effect (increased Na^+ excretion) with decreased K^+ excretion • Reverses adverse effects of aldosterone on the heart
Beta-blockers	Myocardium	Antagonism of cardiac beta-adrenoceptors	• Reduce sympathetic drive to the heart • Oppose neurohormonal adaptation • Antiarrhythmic actions
Digoxin	Myocardium, AV node	Inhibition of Na-pump	• Positive inotropic effects • Induces a degree of AV block
Nitrates	Vascular smooth muscle	Increased cGMP production	• Vasodilatation
Alpha-blockers (prazosin or mixed alpha-betablocker carvedilol)	Sympathetic nervous system	Alpha-adrenoceptor antagonists	• Vasodilatation

ACE, angiotensin-converting enzyme; AV, atrioventricular; cGMP, cyclic guanosine monophosphate.

Diuretics

Thiazides and related agents (e.g. bendroflumethiazide, indapamide, metolazone); loop diuretics (e.g. furosemide (frusemide))

Diuretics are the mainstay of drug treatment in heart failure and provide rapid symptomatic relief. Diuretics reduce circulating volume, thus decreasing preload and afterload and hence cardiac work. In addition, they may have direct vascular effects leading to venodilatation, which further reduces preload. Diuretics provide relief for the symptoms of congestion but do not affect the progression of the disease.

Thiazides act in the distal convoluted tubule to inhibit Na^+/Cl^- reabsorption. Loop diuretics inhibit the $Na^+/K^+/2Cl^-$ cotransporter in the thick ascending limb of the loop of Henle, inhibiting the establishment of a hyperosmotic interstitium and so reducing the ability of the kidneys to produce concentrated urine, leading to profuse diuresis.

Clinical use

The rational use of diuretics includes situations where there is oedema (peripheral or pulmonary). Thiazides induce modest diuresis and are used in mild failure or in the elderly. Loop diuretics, which are more extensively used, cause very pronounced diuresis and are especially useful in causing rapid relief of pulmonary oedema. Indeed, intravenous furosemide rapidly reduces the dyspnoea associated with pulmonary oedema in acute left ventricular failure. This effect precedes the diuresis and is thought to be due to venodilatation reducing preload on the heart.

Why do thiazides and loop diuretics cause hypokalaemia?

Hypokalaemia is a major side-effect of these diuretic agents. By acting on the kidney, largely before the distal tubule, these agents increase the sodium content in the tubular fluid. Under the control of aldosterone, the distal tubule attempts to reabsorb sodium (via amiloride-sensitive sodium channels) but at the cost of excreting potassium. In addition, these agents will also provoke the release of renin and the activation of RAAS, which will further promote the excretion of potassium. By contrast, ACE inhibitors will oppose the aldosterone-sensitive potassium loss and there is a risk of significant hyperkalaemia if the ACE inhibitor is given in addition to potassium supplements or potassium-sparing diuretics (e.g. amiloride, spironolactone).

Spironolactone

This is an aldosterone receptor antagonist, which acts as a weak potassium-sparing diuretic. It is now used at a low dose (25 mg), which does not have pronounced haemodynamic effects but reverses the aldosterone-mediated neurohormonal changes. Even following ACE inhibition, aldosterone levels may still be appreciable and so spironolactone is able to exert substantial beneficial effects. It is thought that spironolactone inhibits aldosterone-induced fibrosis, which otherwise stiffens the heart and is associated with arrhythmias. It may also inhibit the adverse effects of aldosterone on autonomic and baroreceptor function. The RALES trial (Pitt *et al.*, 1999) in which low-dose spironolactone was added to conventional therapies, indicated that this treatment reduced mortality by 30%.

Digoxin

Digoxin used to be the mainstay of therapy and has been in and out of fashion over many years. Its principal action is as a positive inotrope by inhibiting Na^+/K^+ ATPase (which causes a rise in intracellular sodium, which promotes calcium entry, leading to increased force of contraction). However, digoxin also directly and indirectly (via central vagal activation) impairs atrioventricular conduction. This induction of heart block and bradycardia is beneficial in heart failure with atrial fibrillation as it controls ventricular rate. Indeed, it is now widely believed that digoxin should be reserved for heart failure with atrial fibrillation, or when treatment with an ACE inhibitor and a diuretic is inadequate for patients in sinus rhythm.

Clinical usage

Digoxin improves the patient's symptoms, reduces hospitalisation but does not affect all-cause mortality (DIG trial: Digitalis Investigation Group, 1997). Digoxin has a very narrow therapeutic window and is largely renally excreted, which means that renal function should be taken into account, with dose reductions to prevent increased plasma concentrations and toxicity. Digoxin is associated with a range of significant side-effects which include:

- anorexia
- nausea
- gastrointestinal disturbances
- visual disturbances
- arrhythmias

Beta-blockers

Bisoprolol, carvedilol and metoprolol

Beta-adrenoceptor antagonists have traditionally been contraindicated in heart failure, as they reduce sympathetic drive to a failing heart or may precipitate failure in compensated failure. However, there is now evidence that they reduce disease progression, symptoms and mortality (CIBIS-II Investigators and Committee, 1999; MERIT-HF Study Group, 1999). Principally, beta-blockers:

- reduce sympathetic stimulation, heart rate and oxygen consumption
- reduce sudden death by their antiarrhythmic properties
- oppose the neurohormonal activation which leads to myocyte dysfunction

In addition, carvedilol causes vasodilatation as it is also an alpha-blocker, and its antioxidant properties may also be beneficial.

Clinical usage

Metoprolol, bisoprolol and carvedilol are now being increasingly used in patients with stable, moderate heart failure and are especially useful in patients with cardiac ischaemia. However, their use is contraindicated in patients with chronic obstructive pulmonary disease (COPD), which is relatively common in the patient population with the highest incidence of heart failure. Their use would also be contraindicated in hypotension and marked bradycardia.

Beta-blockers should be initiated starting with a low dose under the supervision of a cardiologist or general practitioner (GP) experienced in their usage. The beta-blocker may initially cause a worsening of symptoms but benefit may become apparent after several weeks.

Vasodilators

Nitrates in particular may have a role in CHF as they will cause venodilatation, leading to a reduction in preload. Many patients will also have ischaemic heart disease and so nitrates will also be of benefit in these patients. Nitrates may be suitable for people in whom ACE inhibitors are not tolerated but are contraindicated in hypotension and marked anaemia.

Other vasodilators which may be added on to therapy are alpha-blockers such as prazosin, which will reduce peripheral resistance by opposing sympathetic activity. They are of no proven benefit. The arterial vasorelaxant hydralazine is also used as an add-on drug or for those intolerant of ACE inhibitors.

Other positive inotropes

In addition to digoxin, phosphodiesterase inhibitors (PDEIs) such as milrinone have a limited role. These drugs act to potentiate cyclic adenosine monophosphate (cAMP) in myocytes and so have positive inotropic effects and are used in end-stage failure on a short-term basis in hospital. It should be noted that their long-term use is associated with increased mortality.

Amines such as dobutamine, which acts as a beta-agonist, similarly may have a role in the management of acute failure and end-stage failure in the context of specialist hospital care.

Choice of drugs

This is largely stage (New York Heart Association)-dependent:

- Stage I (asymptomatic)
- Stage II (slight limitations through breathlessness/fatigue on normal exertion)
- Stage III (marked limitations through breathlessness/fatigue on normal exertion)
- Stage IV (breathless at rest)

NICE released guidance in July 2003 that should be consulted and points to ACE inhibitors being used in all cases of left ventricular systolic dysfunction, diuretics where there is oedema and beta-blockers are now recognised as having an important role.

Concurrent disease

Additional considerations when prescribing in CHF

- Renal impairment may preclude the use of ACE inhibitors and thiazides and lead to a dose reduction with digoxin. In moderate failure higher doses of loop diuretics are required and in anuria their use would be precluded.
- Liver function: close monitoring with ACE inhibitors is important in liver disease. Warfarin and carvedilol should be avoided and a reduced dose of metoprolol may be required. The use of potassium-sparing diuretics may be necessary. This is due to the risk of precipitating coma if hypokalaemia develops during treatment with loop and thiazide diuretics. There is also an increased risk of hypomagnesaemia in alcoholic cirrhosis. Thiazides should be avoided in severe liver disease.
- Atrial fibrillation would be a compelling reason to use digoxin and an indication for an anticoagulant (Chapter 15). Amiodarone may also be required.
- COPD and asthma would preclude the use of a beta-blocker. The Committee on Safety of Medicines advises that beta-blockers should not be given to patients with a history of asthma or bronchospasm. In very rare situations where no alternative is available, a cardioselective beta$_1$-blocker may be used with extreme caution and under specialist supervision.
- Diabetes mellitus may be a reason not to use a thiazide (due to risk of hyperglycaemia) but may be a compelling reason to use an ACE inhibitor (Chapter 33). Blood pressure and plasma glucose concentration should be monitored regularly.
- History of stroke would be an indication for perindopril alone or in combination with indapamide. The PROGRESS Collaborative Group trial (2001) has indicated that perindopril alone or in combination with indapamide reduces the incidence of stroke (both haemorrhagic and thromboembolic) in patients who have previously suffered any type of stroke. It remains to be determined if this is specific to perindopril and indapamide or whether it applies to any ACE inhibitor plus a thiazide. Cerebral haemorrhage would be a contraindication for the use of nitrates.
- Ischaemic heart disease would be a reason to add a beta-blocker and nitrates. Attention should also be paid to primary or secondary prevention with antiplatelet agents and correction of hyperlipidaemia (Chapter 12).
- Risk of infection from influenza and pneumonia would be a reason to consider vaccination with influenza and pneumococcal polysaccharide vaccines respectively.

Additional considerations are: Wolff–Parkinson–White syndrome (contraindication for digoxin); closed-angle glaucoma (contraindication for nitrates); Addison's disease (contraindication for thiazides); gout (contraindication for thiazides).

CHF may itself influence drug choice in unrelated conditions: important examples are summarised in Table 14.2.

Drug interactions

In the context of drug choice, the interactions between drugs used in CHF should be considered (Table 14.3).

General counselling

One approach to explaining CHF to a patient is that the heart is simply not able to pump the blood as well as it used to, making exercise more difficult. Patients may notice that they have become increasingly breathless and may notice that their ankles swell. In some cases it may be appropriate to avoid mentioning failure and using terms such as 'congestion' may be helpful. The purpose of the drug treatment is either to reduce the work of the heart or to make it beat more forcefully. Other points to consider:

- General counselling would follow the lifestyle advice outlined in Chapters 3 and 11.
- Use of the term 'failure' may be alarming.
- If the patient is taking diuretics, it would be worth suggesting cutting out excess salt in the

Table 14.2 Examples of how chronic heart failure (CHF) may influence drug choice in other conditions

Condition	Drugs	Comments
Migraine	5HT$_1$ agonists – triptans and ergotamine	Coronary vasoconstriction. CSM warning against use in ischaemic heart disease or Prinzmetal's angina. Also contraindicated with nitrates
Glaucoma	Timolol eye drops	Systemic effects of beta-blockade
Thyroid disease	Levothyroxine	Risk of rapid increase in metabolism and activation of sympathetic nervous system
Bipolar affective disorder	Lithium	Lithium concentrations increased by ACE inhibitors and diuretics
Depression	Tricyclic antidepressants	Prolongation of QT interval. Risk of arrhythmias and sudden death
Pain	NSAIDs. Sodium load from soluble paracetamol	Risk of Na$^+$ and fluid retention, renal failure with ACE inhibitor
Indigestion	Antacids	Na$^+$ content should be considered. Absorption of prescribed drugs may be affected
Infection	Erythromycin, clarithromycin	Prolongation of QT interval. Risk of arrhythmias and sudden death. Macrolides interact with amiodarone, warfarin, digoxin and antihyperlipidaemic agents
Menopause	HRT (also oral contraception)	Contraindicated in thromboembolic disorders
Angina, hypertension, Raynaud's phenomenon	Verapamil, diltiazem, nifedipine	May cause or worsen CHF (bradycardia)
COPD	High doses and chronic use of beta$_2$-adrenoceptor agonists	CSM warning of serious hypokalaemia. Regular monitoring required
Psychosis	Thioridazine and other antipsychotic agents	Prolongation of QT interval. Risk of arrhythmias and sudden death

CSM, Committee on Safety of Medicines; ACE, angiotensin-converting enzyme; NSAIDs, non-steroidal anti-inflammatory drugs; HRT, hormone replacement therapy; COPD, chronic obstructive pulmonary disease.

Table 14.3 Summary of important interactions within drugs used in chronic heart failure

Interaction	Consequences	Comment
ACE inhibitor with potassium-sparing diuretics or potassium supplements	Hyperkalaemia	ACE inhibitors and potassium-sparing diuretics both oppose aldosterone, leading to potassium retention
Loop diuretics or thiazides with digoxin	Enhanced effects of digoxin	Diuretic-induced hypokalaemia will enhance the actions of digoxin
Digoxin with captopril, telmisartan, amiodarone or spironolactone	Increased plasma concentrations of digoxin	Pharmacokinetic interaction
Digoxin with beta-blockers	Bradycardia, increased AV block	Addition of actions
Diuretics with vasodilators	Hypotension	Addition of actions

ACE, angiotensin-converting enzyme; AV, atrioventricular.

diet, as this would undo the beneficial effects of the diuretic.

- Patients are at risk of developing secondary depression as a consequence of reduced quality of life or with the realisation of the seriousness of their condition. The GP should be alert to this and may wish to consider anti-depressant therapy.
- In the presence of orthopnoea, patients would be advised to prop themselves up with pillows in bed at night.
- Patients taking ACE inhibitors, diuretics, alpha- and beta-blockers and nitrates should be alerted to the problems of hypotension and orthostatic hypotension and the possibility of having a fall. They should be advised to stand up slowly.
- Patients should be advised to report muscle cramps, pain, nausea or vomiting which may indicate hypokalaemia. Confusion may point to hyponatraemia.
- Patients should be alert for changes in heart rate and palpitations.

Specific counselling

ACE inhibitors

- Patients may experience pronounced first-dose hypotension; it is best to take the first doses of the ACE inhibitor immediately before retiring to bed at night. First-dose hypotension may be worse if the patient is also taking diuretics and the diuretic may be stopped for a few days before the ACE inhibitor is initiated.
- Discuss any cough with the GP. Patients should be encouraged to persist with the ACE inhibitor, as this is the most effective treatment. The ACE inhibitor could be changed or an angiotensin-receptor antagonist used. Recent evidence points to iron supplements being of benefit.
- Consult a pharmacist before purchasing other medicines or supplements. For example, avoid use of potassium salts (salt substitute, effervescent preparations, cystitis treatments), and caution with NSAIDs.

Diuretics

- Male patients should be informed of possible impotence as a side-effect.

- Diuretics (or 'water tablets') will cause an increase in urine flow, usually after 2 h of taking the dose. This may subside after a couple of weeks. In the case of furosemide, it may be worth pointing out that diuresis may be pronounced.
- It is best to take the diuretic in the morning to limit sleep disturbance. A dose may be taken later in the day to avoid the need for urination interfering with social engagements during the day. If two daily doses are required, then they may be taken at 7 a.m. and 1 p.m.
- Omit a dose during periods of diarrhoea and vomiting to prevent dehydration and electrolyte disturbances.
- If appropriate, correction of oedema may be monitored by the patient's weight.
- Sunscreen advice may be appropriate to avoid photosensitivity reactions.

Digoxin

- Patients should be advised to report signs of toxicity, e.g. nausea, vomiting, diarrhoea, disturbances of vision or loss of appetite.
- Since digoxin may cause arrhythmias, patients should also report dizziness, an irregular heartbeat or palpitations.
- Ensure the pulse does not fall below 60 beats/min. If this occurs, the patient should omit the next dose.

Beta-blockers

- Beneficial effects may not be immediate and there may be a worsening of symptoms.
- Male patients may experience impotence.
- Report any additional breathlessness (due to worsening of symptoms or blockade of bronchial beta$_2$-adrenoceptors); cold extremities or peripheral weakness may reflect blockade of vasodilator beta$_2$-adrenoceptors.
- Do not stop taking the tablets suddenly.

Nitrates

Patients may experience a throbbing headache, which should be relieved with paracetamol.

Spironolactone

Male patients may be advised of the small risk of breast enlargement (gynaecomastia), which in itself is harmless.

Hydralazine

Patients should report any weight loss, arthritis or ill health as this may suggest systemic lupus erythematosus.

Alpha-blockers

- Patients should be alert to first-dose hypotension.
- Patients may also experience urinary incontinence.

Monitoring

Renal function (creatinine)

- This should be monitored prior to treatment to determine glomerular filtration rate, as this may be impaired through age or CHF. This is important, as thiazides (except metolazone, which is rarely used) are ineffective in moderate renal failure. Furthermore, digoxin is largely, but not entirely, excreted renally and so in renal impairment there should be a dose reduction or digitoxin, which is not renally excreted, should be used instead.
- ACE inhibitors are contraindicated in renovascular disease.
- Creatinine and urea may rise slightly after initiating an ACE inhibitor or diuretic and this may require dose reduction. Creatinine, urea and electrolyte levels should then be checked after 2 weeks and after each dose change.

Electrolytes

Ideally, potassium levels should be monitored a week after starting diuretic treatment or adjusting treatment and then at least annually once the regimen is stabilised. Sodium may also be affected, presenting as hyponatraemia in which the patient may become confused. Thiazides are also associated with hypomagnesaemia and hypercalcaemia.

Hyperkalaemia

ACE inhibitors, by inhibiting the production of angiotensin II and aldosterone, will tend to cause potassium retention, leading to hyperkalaemia. This may become significant if the ACE inhibitor is taken with a potassium-sparing diuretic or potassium supplements, and their concurrent use is contraindicated or they should be used with great care (e.g. regular monitoring).

Hypokalaemia

Thiazides (especially) and loop diuretics cause hypokalaemia, which is associated with increased fatal arrhythmias. Hypokalaemia is less of a problem if ACE inhibitors are also used as they have the opposite effect (as mentioned above). Hypokalaemia is especially problematic in patients taking digoxin, as hypokalaemia potentiates its pharmacological actions and may lead to toxicity. If hypokalaemia occurs in patients not receiving an ACE inhibitor (unlikely nowadays), the patient may benefit from the addition of a potassium-sparing diuretic or, less commonly, potassium supplements. Digoxin should be withheld until the hypokalaemia is corrected.

Digoxin

Ideally, plasma levels should be measured on a regular basis, although this does not often happen in practice. Plasma concentrations of digoxin should be measured (6–12 h postdosing, Chapter 6) at regular intervals as toxicity is a common occurrence. As commented above, patients or their carers should be told to ensure that their heart rate does not fall below 60 beats/min, this will also act as a rough therapeutic monitor.

Over-the-counter considerations (Table 14.4)

The main problems with over-the-counter (OTC) products result from sodium or potassium content, sodium retention or sympathomimetic activity. Due to the complex nature of CHF treatment there is also a great potential for drug interactions. The pharmacist is ideally placed to identify concordance problems, side-effects of prescribed medicines or worsening symptoms, and can advise the patient accordingly. For example, a classic side-effect of ACE inhibitors is a persistent cough, which may result in failure of

Table 14.4   Over-the-counter (OTC) medicines to avoid in chronic heart failure

OTC products	Comments
Na^+: table salt, high-salt foods (bacon, crisps etc.), soluble preparations, indigestion remedies (Na^+-free alternatives are available), cystitis treatments	Increased Na^+ will reduce the effect of treatment or enhance renal impairment with ACE inhibitors
K^+: salt substitute, cystitis treatments (low-sodium or potassium citrate mixture), some indigestion remedies	Interaction with ACE inhibitors and K^+-sparing diuretics with a risk of hyperkalaemia
Cough and cold remedies containing decongestants (pseudoephedrine, phenylpropanolamine)	Decongestants may increase blood pressure due to sympathomimetic activity
NSAIDs (aspirin, ibuprofen, ketoprofen) in oral and topical analgesics	In addition to drug interactions, the use of NSAIDs may exacerbate heart failure. Gout may be a side-effect of thiazides and ibuprofen would be unsuitable
Laxatives (senna, lactulose)	Chronic use of laxatives may cause electrolyte disturbances
Caffeine (analgesic preparations)	Caffeine may cause myocardial ischaemia

ACE, angiotensin-converting enzyme; NSAIDs, non-steroidal anti-inflammatory drugs.

treatment due to poor patient concordance. Patients should be encouraged to continue with the ACE inhibitor despite the cough, as alternative treatments may be less effective.

Alternative medicine

In an attempt to avoid polypharmacy and in the absence of reliable clinical trial data, the concurrent use of herbal drugs and conventional medicines should be discouraged. Many herbal drugs exhibit pharmacological activity and therefore have the potential to produce the undesirable side-effects outlined with conventional medicines above. For example, there is some evidence that herbal medicines may exhibit sympathomimetic activity, diuretic or antiplatelet effects. Food supplements may also interact with conventional medicines (Chapters 3 and 4).

Future developments

Endothelin ET_A receptor antagonists, such as darusentan, are currently under trial for the treatment of CHF and would be expected to improve the patient's haemodynamics and oppose the actions of endothelins in neurohormonal adaptation. Vasopeptidase inhibitors (such as omapatrilat) which inhibit both ACE and neutral endopeptidases (involved in the breakdown of ANP and bradykinin and the production of endothelins) are also currently under trial.

Practice points

- Be observant for symptoms suggestive of heart failure, particularly in high-risk patients such as after myocardial infarction.
- Treatment should be aimed at relieving symptoms and reducing the risk of death.
- Take steps to prevent readmission to hospital: ensure good symptom control, improve concordance with medicines and diet, reduce alcohol consumption, recognise psychological problems and lack of social support.

→

Practice points (continued)

- Lower doses of diuretics should be used initially in the elderly due to an increased risk of side-effects.
- ACE inhibitors improve both symptoms and prognosis and have a major role in the management of CHF.
- Regular monitoring is essential, particularly for patients taking digoxin. Potassium-sparing diuretics can cause severe hyperkalaemia in a patient taking an ACE inhibitor.
- Angiotensin AT_1 receptor antagonists may have an important role in patients intolerant to ACE inhibitors.
- Beta-blockers are now recognised as having an important role in improving quality of life and reducing mortality.
- People with CHF are at high risk of developing arrhythmias and of sudden death. Arrhythmias should be investigated and treated as appropriate.
- Be vigilant of the use of OTC medicines and supplements in patients with CHF.
- Patients should be warned about first-dose hypotension with ACE inhibitors and alpha-blockers (extra caution in combination with diuretics).

 CASE STUDY

Last year Mr AH (65 years) found himself increasingly short of breath whilst walking to the shops and he was referred by his GP for cardiological investigations. A physical examination did not reveal any abnormalities but a chest X-ray revealed cardiomegaly without evidence of pulmonary oedema. A subsequent echocardiogram revealed a reduction in ejection fraction. A diagnosis of chronic heart failure was made and the cardiologist prescribed lisinopril starting at 2.5 mg daily (o.n.) and this was increased over several weeks by his GP to 20 mg daily.

1. Comment on the clinical findings.

- His shortness of breath is a symptom of CHF.
- Cardiomegaly is an enlarged heart, and is consistent with CHF.
- Reduced ejection fraction on an echocardiogram is diagnostic of CHF.

2. What is the purpose of the lisinopril?

- The ACE inhibitor will inhibit angiotensin II production and aldosterone release.
- It reduces cardiac work.
- It opposes neurohormonal changes in the heart.

3. How should the patient be counselled with respect to taking the lisinopril for the first time?

- The patient should be warned of first-dose hypotension and advised to take the first dose before retiring to bed.
- The patient may develop a cough. This should be reported to the GP but the benefits of the drug outweigh the cough so he should be encouraged to persist with the medicine if possible.
- He should report any rashes or swellings, which may be due to angioedema.

continued

◖ CASE STUDY (continued)

After his initial treatment, Mr AH felt substantially better. However, after 6 months he was admitted to hospital with breathlessness, which had become worse while taking bed rest. This time a physical examination and chest X-ray revealed pulmonary oedema and the patient rapidly responded to diamorphine (5 mg IV stat) and was started on furosemide (40 mg o.m.).

4. Comment on the use of diamorphine and furosemide.

- Diamorphine induces a degree of euphoria. It opposes dyspnoea and cough associated with pulmonary oedema.
- Furosemide will cause venodilatation to reduce preload. It induces diuresis, reducing fluid and relieving pulmonary oedema.

Several days later, although his condition has improved, the cardiologist also adds spironolactone (25 mg daily) to the patient's discharge medication.

5. What is the purpose of the addition of spironolactone?

- It opposes the effects of aldosterone on the heart.
- It may reverse cardiac enlargement.
- It reduces the incidence of arrhythmias.
- It reduces mortality.

6. In view of his current medication, what precautions must be taken with the addition of spirono-lactone? Why?

- There is an interaction between spironolactone and lisinopril.
- Both may cause hyperkalaemia (although there is concomitant furosemide with an opposing effect).
- Potassium levels should be monitored.

Mr AH's condition is currently well-managed but he is admitted to hospital once again to monitor his progress. This time his GP is concerned with a new addition made by the consultant to the patient's prescription. The addition is for bisoprolol (1.25 mg o.m.). The GP remembers from medical school something about beta-blockers being contraindicated in CHF, and comments: 'surely the consultant means bisacodyl?'

7. How do you respond to the GP?

- The consultant is indeed correct. The bisoprolol may be given. Previously it was thought that beta-blockers were contraindicated due to negative inotropic effects but now evidence points to cardioselective ones being safe in stable CHF. Start with a low dose.

8. What is the rationale for the consultant's new addition?

- To oppose the neurohormonal maladaptation due to catecholamines. Also it is antiarrhythmic.

References

CIBIS-II Investigators and Committee (1999). The Cardiac Insufficiency Bisoprolol Study II (CIBIS-II): a randomised trial. *Lancet* 353: 9–13.

Cohn J N, Tognoni G (2001). A randomized trial of the angiotensin receptor blocker valsartan in chronic heart failure. *N Engl J Med* 345: 1667–1675.

Digitalis Investigation Group (1997). The effect of digoxin on mortality and morbidity in patients with heart failure. *N Engl J Med* 336: 525–533.

Greene R J, Harris N D (2000). *Pathology and Therapeutics for Pharmacists*. London: Pharmaceutical Press.

MERIT-HF Study Group (1999). Effect of metoprolol CR XL in chronic heart failure: Metoprolol CR XL Randomised Intervention Trial in Congestive Heart Failure (MERIT-HF). *Lancet* 353: 2001–2007.

NICE (2003). Chronic heart failure: management of chronic heart failure in adults in primary and secondary care. Clinical guidance 5. London: National Institute for Clinical Excellence.

Pitt B, Zannad F, Remme W J *et al.* (1999). The effect of spironolactone on morbidity and mortality in patients with severe heart failure. *N Eng J Med* 341: 709–717.

Pitt B, Poole-Wilson P A, Segal R *et al.* (2000). Effect of losartan compared with captopril on mortality in patients with symptomatic heart failure: randomised trial – the Losartan Heart Failure Survival Study ELITE II. *Lancet* 355: 1582–1587.

PROGRESS Collaborative Group (2001). Randomised trial of a perindopril-based blood-pressure-lowering regimen among 6105 individuals with previous stroke or transient ischaemic attack. *Lancet* 358: 1033–1041.

Swedeberg K (1987). Effects of enalapril on mortality in severe congestive-heart failure – results of the Cooperative North Scandinavian Enalapril Survival Study (CONSENSUS). *N Engl J Med* 316: 1429–1435.

Further reading

Cleland J G F, Swedberg K, Poole-Wilson P A (1998). Successes and failures of the current treatment of heart failure. *Lancet* 353 (suppl): 19–28.

Cowie M R, Zaphiriou A (2002). Management of chronic heart failure. *BMJ* 325: 422–425.

Perry G, Brown E, Thornton R *et al.* (1997). The effect of digoxin on mortality and morbidity in patients with heart failure. *N Engl J Med* 336: 525–533.

Seed A, McMurry J (2001). Current approaches to treating heart failure. *Prescriber* 12: 75–95.

Online resources

www.bhf.org.uk is the website of the British Heart Foundation, providing patient information (accessed 4 December 2002).

www.doh.gov.uk/nsf/ is the website of the Department of Health and contains the NSF for Coronary Heart Disease (accessed 4 December 2002).

15

Thromboembolic prophylaxis

Thrombosis

Thrombosis is the unwanted formation of blood clots and may be venous or arterial. Venous thrombosis is associated with stasis of blood: the major problem is that the clot may become dislodged and travel to the lungs, leading to a life-threatening pulmonary embolism. By contrast, thrombosis formed at an atherosclerotic site may lead to arterial blockage in the heart (myocardial infarction; Chapter 13), cerebral vessels or the peripheral circulation, resulting in ischaemia and infarction. Additionally, atrial fibrillation is associated with the stasis of blood and the formation of thrombi in the left atria, which may become dislodged and result in embolism of cerebral vessels, leading to a cerebrovascular accident. Other important thrombogenic sites include artificial mechanical heart valves.

Venous thrombosis is largely associated with an inappropriate activation of the clotting cascade; the thrombi formed have a high fibrin but low platelet content. Once again, arterial thrombosis has different characteristics, with platelet activation playing a central role. This has a bearing on prevention, as venous thrombosis is largely managed by anticoagulants and arterial thrombosis largely by antiplatelet agents (Chapter 13), although anticoagulants may also have a role in limiting recruitment of the clotting cascade in arterial thrombosis. Thrombosis associated with atrial fibrillation involves activation of both clotting factors and platelets, hence anticoagulants are predominantly used, but aspirin may also be effective as prophylaxis in low-risk patients.

Risk factors for venous thrombosis include oral contraceptives, hormone replacement therapy, a history of thrombosis, recent surgery, immobility, obesity, pregnancy, malignancy and previous myocardial infarction. Risk factors for arterial thrombosis are detailed in Chapter 13.

Goals of treatment

The goals of treatment are prophylaxis against either arterial or venous thrombosis, and the preventive treatment is targeted at those at risk. Specific targets for treatment with anticoagulants are detailed in Table 15.1.

Table 15.1 Target international normalised ratios (INRs) for various indications for warfarin

Indication	Target INR	Duration of treatment
Pulmonary embolism	2.5	6 months
Proximal deep vein thrombosis	2.5	6 months
Calf vein thrombosis (non-surgical)	2.5	3 months
Postoperative calf vein thrombosis	2.5	6 weeks
Recurrence of deep vein thrombosis or pulmonary embolism in patients not taking warfarin	2.5	Indefinite
Recurrence of deep vein thrombosis or pulmonary embolism in patients already taking warfarin	3.5	Indefinite
Atrial fibrillation	2.5	Long-term
Mural thrombosis after an MI	2.5	3 months
Mechanical prosthetic heart values	3.5	Lifelong

Information obtained from the Oral Anticoagulant guidelines of the British Society for Haematology (1998).
MI, myocardial infarction.

Pharmacological basis of management

Anticoagulants

Injectable anticoagulants

Unfractionated heparin and low-molecular-weight heparins (e.g. dalteparin, enoxaparin, tinzaparin)

Heparin is a mucopolysaccharide found naturally in mast cells and the vascular endothelium. Due to the size of this polymer, heparin is poorly absorbed from the gastrointestinal tract and is therefore given by subcutaneous or intravenous injection. Heparin activates antithrombin III, a natural protein, which inactivates some clotting factors and thrombin by complexing with their serine protease component. Accordingly, the effects of heparin are rapid in onset and are given when anticoagulation is required immediately. Heparin is available as either unfractionated heparin (average molecular weight 15 kDa) or low-molecular-weight heparins (LMWH) (average molecular weight 4.5 kDa). Compared to unfractionated heparins, LMWHs have greater activity against factor Xa and less against thrombin. Unfractionated heparins may also reduce platelet aggregation, which does not occur with LMWHs.

Oral anticoagulants

Warfarin

Warfarin is a vitamin K antagonist, which inhibits the enzyme vitamin K reductase required for vitamin K to act as a cofactor in the production of clotting factors. In this regard, vitamin K is essential for the posttranslational modification by carboxylation of glutamic acid residues of prothrombin and factors VII, IX and X. Accordingly, warfarin inhibits the hepatic synthesis of these clotting factors and its action is only apparent after several days, once the existing clotting factors have been replaced by these newly synthesised, defective factors. The inhibition persists for 4–5 days after the withdrawal of warfarin.

Antiplatelet drugs

Aspirin and clopidogrel are dealt with in Chapter 13, in the context of their major role in the primary and secondary prevention of myocardial infarction and cerebrovascular accidents.

Clinical use of anticoagulants

Oral anticoagulants have a number of indications to prevent thrombosis, which are listed in Table

15.1. To initiate treatment with warfarin it must be borne in mind that it will take several days for full effects to become apparent, while in the meantime there may be an increased chance of clotting due to lowering of the levels of protein C (a protein generated from a vitamin K-dependent precursor, which destroys certain clotting factors). Therefore, heparin is started at the same time to 'anticoagulate' the patient and this should be continued until the target international normalised ratio (INR) has been achieved and maintained for 2 days.

Use of heparin

Heparin may be used to initiate anticoagulant treatment or is given for a short, defined period for the prevention of postoperative thromboembolism, e.g. after surgery and in particular after orthopaedic surgery. In terms of clinical use, LMWHs have the advantage of once-daily administration by subcutaneous injection.

The anticoagulant effects of unfractionated heparin are monitored daily by the activated partial thromboplastin time (APTT), with a target value of 1.5–2.0, and the dose is altered to maintain this. By contrast, LMWHs do not require monitoring as their effects are predictable (and they do not prolong APTT). In addition, the use of heparin is associated with thrombocytopenia (less so with LMWH) and with sustained use (greater than 5 days) the platelet count should be monitored.

Initiation of warfarin

Before starting warfarin, it is appropriate to monitor liver function and the INR. The INR is the key anticoagulant screen for warfarin and is the prothrombin time (the normalised time for thromboplastin to cause clotting when added to citrated plasma). The INR is measured during initiation to achieve a target, which is dependent on the indication (Table 15.1), and should be maintained at this level by altering the dose of warfarin. The INR should be determined daily or on alternate days and then at longer intervals depending on response (unless a change in clinical condition or administration of other drugs dictates otherwise). Once stabilised, the INR should be monitored at least every 12 weeks.

Warfarin is not indicated for ischaemic stroke without atrial fibrillation. Following coronary artery thrombosis, coronary artery bypass grafting or coronary angioplasty, low-dose aspirin (Chapter 13) and/or heparin should be considered. Heparin is also considered for unstable angina.

When initiating treatment, the patient is often loaded with warfarin doses of 10 mg, 10 mg, and then 5 mg on 3 consecutive days and the INR should be reviewed on day 4 to determine the maintenance dose. In patients who initially have a higher INR (>1.2), for example through age, liver disease, or warfarin-potentiating drugs, the loading doses should be reduced.

For patients whose anticoagulant therapy is poorly controlled and who have an elevated INR, a number of procedures may be carried out. These are given in more detail in the *British National Formulary* (section 2.8.2) but, depending on the extent of increase, involve dose reduction or withholding doses, oral or intravenous vitamin K and, in the presence of severe bleeding, the administration of clotting factors or, failing that, fresh frozen plasma. Heparin is reversed with protamine, although it is less effective against LMWHs.

Drug choice

Before initiating warfarin treatment, patients must be identified as able to adhere strictly to the regimen and sufficiently motivated and compliant to ensure that their INR is monitored regularly.

Pregnancy

Warfarin is teratogenic if it is given during the first trimester and particularly after 6 weeks of gestation. During the last few weeks of pregnancy and during delivery warfarin may cross the placenta, leading to a risk of placental or fetal haemorrhage. Vitamin K deficiency of neonates may also be an issue. Warfarin should therefore be avoided during pregnancy and in particular during the first and third trimesters. Heparin does not cross the placenta into the fetus and may be used under expert supervision, although prolonged use is associated with osteoporosis.

Non-rheumatic atrial fibrillation

The prevention of stroke in this condition is subject to various views. The Oral Anticoagulant guidelines of the British Society for Haematology (1998) suggest that warfarin is appropriate in moderate- and high-risk patients (those with hypertension, previous thromboembolism, heart failure or left ventricular dysfunction). Prodigy guidance (see www.prodigy.nhs.uk) suggests that warfarin should be prescribed to patients over 65 years of age or those under 65 years of age with risk factors (hypertension, diabetes mellitus, previous thromboembolism, heart failure or left ventricular dysfunction). In regard to the benefits of using warfarin in atrial fibrillation, some evidence-based guidelines have been produced by Thomson *et al.* (2000). In low-risk patients (with no risk factors), low-dose aspirin alone may be sufficient. Aspirin should also be considered for patients who are unsuitable for warfarin. In general, warfarin reduces the incidence of stroke by two-thirds and aspirin by about one-fifth. Patients with permanent atrial fibrillation who are candidates for electrical cardioversion should receive warfarin for 3 weeks prior to this procedure.

Atrial fibrillation in rheumatic heart disease

This presents a much higher risk for stroke and the current guidelines of the British Society for Haematology recommend warfarin for all patients.

Deep vein thrombosis (DVT)

This is associated with immobility leading to stasis of blood and hypercoagulability: pregnant and postoperative patients are at an increased risk. The major complication is that the thrombus may dislodge and lead to a life-threatening pulmonary embolism. Patients with DVTs should be heparinised and non-pregnant patients should then be initiated on warfarin.

'Economy-class syndrome'

This has received much attention recently. The term describes DVT leading to pulmonary embolism associated with prolonged travel; whether it is exacerbated by air travel has yet to be established. It is associated with immobility, and so exercise and wearing compression stockings may be effective. Recommended exercises include short walks, bending and straightening legs, feet and toes and pressing feet on the ground. Passengers should also avoid excess alcohol and becoming dehydrated. Passengers with a moderate risk for DVT (e.g. pregnancy, heart disease, family history of DVT, hormonal contraception, hormone replacement therapy) may consider low-dose aspirin and support stockings. Recommending low-dose aspirin to all passengers seems unwise, as the risk of gastric bleeding in the general population is greater than the risk of DVT. The Department of Health (2001) has advised that patients at high risk due to previous DVT, clotting tendency (thrombophilia), a history of cancer, major surgery in the past 3 months (including hip or knee replacement) or stroke should consult their GP. High-risk patients may be prescribed an LMWH and/or advised to wear compression stockings.

Concurrent disease

Warfarin is contraindicated in peptic ulcer disease, severe hypertension and bacterial endocarditis and should not be used in cerebral thrombosis or peripheral arterial occlusion as first-line therapy. It should be used with caution following recent surgery. Warfarin itself is associated with a significant risk of haemorrhagic stroke.

Heparin is also contraindicated in patients with peptic ulcer, severe hypertension in addition to haemophilia and other haemorrhagic disorders, thrombocytopenia, recent cerebral haemorrhage, severe liver disease including oesophageal varices, major trauma or recent surgery.

Hepatic disease

Oral anticoagulants should be avoided in severe liver disease, particularly if the prothrombin time is already prolonged. The dose of heparin should be reduced in severe liver disease.

Renal disease

Oral anticoagulants should be avoided in severe renal impairment. There is an increased risk of bleeding when heparin is given in severe renal impairment.

Monitoring

INR, APTT and platelets

See earlier.

Electrolytes

Heparin inhibits aldosterone secretion and may possibly result in hyperkalaemia. The risk increases with prolonged therapy and in patients with diabetes mellitus, chronic renal failure, acidosis and those taking drugs that increase plasma potassium (such as potassium-sparing diuretics and angiotensin-converting enzyme (ACE) inhibitors; Table 2.2; Chapters 11 and 14). The Committee on Safety of Medicines recommends potassium monitoring before starting heparin in patients at risk and regularly throughout treatment, particularly if the treatment period is longer than 7 days.

Drug interactions

Potentiation

Warfarin shows a notoriously wide range of drug interactions, which are of clinical importance due to its narrow therapeutic index. The most common interactions usually result in the enhancement of anticoagulant activity, and this appears largely to be due to competition or inhibition of hepatic metabolism, but is sometimes through displacement from protein-binding sites. The enhancement may lead to increased bleeding. Inhibitors of metabolism are likely to have rapid effects on the levels of warfarin. However, this alteration will take several days to have an effect on the INR and these effects will reverse on stopping the inhibitor, although in the case of drugs with long half-lives, such as amiodarone, they may persist for some time. The dose of warfarin may then need to be altered.

In choosing drugs for patients who are taking warfarin the ideal is to select drugs which do not interact. When starting drugs known to interact with warfarin the British Society for Haematology (1998) recommends:

- For drug changes lasting less than 5 days with a known potentiating drug: no change, minor dose reduction for warfarin or omit one dose of warfarin.
- For longer drug changes: monitor INR after 1 week and alter warfarin dose accordingly.

In addition, when warfarin is initiated in a patient who is already taking a known interacting drug, the loading dose may need to be altered.

Some important drugs which may enhance the actions of warfarin:

(D indicates that a dose reduction of warfarin is likely)

- allopurinol
- amiodarone – may persist after discontinuation of amiodarone due to its long half-life (D).
- azapropazone (contraindicated)
- azoles – fluconazole, ketoconazole, miconazole
- clarithromycin
- co-trimoxazole (D)
- cytotoxic agents (carboplatin, mustine, cyclophosphamide, doxorubicin, etoposide, 5-fluorouracil, ifosfamide/mesna, methotrexate, procarbazine, vincristine and vindesine)
- dextropropoxyphene
- disulfiram (D)
- erythromycin
- fibrates (D)
- H_2-antagonists, cimetidine (famotidine, nizatidine and ranitidine are less likely to interact)
- hydrocodone (rarely)
- interferon
- isoniazid (rarely)
- lansoprazole (rarely)
- levothyroxine (D)
- metronidazole (D)
- phenylbutazone (avoid)
- non-steroidal anti-inflammatory drugs (NSAIDs) – diclofenac and flurbiprofen may increase INR
- omeprazole
- paracetamol – monitoring is required if taken regularly, but safer than aspirin
- penicillins (occasionally)
- quinolones
- selective serotonin reuptake inhibitors: fluoxetine (rarely)
- statins
- sulfinpyrazone (D)

- sulphonamides (D)
- tamoxifen (D)
- tetracyclines (rarely)
- tricylic antidepressants
- zafirlukast (D)

In addition the anticoagulant effects of warfarin may lead to enhanced bleeding with antiplatelet drugs (aspirin, clopidogrel, dipyridamole) or drugs which lead to gastric bleeding. Aspirin may be combined with warfarin but there is an increase in bleeding tendency, although this is less marked with low doses. Warfarin may also lead to gastric bleeding with aspirin and other NSAIDs. Patients should be advised to use para-cetamol for pain relief.

Reduced activity

Less frequently agents will reduce the activity of warfarin and this appears to be due to induction of its metabolism. In dealing with inducers, they take several days to alter the concentrations of warfarin and longer to alter the INR, but these effects are likely to persist for some time after an inducer is stopped. The dose of warfarin may then need to be altered.

Some important drugs which may reduce the actions of warfarin:

- barbiturates
- carbamazepine – oxacarbazepine appears safe
- colestyramine – separate doses
- cytotoxic agents (azathioprine, cyclophos-phamide, mercaptopurine and mitotane)
- disopyramide
- griseofulvin
- phenytoin – monitoring of both warfarin and phenytoin is required (Chapter 22)
- rifampicin – the dose of warfarin may need to be increased (two- to threefold) several days after rifampicin is started
- St John's wort (avoid)
- vitamin K supplements and diet (including spinach, Brussels sprouts, broccoli, liver, lettuce)
- oral contraceptives – contraindicated in thromboembolic disorders

The above lists have largely been compiled from *Drug Interactions* by Stockley (2002). The list gives some important examples but more complete information should be sought from more detailed sources, including *Drug Interactions*.

Over-the-counter considerations

Health professionals should be aware of products containing vitamin K, which may antagonise the effect of warfarin, for example, multivitamin supplements and liquid dietary supplements. Herbal drugs also have the potential to interact with warfarin (Chapter 4). For example, close monitoring is required with garlic supplements. The dose of warfarin may need to be adjusted.

General counselling

In talking to patients, warfarin ('rat poison') is usually referred to as 'thinning the blood'. It should be made absolutely clear to patients that they must stick to their dosage regimen and take it at the same time of day, conventionally at 6 p.m. If they miss a dose then they should not take two doses together and they should inform their doctor at the next blood test.

- Patients should be informed that they must tell any doctor, dentist or pharmacist who treats them that they are receiving warfarin. The need to mention their treatment is essential whilst purchasing over-the-counter medicines (including creams and gels, e.g. antifungal imidazoles) and supplements. Preparations containing vitamin K should be avoided.
- Females of child-bearing age should be advised not to become pregnant while taking warfarin.
- Alcohol may be consumed in moderation but not in excess.
- Patients should avoid excessive consumption of green vegetables (particularly spinach, Brussels sprouts, lettuce, broccoli) and beetroot and liver. Changes to diets rich in vitamin K should be discussed with a healthcare pro-fessional, as a dose change of warfarin may be

required. Warfarin therapy may also be altered following the consumption of regular or large quantities of foods such as avocado, icecream, soybean protein and the sweetener aspartame.

Patients should report:

- haemoptysis
- blood in faeces
- blood in urine
- nose bleeds
- easy bruising
- skin changes (necrosis)

and consult their doctor if they have diarrhoea or vomiting for 2 days or more.

Practice points

- Patients require extensive counselling to ensure compliance.
- Guidelines on oral anticoagulation in *Br J Haematol* 101: 374–387 should be consulted.
- Warfarin interacts with many drugs and the pharmacist should be vigilant of this and look for signs of enhanced actions of warfarin.
- Consider all requests for over-the-counter medicines (especially NSAIDs) as a potential for drug interactions.

 CASE STUDY

A 70-year-old man who has permanent atrial fibrillation associated with left ventricular failure is currently receiving:

Lisinopril 10 mg o.d.
Furosemide (frusemide) 40 mg o.m.
Digoxin 62.5 µg o.d.
Amiodarone 200 mg o.d.

Make a recommendation for thromboembolic prophylaxis.

- The patient is over 65 years old, and has heart failure, which means that he is at moderate risk of thromboembolic complications. Given his moderate risk, he is likely to receive warfarin (if anticoagulation is required immediately then he might also receive heparin). However, it should be noted that amiodarone will enhance the actions of warfarin, so unless an alternative antiarrhythmic (sotalol) or digoxin alone is considered sufficient, his loading dose may need to be reduced and his INR (target 2.5) will need to be closely monitored with a view to dose reductions. Note the low maintenance dose of digoxin, which has been used as amiodarone increases the plasma concentrations of digoxin.

He is stabilised on warfarin but develops a bacterial chest infection. Comment on antibiotic treatment.

- Amoxicillin is first choice and, according to Stockley's *Drug Interactions*, only rarely interacts with warfarin. Monitoring is however advisable, at least before the antibiotic is added. Second-line agents include erythromycin, which may enhance the actions of warfarin.

References

Department of Health (2001). *Advice on Travel-related Deep Vein Thrombosis*. London: Department of Health (www.doh.gov.uk/dvt/index.htm).

Guidelines on oral anticoagulation: third edition (1998). *Br J Haematol* 101: 374–387.

Mehta D K (ed.) *British National Formulary*, latest edition. London: British Medical Association and Royal Pharmaceutical Society of Great Britain.

Stockley I H (2002). *Drug Interactions*, 6th edn. London: Pharmaceutical Press.

Thomson R, Parkin D, Eccles M *et al*. (2000). Decision analysis and guidelines for anticoagulant therapy to prevent stroke in patients with atrial fibrillation. *Lancet* 355: 956–962.

Further reading

Heck A M, DeWitt B A, Lukes A L (2000). Potential interactions between alternative therapies and warfarin. *Am J Health Syst Pharm* 13: 1221–1227.

Hoffbrand A V, Pettit J E, Moss P A H (2001). *Essential Haematology*, 4th edn. Oxford: Blackwell Science.

Lip G Y H, Lowe G D O (1996). ABC of atrial fibrillation: antithrombotic treatment of atrial fibrillation. *BMJ* 312: 45–49.

16

Anaemias

As with several medical specialities, haematology encompasses both minor and serious conditions. Of relevance to the pharmacist are the anaemias, as these are important conditions which are encountered on a regular basis: simple iron-deficiency anaemia is of particular importance.

Anaemias are characterised by reduced levels of haemoglobin and occur when the haemoglobin is less than 13.5 g/dL in males and 11.5 g/dL in females. The signs and symptoms depend on the severity but are related to impaired oxygen transport and delivery due to reduced levels of haemoglobin. Key symptoms include:

- weakness
- lethargy
- impaired exercise tolerance
- shortness of breath

whilst cardiovascular adaptations, coupled to reduced blood viscosity, may result in tachycardia. In severe anaemia, particularly in more elderly subjects, there may be angina due to impaired delivery of oxygen to the cardiac muscle and anaemia may also lead to heart failure. Skin colour is not a reliable sign, as this is determined by blood flow, but pale nail beds and conjunctiva may be present. In haemolytic anaemias, jaundice may be present.

Iron-deficiency anaemia

As the name implies, it is due to impaired iron balance and for this to occur the bone marrow's iron stores must be depleted. The deficiency in iron leads to impaired synthesis of haemoglobin and the production of smaller red cells, which have a reduced mean corpuscular volume (MCV <75 fl; Chapter 2), and this is referred to as microcytic anaemia. In addition to the above features, the patient may also have:

- spoon nails (koilonychia)
- sores on the corner of the mouth (angular stomatitis)
- painful, red tongue (glossitis)
- unusual food cravings

As commented above, for iron-deficiency anaemia to develop the iron stores must be depleted. As the diet normally provides the body's requirement for iron, coupled with the fact that iron is efficiently recycled from destroyed red cells, iron-deficiency anaemia is a chronic condition which occurs when input is impaired, output is increased or there are increased demands.

Input is reduced with:

- poor diet (in infants)
- surgical removal of stomach
- malabsorption (coeliac disease, Crohn's disease)

Clinically the main cause is when there is chronic and excessive blood loss through:

- gastrointestinal bleeding (often from ulcers and chronic non-steroidal anti-inflammatory drug (NSAID)-induced damage, also from colitis, carcinoma, haemorrhoids)
- chronic heavy menstruation (menorrhagia); hence iron-deficiency anaemia is commoner in women due to a more precarious iron balance

Demand is increased in pregnancy due to the fetal requirements and the expansion in the maternal circulating volume, and anaemia, to varying degrees, is very common.

Goals of treatment

These are twofold: to identify and treat the underlying cause and to restore both the iron stores and the level of haemoglobin.

Pharmacological management

The most straightforward approach to restoring iron stores is to give ferrous iron. This is generally in the simple and inexpensive form of oral ferrous sulfate, although this may be poorly tolerated due to gastric irritation and other forms may be used, such as ferrous fumarate. Slow-release preparations have lower bioavailability, as the iron is released in the lower small intestine, where it is not absorbed. The ferrous sulfate is given as 200 mg up to three times daily (once or twice daily in less severe anaemia) with a view to building up the iron stores and increasing the haemoglobin at a rate of approximately 1 g/dL per week. The first response which may be measured is an increase in the reticulocyte count, due to newly formed maturing red blood cells. Once the haemoglobin has returned to normal, iron therapy should be continued for 3 months to build up the iron stores. In prophylaxis of anaemia in pregnancy, the iron may be combined with low doses of folic acid, to ensure an adequate supply of folate.

Interactions with iron therapy

Iron preparations exhibit a range of interactions, largely related to the reduced absorption of the iron or the interacting drug from the gastro-intestinal tract. Some important examples are detailed in Table 16.1.

Counselling

The patient should be counselled that the anaemia is likely to be a symptom of another condition, which should be identified and treated. If patients request iron tablets without a diagnosis, they should be referred to their general practitioner for a blood test, and, if appropriate, identification of the underlying cause.

Iron

Clearly, counselling should be directed towards ensuring compliance and completing the course of iron until stores are replenished. The doses should be evenly spaced or at least 6 h apart as absorption may be reduced by the previous dose. Patients should also be alerted to any important interactions and advised not to take over-the-counter antacids at the same time as the iron salt. The patient should also be made aware of the side-effects of iron; these largely affect the gastrointestinal tract and include:

- gastric irritation, which may be reduced by taking the iron with food. However, this may reduce its absorption
- nausea
- altered bowel habits with constipation or diarrhoea
- the stools will be darkly coloured
- excessive iron is toxic in children

Table 16.1   Clinically significant interactions of iron preparations with other drugs

Interacting drugs	Consequences	Comments
Ferrous salts with antacids	Antacids reduce the absorption of ferrous salts	Their administration should be separated. H₂-antagonists do not significantly affect the absorption of ferrous salts
Ferrous salts with colestyramine	Colestyramine binds ferrous salts and may reduce their absorption	Their administration should be separated
Ferrous salts with neomycin	Neomycin may increase or decrease the absorption of ferrous salts	
Ferrous salts with quinolones	Ferrous salts decrease the absorption of quinolones	The quinolone should be taken at least 2 h before the ferrous salt
Ferrous salts with tetracyclines	Concomitant administration of these agents reduces the plasma concentrations of both iron and tetracyclines	Their doses should be separated
Ferrous salts with levodopa or carbidopa	Ferrous sulfate reduces the bioavailability of these antiparkinson drugs	Their doses should be separated and the control of Parkinson's disease monitored
Ferrous sulfate with levothyroxine	Ferrous sulfate reduces the effects of levothyroxine	Their doses should be separated

Megaloblastic anaemia

This is a rarer form of anaemia due to abnormal red blood cell maturation as a result of defective DNA synthesis, and the bone marrow contains megaloblasts, abnormal precursor cells in which nuclear maturation is impaired in relation to that of the cytoplasm. The abnormal production of red cells results in increased cell volume and is referred to as macrocytic anaemia (MCV >95 fL); there is also a reduced level of haemoglobin. An increased MCV without anaemia may be due to alcohol misuse – a common cause of macrocytosis, which is unrelated to megaloblastic anaemia. However, in severe alcoholism, the toxic effects of alcohol on the bone marrow may lead to megaloblastic anaemia.

In megaloblastic anaemia the symptoms are that of mild anaemia and may also include jaundice, as the enlarged red cells are more likely to undergo haemolysis, raising the level of bilirubin. Megaloblastic anaemia is due to either a deficiency of vitamin B_{12} or folate, and this may be associated with a painful, red tongue (glossitis), sores at the corner of the mouth (angular stomatis) and neuropathy (in vitamin B_{12} deficiency).

Vitamin B_{12} (as a cofactor) and folate (as component) are essential for DNA synthesis, and a deficiency of either impairs synthesis. As there is a substantial rate of red blood cell production with a high requirement for DNA synthesis, then impaired DNA synthesis results in the formation of megaloblasts in the bone marrow. In severe forms impaired DNA synthesis may lead to reduced production of white blood cells and/or platelets.

Deficiencies of vitamin B_{12} can be due to:

- vegan diet
- Crohn's disease, which leads to impaired absorption of vitamin B_{12}
- gastrectomy, which leads to the loss of the intrinsic factor for the absorption of vitamin B_{12}
- metformin, which may reduce the absorption of vitamin B_{12}

In addition, pernicious anaemia is a special subset and is due to an autoimmune destruction of the intrinsic factor which is released by the stomach to facilitate the absorption of vitamin B_{12}.

Folate deficiency may be due to:

- dietary deficiency in alcoholics
- pregnancy due to increased demand
- malabsorption in coeliac disease
- chronic inflammatory conditions such as Crohn's disease, rheumatoid arthritis, tuberculosis
- drug-induced. Methotrexate and trimethoprim are folate antagonists by inhibition of dihydrofolate reductase; phenytoin and phenobarbital may also cause deficiency, possibly due to enzyme induction increasing the requirement for folate

Pharmacological management

This clearly depends on the cause. If a deficiency of vitamin B_{12} is identified as the cause then hydroxocobalamin is given intramuscularly, which avoids the need for absorption from the gastrointestinal tract, as this may be impaired. Oral vitamin B_{12} may of course be used in otherwise healthy vegans. Once the stores have been

replaced, maintenance treatment may need to be continued for life. Hydroxocobalamin (i.m.) is also appropriate as prophylaxis in patients who have had gastrectomy or ileal resection.

Folate deficiency is simply treated by oral folic acid (5–15 mg daily) and this, depending on the cause, may need to be lifelong.

Drug interactions

The drugs used to treat megaloblastic anaemia have a limited number of interactions (Table 16.2).

Other anaemias

There are a range of other anaemias which are beyond the scope of this book. However, a brief description of some of them may be appropriate.

Renal anaemia (Chapter 17)

The kidney is the source of the hormone erythropoietin, which is released in hypoxia (secondary

Table 16.2 Clinically significant interactions of folic acid or vitamin B_{12} with other drugs

Interacting drugs	Consequences	Comments
Folic acid with phenytoin, phenobarbital	As commented above, these anticonvulsants may lead to folate deficiency	In patients treated with folate, the concentrations of the anticonvulsants may fall, leading to impaired seizure control. Monitoring and dose adjustment may be required
Folic acid with trimethoprim, co-trimoxazole	The weak antifolate actions of trimethoprim may substantially reduce the effectiveness of folic acid	They should not be used together
Folic acid with magnesium trisilicate	The absorption of folic acid is reduced	
Folic acid with sulfasalazine	The absorption of folic acid is reduced	
Vitamin B_{12} with H_2-antagonists	H_2-antagonists reduce the absorption of oral vitamin B_{12}	Analogues given by injection are not affected

to anaemia, climbing to altitude and chronic obstructive pulmonary disease, for example) and acts on the bone marrow to increase the production of red blood cells. Renal failure is associated with reduced levels of erythropoietin, which leads to normocytic anaemia. Patients with renal failure and those on dialysis accordingly receive erythropoietin. They may also receive prophylactic iron and folic acid (Chapter 17).

Haemolytic anaemias

This is a class of anaemia and is due to excessive destruction of red cells, which leads to reduced haemoglobin levels. The increased breakdown of red blood cells leads to raised bilirubin levels and this results in jaundice. This may occur in megaloblastic anaemia. The increased erythropoiesis required to replace the cells may actually lead to folate deficiency. Examples of this include:

- spherocytosis – a genetic and abnormal reduction in the red blood cell membrane protein, spectrin, which leads to fragile cells
- sickle cell anaemia – duc to the haemolysis of the sickle-shaped cells
- in glucose-6-phosphate dehydrogenase (G6PD) deficiency, where certain drugs may cause red cell damage (see Chapter 5)
- infections such as malaria

Aplastic anaemia

This is a serious condition in which there is insufficient production of red blood cells, white blood cells and platelets (pancytopenia). The patient has decreased resistance to infections, increased bleeding and the symptoms of anaemia. Most cases are acquired due to viral infection, radiation or drugs (including cytotoxic agents, chloramphenicol, sulphonamides and insecticides). Treatment is via antilymphocyte globulin to prevent suppressor killer T-cells from damaging the stem cells, ciclosporin and sometimes bone marrow transplantation for cure.

Drug-induced haematological changes

See Chapter 5.

Practice points

- Iron-deficiency anaemia is a common occurrence and its underlying cause should be identified and treated.
- Iron-deficiency anaemia may be a presenting feature of NSAID-induced gastric damage.
- Iron preparations have a range of drug interactions.

Further reading

Hoffbrand A V, Pettit J E, Moss P A H (2001). *Essential Haematology*, 4th edn. Oxford: Blackwell Science.

17

The renal patient

This chapter deals specifically with the management issues surrounding patients with renal impairment, which may be associated with other conditions such as diabetes mellitus, hypertension and chronic heart failure. Renal failure has important implications for drug treatment but is a condition in its own right, which must be managed with a view to preserving renal function and dealing with its complications such as anaemia, bone disease, hypertension and uraemia. The focus of this chapter is on renal impairment and chronic renal failure, which are likely to be encountered in primary care, whilst acute renal failure is largely beyond the scope of this book.

Renal function is reflected by the glomerular filtration rate (GFR), which may be estimated from plasma creatinine levels (Chapter 2). In terms of renal function, the following classes are used:

GFR: 125 mL/min – normal
GFR: 60–30 mL/min – renal impairment
GFR: <30 mL/min – renal failure
GFR: <10 mL/min – end-stage failure

Renal failure may be acute or chronic and is classified according to cause:

- Prerenal: this involves reduced renal perfusion, as occurs acutely in hypovolaemia, and secondary to heart failure or renal artery stenosis.

- Intrinsic: this represents pathological damage to the tubular, interstitial or glomerular regions that occur in the kidney itself and may be due to diabetic nephropathy, hypertension, glomerulonephritis (which is largely an immunological disease), pyelonephritis (associated with infection) or nephrotoxic damage, for example due to drugs (Chapter 5).
- Postrenal: this is secondary to impaired renal outflow as occurs with renal stones, tumours and prostatism.

Acute renal failure

Management of acute renal failure

This topic is beyond the scope of this book but the mainstays of therapy are diuretics and the use of dopamine as a renal vasodilator, coupled with the correction of potassium levels.

Chronic renal failure

Chronic failure represents a long-term deterioration in renal function with the progressive loss

215

of nephrons and impaired renal function over many years. The most common cause is diabetic nephropathy, followed by hypertension. Other causes include chronic glomerulonephritis and atherosclerosis of the renal arteries. The consequences of chronic renal failure are related to the extent of impairment. Characteristically there is protein loss in the urine (proteinuria), which leads to less protein in the plasma (hypoalbuminaemia). This resulting reduction in colloidal osmotic pressure in the plasma, coupled with reduced water excretion, leads to tissue oedema. Impaired excretion of toxins leads to uraemia which represents the build-up of urea, phosphate, guanidines, phenols and organic acids in the blood and leads to the following clinical features:

- skin coloration (lemon tinge)
- itching
- nausea and vomiting
- constipation
- pericarditis
- neurological changes, which may include personality changes and cognitive impairment
- fatigue, which is an important presenting complaint

The impaired renal function leads to significant changes in blood biochemistry which may include:

- increased creatinine and urea
- hyperkalaemia
- hyponatraemia or normal sodium levels
- hypocalcaemia
- hyperphosphataemia
- acidosis

In addition, chronic renal failure is associated with the following complications.

Complications

Anaemia

Normocytic anaemia occurs secondary to chronic renal failure, as the kidneys produce erythropoietin (EPO) which regulates red cell production (Chapter 16) and its absence will reduce red cell synthesis. In addition, the uraemic toxins may cause bone marrow suppression and further depress red cell synthesis.

Renal bone disease (renal osteodystrophy)

The kidneys play a major role in calcium balance and renal failure also has consequences for bone mineralisation. In this respect the kidney is involved in the activation of vitamin D_3 (colecalciferol). Specifically, dietary and endogenously synthesised colecalciferol is converted by the liver to 25-hydroxycolecalciferol, which is then converted by renal 1α-hydroxylase to 1,25-hydroxycholecalciferol. This more active derivative is involved in promoting calcium uptake from the gastrointestinal tract, and is consequently impaired in renal failure. This reduction in calcium absorption leads to less calcium for bone mineralisation. Furthermore, the reduced levels of 1,25-hydroxycholecalciferol lead to an increase in the release of parathyroid hormone (PTH) from the parathyroid gland as negative feedback in response to reduced levels of 1,25-hydroxycholecalciferol. Additionally, low calcium also stimulates the release of PTH and this results in hyperparathyroidism, which is associated with increased osteoclastic resorption of bone and calcium release. The calcium may be deposited at sites other than skeletal muscle such as blood vessels. In addition, phosphate excretion is impaired in renal failure, leading to increased phosphate in the plasma, which also promotes calcium loss from the bones. Consequently, renal failure is associated with impaired bone mineralisation, which carries the risk of fractures.

Hypertension

Hypertension is associated with renal failure as renal ischaemia leads to activation of the renin–angiotensin–aldosterone system, resulting in salt and fluid retention together with vasoconstriction. These in turn lead to hypertension and an ensuing vicious circle, which causes further renal damage. Both the hypertension and fluid overload may precipitate heart failure.

Renal failure and impaired drug excretion

Many drugs and/or their metabolites are excreted by the kidneys, especially via the weak acid and base transporters in the proximal tubule.

Consequently, in renal impairment and chronic renal failure, drugs may accumulate and reach toxic levels. Therefore, for renally excreted drugs, impairment should be determined by measuring plasma creatinine levels and estimating the GFR. The *British National Formulary* contains an extensive section dealing with the use of drugs in renal impairment. More specialist and detailed literature includes *The Renal Drug Handbook* (Bunn and Ashley, 1999) and *Drug Prescribing in Renal Failure* by Aronoff *et al.* (1999), which detail how specific regimens should be altered. Generally, the approaches to renal impairment are dose reduction of the maintenance dose, increasing the dosing interval or choosing an alternative drug which is not extensively cleared by the kidneys. For example, digoxin is largely renally excreted and plasma levels will rise in renal impairment. This is dealt with by either reducing the maintenance dose of digoxin or using digitoxin as an alternative which largely undergoes hepatic elimination. When a loading dose is required, and the patient has a 'normal' extracellular volume, then the initial dose is unaffected (Chapter 6) but it may need to be increased if the volume is increased due to oedema or ascites.

Patients with impaired renal function may be more sensitive to the pharmacological actions and side-effects of certain drugs. For example, in the volume-depleted state, alpha-blockers such as prazosin have enhanced hypotensive effects.

Although impaired renal function may lead to drug toxicity through impaired excretion, this may reduce the effectiveness of drugs which require renal excretion for their actions. Examples of these include thiazide diuretics, drugs used in urinary tract infections which require excretion into the bladder to act (e.g. nalidixic acid, nitrofurantoin) and uricosuric agents which promote excretion of uric acid (e.g. probenecid).

Goals of treatment

These are to reduce the progressive loss of renal function, to limit or reverse complications such as anaemia, hypertension and renal bone disease, to reduce uraemia and provide symptomatic relief and to normalise the electrolytic balance of the body.

Management of chronic renal failure

The degree of intervention required is governed by the degree of renal impairment. Detailed guidance produced by the Renal Association may be obtained online (see Online resources, below).

Management of early chronic renal failure

Early chronic renal failure may be managed with diuretics (Chapters 11 and 14) and a diet which is low in sodium, potassium and protein. In choosing a diuretic, attention must be paid to renal function, as thiazides and thiazide-like agents (except metolazone) are ineffective in moderate renal failure since they are themselves renally excreted to enable them to act at their site of action, the distal tubule. Loop diuretics may be used in moderate and severe renal impairment but high doses may be required. The object of the low-protein diet is to slow down the accumulation of nitrogenous end-products of protein metabolism. A low-protein diet is, however, associated with malnutrition and the loss of muscle mass and reduced immune responses which are adverse to health.

Management of itching due to uraemia

Chlorphenamine may be used to relieve itching associated with uraemia.

Management of nausea

See Chapter 8.

Management of hypertension

As commented above, hypertension may lead to renal damage and may also be induced in renal damage as a consequence of activation of the renin–angiotensin–aldosterone system. What is clear is that reducing blood pressure with antihypertensive drugs will reduce the rate of loss of renal function, as assessed by a reduction in the rate of decline of GFR and protein excretion. A target blood pressure of 130/80 mmHg or less is aimed for in patients with stable renal failure and a target of 125/75 mmHg in patients with progressive disease with proteinuria.

The Ramipril Efficacy In Nephropathy (REIN) trial by the GISEN Group (1997) reported that ramipril was more effective than blood pressure lowering alone at reducing proteinuria and the rate of decline in GFR in non-diabetic nephropathy. The implication from this is that ramipril, and perhaps other angiotensin-converting enzyme (ACE) inhibitors, may be renally protective in renal failure and that ACE inhibitors should therefore be used to treat the hypertension associated with renal failure. Although it should be noted that ACE inhibitors may themselves lead to renal impairment (especially in renovascular disease) and renal function should be monitored, ACE inhibitors may increase potassium and this may enhance hyperkalaemia associated with renal failure. ACE inhibitors may also reduce the release of EPO and this may compound the associated anaemia. Angiotensin receptor antagonists can substitute for ACE inhibitors in type 2 diabetes for renal protection (Chapter 33), but whether this is the case for patients who are not diabetic remains to be determined.

Aside from the above issues, the choice and dose of antihypertensives should take account of any reductions in elimination due to renal impairment. It may also be the case that more than one agent is required to reach the target blood pressures.

Hyperlipidaemia

There is an association of hypercholesterolaemia and hypertriglyceridaemia with renal failure and statins are often prescribed (Chapter 12) to lower plasma cholesterol and reduce the cardiovascular risk. The dose of statin should take account of the level of renal impairment with appropriate reductions, and fluvastatin should be avoided in severe renal impairment.

Management of renal anaemia

Oral iron is often given initially to build up iron levels prior to treatment with erythropoietin (EPO). EPO may then be given subcutaneously or intravenously, with the dose adjusted to restore haemoglobin levels to a target of greater than 10 g/dL. The treatment of anaemia should improve exercise tolerance and reduce the risk

of precipitating heart failure. EPO is, however, associated with an increase in blood pressure in a number of patients. There are also rare reports of pure red cell aplasia (failure of red cell production) in patients receiving EPO-alpha by the subcutaneous route. This is believed to be due to the production of antibodies to EPO and treatment with EPO should be stopped. This is why it is recommended that Eprex is no longer used via the subcutaneous route.

Management of renal bone disease

1α-hydroxycholecalciferol (alfacalcidol) and calcitriol are hydroxylated derivatives of vitamin D and are given in renal failure to compensate for impaired endogenous production. Patients taking these agents should have their calcium levels measured to avoid hypercalcaemia and the dose is chosen to correct the increased PTH levels.

The additional problem contributing to renal bone disease is phosphate, as its elimination is impaired in renal failure. To reduce this problem, phosphate binders are taken with meals to bind phosphate in the gastrointestinal tract and prevent its absorption. Foods rich in phosphate include protein-rich foods, dairy products, cereals, nuts, chocolate and cola drinks. Phosphate binders used are aluminium hydroxide and calcium salts (carbonate or acetate). Calcium carbonate is the preferred agent, as, although it is less effective, it is safer than aluminium and may also provide a calcium supplement. Aluminium hydroxide has the problem that aluminium may build up in the plasma, with the risk of toxicity, including dementia and aluminium bone disease. Sevelamer is a phosphate binder which is available for patients on haemodialysis.

Aluminium and calcium-based phosphate binders show a range of interactions by increasing gastric pH and altering the absorption of certain drugs (see Chapters 5 and 7 dealing with antacid interactions). For agents affected in this way, the dose should be separated in time from the phosphate binder. A particularly important interaction is between citrate (in vitamin supplements and effervescent drug formulations) and aluminium hydroxide, which leads to an increase in aluminium levels in the blood and the possibility of encephalopathy. Accordingly, the combination of citrate and aluminium should be avoided.

Management of constipation

Constipation may occur as a result of fluid restriction and the use of aluminium as a phosphate binder, and this may be managed by lactulose and/or senna.

Hyperkalaemia

Increased plasma levels of potassium occur in renal failure and are potentially life-threatening if they rise too high. Hyperkalaemia may be prevented by polystyrene sulfonate ion exchange resins such as calcium polystyrene sulfonate, which is given orally or rectally. Sodium polystyrene sulfonate exchanges sodium for potassium in the gastrointestinal tract and is excreted rectally. Sodium polystyrene sulfonate may lead to sodium overload, which should be avoided. These resins are also constipating and a laxative should be given.

Severe hyperkalaemia is treated with insulin (given with glucose to prevent hypoglycaemia), which promotes cellular uptake of potassium.

Dialysis

Once renal function is substantially impaired and pharmacological and dietary means alone do not control the condition, then renal function must be replaced by artificial means, involving either peritoneal dialysis or haemodialysis, prior to transplantation.

Continuous ambulatory peritoneal dialysis

A permanent indwelling catheter is implanted through the abdominal wall. Sterile salt solution (2–3 L), similar to plasma but with no protein or potassium, is repeatedly run into the peritoneal cavity where it lies next to the mesenteric blood vessels. Uraemic substances accumulating in the blood enter the fluid and approach equilibrium. The solution is then discarded and replaced, and this crudely performs the main functions of the kidney. As the dialysate has zero potassium, it equilibrates with plasma and so draws potassium off down its diffusion gradient. For example, if the plasma potassium concentration is 4 mmol/L

then 10 L of dialysate fluid per day transfers 40 mmol of potassium per day. Therefore, dietary potassium must not exceed this or hyperkalaemia will occur. Adding osmotic solute (glucose) to the peritoneal dialysate can produce 1–1.5 L/day of peritoneal water loss by osmosis and the intake must be controlled to match this. This method of dialysis carries a significant risk of peritoneal infection.

Haemodialysis

This involves the exchange of substances from the blood with dialysate across an artificial semi-permeable membrane outside the body using a machine. Once again, substances diffuse into the dialysate and altering potassium and glucose concentrations may enable regulation of potassium and circulating volume. Patients receiving haemodialysis are usually anticoagulated with heparin to prevent activation of clotting triggered by the foreign surfaces of the machine.

Drug choice and dialysis

Both CAPD and haemodialysis provide routes for drug elimination and certain drugs may be efficiently removed from the body via these routes. The elimination will be determined by their permeability across the natural or artificial membranes, protein binding (drugs with high binding are less likely to be eliminated), the degree of hepatic elimination and water solubility. Hence in choosing drugs for patients on dialysis it is important to establish how the particular form of dialysis (as they may handle drugs differently) will affect drug elimination. In addition, antihypertensive drugs may be omitted or delayed on the day of haemodialysis to prevent hypotension. Accordingly, specialist advice and literature should be consulted when prescribing for patients on dialysis. Specialist books which detail how regimens for an extensive range of drugs should be altered in dialysis include *The Renal Drug Handbook* (Bunn and Ashley, 1999) and *Drug Prescribing in Renal Failure: Dosing Guidelines for Adults* (Aronoff *et al.*, 1999).

Renal transplantation

Renal transplant of kidneys from a living donor or cadaveric donor represents the best chance of a cure in end-stage renal failure. Replacement of the kidney will restore renal function, including vitamin D_3 activation and the production of EPO and their replacement will no longer be required. However, to prevent an immunological rejection of the transplanted kidney, lifelong immunosuppression will be required (except in donations from an identical twin).

Immunosuppression

A range of immunosuppressants are used in various combinations: triple therapy of ciclosporin, prednisolone and azathioprine is commonly used. The immunosuppressants are summarised in Table 17.1.

Over-the-counter considerations

Renal impairment and failure represent an important consideration for providing over-the-counter (OTC) medicines as certain products may not be suitable. An important example of this are the non-steroidal anti-inflammatory drugs (NSAIDs) which are available OTC (aspirin and ibuprofen either as tablets or as topical preparations) as they may cause sodium retention and also a deterioration in renal function and should be avoided. Paracetamol is considered a safe alternative. Similarly, effervescent products should not be used due to their appreciable content of sodium, which may lead to fluid overload in renal impairment.

Other considerations include avoiding oral rehydration therapy for diarrhoea, which will also increase the salt load; antidiarrhoeal agents such as loperamide would be a better alternative. The load of electrolytes should also be considered when using antacids, and OTC H_2-antagonists are suitable alternatives for dyspepsia. Also aluminium and calcium salts used as phosphate binders will provide relief.

Herbal medicines

It is especially important that renal patients report their usage of herbal medicines, as some herbal preparations such as cat's claw and juniper berries may cause renal damage. Furthermore,

Table 17.1 Summary of actions and adverse effects of some immunosuppressant agents

Immunosuppressant	Mechanism of action	Comments
Azathioprine	Inhibits nucleic acid synthesis and prevents lymphocyte production	May lead to bone marrow suppression with reductions in red cell, platelet and white blood cell production
Ciclosporin	Prevents activation of T-lymphocytes	Ciclosporin has many drug interactions; its metabolism may be inhibited by cytochrome P450 inhibitors such as macrolides, imidazoles, diltiazem, verapamil and cimetidine. Its metabolism may be induced by antiepileptic drugs, rifampicin and St John's wort. It is nephrotoxic and may cause hypertension
Corticosteroids	A range of immunosuppressant actions	Widespread steroid side-effects (Chapter 20)
Tacrolimus	Prevents the activation of T-lymphocytes	
Mycophenolate mofetil	Is converted to mycophenolic acid which has a more selective action than azathioprine and inhibits DNA synthesis	May cause gastrointestinal side-effects such as diarrhoea and vomiting. It is less likely than azathioprine to cause leucopenia

herbal remedies may interact with prescribed medicines. For example, St John's wort induces the metabolism of ciclosporin, and could of course render the immunosuppressant less effective and potentially lead to rejection of a transplanted kidney.

Counselling

Phosphate binders

- These should be taken 10–15 min before meals.
- They should also be taken with snacks containing protein.
- Alu-Caps, Renagel and Phosex should be swallowed whole; Calcichew and Titralac may be chewed.
- They should not be taken with antacids which contain aluminium or calcium.
- Aluminium salts may cause constipation.
- Phosphate binders should not be taken at the same time as iron tablets.

Immunosuppressants

- These must be taken continuously or the transplanted kidney may be rejected; patients should only stop taking them if advised by their doctor.
- Patients should ensure that they have adequate supplies.
- Patients taking immunosuppressants should not receive live vaccinations.
- Patients taking steroids should consult their general practitioner (GP) if they come into contact with chickenpox.
- Patients taking immunosuppressants are more susceptible to infections and are regarded as a 'special group', who should have a lower threshold for referral.
- Patients taking tacrolimus, sirolimus or ciclosporin should avoid grapefruit and grapefruit juice for 1 h before taking the drug.
- Patients taking tacrolimus may develop headaches, nausea and trembling and should consult their GP.
- Patients taking azathioprine or mycophenolate mofetil should consult their GP if there is easy bruising or signs of infection which may be due to bone marrow suppression.

- Patients should always take the same brand of ciclosporin.
- The administration of ciclosporin and sirolimus requires counselling (see *British National Formulary*).
- Tacrolimus has been associated with cardiomyopathy, which should be monitored.
- Immunosuppressants (except corticosteroids) are associated with an increased risk of skin cancer and patients taking them should wear sunblock in sunny weather.
- Tacrolimus has been reported to interact with ibuprofen (and this may also occur with other NSAIDs), leading to renal impairment.

Practice points

- Many patients with chronic renal failure also have diabetes mellitus and the treatment of these conditions should occur in tandem. *Metformin should be avoided.*
- Blood pressure should be at or below the target levels.
- Renal patients are likely to be taking many different drugs, which should be reviewed regularly.
- Patient compliance may be improved by producing a list of drugs to take and when.
- Patients with chronic renal failure should be considered for the management of anaemia, renal bone disease (involving phosphate binders and vitamin D) and hypertension.
- Renal impairment and failure and also dialysis have implications for the use of many prescription and OTC drugs.
- *The Renal Drug Handbook* (Bunn and Ashley, 1999) is an essential resource.

References

Aronoff G R, Berns J S, Brier M E *et al.* (1999). *Drug Prescribing in Renal Failure: Dosing Guidelines for Adults*, 4th edn. Philadelphia: American College of Physicians.

Bunn R, Ashley C (eds) (1999). *The Renal Drug Handbook*. Oxford: Radcliffe.

GISEN Group (1997). Randomised placebo-controlled trial of the effect of ramipril on decline of glomerular filtration rate and risk of terminal renal failure in proteinuric, non-diabetic nephropathy. *Lancet* 349: 1857–1863.

Mehta D K (ed.) *British National Formulary*, latest edition. London: British Medical Association and Royal Pharmaceutical Society of Great Britain.

Online resources

Renal Association (2002). *Treatment of Adult Patients with Renal Failure: Recommended Standards and Audit Measures*, 3rd edn. Published online at www.nephronline.org (accessed 4 December 2002).

www.kidney.org.uk is the website of UK National Kidney Foundation, which provides patient information (accessed 4 December 2002).

www.nephrologypharmacy.com is the website of Nephrology Pharmacy Associates and provides extensive resources, including dialysis of drugs (accessed 4 December 2002).

www.nephrononline.org provides professional advice regarding the management of renal failure (accessed 4 December 2002).

www.renalpharmacy.org.uk is the website of the UK Renal Pharmacy Group (accessed 4 December 2002).

Part E

Respiratory diseases

18

Coughs and colds

This is clearly a key topic in community practice, with many patients having consultations for a range of related illnesses. Nevertheless, this can be a controversial area as some commonly used remedies are of questionable value.

Colds or acute coryza

This is a very common occurrence, usually due to either rhino- or adenovirus infections, which produce symptoms of a runny nose (rhinorrhoea), sneezing and pyrexia. The common cold is often referred to as a 'flu-like' illness but it should be noted that influenza is an entirely different and more serious infection. Infants may have around 12 colds per year and adults can expect to have 1–2 per year. Colds are self-limiting with a typical course of 1 week. However, there are a number of complications, including sinusitis, otitis media and secondary chest infections.

Treatment of a cold

Treatment of the cold is generally directed at symptomatic relief. The mainstay of treatment should be regular ibuprofen and/or paracetamol to reduce the increased temperature. Recent evidence has suggested that zinc lozenges (15 mg, 5 times daily) are effective at reducing the length and severity of a cold, provided they are taken at the onset of symptoms. This action has been attributed to the prevention of viral particles entering the epithelial cells of the upper respiratory tract. Additional simple measures include steam inhalation, which appears to hydrate the airways and promote the removal of mucus.

Nasal decongestants

Topical nasal decongestants are also effective at reducing the symptoms of excessive mucus production. Topical decongestants, such as xylometazoline and oxymetazoline, are alpha-adrenoceptor agonists which cause nasal vaso-constriction and so reduce the flow of mucus. The only major problem is that prolonged use (5–7 days) may lead to rebound congestion (rhinitis medicamentosa).

Systemic decongestants are also widely used but are probably less effective than topical agents and their systemic administration may be associated with side-effects. Systemic agents include phenylephrine, which has direct sympathomimetic activity, while pseudoephedrine and phenylpropanolamine both have direct and indirect sympathomimetic vasoconstrictor actions, leading to nasal vasoconstriction. Their sympathomimetic activity also means that they are unsuitable for patients with:

- severe ischaemic heart disease
- uncontrolled hypertension
- hyperthyroidism
- diabetes

Indeed, phenylpropanolamine, when used at higher doses than those in the UK, has been implicated in causing stroke in patients in the USA. The Committee on Safety of Medicines (CSM) has now indicated that the daily dose of phenylpropanolamine should not exceed 100 mg. In theory, pseudoephedrine should cause bronchodilation via activation of $beta_2$-adrenoceptors on the bronchial smooth muscle, which may be of benefit in infections which involve the airways. Sympathomimetics show a range of interactions and in particular will be potentiated by monoamine oxidase inhibitors (MAOIs), which precludes their concurrent use. Some important interactions are detailed in Table 18.1.

Cough mixtures

Antitussives, e.g. codeine, dextromethorphan, pholcodine; expectorants, e.g. guaifenesin, ipecacuanha, ammonium chloride

Although a cough is a symptom and not an illness, it is appropriate to consider cough mixtures here as they are widely used in colds. Cough mixtures are divided into antitussives (cough suppressants) and expectorants. In general, cough mixtures are of doubtful medicinal value but do provide an appreciable placebo effect, from which patients may derive benefit. Antitussives contain opioids which act on the cough centres in the brain to suppress the cough. Codeine in particular

has the potential for dependence and pronounced opioid side-effects such as constipation. These agents will suppress the cough and remove the symptoms. However, the cough serves the purpose of clearing the lungs and cough suppression may be inappropriate. Indeed, retention of sputum means that they are harmful in chronic obstructive pulmonary disease (COPD) and asthma, and may also mask worsening symptoms. Expectorants are intended to facilitate mucus removal but there is no convincing evidence to support this occurring at the doses used.

Given the apparent lack of efficacy of cough mixtures, a simple linctus may be beneficial by a soothing action and a placebo effect.

Compound preparations

Many proprietary compound preparations are available and typically contain some of the following: an antitussive, an antipyretic (paracetamol or ibuprofen), a systemic decongestant and an antihistamine. The effectiveness of each agent has been considered above, except antihistamines. Sedating (or old) antihistamines such as promethazine will promote sleep (which could be disturbed by the cough) and their antimuscarinic side-effects will help dry up the secretions.

Echinacea

Echinacea is widely used to shorten the duration and reduce the severity of cold symptoms. To date, there have been trials which both confirm and question its efficacy.

Influenza

As commented above, this must be distinguished from flu-like illnesses. Influenza is an upper respiratory tract infection which has a more severe course and is associated with more complications and significant mortality. Indeed, more people died in the epidemic of Spanish flu (1918–1919) than were killed in the First World War. It is caused by influenza viruses A, B or C. The associated symptoms include pyrexia, chills, headache, muscle aches, backache, sore throat, cough and

Table 18.1 Some interactions of drugs with oral sympathomimetic agents

Drugs	Consequences	Comments
Phenylephrine with monoamine oxidase inhibitors (MAOIs)	The pressor activity of phenylephrine is substantially enhanced by MAOIs	This is largely because phenylephrine is normally metabolised by MAO and only small amounts enter the circulation. This may lead to a fatal hypertensive crisis. Their concurrent use should be avoided
Indirectly acting sympathomimetic agents (e.g. phenylpropanolamine, pseudoephedrine) with MAOIs	This combination may lead to a fatal hypertensive crisis	Their concurrent use should be avoided
Indirectly acting sympathomimetic agents (e.g. phenylpropanolamine, pseudoephedrine) with tricyclic antidepressants	The actions of indirectly acting sympathomimetic agents would be expected to be reduced by tricyclic antidepressants	This is not believed to be significant
Phenylephrine with tricyclic antidepressants	The pressor actions of phenylephrine would be expected to be increased by tricyclic antidepressants	This is not believed to be significant
Phenylephrine/ phenylpropanolamine with beta-blockers	No significant interaction between OTC phenylephrine and beta-blockers occurs	Phenylpropanolamine has been shown to cause a pressor effect in patients taking beta-blockers but this is not regarded as clinically significant. The CSM has advised that phenylpropanolamine should not be taken by patients with hypertension, heart disease or hyperthyroidism
Phenylpropanolamine with caffeine	The pressor effects of phenylpropanolamine are enhanced by caffeine and this may result in hypertension in susceptible patients	

OTC, over-the-counter; CSM, Committee on Safety of Medicines.

runny nose and it is followed by postviral debilitation which may persist for several weeks after the infection.

Treatment of uncomplicated influenza is directed towards symptomatic relief, including ibuprofen and/or paracetamol for pain relief and reduction of pyrexia. A recent development has been the introduction of viral neuramidase inhibitors, such as zanamivir, which prevent the entry and release of viral particles from host cells. These drugs are effective against influenza A and B. It is given by inhalation and this has occasionally been associated with bronchospasm and so should be used with caution in asthma (a bronchodilator should be available) and avoided in severe asthma. In 2002, the National Institute of Clinical Excellence (NICE) released guidance recommending that zanamivir was not for use in normally healthy patients but was appropriate for:

- patients over 65 years of age
- patients with chronic respiratory diseases
- patients with cardiovascular disease (but not hypertension)
- immunocompromised patients
- patients with diabetes mellitus

It is now extended to chronic renal disease and must be started within 48 h of the start of symptoms.

Amantadine (an antiparkinson drug) also has a limited role in the prevention of influenza A and acts by inhibiting viral DNA replication. It is best used as prophylaxis in patients who are at risk but who cannot be vaccinated or while vaccination takes effect (2 weeks).

Vaccination now plays an important role in the prevention of influenza in vulnerable patients and annual vaccination is recommended for:

- patients over 65 years of age
- people in residential care homes
- patients with:
  - chronic respiratory conditions
  - chronic heart disease
  - chronic renal failure
  - diabetes mellitus
  - immunosuppression due to drugs, disease or following a splenectomy

Acute bronchitis

A potential complication of an upper respiratory infection is acute bronchitis, which may be viral or bacterial. A viral infection may give rise to a dry cough, while a secondary bacterial infection is more often associated with the production of thick green sputum. Additional symptoms may include a wheeze and breathlessness.

In healthy patients acute bronchitis usually resolves spontaneously in 1–2 weeks but may exacerbate asthma and COPD (Chapter 20) and there is a risk of bronchopneumonia. As mentioned in Chapter 20, patients with asthma may have a steroid introduced or the dose of an existing steroid increased; patients with COPD may be given prophylactic antibiotics to take at the start of an exacerbation, and if appropriate may receive a steroid. In normally healthy patients symptomatic relief may be all that is required. Elderly patients or those with concurrent illnesses such as heart disease or diabetes may be treated with amoxicillin; in patients who are penicillin-allergic, tetracycline or erythromycin may be prescribed. Failure of initial treatment with amoxicillin may be followed by the use of co-amoxiclav, tetracycline or a macrolide.

Pneumonia

Pneumonia involves infection of the alveoli as opposed to the bronchi. This may lead to sputum (which may be blood-stained, and is often rusty in appearance), breathlessness, pleuritic chest pains and fever. In pneumonia acquired in the community (as opposed to hospital) the principal causative agents are *Streptococcus pneumoniae* (most), *Haemophilus influenzae* and *Chlamydia pneumoniae*, while *C. psittaci* is associated with contact with birds. Given the potential seriousness of pneumonia, antibacterial treatment is appropriate with amoxicillin (or erythromycin if penicillin-allergic) being used first-line for mild, community-acquired infections. Depending on response and the strain of bacteria, other agents which may be used include: tetracycline, flucloxacillin, erythromycin, clarithromycin, cefuroxime, cefotaxime, and gentamicin, alone or in various combinations. For example, *C. psittaci* and *C. pneumoniae* are treated with a macrolide or tetracycline, and *H. influenzae* with cefaclor (Chapter 30).

Acute sinusitis

This is infection of the facial sinuses, and is usually bacterial, with *S. pneumoniae*, *H. influenzae* and *Staphylococcus aureus* being the common causative organisms. Sinusitis is associated with discomfort and purulent discharge. Treatment may include nasal decongestants and analgesics to provide symptomatic relief. Sinusitis should normally resolve spontaneously but, in severe or poorly resolving cases, systemic antibiotics (amoxicillin, co-amoxiclav, erythromycin or doxycycline) are appropriate. There is no evidence that topical antibacterial agents are effective.

Otitis media

This is earache due to middle-ear infection and is very common in children, often following a cold or sore throat. On examination the eardrum is bulging and inflamed. The cause is often viral but may also be bacterial (mostly due to *Streptococcus* pneumoniae, *H. influenzae*, *Moraxella catarrhalis* and, less commonly, *S. pyogenes*) and there is no way of identifying the causative agent unless the eardrum is perforated and a swab taken for culture.

The initial management is for pain relief with either paracetamol and/or ibuprofen and this is certainly appropriate for the first day or so as most cases will resolve spontaneously. Further treatment with antibiotics is controversial as many cases are viral. Some practitioners prescribe antibiotics blind and amoxicillin is used, but 15% of *H. influenzae* are resistant due to beta-lactamase production and so co-amoxiclav or cephalosporins may be more appropriate; macrolides may also be considered. However, evidence indicates that antibiotics only shorten the course of the infection by a couple of days, and then only in approximately 15% of patients, so their empirical use is often unnecessary (Damoiseaux *et al.*, 2000). Furthermore the use of antibiotics is associated with side-effects (such as diarrhoea and nausea) and overuse has been implicated in secretory otitis media ('glue ear').

Sore throats – pharyngitis and tonsillitis

Pharyngitis, other than that due to irritation (e.g. smoke) is mostly viral in origin and thus requires symptomatic relief. This typically involves paracetamol or ibuprofen. Interestingly, antibacterial lozenges are of no value and may in fact irritate the inflamed mucosa, while local anaesthetic lozenges may sensitise the mucosa. Indeed, simple sugar-free boiled sweets may provide relief.

Some sore throats are bacterial, generally due to infection with group A beta-haemolytic streptococci. It is particularly difficult to distinguish a bacterial sore throat from a viral infection. Some features which may point to a bacterial infection are an inflamed pharynx with yellow/white exudates on the tonsils, enlarged, tender cervical lymph nodes and a sore throat in isolation not accompanied by upper respiratory tract infection. Bacterial sore throats may be treated with antibiotics when there is proven streptococcal infection, when they fail to resolve spontaneously, when the symptoms are severe and may involve systemic symptoms such as scarlet fever or in children with diabetes mellitus. Currently phenoxymethylpenicillin for 10 days is the standard first-line drug treatment for infections by beta-haemolytic streptococci but cephalosporins and macrolides are also effective. Amoxicillin and ampicillin should not be used blind, as in glandular fever they frequently lead to a maculopapular rash.

Previously rheumatic fever and glomerulonephritis were occasional complications of streptococcal throat infections. This is because *S. pyogenes* antigens cross-react with human connective tissue. Group A streptococci share antigenic properties with heart valve glycoprotein leading to damage, nephritis and also arthritis. This complication is very rare nowadays but patients who have previously had endocarditis, who have a history of nephritis or who have artificial heart valves should receive antibiotics during throat infections.

Sore throats are a common occurrence in patients with drug-induced neutropenia and patients who are taking:

- carbamazepine
- phenytoin
- clozapine
- mianserin
- gold salts
- carbimazole
- 5-aminosalicylates
- azathioprine

should be counselled to report sore throats as this may indicate neutropenia and a white blood cell count is required. Inhaled steroids may also promote candidial infections of the throat (Chapter 20).

Cough

A cough is not an illness but a symptom of a range of other conditions, ranging from trivial to serious (Chapter 1).

Counselling and practice points

It is impossible to provide generic counselling for the infections described above; however, there are several important points which should be borne in mind:

- Simple analgesia and antipyretic treatment with paracetamol and/or ibuprofen has a major role in many of these conditions. Paracetamol tends to be used first line in pyrexia and is favoured as it has limited adverse drug reactions (ADRs) and interactions; ibuprofen may be added in resistance.
- Symptomatic relief has a major role in colds, sore throats, otitis media and sinusitis. Reassurance of parents plays an important role with children.
- Cough mixtures generally lack efficacy but have an appreciable placebo effect.
- Antitussive agents may cause sputum retention which is potentially harmful in COPD and asthma.
- Sympathomimetic agents are best via the topical route; with the oral route there is the potential for systemic effects and life-threatening interactions with concurrent MAOIs.
- In pharyngitis and otitis media, most cases are viral and it is difficult to identify bacterial infections. Antibiotic treatment is appropriate on the suspicion of a bacterial infection, in a poorly resolving infection or in patients who are at risk.
- Be alert for pharyngitis as a symptom of neutropenia as an ADR.
- Be alert for cough as a symptom of a range of diseases (Chapter 1).
- When a course of antibiotics is prescribed, the importance of completing the course should be emphasised and instructions given when to take the agent in relation to food.
- In influenza, zanamivir has been recommended for use in vulnerable patients, but must be started within 48 h of the appearance of symptoms. It carries the risk of bronchospasm and patients with asthma should have a bronchodilator available.
- Given the need for prompt initiation of zanamivir, systems should be in place to ensure that it is available for immediate dispensing.
- Vaccination against influenza is recommended for patients at a high risk of complications.

 CASE STUDIES

Case 1
Mr NC (35 years old), who has previously been in good health, visits his general practitioner (GP) complaining of a 'nasty, painful and irritating cough'. On questioning, the GP establishes that the patient has retrosternal pain on coughing and that the cough is non-productive. The GP recommends paracetamol if there is any fever.

The GP's next patient is Mr CC (65 years), who has previously been in good health and is complaining of a 'nasty cough', is slightly breathless and has been coughing up thick green sputum for 5 days. On auscultation the GP hears wheezing in a previously healthy chest. The GP prescribes amoxicillin 250 mg t.d.s. to be taken for 1 week and recommends paracetamol if required.

Why has the GP treated these patients differently?

- Mr NC probably has a viral infection leading to a non-productive painful cough, whereas Mr CC appears to have acute bronchitis, which may well be secondary to a recent bout of viral tracheitis – the bacterial infection is indicated by the cough productive of green sputum. Antibiotics may be appropriate, although less so in a previously healthy chest.

How would you counsel Mr CC?

→

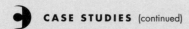 **CASE STUDIES** (continued)

- He should complete the course, even if the cough clears up, as there may still be bacteria present (especially the more resistant strains), so the complete course is required for full eradication.
- He should take the antibiotic three times a day: breakfast, lunch and bedtime is a traditional and convenient spacing.
- As a common side-effect of antibiotic treatment, he might get diarrhoea.

Case 2

Mrs PT visits the above GP complaining of a sore throat and a raised temperature. Following an examination, the GP recommends that she takes either paracetamol or ibuprofen, rests and takes plenty of fluids.

Mrs SP is the next patient and complains of the same symptoms. Following a throat examination the GP observes pus exudates, and enlarged cervical lymph nodes. Phenoxymethylpenicillin 500 mg q.d.s. was prescribed for 10 days.

Why has the GP treated these patients differently?

- Most cases of pharyngitis are viral and thus require symptomatic relief. Some infections are bacterial (streptococcal) and present with similar symptoms. On examination, the bacterial infection may be suggested by an inflamed pharynx with yellow/white exudates visible on the tonsils. The patient may have enlarged, tender cervical lymph nodes. Mrs PT has a viral infection and Mrs SP a presumed bacterial infection.

Comment on the choice of antibiotic.

- Phenoxymethylpenicillin is recommended first-line. Amoxicillin and ampicillin should not be used blind in a sore throat because in glandular fever they generally lead to a maculopapular rash.

Case 3

An 18-year-old female student visits her GP complaining of a sore throat and general tiredness. Following a limited consultation the GP gives her a prescription for amoxicillin 250 mg t.d.s. The following day, the student develops a maculopapular rash and seeks your advice.

How might you respond to the rash?

- She should stop taking the amoxicillin. She should take an antihistamine (loratadine 10 mg daily or chlorphenamine 4 mg q.d.s., but sedation may be a problem) for relief of the rash.

What are the likely causes of the rash?

- penicillin allergy
- glandular fever; amoxicillin should not be given blind for a sore throat as 90% of patients with glandular fever develop a rash. This does not mean a lifelong allergy to penicillins

What further tests and treatment may be appropriate for this patient?

- A blood test (Monospot or Paul–Bunnell test) for glandular fever. If she has glandular fever then symptomatic relief is required and she should avoid alcohol.
- If she has a penicillin allergy, then she should be prescribed a non-penicillin, non-cephalosporin such as erythromycin (250 mg q.d.s.) and the allergy documented on her medical records.

References

Damoiseaux R A M J, van Balen F A M, Hoes A W *et al.* (2000). Primary care based randomised, double blind trial of amoxicillin versus placebo for acute otitis media in children aged under 2 years. *BMJ* 320: 350–354.

NICE (2002). Guidance of the use of zanamivir (Relenza) in the treatment of influenza. Technology Appraisal Guidance no. 15. London: National Institute for Clinical Excellence (via www.nice.org.uk).

Further reading

Brooks A, Ryan R (2001). Diagnosis and treatment of otitis media in children. *Prescriber* 12: 84–91.

Jewes L (2000). When and how to treat URTI with antibiotics. *Prescriber* 11: 97–109.

Rice P (2002). Influenza – recommended treatment and prevention. *Prescriber* 13: 48–57.

Schroeder K, Fahey T (2002). Systematic review of randomised controlled trials of over the counter cough medicines for acute cough in adults. *BMJ* 324: 329–331.

Wilkinson M (2001). Chest infections: causes and when to treat. *Prescriber* 12: 25–32.

19

Allergy

Allergy may be viewed as an inappropriate immune response provoked by a foreign agent, the allergen, which leads to a troublesome pathophysiological response; in the extreme there may be life-threatening anaphylaxis.

In an allergic response an antigen (allergen) leads to increased immunoglobulin E (IgE) synthesis. The IgE becomes attached to mast cell surfaces and the cross-linking of IgE by the allergen leads to calcium entry. This is followed by mast cell degranulation and the release of inflammatory mediators (including histamine and leukotrienes) leading to increased vascular permeability, chemotaxis, increased production of mucus and oedema (due to increased vascular permeability and vasodilatation in response to histamine).

There are a number of conditions associated with allergic responses and these include allergic rhinitis, allergic asthma, contact dermatitis (Chapter 32), drug-induced skin reactions (Chapter 5) and anaphylaxis.

Allergic rhinitis

Disease characteristics

Allergic rhinitis may be perennial (throughout the year), seasonal (as in hayfever) or occupational, resulting from exposure to chemicals, dusts and animal dander and urine. The clinical features include:

- nasal itching
- rhinorrhoea
- sneezing
- itchy throat
- wheezing
- conjunctival symptoms which involve itchiness and bilateral red eye, worsened by irritants such as smoke.

The precise balance of symptoms may vary between the causes, with the perennial disease having less prominent eye symptoms.

In response to allergen exposure, mast cells and T-lymphocytes are activated with tissue recruitment of basophils and eosinophils. Histamine is the primary mediator from mast cells and basophils and acts largely on H_1-receptors to evoke the characteristic symptoms, while actions at H_2- and H_3-receptors also occur, leading to nasal obstruction. In addition, leukotrienes, prostaglandins and kinins also contribute to the inflammatory response.

Goals of treatment

These are to provide symptomatic relief with the minimum of side-effects.

Management

The first approach is to minimise exposure to allergens such as grass pollen in the spring, tree pollen at other times and house dust mites; simple measures such as vacuuming the house, washing bed clothes at 60°C and freezing pillows may help.

Antihistamines

Initial pharmacological treatment is directed against histamine and involves H_1-receptor antagonists or antihistamines. These agents remove the symptoms of rhinorrhoea, itching, conjunctivitis and sneezing but not nasal obstruction. Older sedating agents include:

- chlorphenamine (Piriton)
- promethazine (Phenergan)
- alimemazine (Vallergan)

Some antihistamines (especially promethazine) have prominent antimuscarinic effects, which may limit their use. More recently, non-sedating agents have been introduced which have a better side-effect profile which favours their use. Examples of non-sedating antihistamines include:

- acrivastine (Benadryl)
- cetirizine (Zirtek)
- fexofenadine (Telfast)
- loratadine (Clarityn)

- desloratadine (Neoclarityn), which is a metabolite of loratadine

and all, except acrivastine, can be used once daily.

Topical antihistamines

Antihistamines such as levocabastine are available as topical nasal and eye drops for the rapid relief of nasal and eye symptoms. Patients are probably better maintained on oral antihistamines but topical antihistamines may have a limited role as 'on demand' treatment against a background of continuous oral drug treatment. In addition, ocular antihistamines may be of use for the relief of occasional symptoms. Some ocular preparations may also contain sympathomimetic vasoconstrictors such as xylometazoline to reduce the red eye.

Topical intranasal corticosteroids

e.g. Beclometasone, budesonide, fluticasone and triamcinolone

Corticosteroids reduce the production of cytokines and chemokines and reduce infiltration of antigen-presenting cells, T-cells, eosinophils in the tissue and mast cells in epithelial mucosa. Clinical trials have shown that they are superior to oral or topical antihistamines for nasal symptoms but take several days for an effect, during which time an oral antihistamine is appropriate.

Administration via the nasal route reduces the side-effects associated with corticosteroids, such as the risk of hypothalamic pituitary–adrenal axis suppression, but in children their height should be monitored for height suppression. Patients with allergic rhinitis may also be asthmatic, and although the topical nasal steroids may be used in addition to inhaled steroids, there is an increased risk of side-effects. Intranasal steroids should be avoided during nasal infection.

Oral steroids are not recommended as first-line treatment but can be used for short periods (<2 weeks) in severe disease or when control of symptoms is essential, for example during examination times. Indeed, by reducing mucus production in severe disease, they may enable topical agents to penetrate more easily.

Topical cromones

Sodium cromoglicate and nedocromil sodium

The action of cromones is poorly defined but they may inhibit cytokine release from mast cells, possibly by blocking calcium channels. They may also inhibit sensory nerve activity and suppress local reflexes. Their effects are weak but they are devoid of side-effects and are largely for seasonal disease. Eye drops containing cromones may also be effective for conjunctival symptoms. In both cases it may take several days for cromones to exert an effect.

Muscarinic antagonists

Ipratropium

The muscarinic antagonist ipratropium is available as a nasal spray and will reduce the rhinorrhoea but will not affect other nasal symptoms such as itchiness. The older antihistamines also have appreciable antimuscarinic activity, which will contribute to their actions.

Decongestants

e.g. Oxymetazoline, xylometazoline

These sympathomimetic agents are dealt with in Chapter 18. In the context of allergic rhinitis, these are applied topically and provide relief from nasal obstruction but once again their use should be limited to a week due to rebound congestion.

Hyposensitisation

This involves desensitisation of a patient towards an allergen but is very rarely carried out these days. To achieve this the patient is challenged with increasing doses of the allergen over time, starting with a very low dose, and this is believed to reduce the IgE response. This may be effective for severe allergic rhinitis when the allergen is identified and conventional treatment has failed, and may also be appropriate for wasp and bee venom stings. However, the process carries a significant risk of anaphylaxis and so hyposensitisation for allergic rhinitis is contraindicated in asthmatics, although in the case of bee and wasp stings, the allergic response may be fatal and so asthma is not an absolute contraindication.

Choice of drugs

Oral antihistamines and/or intranasal steroids seem to be the mainstay of therapy, with other agents being added to treatment in response to symptoms. Oral antihistamines tend to be used for mild or intermittent disease, while intranasal steroids are perhaps best used for persistent, moderate and severe disease, especially with nasal symptoms. Combining oral antihistamines and regular intranasal steroids would probably be the best approach in more severe disease. Other considerations are detailed in Table 19.1.

Drug interactions

The most significant interactions in the past have resulted from the increase in plasma concentrations of terfenadine due to various inhibitors of cytochrome P450, including macrolides. Inhibition of cytochrome P450-dependent metabolism prevents the breakdown of terfenadine to its active metabolite (fexofenadine) and the augmentation of terfenadine levels is associated with QT prolongation and fatal arrhythmias. In 1997 this resulted in terfenadine being changed from an over-the-counter (OTC) medicine to a prescription-only medicine (POM) and the introduction of fexofenadine. Terfenadine should not be used with other drugs which cause QT prolongation or affect its metabolism. Other specific interactions are detailed in Table 19.2.

Counselling

General counselling may be directed at avoiding contact with allergens and limiting them in the home. Patients with hayfever may benefit from wearing sunglasses and should avoid going outdoors and keep the windows closed when the pollen count is high. For occupation-related allergies the patient should be advised to wear suitable protective clothing.

Antihistamines

- Patients taking sedating antihistamines should be advised that their ability to drive or operate

Table 19.1   The effects of concurrent conditions on drug choice in allergy

Condition	Effect on drug choice	Comments
Symptoms affecting sleep	This would favour the use of a sedating antihistamine	
Patient must be alert (e.g. driving, exams)	This would preclude the use of a sedating antihistamine. Non-sedating antihistamines would be appropriate or nasal or, rarely, oral steroids	The sedating effects are enhanced by alcohol. There is no evidence that alcohol enhances the effects of the newer, non-sedating antihistamines but patients should exercise caution
Glaucoma, prostatic hypertrophy, urinary retention	Ipratropium is best avoided. Antimuscarinic side-effects of certain older antihistamines mean that they should be used with caution in these conditions. Nasal steroids may rarely affect glaucoma. Vasoconstrictors, such as xylometazoline, should be avoided in angle-closure glaucoma	Newer, non-sedating antihistamines are generally devoid of antimuscarinic actions and would be appropriate. The use of other drugs with antimuscarinic effects should be taken into account
QT prolongation	Avoid terfenadine and mizolastine	Terfenadine and mizolastine are associated with QT prolongation, leading to arrhythmias
Epilepsy	Antihistamines may occasionally lead to convulsions	Caution should be exercised
Porphyria	Avoid certain antihistamines	Cetirizine, chlorphenamine, cyclizine, diphenhydramine, doxylamine, loratadine and alimemazine are considered safe. Refer to the *British National Formulary*
Asthma	Steroids and leukotriene receptor antagonists are also used for asthma. Antihistamines are of no clear benefit in asthma	Intranasal steroids may be used concurrently with inhaled steroids taken for asthma, but this may increase the chances of an ADR. Leukotriene receptor antagonists reduce the symptoms of allergic rhinitis and this may be a reason to choose them in concurrent asthma
Risk of anaphylaxis	This may be a reason to avoid continuous use of antihistamines	Antihistamines may mask the early warning symptoms
Renal impairment	Avoid acrivastine in moderate impairment. Chlorphenamine is used for pruritus associated with renal failure	

ADR, adverse drug reaction.

machinery may be impaired. The sedation will be enhanced by alcohol.
- Non-sedating antihistamines rarely affect skilled tasks in this way but patients should be advised to exercise caution.

Topical antihistamines

- Nasal antihistamines would be best used as an add-on to oral treatment with worsening symptoms.

Table 19.2   Some important interactions with antihistamines

Drugs	Consequences	Comments
Alcohol with sedating antihistamines	The sedating effects are enhanced by alcohol	There is no evidence that alcohol enhances the effects of the newer non-sedating antihistamines but patients should exercise caution
Zafirlukast with terfenadine	Terfenadine significantly reduces the plasma concentrations of zafirlukast	
Loratadine with cimetidine, clarithromycin, erythromycin or ketoconazole	The plasma concentration of loratadine is substantially increased by the concomitant administration of the drugs listed	This is not believed to be clinically significant
Mizolastine with erythromycin, ketoconazole or antiarrhythmics (class I and III) which prolong QT interval	Concomitant use should be avoided due to the risk of potentially fatal torsade de pointes arrhythmias	Caution with cimetidine, ciclosporin and nifedipine
Older antihistamines with antimuscarinic agents (e.g. tricyclic antidepressants, certain antipsychotics)	Potentiation of antimuscarinic side-effects	

Decongestants

- These should only be used for 5–7 days due to the risk of rebound congestion.

Ocular agents

- Ocular antihistamines are best used for occasional eye symptoms.
- Long-term use of eye drops containing xylometazoline should be avoided due to vasoconstrictor effects on the eye.
- Contact lenses should not be worn during conjunctival symptoms or following the application of drugs.

Topical corticosteroids

- In seasonal rhinitis treatment should be started a week or two before the appearance of pollen.
- These drugs will take several days to act and in the meantime an oral antihistamine may be used for relief.
- They should be used continuously, even if the patient feels better.

Cromones

- They will take a few days for an effect to occur.
- They should be used continuously, even if symptoms resolve.

Intranasal agents

- Correct application is important. The patient should shake the container, close the other nostril with a finger, bend forward, spray and inhale, but avoid sniffing.

Allergy and anaphylaxis

Many foreign substances can elicit an allergic response, affecting many systems, including the skin and airways. Examples of important allergens include:

- drugs (especially penicillins, streptokinase, non-steroidal anti-inflammatory drugs (NSAIDs) including aspirin, monoclonal antibodies, vaccines, radiological contrast media)

- food (particularly nuts and seafood) but should be distinguished from food intolerance
- insect bites
- snake venom
- latex
- household chemicals or pollutants

Drug-induced allergy

This is a serious type B adverse drug reaction and affects a minority of patients on second exposure to the drug, even to minute doses, and manifests as an allergic response. Allergic drug reactions are dealt with in more detail in Chapter 5.

Management of allergic reaction

Regardless of the cause, the first measure is to remove the patient from exposure to the allergen or prevent exposure. In an allergic reaction leading to a maculopapular rash or urticaria, an oral antihistamine should be considered the mainstay of treatment. In local allergic responses to insect stings, an oral antihistamine should be given and topical hydrocortisone may be applied. In both cases, topical antihistamines such as mepyramine should be avoided as they may irritate the tissue. As a secondary measure for more severe reactions, an oral steroid may be appropriate.

Prophylaxis

When it is anticipated that medical treatment, such as the use of radiological contrast media or monoclonal antibodies, may lead to an allergic response, patients may receive a prophylactic oral antihistamine and possibly a corticosteroid.

Anaphylaxis

Anaphylactic shock is a serious life–threatening allergic reaction due to production of IgE and involves high yields of mediators, especially histamine. Anaphylactoid shock is related to anaphylaxis but does not involve IgE. Anaphylaxis may manifest within 30 min of exposure and symptoms include:

- angioedema (including swollen lips, eyelids and tongue)
- shortness of breath
- wheezing
- generalised itch
- hypotension

Oedema is an important feature, with extravasation of fluid from the circulation leading to hypotension and airway obstruction. Antihistamines may mask the early symptoms of anaphylaxis and so they should be avoided as continuous treatment in patients at risk.

Treatment of anaphylaxis

Basic life support measures are essential and involve maintaining airways and laying the patient flat. Treatment is aimed at bronchodilation, supporting the circulation and suppressing the immune response. To this end 'shock boxes' containing adrenaline (epinephrine), chlorphenamine and hydrocortisone are available.

Initially adrenaline is given intramuscularly and this may be repeated at 10-min intervals according to blood pressure and respiration. The purpose of administering adrenaline is to restore blood pressure by increasing cardiac output, via activation of cardiac beta$_1$-adrenoceptors, and vasoconstriction via alpha-adrenoceptors. The adrenaline will also act on bronchial beta$_2$-adrenoceptors to oppose the bronchospasm. In patients who are receiving non-selective beta-blockers, the effects of adrenaline will be reduced and so intravenous salbutamol should also be considered. Further measures include oxygen, an inhaled beta$_2$-agonist if there is a wheeze, a saline infusion to restore circulating volume in hypotension and intravenous antihistamine (e.g. chlorphenamine) to oppose the effects of histamine.

As a secondary measure to suppress the immune response, hydrocortisone may be given intravenously.

Adrenaline for self-administration

Patients at risk of anaphylaxis may be given adrenaline for self-administration via intramuscular injection as required, for example following a bee-sting. These patients require instructions in the use of the adrenaline administration devices and should be advised to wear a 'medic alert' bracelet.

Drug interactions with adrenaline

As commented above, adrenaline may be less effective in patients taking beta-blockers and higher doses of adrenaline or intravenous salbutamol should be used. The interaction between non-selective beta-blockers (such as propranolol) and adrenaline in normotensive patients is discussed in Chapter 5. Topical beta-blockers such as timolol eye drops for glaucoma may also interact with adrenaline. In patients who are at risk of anaphylaxis it may be sensible, if possible, to swap from beta-blockers to alternative drugs.

The effects of adrenaline are enhanced by tricyclic antidepressants which prevent the uptake of adrenaline and so increase its concentrations.

Accordingly, lower doses of adrenaline should be used in patients who are taking tricyclic antidepressants. Alternatively, the antidepressant may be changed to a selective serotonin reuptake inhibitor, which should not interact with adrenaline.

Practice points

- Oral antihistamines and/or nasal steroids should be regarded as the mainstay of therapy for allergic rhinitis.
- Prompt recognition of the symptoms of anaphylaxis is essential.
- Patients at risk of anaphylaxis should be counselled on how to use an adrenaline autoinjector.

 CASE STUDY

A 40-year-old lorry driver visits his community pharmacy complaining of hayfever, which he had as a child but remembers the drugs he took as being 'awful' as they made him feel worse than the hayfever.

Past medical history: asthma
Drugs: Salbutamol 200 µg p.r.n.
Beclometasone 200 µg b.d.

1. What symptoms is the patient likely to have?

- nasal itching, rhinorrhoea, sneezing and conjunctival symptoms, which are worsened by irritants

2. He would like something that will clear up his hayfever; what do you suggest?

- A non-sedating H_1-receptor antagonist such as loratadine or acrivastine may be recommended. These are available OTC and should not interfere with his ability to drive.

3. He is somewhat disturbed by the cost of the tablets you suggest. What advice can you give him?

- He should see his general practitioner for a prescription.

Several weeks later he complains that, although he is much better, his nose is still blocked and his eyes are still watery.

continued

CASE STUDY (continued)

4. What OTC medication might you prescribe?

Possibilities include:

- a topical nasal steroid such as beclometasone for prophylaxis and treatment. It may be added in addition to the inhaled steroid
- sodium cromoglicate nasal spray or eye drops, but these will take several days to act. He should not drive immediately after the drops if his vision is blurred
- antihistamine eye drops for fast relief

Reference

Mehta D K (ed.) *British National Formulary*, latest edition. London: British Medical Association and Royal Pharmaceutical Society of Great Britain.

Further reading

Croom A (2002). Anaphylaxis: prevention and acute treatment. *Prescriber* 13: 18–28.

Rusznak D, Davies R J (1998). ABC of allergies. Diagnosing allergy. *BMJ* 316: 686–698.

20

Respiratory diseases: asthma and chronic obstructive pulmonary disease

Asthma

Disease characteristics

Asthma is a common clinical condition affecting 5–10% of the population and appears to be on the increase. It is especially prevalent in children but also has a high incidence in more elderly patients. Asthma is defined as reversible increases in airway resistance, involving both broncho-constriction and inflammation.

Underlying pathology

In order to appreciate the causes and treatment of asthma, it is important to understand the control of bronchial calibre, and hence airway resistance. Parasympathetic innervation results in acetylcholine acting on bronchial M_3-muscarinic receptors, which cause bronchoconstriction and increased mucus secretion. The bronchial smooth-muscle cells also contain $beta_2$-adrenoceptors, which are linked via cyclic adenosine mono-phosphate (cAMP) to bronchodilation. The $beta_2$-adrenoceptors have no direct innervation but are responsive to circulating adrenaline (epinephrine), which stimulates bronchodila-tion. In addition, the mucous glands contain $beta_2$-adrenoceptors which inhibit mucus secre-tion. There are also a limited number of sympathetic fibres which release noradrenaline (norepinephrine), acting on $beta_2$-adrenoceptors at parasympathetic ganglia to inhibit trans-mission. Non-adrenergic non-cholinergic (NANC) fibres also play a role in which nitric oxide and vasoactive intestinal polypeptide are inhibitory transmitters and substance P is an excitatory transmitter. These sensory nerve fibres are thought to play a role in local reflex responses to irritant stimuli.

An asthmatic attack may comprise an early (immediate) phase with bronchospasm which may be followed by a late phase, characterised by both increased airways resistance and inflammation. Other variations include an immediate phase alone, a late phase without an immediate phase and recurrent late phases.

An asthmatic attack is often provoked by allergens, cold air, viral infections, smoking, certain foods or exercise. It should also be noted that asthma has a genetic component and is associated with atopy. The immediate phase of the attack is associated with the release of spasmogens (histamine, prostaglandin D_2, leukotrienes C_4 and D_4, and platelet-activating factor (PAF)) from mast cells and mononuclear cells, which lead to rapid bronchospasm (Figure 20.1). Chemotaxins (including leukotriene B_4 and PAF) then attract leukocytes (especially eosinophils and mononuclear cells), which lead to inflammation and airway hyperactivity, associated with the late phase. This second phase occurs some 3–6 h after the initial release of the mediators.

Long-term growth changes in the bronchial smooth muscle in asthma lead to hyperplasia, with associated increases in airway responsiveness. This is referred to as remodelling.

Drug-induced asthma

Non-steroidal anti-inflammatory drugs (NSAIDs) may provoke asthma in a number of sensitive individuals (about 15% of asthmatics). This is achieved by inhibition of cyclooxygenase, and is thought to lead to more arachidonic acid being available as substrate, resulting in increased leukotriene production (Figure 20.2).

Beta-blockers may also induce bronchospasm, by blocking the beta$_2$-adrenoceptors on the bronchial smooth muscle. It is for this reason that beta-blockers (even in eye drops for glaucoma) are contraindicated in asthma (and chronic obstructive pulmonary disease (COPD)). Beta$_1$-adrenoceptor antagonists should only be used in *extreme* circumstances in asthmatics (and also patients with COPD) and under supervision.

Clinical features

The leading clinical features are wheezing, breathlessness, a tight chest and cough, which are intermittent and may be worse at night or on exercise.

Asthma is due to reversible increases in airway resistance, characterised by reversible decreases in the ratio of forced expiratory volume in the first second (FEV_1) to the forced vital capacity (FVC). A value of less than 70% suggests increased airway resistance and in asthma the change should be reversed by a beta$_2$-adrenoceptor agonist. In diagnosis, the following point to asthma (British Thoracic Society (BTS) and Scottish Intercollegiate Guidelines Network (SIGN) joint British guidelines (2003)):

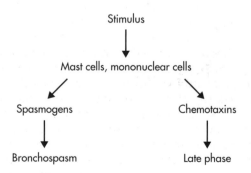

Figure 20.1 Summary of the different phases of an asthmatic attack.

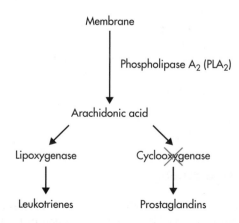

Figure 20.2 The arachidonic acid pathway, showing the potential for increased production of leukotrienes following inhibition of cyclooxygenase.

- a variation of peak expiratory flow (PEF) of greater than 20% on 3 days or more in a week over 2 weeks

or

- an FEV_1 which improves by more than 15% with an inhaled beta$_2$-adrenoceptor agonist

or

- an FEV_1 which improves by more than 15% after a 14-day trial of oral steroids (30 mg prednisolone per day)

or

- an FEV_1 which decreases by more than 15% after 6 min of exercise (running)

In asthmatics the airway resistance may also show variations throughout the day and typically increases in the morning; this is termed 'morning dipping'. In children, the diagnosis is often based on a history which may include wheezing, cough (a persistent dry nocturnal cough may be the only feature), exacerbations on infection and a family association. Asthma is associated with atopy and individuals are likely to have a history of eczema and hayfever.

Asthma is further divided into episodic asthma and chronic asthma. Episodic asthma tends to occur in atopic individuals who have periods of attacks associated with provoking factors such as viral infection, allergens or exercise. The attacks include wheezing and breathlessness but the patient shows no symptoms between attacks. Chronic asthma runs a course of prolonged periods of breathlessness and wheezing, with a cough and wheezing at night. The cough is often productive of mucoid sputum. Severe acute asthma (status asthmaticus) is a serious and potentially life-threatening occurrence which involves severe bronchospasm: its management is considered later.

Goals of treatment

Given the two key phases of an asthmatic attack, treatment is divided into relief of symptoms, which is achieved by bronchodilators (relievers), which may reverse the early phase, and prevention using anti-inflammatory agents (preventers).

Pharmacological basis of management

Beta-adrenoceptor agonists

e.g. Salbutamol, terbutaline

These are the agents of first choice and act on beta$_2$-adrenoceptors on the bronchial smooth muscle to increase cAMP, leading to rapid bronchodilation and reversal of the bronchospasm associated with the early phase. Prolonged use is associated with receptor down-regulation, making them less effective. However, there is some evidence that concomitant treatment with corticosteroids may reduce receptor down-regulation.

Long-acting beta-adrenoceptor agonists

Formoterol (eformoterol), salmeterol

Although these are also beta$_2$-adrenoceptor agonists, which cause bronchodilation, their rate of onset is slow and, more importantly, by lipophilic properties the molecule is retained near the receptor for a prolonged period, which means that its action persists. Accordingly, they are not used to reverse an attack but cause prolonged bronchodilation, which is preventive. They are more effective than xanthines or cromones.

Xanthines

Aminophylline, theophylline

These are also bronchodilators, but are not as effective as beta$_2$-adrenoceptor agonists and are given orally (theophylline or aminophylline, which is theophylline with ethylenediamine) or occasionally intravenously (aminophylline which has improved solubility). Pharmacologically, their actions are less clear; they are phosphodiesterase III and IV inhibitors and so will potentiate cAMP by preventing its breakdown, which leads to bronchodilation. Additional therapeutic actions may include blockade of adenosine receptors, which leads to bronchial smooth-muscle relaxation, and anti-inflammatory actions through a reduction in mediator release. Xanthines show a narrow therapeutic window (Chapter 6), with toxic concentrations leading to nausea and central nervous system (CNS) stimulation as side-effects.

Muscarinic M-receptor antagonists

Ipratropium

Ipratropium is given by inhalation and blocks parasympathetic-mediated bronchoconstriction with only limited systemic side-effects. Tiotropium bromide is a new long-acting member and may be given once a day. The bronchodilator effects of muscarinic antagonists are less than those of beta$_2$-adrenoceptor agonists. Indeed, BTS/SIGN guidelines (2003) indicate that they are of little or no value in the treatment of asthma.

Corticosteroids

Inhalation (beclometasone, budesonide, fluticasone) and oral (prednisolone)

These agents have an anti-inflammatory action via activation of intracellular receptors, leading to altered gene transcription. This results in decreased cytokine production and the synthesis of lipocortin, which inhibits phospholipase A$_2$, and the production of prostaglandins and leukotrienes (Figure 20.3).

Fungal oral infections occur as a common side-effect with inhalation, due to local immuno-suppression. Laryngeal myopathy may also lead to hoarseness. Systemic steroid effects, including adrenal suppression and bone resorption, occur with high-dose inhalation or oral dosing.

Cromones

Nedocromil sodium, sodium cromoglicate

Sodium cromoglicate prevents both the early and late phases of an attack. Its action is uncertain but may include a reduction in sensory nerve reflexes, stabilisation of mast cells and a reduction in the release of PAF and cytokines. Cromones are only effective in a few patients: prevention of bronchoconstriction is an early effect and prevention of the late phase may require up to a month of treatment to occur. The BTS/SIGN guidelines do not support the use of cromoglicate in children. Nedocromil sodium is only of benefit in children aged 5–12 years, although cromones may be affective in exercise-induced asthma.

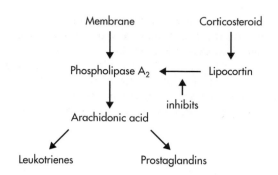

Figure 20.3 The arachidonic acid pathway, showing the inhibition of leukotriene and prostanoid synthesis following inhibition of phospholipase A$_2$.

Leukotriene receptor antagonists

Montelukast, zafirlukast

This is a new class of orally active drugs which block leukotriene receptors and so will oppose the bronchoconstrictor and inflammatory actions of leukotrienes. However, the Committee on Safety of Medicines (CSM) has warned that they should not be used to reverse an attack and they should be used as a 'preventer'.

IgE antibodies

Omalizumab

This novel agent has a role in treatment-resistant asthma. It is a monoclonal antibody which is directed against free immunoglobulin E (IgE), but not bound IgE, and prevents IgE from binding to immune cells which would otherwise lead to allergen-induced mediator release in allergic asthma.

Choice of drugs

The initial approach is to educate the patient to recognise and avoid trigger factors such as dust, animals, smoke and cold air. Lifestyle advice regarding weight reduction may be beneficial in overweight patients. Breast-feeding of infants is also recommended as it is protective against the development of asthma.

Drugs have a major role in the management of asthma but two major problems limit their effectiveness: undertreatment and poor patient compliance, largely due to poor inhaler technique. The pharmacological basis of the treatment of asthma is well-established and described in the BTS and SIGN joint British guidelines (2003) and has a stepped-care approach (Table 20.1). These guidelines differ from previous recommendations by favouring the use of alternative drugs before increasing the dose of inhaled steroids. Another important feature is the emphasis that inhaled steroid dosages should be the minimum required for control.

The treatment should be reviewed regularly (3 months) and a step-down considered in patients who are stabilised. If a reduction in the dose of the inhaled drug is appropriate then it should be reduced by 25–50%, with further reductions considered thereafter at 3-month intervals.

The role of leukotriene receptor antagonists has now been established in the BTS/SIGN guidelines. In addition, their pharmacological action suggests that they would oppose NSAID-induced asthma, by blocking the actions of leukotrienes, which are implicated in this adverse drug reaction.

Long-acting $beta_2$-adrenoceptor agonists have a valuable role in addition to, and not in place of, inhaled steroids. Their prolonged action means that they are of particular benefit in nocturnal asthma but it is important that their effectiveness does not lead to reduced compliance with inhaled steroids.

There has been some concern in the USA that long-acting $beta_2$-adrenoceptor agonists have been associated with increased mortality but it is believed that this may be due to their use in the absence of inhaled steroids, which is not what is recommended in the BTS/SIGN guidelines.

Intercurrent infections: the previous BTS guidelines (1997) suggested that the dose of inhaled steroid should be doubled in asthmatic patients during acute exacerbation in infections. Evidence for the effectiveness is unproven and the current BTS/SIGN guidelines (2003) comment that this increased dose is only of benefit at low dosages of steroids. Vaccinations against pneumococcal infection and influenza are appropriate for patients with asthma.

In severe disease, and to reduce the need for steroids ('steroid-sparing'), immunosuppression with ciclosporin or methotrexate is used in some patients.

Children

In children there is also a stepped-care approach with different BTS/SIGN guidelines for those

Table 20.1 Summary of the BTS/SIGN British guidelines (2003) for the management of asthma in adults

Stage	Management
Step 1	Occasional bronchodilator (inhaled short-acting $beta_2$-adrenoceptor agonist) as required. Move up to step 2 if the $beta_2$-adrenoceptor agonist is required frequently
Step 2	Short-acting $beta_2$-adrenoceptor agonist as required and regular inhaled steroid in the range 200–800 μg beclometasone dipropionate (BDP) equivalent per day, depending on the disease: 400 μg is a recommended starting point
Step 3	Step 2 plus add-on therapy with a trial of a long-acting $beta_2$-adrenoceptor agonist. If there is benefit but not full control the steroid may be increased (to 800 μg BDP equivalent per day). If there is no response to the long-acting $beta_2$-adrenoceptor agonist then other agents (e.g. leukotriene receptor antagonists, modified-release theophylline) may be tried
Step 4	Consider increasing the dose of steroid up to 2000 μg BDP equivalent per day or addition of a 4th drug (e.g. leukotriene receptor antagonist)
Step 5	Oral steroids may be added (at the lowest adequate dose) to existing therapy, with high dose inhaled steroids maintained at 2000 μg BDP equivalent per day

BTS, British Thoracic Society; SIGN, Scottish Intercollegiate Guidelines Network. (*Thorax* (2003) 58(suppl 1): i1–i94; adapted and reproduced with permission from the BMJ Publishing Group.)

under 5 years of age (Table 20.2) and those aged between 5 and 12 (Table 20.3).

During treatment, the BTS/SIGN guidelines (2003) recommend that the child's height should be monitored in relation to the adverse effects of uncontrolled asthma on height and steroid-induced growth retardation.

In very young children under 18 months, it is unclear whether the beta$_2$-adrenoceptors are fully functional. Beta$_2$-adrenoceptor agonists have been viewed as being less effective and ipratropium has been used in their place. However, the recent BTS/SIGN guidance (2003) supports the use of beta$_2$-adrenoceptor agonists while muscarinic receptor antagonists are not recommended.

Exercise-induced asthma

The BTS/SIGN guidelines indicate that beta$_2$-adrenoceptor agonists (long- and short-acting), inhaled steroids, xanthines, leukotriene receptor antagonists and cromones protect against

Table 20.2 Summary of the BTS/SIGN British guidelines (2003) for the management of asthma in children under 5 years of age

Stage	Management
Step 1	Occasional bronchodilator (inhaled short-acting beta$_2$-adrenoceptor agonist) as required
Step 2	Short-acting beta$_2$-adrenoceptor agonist as required plus regular inhaled steroid (200–400 µg BDP equivalent per day). If an inhaled steroid is inappropriate then a leukotriene receptor antagonist may be added
Step 3	In children aged 2–5, a leukotriene receptor antagonist may be trialled in addition to a short-acting beta$_2$-adrenoceptor agonist and a regular inhaled steroid. In children under 2, referral to a respiratory physician should be considered
Step 4	Referral to respiratory physician

BTS, British Thoracic Society; SIGN, Scottish Intercollegiate Guidelines Network; BDP, beclometasone dipropionate. (*Thorax* (2003) 58(suppl 1): i1–i94; adapted and reproduced with permission from the BMJ Publishing Group.)

Table 20.3 Summary of the BTS/SIGN British guidelines (2003) for the management of asthma in children aged 5–12 years

Stage	Management
Step 1	Occasional bronchodilator (inhaled short-acting beta$_2$-adrenoceptor agonist) as required
Step 2	Short-acting beta$_2$-adrenoceptor agonist as required plus regular inhaled steroid (200–400 µg BDP equivalent per day, depending on disease: 200 µg BDP equivalent per day is a typical starting dose). If an inhaled steroid is inappropriate then other drugs (e.g. leukotriene receptor antagonists, modified-release theophylline) may be considered
Step 3	Step 2 plus add-on therapy with a trial of a long-acting beta$_2$-adrenoceptor agonist. If there is benefit but not full control the steroid may be increased (to 400 µg BDP equivalent per day). If there is no response to the long-acting beta$_2$-adrenoceptor agonist then other agents (e.g. leukotriene receptor antagonists, modified-release theophylline) may be tried, with the inhaled steroid used at 400 µg BDP equivalent per day
Step 4	Increase inhaled steroid up to 800 µg BDP equivalent per day
Step 5	Oral steroids may be added (at the lowest adequate dose) to existing therapy, with high-dose inhaled steroids maintained at 800 µg BDP equivalent per day. Referral to respiratory physician

BTS, British Thoracic Society; SIGN, Scottish Intercollegiate Guidelines Network; BDP, beclometasone dipropionate. (*Thorax* (2003) 58(suppl 1): i1–i94; adapted and reproduced with permission from the BMJ Publishing Group.)

exercise-induced asthma whereas antimuscarinic agents do not. The guidelines also suggest that exercise-induced asthma may indicate poor management of asthma and that treatment should be reviewed.

Pregnancy

During pregnancy control of asthma is important. The BTS/SIGN guidelines (2003) recommend that beta$_2$-adrenoceptor agonists and inhaled steroids are used as normal and that oral steroids may be used as normal in severe asthma. Leukotriene receptor antagonists may be continued if they were essential for control prior to pregnancy but should not be introduced.

Choice of inhaler

The choice of an inhaler device is crucial for effective delivery of the drugs. Metered dose inhalers (MDIs) are the most commonly used; however, it should be recognised that many patients have a poor inhaler technique and require counselling in their use. To overcome problems of coordination of breathing with administration, a spacer may be used in which the drug is distributed for inhalation. This may also reduce steroid-induced oral candidiasis.

In addition, in the selection of an inhaler the following should be taken into account:

- The age of the patient: for children under 5 years of age, the National Institute of Clinical Excellence (NICE) (2000) recommends that inhaled therapy should be via a pressurised MDI and spacer, with a mask if required. When this is not possible or effective, then nebulised therapy is appropriate; a dry powder inhaler may also be considered for 3–5-year-olds. NICE guidelines (2002) recommend that, for children aged 5–15 years, a pressurised MDI and spacer are used for regular corticosteroid therapy, unless adherence is problematic. For other inhaled therapy, especially bronchodilators, the device that best allows spontaneous use should be chosen. The inhaler requirements should be reviewed at least annually.
- Impaired respiratory function: this may make a breath-activated device impossible to use.

- The lifestyle of the patient: can the inhaler be used at school or work?
- The physical ability of the patient: e.g. patients with arthritis may not be able to activate the pressurised inhalers or refill devices. Patients with poor eyesight may be unable to read the dose counters.

When patients are changed to newer inhalers with chlorofluorocarbon (CFC)-free propellant, the dose of steroid (but not beta$_2$-adrenoceptor agonists) may need to be reduced in well-managed asthma. For the Qvar inhaler the *British National Formulary* recommends that in stable asthma, a 100 µg dose of beclometasone dipropionate is used in place of 200–250 µg beclometasone dipropionate or 200–250 µg budesonide. In poorly controlled asthma, a dose-for-dose change is recommended.

Adverse drug reactions and interactions

Asthma therapy largely involves inhalation, which limits systemic effects. Having said that, overadministration or absorption may of course lead to side-effects. Systemic effects of beta$_2$-adrenoceptors agonists include tremor and tachycardia, due to activation of peripheral beta$_2$-adrenoceptors and cardiac beta-adrenoceptors respectively. The sympathomimetic actions of beta$_2$-adrenoceptor agonists mean that they should be used with caution in conditions where increased sympathetic activity would be undesirable, such as in hyperthyroidism, arrhythmias, hypertension and diabetes mellitus. Prolonged overuse of beta$_2$-adrenoceptor agonists is also associated with hypokalaemia, due to activation of the sodium pump leading to cellular uptake of potassium.

Systemic side-effects of ipratropium are antimuscarinic in nature but are limited. When using nebulised ipratropium, the drug should not come into contact with the eyes as this may lead to glaucoma.

Xanthines are given either orally or intravenously and will of course have systemic effects. This is important as xanthines have a narrow therapeutic window and toxicity may lead to gastrointestinal and CNS side-effects. Accordingly, monitoring of its plasma levels and side-effects is important.

Side-effects of inhaled corticosteroids are dose-related and are more pronounced at the higher doses (greater than 800 µg of BDP equivalent in adults and 400 µg of BDP equivalent in children). These include height suppression in children (which should be monitored), adrenal suppression, osteoporosis, skin thinning, cataracts and anti-insulin effects leading to diabetes. Inhalation of the steroid may lead to impaction on the throat, which may promote local candidiasis. In 2002, the CSM brought to the attention of practitioners the need to be vigilant of adrenal suppression in children. The CSM pointed out that adrenal suppression was a recognised adverse effect of inhaled steroids and may present as non-specific symptoms such as weight loss, nausea, hypoglycaemia, and reduced consciousness. To avoid these problems, the maximum licensed doses should not be exceeded and the lowest effective dose should be used. Oral corticosteroids are more likely to lead to systemic effects and are associated with gastric damage (Chapter 7).

Leukotriene receptor antagonists have been associated with Churg–Strauss syndrome (lung vasculitis), which may be accompanied by a rash. This may be more likely to occur when oral steroid therapy is reduced or stopped.

In terms of drug interactions, there are no obvious intergroup interactions which would have a significant bearing on therapy. However, xanthines, by preventing the breakdown of cAMP will potentiate the actions of beta$_2$-adrenoceptor agonists. This is generally considered desirable but the side-effects of beta$_2$-adrenoceptor agonists (including risk of hypokalaemia) may also be enhanced. The hypokalaemic effect of beta$_2$-adrenoceptor agonists and xanthines will also be potentiated by concomitant corticosteroids and potassium-losing diuretics (loop diuretics and thiazides). The CSM has advised that plasma potassium levels should be monitored in patients with severe asthma.

Theophylline, in particular, has a number of significant interactions. These interactions are largely at the level of cytochrome P450, with some inducers of cytochrome P450 reducing the concentrations of theophylline, whilst some inhibitors may augment the plasma levels. In view of its narrow therapeutic window, theophylline should be used with caution and monitored appropriately and the dosage altered if necessary. Some drugs which may influence plasma levels of theophylline are summarised in Table 20.4.

In addition, theophylline may enhance renal excretion of concomitant lithium therapy, leading to reductions in its plasma concentrations, which should be monitored and the dosage increased if necessary.

Beta$_2$-adrenoceptor agonists and corticosteroids used in combination are particularly effective in the control of asthma. A recent

Table 20.4   Some drugs which may influence plasma levels of theophylline

Drugs which may increase plasma levels of theophylline	Drugs which may decrease plasma levels of theophylline
• Aciclovir	• Aminoglutethimide
• Amiodarone (rare)	• Barbiturates
• Oral contraceptives (but not thought to lead to toxicity)	• Carbamazepine
• Disulfiram	• Rifampicin
• Erythromycin; this is much less of a problem with clarithromycin	• Ritonavir
• Fluvoxamine	• Tobacco smoke
• Cimetidine	• Levothyroxine
• Phenylpropanolamine	• Ketoconazole (isolated reports)
• Ciprofloxacin	
• Carbimazole	
• Nifedipine, verapamil and fluconazole (isolated reports)	

laboratory-based study by Roth *et al.* (2002) has demonstrated that beta$_2$-adrenoceptor agonists and corticosteroids interact at the cellular level to enhance gene transcription. It was proposed that this might contribute to their antiproliferative effects on the bronchial smooth muscle.

Over-the-counter considerations

Respiratory complaints form a large proportion of requests for over-the-counter (OTC) medicines such as cough mixtures and sympathomimetics (Chapter 18). This raises issues for patients with asthma or COPD. In both conditions a cough may suggest poor control or an exacerbation and a referral is appropriate. Furthermore, as commented above, a nocturnal cough in a child may arouse the suspicion of asthma. Of particular importance, antitussive agents are contraindicated in COPD as they may lead to sputum retention.

Despite many people's perceptions, asthma alone is not a sound reason to avoid sympathomimetics. However, on theoretical grounds they would be expected to enhance the sympathetic actions and side-effects in patients taking beta$_2$-adrenoceptor agonists and should be used with caution. Topical agents are less likely to have systemic effects and are preferred to oral ones (Chapter 18), although, once again, the request for a sympathomimetic may indicate an intercurrent infection. Caution should also be exercised with preparations which contain theophylline, as they will alter plasma levels in patients stabilised on xanthines.

Counselling

Counselling has a major role in ensuring patient compliance and correct inhaler technique. General counselling should include advice to avoid precipitating factors, including caution with NSAIDs and avoidance in patients with a known sensitivity to them. Smoking and smoky atmospheres must be avoided. Patients should always have a short-acting beta$_2$-adrenoceptor agonist inhaler available and should ensure that they do not run out of supplies. Attention should be paid to inhaler technique as a significant number of patients are incapable of using a pressurised inhaler or have a poor technique leading to failure of treatment. Patients should monitor their own PEF and may require counselling in the use of peak flow meters. Specific advice is as follows:

Spacers

- The device should be washed out weekly and left to air-dry after use to prevent static electricity from causing the drug particles to stick to it.

Short-acting beta$_2$-adrenoceptor agonists

- They should be used as required to relieve an attack.
- They may be used prior to an event which may trigger asthma such as exercise.
- If they are required more than once a day, patients should consult their general practitioner (GP) with a view to moving up the ladder of care.
- Patients should not exceed the maximum dose or frequency in 24 h.
- CFC-free inhalers may taste and feel different to CFC-containing preparations.

Long-acting beta$_2$-adrenoceptor agonists

- These will not relieve an attack but are used to prevent an attack.

Inhaled corticosteroids

- The judicious use of steroids outweighs any adverse effects, even in children.
- Inhalation limits their systemic effects.
- These will take several days to have an effect.
- If taking with a beta$_2$-adrenoceptor agonist, the beta$_2$-agonist should be taken first to dilate the airways, which will aid deposition of the steroid.
- They may cause a sore throat: to reduce the chances of this occurring, patients should rinse their mouth or gargle after use.
- High-dose steroids from an MDI should be administered with a spacer device, to prevent impaction on the throat.

- These are preventive and should be taken even when the patient is stabilised with few or no attacks.
- Patients may have previously been advised by their GP to double the dose in acute exacerbations of asthma. However, BTS/SIGN guidelines (2003) indicate that the benefit of this has yet to be established.
- Steroid cards should be issued to those with high-dose inhalers.
- With doses exceeding 800 µg beclometasone (or equivalent) per day, there is a risk of osteoporosis. Measures to avoid this should be encouraged, such as exercise, adequate calcium and vitamin D intake, smoking cessation and hormone replacement therapy, if appropriate.

Oral steroids

- These may have an important role in poorly controlled asthma.
- They should be taken in the morning.
- Any indigestion should be reported.
- The patient should not stop taking the steroid suddenly if the course is longer than 3 weeks.
- If patients have never had chickenpox, they should avoid contact with the virus and consult their GP if they are exposed to it.

Xanthines

- Patients should be vigilant for signs of toxicity such as tremor, palpitations, nausea and CNS stimulation.
- Patients should avoid excess caffeine.
- Patients should not change from brands on which they are stabilised.

Cromones

- They may themselves cause wheezing due to the irritant effects of the powder on the airways.

Leukotriene receptor antagonists

- These should not be used for an acute attack.
- They may cause a headache.
- Any rash whilst taking them should be reported.
- Patients taking zafirlukast should report nausea, jaundice or other signs of liver damage.

Acute severe asthma

Although acute asthmatic attacks are largely beyond the scope of this book, a brief description of their features and management is appropriate. It should be recognised that asthma may be life-threatening and prompt recognition of clinical features is important. In a severe attack the following may be present:

- The patient is unable to complete a sentence.
- There may be tachycardia (>110 beats/min; greater in children).
- There may be tachypnoea (>25 breaths/min; greater in children).
- Peak flow >35 – <50% of predicted.

Signs and symptoms of life-threatening attacks include:

- a silent chest
- cyanosis
- bradycardia
- exhaustion
- peak flow <35% of predicted

In a severe acute attack the treatment is:

- oxygen (40–60%)
- nebulised beta$_2$-adrenoceptor agonist (e.g. salbutamol or terbutaline) as soon as possible
- oral prednisolone or intravenous hydrocortisone. Prednisolone (40–50 mg) should be continued for at least 5 days

In a life-threatening attack the following may be added:

- nebulised ipratropium
- intravenous magnesium sulfate
- intravenous aminophylline, provided the patient is not already receiving a xanthine

Chronic obstructive pulmonary disease

Disease characteristics

COPD encompasses both chronic bronchitis and emphysema and is typically a disease of late onset with a very close association with a history of smoking. Some smokers are more susceptible to developing COPD than others, whilst a smoker's cough may be an early manifestation of the disease. COPD may also appear in former smokers decades after they have stopped smoking. In most patients, COPD is generally a combination, to varying degrees, of both chronic bronchitis and emphysema.

In the past chronic bronchitis was defined as sputum production for 3 months of the year for 2 consecutive years. A more helpful definition of COPD is a chronic reduction in the predicted FEV_1, with the following grades (Table 20.5).

The FEV_1/FVC ratio is likely to be less than 70% and, unlike asthma, there is little variation in PEF. Absolute PEF measurements tend to underestimate the extent of COPD, and FEV_1 is the measurement recommended by the BTS for diagnosis and monitoring.

Chronic bronchitis is an inflammatory response (usually following many years of smoking), leading to proliferation of goblet cells with excess mucus production, which leads to airway obstruction. The chronic inflammation, oedema and fibrosis also lead to increases in airway tissue thickness. These changes lead to the symptoms of a productive cough, wheeze, dyspnoea and acute exacerbations with infections. In more severe disease, the dyspnoea is disabling, there may be secondary polycythaemia and pulmonary hypertension may lead to right-sided heart failure (cor pulmonale). Emphysema is similarly linked to smoking, although in a very small proportion of patients it is due to a genetic deficiency of alpha$_1$-antitrypsin. There is marked destruction of the alveoli, leading to dilation, with reduced elastic recoil of the airways and so the airways are held open during expiration.

Goals of treatment

The prognosis of COPD depends on severity but is generally poor with progressive deterioration. The key goal of treatment is to improve respiratory function.

Management

The treatment of COPD was reviewed by the BTS in 1997 and their guidelines should be consulted. In the first instance, smoking cessation must be emphasised, as this may lead to a slowing of the disease process and a reduction of carboxyhaemoglobin. The pharmacological management is based on the drugs used in asthma, described above.

Bronchodilators

In general, patients with COPD are less responsive to bronchodilators as bronchospasm is not a feature of COPD. However, some patients do benefit from beta$_2$-adrenoceptor agonists and they are widely prescribed for the relief of symptoms and for use before exercise. Traditionally, muscarinic antagonists such as ipratropium have also been used to oppose vagally mediated

Table 20.5 The British Thoracic Society (1997) definitions of grades of chronic obstructive pulmonary disease

Grade	FEV$_1$	Symptoms
Mild	80–60% of predicted	Typically 'smoker's cough' with little or no breathlessness. The initial presentation may be of a productive cough or an acute chest infection
Moderate	59–40% of predicted	Breathlessness on moderate exertion, possibly with wheezing and a cough with or without sputum
Severe	Less then 40% of predicted	Breathlessness at rest or on mild exertion, usually with a wheeze and cough

FEV$_1$, forced expiratory volume in 1 s.

bronchoconstriction and appear to be as effective as beta$_2$-adrenoceptor agonists, but have a slower rate of onset and so are less effective as relievers. The combination of a beta$_2$-adrenoceptor agonist and muscarinic antagonist may give an even better response.

The BTS guidelines suggest that all patients with COPD should receive a bronchodilator reversibility test. Here a positive response is defined as a greater than 200 mL increase in FEV$_1$ and a greater than 15% increase of the baseline value in response to inhaled bronchodilators. This should identify patients who would benefit most from bronchodilator therapy. Responses with a greater than 500 mL increase in FEV$_1$ may, in fact, reveal asthma.

The current position of long acting beta$_2$-adrenoceptor agonists in COPD therapy has yet to be defined. However, in some patients they do appear to cause some relief and are once again of benefit for nocturnal symptoms. A recent comparison between ipratropium and formoterol has indicated that formoterol produced greater improvements in respiratory function and symptom control (Dahl *et al.*, 2001).

Xanthines have less of a role in COPD due to their narrow therapeutic window and offer no advantages over beta$_2$-adrenoceptor agonists or muscarinic antagonists. However, some patients may empirically show an improvement with xanthines.

The role of corticosteroids

Despite the inflammatory nature of COPD, corticosteroids are relatively ineffective in most patients. However, approximately 15% of patients respond to corticosteroids (perhaps due to a high asthmatic component of their disease) and it is important that these patients are identified and treated. This may be achieved by monitoring the response of lung function to a 'trial of steroids', which involves the patients receiving oral prednisolone (typically 30 mg daily) for 2 weeks. Patients who show a favourable response may then receive inhaled steroids. Despite only a small proportion of patients demonstrating a positive response to

steroids, a substantial number of patients who do not respond to steroids are actually prescribed these drugs. The BTS suggests that their treatment should be reviewed, and if appropriate, their steroid treatment should be discontinued.

Choice of drugs

The BTS guidelines suggest the following approach to treatment:

- Mild COPD: bronchodilator drugs (beta$_2$-adrenoceptor agonists or antimuscarinic agents) as required.
- Moderate COPD: bronchodilator drugs (alone or in combination) plus a trial of steroids.
- Severe COPD: regular bronchodilators, a trial of steroids and consider nebuliser use at home (after assessment by a respiratory physician).

Other considerations

The BTS recommends that patients with COPD should be vaccinated against influenza and pneumococcal infection, although evidence for the effectiveness of the latter is yet to be fully established. Depression should be identified and treated.

Long-term oxygen therapy is the only treatment known to improve the outlook in patients with severe COPD. By providing 24–28% oxygen for at least 15 h a day the consequences of hypoxia (e.g. pulmonary hypertension, cor pulmonale and polycythaemia) are reduced. The oxygen concentration should not exceed 28%, as higher concentrations will lead to carbon dioxide trapping.

In the presence of cor pulmonale, leading to peripheral oedema, the administration of diuretics is appropriate. Venesection (bleeding the patient) should be considered for polycythaemia.

In an acute exacerbation, the use of bronchodilators may be increased. Oral steroids may also be added for 7 days for patients who are already taking oral steroids, those with a documented positive response to steroids and those who have failed to respond to increased use of bronchodilators. Antibiotics may be of benefit in acute exacerbations and may be given to motivated patients who would be able to initiate treatment at the start of an exacerbation. The BTS recommends that antibiotics are only of value if at least two of the following are present: purulent sputum, increased breathlessness or increased volume of sputum.

Counselling

Smoking cessation must be emphasised as this will slow the progression of the disease. Exercise should be encouraged to improve exercise tolerance.

For drug-specific counselling, see the comments above for the drugs used in asthma.

Practice points for asthma and COPD

- Asthma can kill.
- Many patients with asthma may be undertreated.
- Be alert for the overuse of bronchodilators. In asthma, if a short-acting beta$_2$-agonist is required for relief more than once a day then the patient should be reviewed with a view to stepping up treatment.
- Poor inhaler technique is a major cause of undertreatment.
- In both cases, smoking cessation is essential.
- The BTS provides detailed guidelines for the treatment of both asthma (in conjunction with SIGN) and COPD.
- In asthma a written action plan improves health outcome.
- Some patients with COPD demonstrate a positive response to steroids and these patients should be identified and treated.
- Patients with COPD are often maintained on a number of drugs and it may be difficult to deduce rationally which agents confer the most benefit.

 CASE STUDY

Mr SM (aged 65) has COPD with an FEV$_1$ 55% of predicted. He is a current smoker with a 50-pack-year history (i.e. he has smoked the equivalent of one packet of cigarettes per day for 50 years). He has been prescribed:

Salbutamol 200 µg p.r.n.
Ipratropium 80 µg t.d.s.

How should you counsel this patient?

- He should be advised that giving up smoking will slow down the progression of COPD. He should take salbutamol as required, and before activities which may provoke shortness of breath. Taking salbutamol prior to ipratropium may help more ipratropium get into the lungs.

His consultant would like to give him a 2-week trial of oral prednisolone 30 mg o.m. What is the purpose of this trial?

- Some patients with COPD respond positively to steroids. They are given a trial of high-dose oral or inhaled steroids for several weeks to determine whether they respond. Patients who show a positive response should be maintained on a high-dose steroid inhaler.

continued

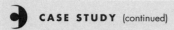

CASE STUDY (continued)

How should you counsel the patient in taking the prednisolone?

- Take each morning after breakfast.
- A steroid card should be issued and he should tell any pharmacist, doctor or dentist treating him that he is taking steroids.
- He should consult his GP if he comes into contact with an infectious disease.
- If he has not had chickenpox, he should avoid contact with it.
- He should report indigestion (as this may indicate gastric damage).
- He should avoid OTC NSAIDs as these may enhance the gastric damage caused by steroids.

Why should the prednisolone be taken in the morning?

- This reduces adrenal suppression, as it mimics the natural rise in cortisol in the morning.

Several months later Mr SM is still taking salbutamol and ipratropium but now with beclometasone (500 µg b.d.). However, he is short of breath and has thick green sputum, which is occasionally streaked with blood. What is the likely cause of this exacerbation?

- The symptoms may point to acute bronchitis.

What treatment may be appropriate?

- An antibacterial such as amoxicillin (250–500 mg t.d.s.) or erythromycin or tetracycline. He should also be advised to increase his use of the bronchodilators and may be prescribed a short course of oral steroids.

Several weeks later the patient's condition has not improved. What tests may be appropriate?

- Further investigations are appropriate. As he is a smoker this may point to other serious pathologies (e.g. lung cancer, tuberculosis) and a chest X-ray is appropriate.

References

British Thoracic Society (1997). BTS guidelines for the management of chronic obstructive pulmonary disease. *Thorax* 52 (suppl. 5): S1–S28.

British Thoracic Society (BTS) and Scottish Intercollegiate Guidelines Network (SIGN) (2003). British guidelines on the management of asthma. *Thorax* 58 (suppl I).

Dahl R, Greefhost L A P M, Nowak D *et al.* (2001). Inhaled formoterol dry powder versus ipratropium bromide in chronic obstructive pulmonary disease. *Am J Respir Crit Care Med* 164: 778–784.

Mehta D K (ed.) *British National Formulary*, latest edition. London: British Medical Association and Royal Pharmaceutical Society of Great Britain.

NICE Technology Appraisal Guidance no. 10 (2000). Guidance of the use of inhaler systems (devices) in children under the age of 5 years with chronic asthma. London: National Institute for Clinical Excellence (via www.nice.org.uk).

NICE Technology Appraisal Guidance no. 38 (2002). Inhaler devices for routine treatment of chronic asthma in older children (aged 5–15 years). London: National Institute for Clinical Excellence (via www.nice.org.uk).

Roth M, Johnson P R A, Rudiger J J *et al.* (2002). Interaction between glucocorticoids and β_2 agonists on bronchial airway smooth muscle cells through synchronised cellular signalling. *Lancet* 360: 1293–1299.

Further reading

Tattersfield A E, Knox A J, Britton J R *et al.* (2002). Asthma. *Lancet* 360: 1313–1322.

Online resources

www.asthma.org.uk is the website of the UK National Asthma Campaign (accessed 4 December 2002).

www.brit-thoracic.org.uk is the website of the British Thoracic Society (accessed 4 December 2002).

Part F

Central nervous system disorders

21

Migraine

This is a common and often debilitating condition, which is frequently undertreated. It is characterised by a severe headache, which may be unilateral and throbbing, and lasts for 4–72 h. There may also be nausea, photophobia, phonophobia and sensitivity to movement. Migraine is more common in women. In 10–25% of migraineurs (patients with migraine) the headache is preceded, by approximately 1 h, by an aura with visual (flashing and zigzag lines) and other sensory disturbances and this is referred to as 'classical migraine'. Most cases of migraine are, however, without an aura and termed 'common migraine'. In terms of diagnosis, migraine must be differentiated from cluster and tension headaches and other causes of headache.

Pathophysiology

Migraine is a neurovascular disease and is thought to be due to an abnormal neuronal discharge, which initiates a train of further neurological activations (Ferrari, 1998; Goadsby *et al.*, 2002). The precise mechanisms underlying an attack are not fully understood and this is an area of much controversy. There is thought to be 'cortical spreading depression', a wave of depolarisation across the cortex, which depresses neuronal activity, and this may lead to an aura. There is also activation of serotonergic (5-hydroxytryptamine, 5-HT) neurons, leading to perivascular inflammation and the release of vasodilator and pain mediators, namely prostanoids, calcitonin gene-related peptide (CGRP) and kinins, resulting in vasodilatation and pain. In summary, there is a humoral response, which leads to a vascular response with disturbed brain function and pain.

Although the precise causes are unclear, migraine may be triggered by a range of influences including emotions (e.g. anxiety, depression and fatigue), hormonal influences (e.g. menstrual cycle, puberty, oral contraceptives, pregnancy and menopause), vision, sound, smoking, smell, unaccustomed exercise and too much or too little sleep. The role of foods such as cheese, red wine, chocolate, citrus fruits and coffee is unclear.

Goals of treatment

These are twofold: prevention and relief of attacks. In the first instance therapy is directed at relief but in recurrent attacks, prophylaxis is introduced.

Pharmacological basis of management

Analgesics

e.g. Aspirin, diclofenac, ibuprofen, paracetamol, tolfenamic acid

These may be used in an acute attack to inhibit the production of the noxious and vasodilator prostanoids. As discussed in Chapter 27, preference for paracetamol or a non-steroidal anti-inflammatory drug (NSAID), will be determined by side-effects and concurrent illness. In addition to the analgesics, antiemetics such as metoclopramide, domperidone, cyclizine or prochlorperazine may be given, as these will reduce any associated nausea. In the case of metoclopramide and domperidone, the prokinetic actions of these drugs will also increase gastric emptying and accelerate the uptake of the analgesics given at the same time. This is particularly important, as migraine is associated with gastrointestinal disturbances, which may reduce transit. Diclofenac may be given as suppositories or intramuscularly when there is vomiting, as absorption via the oral route will be limited.

The use of low doses of codeine in over-the-counter (OTC) preparations may be inappropriate as the doses present only have weak analgesic effects but have marked opioid side-effects (e.g. constipation) and may lead to analgesic or overuse headache with persistent use (Chapter 27).

Triptans

Almotriptan, eletriptan, naratriptan, rizatriptan, sumatriptan, zolmitriptan

Sumatriptan, the prototypic member of this group, was developed to revolutionise the management of migraine. Triptans are 5-HT_{1D} full agonists but they also activate 5-HT_{1B} and 5-HT_{1F} receptors and these actions cause cerebral vasoconstriction to abort an attack. Triptans may also act presynaptically to inhibit neuronal CGRP release, which is associated with inflammation and vasodilatation. In addition, they may act directly on neuronal cells to reduce excitability. The use of 5-HT receptor agonists to manage migraine may seem counterintuitive given the role of 5-HT in migraine, but it should be noted that these agonists are selective for subtypes of 5-HT_1 receptor and are used to abort an attack after its initiation (which is thought to involve 5-HT acting at 5-HT_2 receptors).

The vasoconstrictor action of triptans means that they may cause chest pain and are therefore contraindicated in patients with ischaemic heart disease, peripheral vascular disease or a history of cerebrovascular accident. Sumatriptan tablets have poor bioavailability but may also be given by a nasal spray or subcutaneously by an auto-injector. The newer agents may be given as tablets or in some cases (rizatriptan and zolmitriptan) as wafers, which dissolve on the tongue. If a patient fails to respond to the first triptan used, switching to an alternative triptan may be effective.

Ergotamine

This is a 5-HT_{1D} partial agonist which acts in a similar manner to the triptans but its use is limited by widespread side-effects including nausea, vomiting and gastrointestinal disturbances.

Prophylactic drugs

This class includes pizotifen, an antagonist of both 5-HT$_2$ and histamine H$_1$ receptors. By blocking 5-HT$_2$ receptors, pizotifen will oppose the 5-HT neuronal activation associated with the initiation of migraine attacks and is therefore used as a preventive measure. Methysergide is also a 5-HT$_2$ receptor antagonist but is toxic and its use is limited to prescription by hospital consultants.

Certain beta-blockers (propranolol, metoprolol, atenolol and bisoprolol) are also widely used for prophylaxis. In addition, tricyclic antidepressants (amitriptyline), sodium valproate, calcium channel blockers (verapamil) and the alpha$_2$-adrenoceptor agonist, clonidine, are also used for prophylaxis. The therapeutic action of these diverse agents in preventing migraine is unclear.

Drug choice

Migraine management should be reviewed regularly with a stepped-care approach, moving up the scale when the measures taken are inadequate on several occasions. The guidelines produced by the British Association of the Study of Headache (available at www.bash.org.uk) should be consulted. Some key points are summarised here:

Step 1: for mild and occasional attacks then simple analgesia (paracetamol or ibuprofen) with or without an antiemetic taken as soon as possible. The inclusion of domperidone or metoclopramide as antiemetics will enhance absorption.

Step 2: when step 1 is inadequate, diclofenac suppositories plus domperidone suppositories should be used. This step is not popular with patients and is often avoided and step 3 is used.

Step 3: when step 2 is insufficient and for moderate attacks, which are once a month or less, possibly lasting 2–3 days, then a simple analgesic with an antiemetic plus a triptan

(sumatriptan, rizatriptan and zolmitriptan as first-line) should be used.

Step 4: for severe or frequent attacks (more than two per month) then prophylaxis may be added. Prophylaxis should be used for 4–6 months and then reviewed. Ergotamine may be used in place of a triptan but should be given at least 12 h after the triptan. Despite the addition of prophylaxis, many patients are resistant to this and also find the associated side-effects unacceptable.

Drug choice will be influenced by concurrent illness and conditions; migraine may also influence other drug choices such as oral contraceptives and some considerations are summarised in Table 21.1.

Drug interactions

The interactions of triptans and other antimigraine drugs are complex. Whilst certain drugs are predicted to interact with triptans, evidence for these adverse effects is often lacking or incomplete. The reader is therefore referred to specialised literature such as *Drug Interactions* by Stockley (2002). Some important interactions are summarised in Table 21.2.

Over-the-counter medicines and dietary supplements

OTC considerations include the use of appropriate analgesics and referral to the general practitioner (GP) when simple analgesics have failed to control symptoms. Patient counselling regarding trigger factors is also important.

Supplements requested in the pharmacy for the treatment of migraine include feverfew, riboflavin (vitamin B$_2$) and magnesium. Feverfew is a herbal preparation, riboflavin a water-soluble vitamin and magnesium an essential mineral.

Feverfew

There is some clinical evidence for the efficacy of feverfew in the prevention and treatment of

Table 21.1   Some considerations for the choice of drugs in migraine

Condition	Drugs affected	Comments
Vomiting	Sumatriptan	If vomiting occurs then the subcutaneous route should be used. The nasal spray is not appropriate as ingestion is also involved
Ischaemic heart disease	Triptans and ergotamine	Contraindicated in ischaemic heart disease as these agents may cause coronary vasoconstriction
Ischaemic heart disease or hypertension	Beta-blockers	These would be reasons to choose beta-blockers for prophylaxis
Peripheral vascular disease	Triptans and ergotamine	These should be avoided due to vasoconstriction
Cerebrovascular accidents	Triptans and ergotamine	These should be avoided due to vasoconstriction
Age	Triptans	Triptans are not recommended in patients aged over 65 years
Wolff–Parkinson–White syndrome	Zolmitriptan	This is contraindicated
Asthma or peptic ulceration	NSAIDs should be used with caution or avoided	See Chapters 7 and 20
Contraception	Combined oral contraceptives	• Migraine is associated with an increased risk of ischaemic stroke. As combined oral contraceptives may compound this risk they should be avoided in patients with migraine with aura, in severe migraine and in migraine without aura but with at least one other risk factor (over 35 years of age, smoking, diabetes mellitus, hypertension, hyperlipidaemia, obesity, family history). They should be used with caution in patients with migraine without aura, who do not have any of these risk factors • Patients who develop migraine or who have increased incidences or severity after starting combined oral contraceptives should stop taking them • Progesterone-only contraceptive pills may be used with caution • A current focal migraine attack is a contraindication to emergency hormonal contraception • Migraine is not a contraindication to hormone replacement therapy
Menstrual migraine		This is migraine without aura around the time of menstruation. It may be managed by mefenamic acid or transdermal oestrogen for 3 days before menstruation and for 7 days afterwards
Depression	Amitriptyline	This would be a reason to choose amitriptyline as a prophylactic agent. Similarly, amitriptyline would be appropriate if there are sleep problems
Depression	Clonidine, beta-blockers	This would be a reason to avoid beta-blockers and clonidine as they may aggravate depression

NSAIDs, non-steroidal anti-inflammatory drugs.

Table 21.2   Some important interactions of antimigraine drugs

Interacting drugs	Consequences	Comments
Triptans with nitrates or beta-blockers	Triptans should not be taken with either nitrates or beta-blockers in ischaemic heart disease due to the risk of coronary vasoconstriction	CSM warning (1992)
Triptans with antidepressants	The combination of an SSRI and sumatriptan is contraindicated by the manufacturers due to the possible potentiation of 5-HT	• Stockley (2002) reports that this only occasionally leads to adverse effects • There is no evidence of naratriptan interacting with tricyclic antidepressants or SSRIs • There is no evidence of rizatriptan interacting with paroxetine • There is no evidence of zolmitriptan interacting with fluoxetine
Ergotamine with triptans	These combinations are contraindicated due to enhanced vasoconstrictor effects	Concurrent ergot derivatives and rizatriptan are contraindicated by the manufacturers, who recommend that ergot derivatives should be taken at least 6 h after rizatriptan and that rizatriptan should be taken 24 h after ergots. The manufacturers advise that zolmitriptan and ergotamine should be taken at least 6 h apart
Sumatriptan with lithium	This combination is contraindicated	
Sumatriptan, rizatriptan with MAOIs	MAOs metabolise sumatriptan and rizatriptan and so MAOIs may increase their concentrations	These combinations are contraindicated
Sumatriptan with sibutramine	Possible potentiation of 5-HT effects	This combination is contraindicated but there is no evidence of adverse reactions
Rizatriptan with propranolol	Propranolol doubles the plasma levels of rizatriptan	The dose of rizatriptan should be halved to 5 mg and the doses separated by 2 h
Tolfenamic acid with magnesium hydroxide or aluminium hydroxide	Magnesium hydroxide accelerates the rate of absorption of tolfenamic acid (this will enhance the onset of action) while aluminium hydroxide may slow the rate of absorption	Aluminium hydroxide should be given separately
Ergotamine with erythromycin	Erythromycin may inhibit the metabolism of ergotamine, leading to severe side-effects such as peripheral vasoconstriction	Their concurrent use should be avoided
Ergotamine with tetracycline	Risk of ergotism	Concurrent use should be monitored
Ergotamine with methysergide	Risk of severe vasoconstriction	This combination should be avoided
Pizotifen with triptans	There is no evidence that pizotifen interacts with sumatriptan and zolmitriptan	
Methysergide with tolbutamide	Methysergide has been shown to enhance the actions of tolbutamide	

CSM, Committee on Safety of Medicines; SSRI, selective serotonin reuptake inhibitor; 5-HT, 5-hydroxytryptamine; MAOIs, monoamine oxidase inhibitors.

migraine. This effect is summarised in a systematic Cochrane review (Pittler *et al.*, 2002). The
lack of information, in comparison with that
provided by clinical trials, favours the use of
conventional medicine. When these have failed,
feverfew may be considered. Adverse effects are
rare but a 'post-feverfew syndrome' of nervousness, tension headaches, insomnia, joint pain
and tiredness has been reported on cessation of
treatment. Feverfew is contraindicated in pregnancy and previous hypersensitivity to related
preparations, including camomile, ragweed and
yarrow or a rash on direct contact with the plant.

Riboflavin

Riboflavin is a water-soluble vitamin found in
fortified breakfast cereals, soya milk, lamb's liver
and dairy products. Deficiency is rare in patients
with a healthy diet (Chapter 3). Vegans may
require supplements. There is some evidence that
higher doses may reduce the duration and frequency of migraine. Chronic use of alcohol, barbiturates and oral contraceptives may produce
riboflavin deficiency. Tricyclic antidepressants
and phenothiazines may increase the requirement for riboflavin. It should be noted that the
deficiency of a single B-vitamin in isolation is
unlikely and supplements of vitamin B complex
would be preferred.

Magnesium

Magnesium is an essential mineral found in
tomatoes, breakfast cereals, wholemeal bread,
pasta and rice, nuts and beans. There is limited
evidence that magnesium may reduce the frequency and pain of migraine. A healthy diet, as
recommended in Chapter 3, should provide an
adequate intake of magnesium. Deficiency may
occur following excess alcohol intake and the
administration of diuretics due to increased
excretion of magnesium. Patients requesting a
supplement of magnesium can be reassured that
adverse effects are unlikely. However, patients
with renal impairment should avoid high doses.
Consideration should also be given to absorption
drug interactions such as with tetracyclines and
4-quinolones.

Counselling

The first general advice, which may be effective
in some patients, is the identification and avoidance of trigger factors as mentioned above
(certain foods, emotional stress, changes in sleep
patterns and hormonal changes, including oral
contraceptives). Rest and sleep may provide some
relief from an attack. Specific counselling points
are described below.

NSAIDs and paracetamol

See Chapter 27.

- These should be taken at the start of an attack,
even before the headache develops.
- The use of diclofenac suppositories does not
avoid side-effects, including gastrointestinal
toxicity or hypersensitivity.

Triptans

- Triptans should be taken at the onset of a
headache and not during the aura as they will
not stop the aura and not all auras lead to a
headache.
- Side-effects of triptans include nausea, dizziness, dry mouth, warm sensations and tingling.
- Some patients experience chest symptoms of
tightness, shortness of breath and occasionally
pain. If there is chest pain, patients should
consult their GP.
- Wafers should be placed on the tongue and
allowed to dissolve.
- Triptans may cause drowsiness.
- In a high proportion of patients taking a
triptan, the migraine may recur within 12 h.
- Frequent use may lead to overuse migraine.

Ergotamine

- If patients develop numbness and tingling
of extremities they should stop taking ergotamine and report this to their GP.
- Important side-effects may include nausea,
vomiting, headache and chest pains.

Prophylactic agents

Some of these are covered in Chapters 11 (beta-blockers, clonidine, calcium-channel blockers), 22 (sodium valproate), and 23 (tricyclic anti-depressants).

Pizotifen

- Pizotifen may cause drowsiness and weight gain.

- Pizotifen is best taken at night due to its sedating actions.

Methysergide

- This may cause drowsiness and may affect the ability to operate machinery or drive
- It may cause a range of other side-effects, including nausea, vomiting and rashes.

Practice points

- Pharmacological treatment is via a stepped-care approach, with simple analgesia providing the first effective step.
- Soluble preparations are preferred due to delayed gastric emptying during migraine.
- Triptans are recommended when treatment with simple analgesia with or without antiemetics has failed.
- Nausea and vomiting may make the oral route ineffective.

 CASE STUDY

A 35-year-old woman who has a history of migraine since the age of 15 years now requires further medication, as paracetamol is ineffective at managing her condition.

Her current medication is:

Sertraline 50 mg (o.d.)
Eugynon 30

1. Comment on her current medication.

- First, it should be noted that combined oral contraceptives may lead to increases in migraine. Instead, progesterone-only contraceptives pills may be used. Her age and obesity (revealed later on) would also favour the use of progesterone-only contraceptives pills (with caution) or alternative contraceptive measures.
    Sertraline is a selective serotonin reuptake inhibitor (SSRI) which may lead to headaches and nausea, and so one needs to be certain that her symptoms are not related to the SSRI.

2. What antimigraine treatment would be appropriate in her case?

- The next likely step would be simple analgesic with an antiemetic plus a triptan (sumatriptan, zolmitriptan or rizatriptan as first-line). Step 2 of diclofenac suppositories plus domperidone

continued

CASE STUDY (continued)

suppositories is often unacceptable to patients. If she is maintained on the sertraline then the use of a triptan is contraindicated by manufacturers of sumatriptan due to the possibility of central nervous system (CNS) toxicity through potentiation of the effects of 5-HT. However, Stockley (2002) points out that the combination of sumatriptan and an SSRI only occasionally leads to adverse effects and suggests that they may be used together with caution.

Her depression is compounded by her obesity (body mass index = 35) but she has shown motivation in losing weight and her GP is prepared to prescribe an antiobesity drug.

3. What advice would you give her GP in drug choice?

• The choice of antiobesity drugs is between sibutramine and orlistat. If she is taking a triptan and/or sertraline then sibutramine would be contraindicated, as there is a risk of CNS toxicity through potentiation of the effects of 5-HT. Therefore, orlistat, which acts on pancreatic lipases, would be a safer choice. In terms of future antimigraine treatment, pizotifen should be avoided as this may cause weight gain. She should be encouraged to take regular exercise and maintain a healthy diet.

References

Committee on Safety of Medicines (1992). *Curr Probl* 34: 2.

Ferrari M D (1998). Migraine. *Lancet* 351: 1043–1051.

Goadsby P J, Lipton R B, Ferrari M D (2002). Migraine – current understanding and treatment. *N Engl J Med* 346: 257–270.

Pittler M H, Vogler B K, Ernst E (2002). Feverfew for preventing migraine (Cochrane review). In: *The Cochrane Library* issue 2. Oxford: Update Software.

Further reading

Goadsby P J, Olesen J (1996). Fortnightly review: diagnosis and management of migraine. *BMJ* 312: 1279–1283.

Stockley I H (2002). *Drug Interactions*, 6th edn. London: Pharmaceutical Press.

Online resources

www.bash.org.uk is the website of the British Association of the Study of Headache, providing guidelines for the diagnosis and management of migraine and tension-type headache (accessed 4 December 2002).

www.migrainetrust.org is the website of the Migraine Trust, with professional and patient information on migraine (accessed 4 December 2002).

22

Epilepsy

Disease characteristics

This is the most common serious neurological condition, with 3–5% of the population experiencing some form during their lifetime. There are several forms, ranging from temporary loss of concentration (absences) to full-blown seizures with convulsions and loss of consciousness. The seizures are divided into partial and generalised seizures and the major forms are described below.

Generalised seizures

In generalised seizures, abnormal electrical activity spreads simultaneously throughout the cerebral cortex and there are several forms:

- Tonic-clonic convulsions (or grand mal seizures) involve sudden loss of consciousness; the limbs may stiffen (tonic) and then jerk (clonic). There is often tongue biting and incontinence. On regaining consciousness, the patient is often drowsy and confused.

- Tonic seizures involve going stiff but without loss of consciousness.
- Atonic seizures involve loss of tone and becoming limp.
- Absences (or petit mal epilepsy) often occur in children who go blank and stare for approximately 10–30 s: this may be mistaken for daydreaming.
- Myoclonic epilepsy is characterised by abrupt jerks which may affect the whole body, arms or legs.

Partial seizures

These are focal seizures which are localised to a brain region and produce simple symptoms such as muscle contractions and abnormal sensory changes without collapsing. Simple partial seizures involve changes in activity while complex partial seizures involve changes in awareness. In secondary generalised seizures activity starts in one area and then spreads, which may lead to a full seizure.

Causes

In general, epilepsy is due to abnormal neuronal discharges, which may or may not spread across the brain. The cause may be due to a structural lesion, secondary to trauma or due to some unidentified change. Biochemical changes such as hypoglycaemia, hyperglycaemia, hypo-natraemia or alcohol abuse may also lead to seizures. Infections such as meningitis may also cause seizures. In some cases, particularly those appearing later in life, they may be due to lesions such as brain tumours, which should be excluded. Therapeutic drugs may induce seizures in patients with or without a history of epilepsy and important examples are:

- quinolones
- tricyclic antidepressants
- selective serotonin reuptake inhibitors (SSRIs)
- antihistamines
- amfebutamone
- donepezil
- baclofen
- lithium
- mefloquine
- theophylline
- tramadol

In addition, withdrawal from alcohol, benzodiazepines and barbiturates is associated with seizures.

Goals of treatment

These are to control seizures with the lowest possible dose, and with fewest side-effects.

Pharmacological management

For a first seizure it is important to exclude other pathologies which may have caused the seizure, important examples of which are detailed above. In the absence of any obvious cause, a first or isolated seizure may go untreated, as in a high proportion of patients (up to 50%) they may not recur. However, once a patient has a subsequent seizure, epilepsy may be diagnosed and anti-epileptic drugs (AEDs) are prescribed to prevent further seizures. In general, AEDs either reduce neuronal excitability and so prevent the spread of neuronal discharges or potentiate inhibitory transmitters such as gamma-aminobutyric acid (GABA). Given these depressant actions on the brain, AEDs are associated with a wide range of central side-effects, which are summarised together with their modes of action in Table 22.1.

Vagal nerve stimulation

This involves insertion of a generator into the chest, with electrodes connected to the vagus nerve. The stimulator provides electrical impulses every 3–5 min and during an aura or the early stages of a seizure the patient or an observer can activate the stimulator to stimulate the vagus, which is thought to disrupt attacks. The mechanism by which this occurs is unclear.

Drug choice

The aim of pharmacological therapy is to control seizures and this is ideally achieved by using one drug at an effective dose. If the first drug fails to control epilepsy at its maximum dose, then a second drug is often tried as the first drug is slowly withdrawn. Only after failure of monotherapy is combined therapy used. Currently, sodium valproate and carbamazepine are widely used, with lamotrigine having an increased role and phenytoin and phenobarbital being less widely used. Some choices of AEDs are summarised in Table 22.2.

Currently gabapentin, levetiracetam, tiagabine, topiramate and vigabatrin (except as mono-therapy for infantile spasms) are only licensed as add-on drugs where control is not attained with monotherapy.

In some cases, seizures increase around menstruation and this is termed catamenial epilepsy. In these patients the benzodiazepine clobazam may be used around that time.

In status epilepticus, a prolonged seizure lasting more than 30 min, benzodiazepines such as diazepam, lorazepam or clonazapam may be given to stop the attack. The rectal route may be more practical during a seizure. If this fails to

Table 22.1   Summary of the pharmacological actions and adverse effects of antiepileptic drugs

Antiepileptic drug	Mechanism of action	Adverse effects and comments
Sodium valproate	Acts weakly by potentiating GABA and causing use-dependent blockade of Na^+-channels	• Sedation, ataxia, diplopia, nystagmus, weight gain, nausea, hair loss and tremor • May rarely cause thrombocytopenia and agranulocytosis • Liver dysfunction and failure have occurred • Pancreatitis may also occur
Carbamazepine	Use-dependent blockade of Na^+-channels	• Induces its own metabolism and so the dosage is increased gradually • It is associated with sedation, erythematous rashes, dizziness, and diplopia (double vision) • It is also associated with hyponatraemia, which itself may reduce seizure threshold • May cause agranulocytosis and thrombocytopenia • It is an important enzyme inducer
Oxcarbazepine	Derivative of carbamazepine	As for carbamazepine but causes less enzyme induction and skin rashes. Hyponatraemia is more problematic than with carbamazepine
Phenytoin	Use-dependent blockade of Na^+-channels	• It shows zero-order pharmacokinetics (Chapter 6), therefore achieving therapeutic concentrations is difficult and side-effects such as nystagmus are indicative of toxic effects • It frequently causes adverse effects, including gingival hypertrophy, hair growth, coarsening of facial features, diplopia, sedation and ataxia. It may cause agranulocytosis • Risk of folate deficiency leading to megaloblastic anaemia • It is an important enzyme inducer
Lamotrigine	Use-dependent blockade of Na^+-channels and decreased release of the excitatory transmitter, glutamate	• Less sedating than the older agents but there may be dizziness and ataxia • It is associated with skin reactions, including toxic epidermal necrolysis and Stevens–Johnson syndrome
Gabapentin	Uncertain	Associated with dizziness, ataxia, somnolence, diplopia, nystagmus and nausea
Vigabatrin	Potentiates GABA by inhibiting its metabolism via the GABA-transaminase enzyme	Associated with drowsiness and fatigue. It may cause irreversible visual field defects
Topiramate	Uncertain, but it may act via blockade of sodium channels and/or enhancing the actions of GABA by binding to a modulatory site	CNS side-effects such as confusion, dizziness, fatigue and memory impairment
Ethosuximide	Inhibition of T-type calcium channels	Associated with gastrointestinal side-effects, drowsiness and dizziness
Phenobarbital	Enhances the effects of GABA at opening the GABA receptor-associated chloride channel	• Sedation is a major problem and it is rarely used • It is an important enzyme inducer
Primidone	Metabolised to phenobarbital	As for phenobarbital
Benzodiazepines e.g. clonazepam clobazam diazepam	Enhance the actions of GABA via the benzodiazepine receptor	Sedation and dependence
Levetiracetam	Uncertain	Dizziness, somnolence, diplopia, tremor, depression and headaches
Tiagabine	Inhibitor of GABA reuptake	Dizziness, somnolence, nervousness and tremor

GABA, gamma-aminobutyric acid; CNS, central nervous system.

Table 22.2 Summary of drug choices in the different forms of epilepsy

Form of epilepsy	First-line	Second-line	Antiepileptic drugs to avoid
Absence	Sodium valproate	Ethosuximide	Carbamazepine
Tonic-clonic	Sodium valproate Carbamazepine Phenytoin	Lamotrigine Vigabatrin	
Myoclonic	Sodium valproate	Clonazepam Ethosuximide Lamotrigine	Carbamazepine
Partial seizures	Sodium valproate Carbamazepine Phenytoin	Lamotrigine Gabapentin Vigabatrin Clonazepam	

control the seizure then intravenous phenytoin or phenobarbital may be used.

Other considerations include concurrent diseases or conditions and some important examples are depression and pregnancy.

Affective disorders

Depression is an important consideration, and this may well occur secondary to patients developing epilepsy. The use of antidepressants is associated with decreasing the seizure threshold, which may lead to episodes of epilepsy, and so antidepressants should be used with caution in epilepsy. In concurrent bipolar affective disorder then carbamazepine may be considered as a compelling choice because it is effective in this condition. It should be noted that carbamazepine may be used effectively with lithium, but there have been instances of increased neurotoxicity with this combination.

Pregnancy

Pregnancy is a major issue in patients with epilepsy as the associated physiological changes may increase the incidence of seizures. Furthermore, AEDs are associated with a range of birth defects. For example, carbamazepine and sodium valproate are associated with increased risks of neural tube defects and phenytoin and pheno-

barbital are associated with cleft palates. Other adverse effects may include impaired psychomotor development in the child, cardiac defects and facial abnormalities. Some patients who are seizure free for some time may have their AED withdrawn prior to conception. However, if this is not the case continuing AEDs during pregnancy is considered important as seizures during pregnancy may have serious consequences for both the mother and fetus. To reduce the chances of neural tube defect, patients should receive 5 mg of folic acid daily from the cessation of contraception and for at least the first 12 weeks of pregnancy. In the case of phenytoin and phenobarbital, folic acid may reduce the plasma concentrations of these agents so monitoring may be required. Carbamazepine, phenytoin and phenobarbital are associated with increased neonatal bleeding (including intracranial bleeds) and vitamin K is given to the mother from the 36th week of pregnancy before delivery and to the baby at birth. Experience of the newer agents in pregnancy is limited and so there is little information regarding birth defects. Some practitioners favour the use of lamotrigine in females of child-bearing age, but this may of course change in the light of more information. Older agents such as phenobarbital and phenytoin should be avoided in women of child-bearing age if possible, due to the increased risk of birth defects.

Breast-feeding

Breast-feeding is considered safe for mothers taking carbamazepine, phenytoin and sodium valproate. Breast-feeding whilst taking phenobarbital, primidone, vigabatrin (risk of visual defects) and ethosuximide should be avoided. Breast-feeding is considered safe with newer agents such as lamotrigine, and gabapentin if taken during pregnancy. Non-hormonal methods of contraception may be required during breast-feeding by patients prescribed enzyme-inducing drugs as progestogen-only contraceptives may be less effective.

Contraception

Compounding the issue of pregnancy is the established interaction of the enzyme-inducing AEDs (carbamazepine, oxcarbazepine, phenytoin, phenobarbital and topiramate) with oral contraceptives, which accelerate their metabolism, and this may lead to contraceptive failure. To overcome this problem alternative contraception such as barrier methods should be used. Alternatively a high-dose oestrogen (50 µg ethinylestradiol)-containing pill might be prescribed. For progestogen-only pills the dose should also be increased. As other first-line AEDs such as sodium valproate and lamotrigine do not interact with oral contraceptives, this may be a reason to choose these agents in favour of enzyme-inducing agents.

Young children

It should be noted that young children may require higher doses per kilogram of body weight of antiepileptics, with more frequent doses due to more rapid metabolism of these drugs.

Drug interactions

AEDs show a wide range of interactions and the reader is referred to specialised literature such as *Drug Interactions* by Stockley (2002). However, a few important points to note are that carbamazepine (oxcarbazepine to a lesser extent), phenytoin and phenobarbital induce cytochrome P450, and accelerate the metabolism of other drugs.

Indeed, one reason to favour monotherapy is that many of the AEDs interact with each other, often increasing each other's metabolism. By contrast, sodium valproate inhibits the metabolism of lamotrigine, thus increasing its plasma half-life. Some important examples of other interactions due to induction of metabolism are as follows.

Carbamazepine, phenytoin and phenobarbital may significantly accelerate the metabolism of:

- doxycycline but not other tetracyclines
- warfarin (phenytoin may also potentiate the actions of warfarin)
- indinavir, nelfinavir, saquinavir
- dihydropyridines
- corticosteroids
- oestrogens and progestogens
- theophylline
- levothyroxine
- certain other AEDs

In addition, given the hepatic route of metabolism of some AEDs, there is scope for inhibitors of these pathways to interact with AEDs, resulting in increased concentrations and promoting toxicity. Important examples of this are the interactions of carbamazepine with erythromycin, clarithromycin, dextropropoxyphene, diltiazem, verapamil, certain SSRIs (fluoxetine and fluvoxamine) and cimetidine (transiently). St John's wort may induce the metabolism of carbamazepine, making it less effective. Having commented on the extensive range of drug interactions with AEDs, it should also be noted that gabapentin is not known to have any significant interactions.

Monitoring

AEDs are associated with a range of serious adverse drug reactions (ADRs) affecting the liver (Chapter 5) and haematological system (Chapter 5) and so monitoring is appropriate. Baseline monitoring of haematology and biochemistry is often carried out prior to starting treatment. Liver function testing (LFT) is essential with sodium valproate before treatment and during the first 6 months, including a determination of international normalised ratio. Some of the inducing AEDs may alter LFTs (Chapter 2) via enzyme induction (e.g.

increased levels of gamma-glutamyl transferase (GGT)) and may also promote damage due to the enhancement of drug metabolism, which may give rise to toxic metabolites.

Blood counts should be determined if there are signs of reduced white cell counts (leucopenia due to agranulocytosis) such as increased infections (e.g. sore throats, fevers, mouth ulcers) or thrombocytopenia (increased bruising), which may occur with carbamazepine, ethosuximide, lamotrigine, phenytoin (the manufacturer recommends monitoring of blood counts) and sodium valproate (principally thrombocytopenia). If serious blood disorders such as leucopenia or thrombocytopenia are identified then the AED should be withdrawn under the cover of another agent.

Visual fields should also be measured every 6 months with vigabatrin.

Withdrawing antiepileptic drugs

In many patients it is undesirable that they are maintained indefinitely on AEDs; indeed, the condition which may have led to their seizures may have resolved. Therefore, after a suitable seizure-free period, the patient and doctor may consider withdrawal of therapy. Typically, patients who are seizure-free for 2–4 years are considered, as a substantial proportion will remain seizure-free on withdrawal. Withdrawal of AEDs may itself decrease the seizure threshold, so this should be gradual with a dose reduction over time. Typical reducing regimens are dose reductions (e.g. carbamazepine by 100 mg, sodium valproate by 200 mg) every 4 weeks. Phenobarbital should be withdrawn over several months. During the withdrawal period and for 6 months afterwards, patients should not drive, as the withdrawal may precipitate seizures or the patient's epilepsy may return. When changing medication, the original drug should only be withdrawn once the new drug is established.

Over-the-counter medication and supplements

Over-the-counter (OTC) issues in epilepsy involve screening for ADRs and drug interactions and providing support to patients to aid compliance. Drugs such as cimetidine, a cytochrome P450 inhibitor, should be avoided (see earlier). Female patients should be advised to consult their doctor before planning a pregnancy, for counselling and prescription of folic acid together with a medication review. Patients with epilepsy should not take evening primrose oil or ginkgo biloba due to a risk of seizures with these agents.

Counselling

To achieve adequate control of epilepsy, patients should be informed of the importance of compliance, as omitting doses or abrupt withdrawal may cause a rebound increase in the occurrence of seizures.

Informing family and colleagues about their condition may help as seizures can appear frightening.

Haematological and hepatic adverse effects

Patients taking carbamazepine, oxcarbazepine, ethosuximide, gabapentin, lamotrigine, phenytoin and sodium valproate should be counselled to report promptly signs of blood disorders such as sore throats, mouth ulcers, fevers or easy bruising. In the case of lamotrigine, patients should also report rashes or flu-like illnesses. Patients taking carbamazepine, oxcarbazepine and sodium valproate should report symptoms which may indicate liver damage such as jaundice, itching, nausea and vomiting.

Skin reactions

Many of the AEDs may cause skin reactions (Chapter 5). Although many of these are harmless, some may be serious and so patients should consult their doctor.

Sedation

Many of the AEDs may cause sedation and so patients should be warned of this possibility. When taking carbamazepine, gabapentin, vigabatrin, topiramate, barbiturates and benzodiazepines, patients should be specifically advised that sedation may affect their ability to operate machinery.

Driving

This is subject to clear regulations of the driving licensing authorities (see the *British National Formulary*) and the onus is on patients to report their condition. Patients should also stop driving for 6 months on withdrawal of AEDs. In addition, all of the AEDs may impair driving and so patients should be alerted to this.

Alcohol

Alcohol may enhance central nervous system side-effects such as sedation in some AEDs such as carbamazepine. Excessive fluid intake may also predispose patients taking carbamazepine and oxcarbazepine to hyponatraemia, which itself may lead to seizure. Hence patients should be cautioned against excessive alcohol intake.

Drug interactions

Patients should inform all healthcare professionals that they are taking AEDs.

Pregnancy

Female patients should be advised to discuss with their general practitioner (GP) the issues surrounding pregnancy and epilepsy (see above) before stopping contraception. Advice should be given on the interaction of antiepileptics and oral contraceptives, the risks associated with unplanned pregnancy and the risks/benefits of AED use during pregnancy.

Bone

The enzyme-inducing AEDs (carbamazepine, phenytoin and phenobarbital) have been associated with accelerated metabolism of vitamin D, leading to impaired calcium levels. These effects have been associated with rickets and osteomalacia and so the importance of a balanced diet should be stressed. This may be particularly important in the presence of additional risk factors such as early menopause, and use of corticosteroids.

Side-effects

In addition to the extensive range of side-effects reported above, some other drug-specific counselling points are as follows.

Phenytoin
This may cause increased growth of the gums.

Vigabatrin
This may cause irreversible changes in vision, which should be reported.

Practice points

- Epilepsy is a common condition, which is usually managed by drugs.
- Monotherapy is preferred.
- Pharmacists have an important role in ensuring adherence to AEDs.
- AEDs have a wide range of interactions and the enzyme inducers may cause a failure of oral contraception.
- AEDs are associated with a range of side-effects and may cause birth defects.
- In treatment failure, check that the dose has been increased to an appropriate maintenance dose, and/or check blood levels prior to a new prescription. For example, carbamazepine induces its own metabolism, requiring a gradual dose increase.

CASE STUDY

A 25-year-old woman has been diagnosed with tonic-clonic epilepsy. Antiepileptic treatment was initiated with carbamazepine (100 mg b.d.) and subsequently maintained at a total daily dose of 800 mg.

1. How would you counsel this patient with respect to treatment with carbamazepine?

She should:

- not discontinue her medicine without advice
- report any unexplained sore throats, mouth ulcers, rashes, bleeding or bruising to her GP
- take effective contraceptive measures and seek specialist advice before considering conception

2. What contraceptive measures would be appropriate? Why?

- It is best to use an effective barrier method but, if this is not possible, she should use an oral contraceptive with 50 μg or more oestrogen or tricycling with monophasic tablets (three or four packs without a break).
- Carbamazepine is an enzyme inducer, making oral contraceptives less effective, and in view of the teratogenic effects of carbamazepine, pregnancy should be avoided without specialist advice.

After several weeks she complains to you, as her community pharmacist, of a persistent sore throat.

3. What action should you take?

- She should be referred to her GP.

4. What tests are appropriate? Why?

- She should have a full blood count, as carbamazepine is associated with agranulocytosis which results in reduced white blood cell counts (leucopenia).

5. Considering the different potential outcomes of the test(s), what actions might be taken?

- If there is neutropenia, the carbamazepine should be stopped under the cover of another antiepileptic. Neutropenia is not a class effect and another antiepileptic might be tried. If the white blood count is normal, then the sore throat should be treated. If this is bacterial, then phenoxymethylpenicillin or cephalosporins might be used or if it is viral, then simple linctus or soothing sweets could be recommended.

References

Mehta D K (ed.) *British National Formulary*, latest edition. London: British Medical Association and Royal Pharmaceutical Society of Great Britain.

Stockley I H (2002). *Drug Interactions*, 6th edn. London: Pharmaceutical Press.

Further reading

Brodie M J, French J A (2000). Management of epilepsy in adolescents and adults. *Lancet* 356: 323–329.

Craig J, Sisodiya S (2001). Guide to the management of epilepsy in pregnancy. *Prescriber* 12: 30–36.

Feely M (1999). Drug treatment of epilepsy. *BMJ* 318: 106–109.

Online resources

www.epilepsy.org.uk. is the wesbiste of Epilepsy Action (British Epilepsy Association), a very useful resource for information on epilepsy, with excellent patient information (accessed 4 December 2002).

www.epilepsynse.org.uk is the website of National Society for Epilepsy , a very useful resource for information on epilepsy with excellent patient information (accessed 4 December 2002).

23

Affective disorders

Disease characteristics

Affective (emotion) disorders consist of changes in mood, with the most common manifestation being depressed mood. Typically this is a long-standing condition which may be associated with feelings of low self-esteem, a lack of motivation, an inability to derive pleasure, and sleep may be disturbed, often with early waking. The cause is often difficult to identify and may be multi-factorial with risk factors including creative, per-fectionist and neurotic personality types, stressful life events, history of abuse in childhood, the later stages of pregnancy, following childbirth and with a hereditary link, particularly in bipolar disorder. There is also a close association with chronic illnesses (such as multiple sclerosis, myocardial infarction, stroke, Parkinson's disease, cancer, human immunodeficiency virus (HIV)), and may be precipitated by major events such as bereavement. Depression may complicate or worsen pre-existing disease. In addition certain drugs may lead to or exacerbate depression, for example, isotretinoin, corticosteroids, benzodiazepines and alcohol (Chapter 5). Substance misuse is also a significant cause. For detailed guidance on the management of depression the reader is referred to Anderson *et al.* (2000).

Underlying pathology

The underlying pathology of affective disorders is poorly understood. The most widely accepted theory remains the monoamine theory, which is now 40 years old, but does not, however, satisfactorily account for all of the pathology. This theory links reduction in the monoamine neurotransmitters noradrenaline (norepinephrine) and 5-hydroxytryptamine (5-HT, serotonin) as the main biochemical changes linked to clinical symptoms of depression. The theory was developed following the observation that drug-induced changes in monoamine neurotransmitters either caused or improved symptoms of depression. For example, reserpine used to treat hypertension was withdrawn due to side-effects of depression, which was thought to be due to a reduction in noradrenaline and 5-HT-mediated transmission in the brain. By contrast the anti-tuberculosis drug isoniazid, which increased levels of catecholamines, enhanced mood. Antidepressant drugs were, therefore, designed to increase the availability of noradrenaline and 5-HT in the brain, leading to a clinical response.

Anomalies exist in the theory in that some drugs affect noradrenaline and/or 5-HT activity without evoking changes in mood. For example, methysergide, a 5-HT antagonist, does not produce a depressed mood, as might be predicted. A further discrepancy in the monoamine theory is the delayed onset of antidepressant action despite a rapid change in monoamine levels detectable by analysis of noradrenaline and 5-HT metabolite concentrations in cerebrospinal fluid or urine. A change in receptor numbers has therefore been proposed as an important mechanism since a common and delayed down-regulation of beta-adrenoceptors and 5-HT_2 receptors is observed following prolonged antidepressant treatment.

Despite the anomalies described above, increased availability of monoamines in the brain remains the most effective biochemical manipulation used in the treatment of depression, being common to all antidepressant drugs, with the possible exception of amfebutamone (bupropion).

Classification and clinical features

Depressive illness is classified according to the *Diagnostic and Statistical Manual of Mental Disorders* (DSM-IV) criteria (American Psychiatric Association, 1995) and the *International Statistical Classification of Diseases and Related Health Problems* (ICD-10: World Health Organization, 1992). These classifications are intended to differentiate between normal and pathological states through assessment of behavioural, psychological and biological dysfunction with the aim of classifying disorders, not people. For example, terms such as 'schizophrenic' and 'alcoholic' are no longer used. There is considerable overlap and mutual working between the two classifications. The following section will therefore consider the DSM-IV criteria to prevent repetition.

The previous terminology used in the classification of affective disorders comprised reactive, endogenous, manic, psychotic or neurotic. The terms 'reactive' and 'endogenous' differentiated between depression occurring in response to life events or tending to have a hereditary component without associated life events, respectively. The types of depressive illness are currently classified as postnatal depression, seasonal affective disorder (SAD), dysthymia, unipolar depression (in response to stressful life events) and bipolar depression (previously manic depression). Psychotic symptoms may be present but do not constitute a distinct disorder.

Postnatal depression

The diagnosis of postnatal depression is made if any of the criteria below are met and symptoms occur within 4 weeks of childbirth.

Seasonal affective disorder

It is increasingly recognised that affective disorders may follow a seasonal pattern, with onset during the winter months. Accordingly, the DSM-IV criteria recognise SAD, when a regular and recurrent temporal relationship is observed and seasonal psychosocial stressors are excluded (e.g. unemployment every winter). In addition, two major depressive episodes will have been present in 2 years. Full remission or a switch from depression to mania or hypomania also follows a temporal relationship, such as occurs in springtime. Major depressive episodes should also be absent outside the seasonal episodes. Finally, major depressive episodes with a seasonal onset should outnumber those without seasonal onset during the patient's life.

Dysthymic disorder

The DSM-IV criteria for dysthymic disorder include depressed mood for most of the day for most days for at least 2 years. The symptoms cause significant distress or reduced social or occupational functioning. At least two or more of the following symptoms are present with no more than 2 months without symptoms:

1. poor appetite or overeating
2. altered sleep requirements
3. reduced energy or fatigue
4. low self-esteem
5. poor concentration or indecisiveness
6. feelings of hopelessness

In addition, the criteria require that no major depressive episodes have been diagnosed within the first 2 years. This excludes the possibility of partial remission following a major depressive episode. Full remission would include being symptom-free for 2 months. Diagnosis is made following the exclusion of other mental disorders, drug abuse, medication (Chapter 5) or underlying disease such as hypothyroidism.

Children

Dysthymic disorder may present as irritable mood in children and adolescents, with duration of at least 1 year.

Unipolar affective disorder (major depression)

Unipolar depression is the most common disorder, affecting one in six people. As many as one in three people are likely to suffer an episode of unipolar depression in their lifetime. Diagnosis of a major depressive episode according to the DSM-IV criteria is currently considered when five or more of the following symptoms have been present on most days or nearly every day for 2 weeks and are causing clinical significant distress or impaired functioning. In addition, at least one of the symptoms must include at least one of the first two symptoms listed below. Major depressive disorder is diagnosed following one or more major depressive episodes, including:

1. depressed mood
2. loss of interest or pleasure in all or most activities
3. increased or decreased appetite, particularly associated with significant weight change (more than 5% in a month and not dieting)
4. altered sleep
5. psychomotor agitation or retardation
6. fatigue
7. worthlessness or excessive or inappropriate guilt
8. reduced ability to think or concentrate or indecisiveness
9. recurrent thoughts of death or suicide

The diagnosis is only made following the exclusion of substance abuse, bereavement (see below) or general medical conditions such as hypothyroidism.

Children

In children and adolescents, the symptom of depressed mood (point 1 above) may present as irritable mood. In addition, weight changes may present as a failure to make expected weight gains (see below).

Psychotic depression

A depressive episode may also present with additional psychotic symptoms. The term 'psychosis' is used to describe severe mental illness with loss of contact with reality. Thought processes are often altered and patients suffer hallucinations and delusions (Chapter 26). Psychosis is a component of severe schizophrenia, depression and bipolar affective disorder. For a discussion of the psychotic symptoms associated with antimuscarinic drugs, see Chapter 26.

Severity

The severity of a depressive episode may be mild, moderate or severe. An episode is described as mild if the number of symptoms required for a positive diagnosis is only exceeded marginally. The impact of a minor episode only produces limited effects on social and occupational functioning. By contrast, a severe episode will present with numerous additional symptoms than those required to make a diagnosis, and a marked disruption to normal functioning occurs. Moderate illness falls between the two extremes.

Elderly patients and bereavement

The recognition and treatment of depression in the elderly are important but bereavement and/or dementia may complicate diagnosis. Bereavement is differentiated from depression if symptoms develop within 2–3 weeks of the death of a close friend or relative and resolve spontaneously. Dementia may be excluded depending on the magnitude of decline in memory.

Children

Depression in children and adolescents is now increasingly recognised, often presenting as self-criticism, pessimism about the future, lack of energy, sleep disturbance, stomachache, headache, indecision and difficulty concentrating (see also DSM-IV criteria listed above). Children may lack interest in activities they enjoyed previously. Risk factors include a family history of affective disorders, stress, viral infections and a history of abuse. There is sparse information relating to the treatment of childhood depression but this may involve cognitive behaviour therapy (CBT) and possibly the selective serotonin reuptake inhibitors (SSRIs), fluoxetine and sertraline (unlicensed indications). The side-effect profile precludes the use of tricyclic antidepressants (TCAs) in children aged less than 16 years, although these drugs are licensed for short-term treatment of nocturnal enuresis. Paroxetine should not be used for patients under 18 years.

Goals of treatment

Treatment aims are to improve the quality of life, including the ability to work and function socially, together with the prevention of suicide. This should of course be achieved with the minimum of side-effects. Drug treatment should ideally be used with appropriate CBT or psychotherapy, which may hasten recovery and prevent recurrence. Currently however, CBT and psychotherapy are not widely available in the UK.

Pharmacological basis of management

Treatment should be continued for at least 6 months after symptoms resolve to prevent relapse and recurrence. The recommended length of treatment varies according to the severity of symptoms and the number of episodes suffered. Initially, treatment is recommended for 4–6 months from the resolution of symptoms and at the dose used to achieve this. The duration of treatment of a second episode should be at least 12 months. For recurrent depression such as previous episodes less than 2½ years apart however, treatment may be continued for 5 years or more (Kupfer *et al.*, 1992) at the dose required to achieve remission of symptoms. Bipolar affective disorder has a high risk of recurrence and suicide and therefore long-term prophylactic treatment, usually with lithium, is indicated.

Tricyclic antidepressants

e.g. Amitriptyline, dosulepin (dothiepin), imipramine, lofepramine, nortriptyline

TCAs are similar in structure to phenothiazines (prochlorperazine, thioridazine) and inhibit the neuronal uptake of noradrenaline and 5-HT, leading to augmented concentrations in the synaptic cleft. The increase in catecholamines may lead to down-regulation of presynaptic alpha$_2$-adrenoceptors and 5-HT receptors and postsynaptic beta-adrenoceptors. In addition, TCAs exhibit binding at a range of receptors, including muscarinic receptors, histamine, alpha$_1$-adrenoceptors and 5-HT receptors. The inhibition of muscarinic receptors results in side-effects such as dry mouth, blurred vision, constipation and urinary retention. TCAs vary in the degree of sedation they cause (with amitriptyline and dosulepin having significant effects and lofepramine being less sedating) and this may have a bearing on their use where sedation may be an advantage or unwanted. TCAs may cause cardiac effects such as QT interval prolongation and the potentiation of catecholamines also predisposes to heart block and arrhythmias. The cardiac effects of TCAs (except lofepramine), together with increased effects of alcohol, including respiratory depression, mean that these agents are dangerous in overdose. They are not suitable for patients with ischaemic heart disease, aged over 70 years or those patients who are thought to be at high risk of attempting suicide.

Monoamine oxidase inhibitors (MAOIs)

Isocarboxazid, moclobemide, phenelzine, tranylcypromine

MAOIs are only occasionally used because of their widespread side-effects and drug interactions, including those with tyramine-containing foods. They were the first antidepressants used after the observation that treatment with isoniazid for tuberculosis improved mood. MAOIs inhibit the monoamine oxidases, which metabolise catecholamines. Once again, their action is to increase the concentration of these neurotransmitters. Because of this effect, MAOIs also prevent the breakdown of tyramine, the indirectly acting sympathomimetic amine, which is present in the diet. By preventing the breakdown of tyramine, this amine causes the release of catecholamines and leads to a hypertensive response. Tyramine is present in certain foods such as yeast extracts (including Bovril and Marmite), some wines and beers, avocado, banana, pickled herring and cheese, and this response is known as the 'cheese reaction'. Since the majority of MAOIs inhibit MAO irreversibly, these reactions may persist for 2–3 weeks after the cessation of treatment until new MAO is synthesised.

MAO exists as either MAO-A, which metabolises predominantly noradrenaline and 5-HT, or MAO-B, for which phenylethylamine is a substrate. Tyramine and dopamine are metabolised by both subtypes. In an attempt to reduce side-effects and interactions, selective inhibitors of MAO have been developed. For example moclobemide, a selective reversible inhibitor of MAO-A (RIMA), reduces interactions with food since tyramine is metabolised by MAO-B. The MAO-B inhibitor selegeline is used to treat Parkinson's disease.

Selective serotonin reuptake inhibitors

Citalopram, escitalopram (active isomer of citalopram), fluoxetine, fluvoxamine, paroxetine, sertraline

As the name implies, SSRIs selectively inhibit the neuronal reuptake of 5-HT, thus enhancing synaptic concentrations of 5-HT and down-regulating presynaptic 5-HT receptors. SSRIs have a different side-effect profile compared with TCAs, including nausea, diarrhoea, constipation, dizziness, headache, altered platelet function, anorexia, insomnia, loss of libido and delay or failure of orgasm. Some SSRIs are also licensed for the treatment of anxiety disorders, panic and obsessive-compulsive disorders (Chapter 24).

Noradrenaline reuptake inhibitors (NARIs)

Reboxetine

Reboxetine is one of the newer reuptake inhibitors. It selectively inhibits noradrenaline reuptake, providing an option for patients who cannot take TCAs (Table 23.1) but who are resistant to the effects of SSRIs.

Serotonin–noradrenaline reuptake inhibitors (SNRIs)

Venlafaxine

A relatively new reuptake inhibitor is venlafaxine. The mechanism of action involves the inhibition of both serotonin and noradrenaline reuptake, as with TCAs. SNRIs, however, fail to bind to additional receptors and therefore demonstrate fewer side-effects compared to TCAs, including a lack of sedative and antimuscarinic side-effects, but do cause gastrointestinal side-effects. In addition, a recent analysis of fatal toxicity of antidepressants in the UK reported that venlafaxine toxicity is greater than for other serotonergic agents and similar to some TCAs (Buckley and McManus, 2002).

Noradrenergic and specific serotonergic antidepressants (NaSSAs)

Mirtazapine

Observations of the pharmacological activity of mianserin have been exploited in the development of mirtazapine. This agent exhibits $alpha_2$-adrenocepter antagonist activity, inhibiting negative feedback by these presynaptic receptors and thus producing an increase in noradrenaline and 5-HT transmission. Mirtazapine also inhibits $5-HT_2$ and $5-HT_3$ receptors, preventing sexual dysfunction and nausea, respectively. Sedation predominates in early treatment but antimuscarinic side-effects are limited.

Serotonin receptor modulators (SRMs)

Nefazodone and trazodone

Nefazodone and trazodone are similar in structure and exhibit mixed serotonergic activity, including both inhibition of serotonin reuptake and the selective inhibition of postsynaptic 5-HT receptors. Trazodone also acts at noradrenaline receptors, with nefazodone exhibiting less activity at these receptors.

TCA-related antidepressants

Bupropion, maprotiline, mianserin, viloxazine

In the ongoing search for antidepressants with fewer side-effects, reduced toxicity in overdose and without a delayed onset of action, a number of agents have been developed which do not fit the above classes of MAOI, SSRI or TCA. For example, some agents possess a non-TCA structure but exhibit similar modes of action. The mechanisms thought to be involved in the antidepressant effects of these TCA-related agents include:

- the inhibition of noradrenaline uptake (nomifensine and maprotiline)
- a small reduction of 5-HT uptake and possibly inhibition of dopamine uptake (nomifensine)
- agents that do not affect amine uptake (mianserin, bupropion)
- mechanisms that differ slightly from other antidepressants, inhibiting noradrenaline reuptake but also stimulating serotonin release from neurons (viloxazine)
- inhibition of 5-HT and $alpha_2$-adrenoceptors, thereby inhibiting negative feedback and increasing release of noradrenaline without the conventional effects on the reuptake of noradrenaline and serotonin (mianserin)
- unknown mechanisms – bupropion is efficacious but fails to demonstrate biochemistry in common with conventional antidepressant activity

Benzodiazepines (e.g. clonazepam, lorazepam) and beta-blockers

These are used on a temporary basis in depression with a component of severe anxiety or hyperactivity (Chapter 24). For example, a short-acting benzodiazepine such as lorazepam may be used when antidepressants are initiated, prior to the onset of efficacy. Long-term use may worsen

Table 23.1 Some considerations when choosing the most appropriate antidepressant

Condition	Cautions and contraindications	Compelling drug choices
Cardiovascular disease	All antidepressants, including lithium, should be used with caution due to increased effects of sympathetic and serotonergic systems. Venlafaxine has been associated with dose-related hypertension	SSRIs are preferred
Recent MI	TCAs are contraindicated	SSRIs considered safe, particularly sertraline (Glassman et al., 2002)
Arrhythmias	TCAs are contraindicated. Venlafaxine and antipsychotics may cause QT prolongation. Atypical antipsychotics have not been associated with this but caution is needed if coprescribed with drugs known to prolong the QT interval (Chapter 5)	SSRIs (not fluoxetine) Avoid fluoxetine and trazodone, which can cause atrial fibrillation
Stroke	Avoid MAOIs due to the risk of a hypertensive episode. Use venlafaxine with caution due to dose-related hypertension (see above)	
Insomnia	SSRIs may occasionally cause insomnia. Lofepramine is a less-sedating TCA	Sedating TCAs (e.g. amitriptyline, dosulepin), maprotiline, mianserin or trazodone
Risk of deliberate self-harm or suicide attempt	See text	
Epilepsy	All antidepressants have the potential to lower the convulsive threshold and should be used with caution and avoided in poorly controlled epilepsy	• Carbamazepine and lamotrigine (unlicensed indication) may be considered in bipolar affective disorder • Additional risk factors include diabetes mellitus or concurrent treatment with drugs known to lower the convulsive threshold (Chapter 5, Table 5.9) • Risk of seizure is considered to be greatest with clomipramine, maprotiline and bupropion • Lowest risk has been suggested with fluoxetine, sertraline, paroxetine and fluvoxamine (Knodel et al., 1998)
Bipolar affective disorder – manic phase	TCAs, MAOIs and SSRIs are contraindicated. Antidepressants may trigger bipolar disorder, particularly in patients with hypomania and/or a family history	Mood stabilisers (lithium, neuroleptics, carbamazepine and valproate (see text)). Combining SSRI treatment (avoiding long-acting preparations, e.g. fluoxetine) with a mood stabiliser may reduce the risk of switching to mania (Grunze et al., 2002)
Anxiety disorders	Long-term use of propranolol and/or benzodiazepines should be avoided as these drugs may aggravate depression	For depression with associated anxiety symptoms, refer to Chapter 24

Continued

Table 23.1   Continued

Condition	Cautions and contraindications	Compelling drug choices
Migraine	SSRIs may cause headache (Chapter 5)	TCAs may be appropriate (Chapter 21)
Neuropathic pain		TCAs or carbamazepine
Alcoholism	Avoid isoniazid due to hepatotoxicity. Sedative effects of TCAs enhanced	
Eating disorders		High-dose fluoxetine is indicated for bulimia nervosa
Parkinson's disease treated with co-beneldopa, co-careldopa, levodopa	Irreversible MAOIs should be avoided with drugs used to increase dopamine	
Peptic ulcer disease	Increased risk of GI bleeds, therefore caution with SSRIs. Consider high-risk patients such as those with a history of previous GI bleed and/or aged over 80 years (Chapter 7)	
Urinary problems (prostatism), glaucoma and constipation	Caution with TCAs and maprotiline and mirtazapine due to antimuscarinic side-effects	
Hyperthyroidism	Caution with TCAs due to augmentation of sympathetic nervous system. Lithium should be used with caution and initiated when patients are euthyroid. Regular monitoring of thyroid function is essential (Chapter 2)	

SSRIs, selective serotonin reuptake inhibitors; MI, myocardial infarction; TCAs, tricyclic antidepressants; MAOIs, monoamine oxidase inhibitors; GI, gastrointestinal.

depression and lead to addiction to benzodiazepines and apparent worsening anxiety (withdrawal reactions, Chapter 5).

Flupentixol

Lower doses of flupentixol compared with those used in schizophrenia are indicated for the treatment of depressive illness.

L-tryptophan

L-tryptophan, a precursor for 5-HT, is an amino acid found in food. It has a mild antidepressant effect but use is limited to prescribing by hospital specialists for patients with chronic severe depression who are already taking other antidepressants. This is mainly due to the risk of eosinophilia–myalgia syndrome (increased eosinophils

in blood, with muscle pain) and close monitoring of the eosinophil count and muscle symptoms is required.

Electroconvulsive therapy (ECT)

ECT is reserved for severe and suicidal depression, with greatest efficacy in depression with psychomotor retardation (literally, a slowing of muscular and mental activity), such as depressive stupor. This is a condition of near unconsciousness, apparent mental inactivity and a reduced response to stimulation. The procedure is carried out under general anaesthesia and a convulsion is induced by passing an electric current through the brain. The main side-effects are temporary confusion and memory loss. This treatment should therefore be used with caution in elderly patients with cognitive impairment. Other risks to be considered are those associated with general anaesthesia and the use of ECT during pregnancy. These risks are considered alongside the benefits and potential risks of withholding treatment. The mechanism involved remains unclear but ECT is an effective treatment with rapid onset.

Lithium

Lithium is a useful adjunct in the treatment of resistant depression. It may be added to TCA or SSRI treatment under specialist supervision. The use of TCAs and SSRIs is associated with a risk of switching patients into mania, a particular problem when treating the depressive phase of bipolar disorder. The highest risk is associated with the use of TCAs.

Non-pharmacological therapy

Structured counselling based on theoretical models includes psychotherapy or CBT. Psychotherapy may be of particular benefit to patients with a history of abuse or social history such as stressful life events. CBT has been shown to be effective in mild depression and in combination with antidepressants in moderate depression (Scott *et al.*, 1997). This would seem logical since neurotic, perfectionist, obsessional or anxious personality types may be linked to depression. The negative thought patterns associated with these personality types are identified and addressed during CBT. In addition, increased insight and the avoidance of overly stressful situations contribute to successful treatment. The reader is referred to *Mind over Mood* (Greenberger and Padesky, 1995) for an excellent CBT-based workbook for motivated patients.

Evidence-based guidelines also recommend support, education and problem-solving techniques as an alternative to antidepressants in acute mild depression (Anderson *et al.*, 2000). Patients with SAD may benefit from light therapy (Levitt *et al.*, 2002). Chronobiological intervention may include sleep deprivation and sleep phase advance for patients with a history of a poor response to or poor tolerability of treatment with antidepressants (Grunze *et al.*, 2002).

Choice of drugs in unipolar affective disorder

Studies have shown little difference in the efficacy of antidepressant drugs. For example, a meta-analysis of 102 randomised controlled trials indicated comparable efficacy between SSRIs and TCAs, although SSRIs were not as efficacious for inpatients with severe and/or psychotic depression and when compared against amitriptyline (Anderson *et al.*, 2000). This superior effectiveness of amitriptyline was also confirmed in a systematic review (Barbui and Hotopf, 2001). Amitriptyline is however less well tolerated than other TCAs and SSRIs.

Generally, the choice is between an SSRI and TCA, with the most appropriate drug class being selected, according to:

- sedative properties
- side-effect profile
- previous response
- potential for toxicity in ovderdose
- concurrent disease (Table 23.1)

The first-line choice of a TCA may be amitriptyline, due to proven efficacy and low cost or lofepramine if reduced sedation and lower risk of overdose are preferred. The first-line choice of SSRI is often fluoxetine as it is well established and has cost advantages over newer agents. SSRIs are now the most commonly prescribed antidepressants, due mainly to the absence of cardiac side-effects that render TCAs (except lofepramine) dangerous in overdose. SSRIs also lack the food and drug interactions that limit the prescribing of MAOIs.

Risk of suicide

TCAs are avoided in patients considered to be at risk of committing suicide, such as those with a history of contemplating or attempting suicide. This is due to the toxic effects of TCAs (except lofepramine) in overdose. SSRIs are preferred due to relative safety in overdose, although patients should be monitored closely during early treatment with all antidepressants and particularly SSRIs, due to a possible increased risk of suicide attempts. Alternative treatment includes the use of mirtazapine, nefazodone and reboxetine, which are considered to be relatively safe in overdose. For a discussion of the use of venlafaxine, see SNRIs above.

Treatment failure

Failure of treatment (typically after 4 weeks) may lead to a different class being used. It should be noted that a failure of TCAs may reflect too low a dosage being prescribed, as it has been found that older TCAs are more effective in the 125–150 mg dose range than at lower doses. A subsequent failure with both TCAs and SSRIs may be a reason to consider an MAOI.

It should be noted that many antidepressants have a long half-life and therefore MAOIs should not be started until at least 7–14 days after a tricyclic or related antidepressant is stopped. The following examples are specific recommendations for washout periods prior to initiating MAOIs:

- 2 weeks for paroxetine and sertraline
- 5 weeks for fluoxetine
- 3 weeks for clomipramine or imipramine

When the reverse change is made from an MAOI to an alternative MAOI, SSRI, TCA or related antidepressant, then a washout period of 2 weeks is required (3 weeks for clomipramine or imipramine). For RIMAS, the inhibition is reversible and a delay of only 24 h may therefore be sufficient before initiating an alternative agent.

Bipolar affective disorder

Bipolar depression is characterised by cycling between depression and mania and has a strong hereditary link, although no specific gene(s) has been identified to date. It is less common than unipolar depression, affecting 1 in 100 of the population.

Manic episode

By contrast to the symptoms of depression outlined above, the manic phase of bipolar affective disorder presents as abnormally and persistently elevated expansive or irritable mood. The DSM-IV criteria classify a manic episode when three or more of the following symptoms are significant and present for at least 1 week and/or require hospital admission:

1. inflated self-esteem or grandiosity
2. reduced requirement for sleep
3. rapid speech with pressure to keep talking
4. flight of ideas
5. distractibility
6. increased goal-directed activity or psycho-motor agitation (compare psychomotor retardation in depressive symptoms)
7. reduced inhibitions such as sexual indiscretion and uncontrolled spending

In addition, the criteria state that a diagnosis is made when the above symptoms are sufficient to impair normal occupational and social activities and relationships with others, require hospital treatment to prevent self-harm or harm to others, or psychotic features are present. Again, additional causes such as medication, ECT, light therapy, drug abuse or hyperthyroidism should be excluded.

Hypomania

Hypomania is diagnosed when mood becomes persistently elevated, expansive or irritable compared with normal mood and persistent throughout the day for at least 4 days. The significant presence of three or more of the symptoms listed for a manic episode or four if the mood is irritable may result in a diagnosis of hypomania. Additional requirements are that others observe an uncharacteristic change in mood and functioning. A hypomanic episode differs from mania in that there is minimal effect on social or occupational function, hospital admission is not required and psychotic symptoms are absent. Additional causes such as medication should be excluded, as stated previously.

Rapid cycling

The diagnosis of rapid cycling is made when four episodes of mood disturbance occur, according to the above criteria, during a 12-month period. Partial or full remission occurs for at least 2 months between episodes. Alternatively a switch between a depressive and manic episode may occur.

Treatment

Lithium remains the first-line agent for both acute treatment and prophylaxis of bipolar disorder, although a delay in the onset of action necessitates the concurrent use of neuroleptics (Chapter 26) in acute mania. Lithium is a monovalent cation that mimics the role of sodium ions by permeating fast voltage-sensitive channels responsible for generating action potentials in excitable tissue.

Lithium exerts many effects on neurotransmission and its relatively selective action on the brain and kidney has not been elucidated fully (Williams and Harwood, 2000). The main site of action is the inhibition of recycling by hydrolysis of the intracellular second messenger inositol triphosphate (IP_3) to phosphatidyl inositol (PI) in cell membranes. This reduces the effects of substances which activate receptors (e.g. alpha$_1$-adrenoceptors) linked to IP_3 generation and subsequent Ca^{2+} release from intracellular stores. The extensive distribution of such receptor systems throughout the body suggests many potential effects of lithium. The apparent selectivity has been suggested to result from selective uptake of lithium dependent on sodium channel activity. Other proposed mechanisms of action include inhibition of glycogen synthase kinase-3 (GSK-3), with alterations in gene transcription.

Toxic effects of lithium may result from reduced hormone responses involving the second messenger, cyclic adenosine monophosphate (cAMP). For example, the inhibition of cAMP-mediated antidiuretic hormone (ADH) activity in the kidney results in polyuria and polydipsia. Sodium ions are retained, leading to increased ADH secretion and possible damage of renal tubules. The failure of the thyroid gland to respond to thyroid-stimulating hormone (TSH) may result in an enlarged thyroid gland and hypothyroidism.

Anticonvulsants, e.g. carbamazepine and valproate

Carbamazepine and valproate are used second-line as prophylactic mood stabilisers in bipolar disorder and lack the extrapyramidal effects of the antipsychotic drugs. The mechanism of action has not yet been fully elucidated but is thought to involve effects on ion channels, increasing the release of the inhibitory and excitatory neurotransmitters, gamma-aminobutyric acid (GABA) and glutamate, respectively. The anticonvulsants lamotrigine and gabapentin have an unlicensed role in bipolar affective disorder when other treatments have failed.

Antipsychotics, e.g. haloperidol and chlorpromazine

Antipsychotics such as haloperidol and chlorpromazine may be used to control psychotic symptoms, which may be associated with depression and particularly during the manic phase of bipolar disorder. They have a rapid rate of onset and so may be initiated concurrently with lithium, controlling the manic phase until the lithium begins to exert its effects in patients with bipolar disorder. The blockade of dopamine D_2 receptors is thought to be the predominant mode of action. Haloperidol is often preferred due to reduced sedative and cardiovascular effects compared with chlorpromazine. The atypical antipsychotic olanzapine has been licensed for use in bipolar disorder and is less likely to cause extrapyramidal effects compared with the older agents (Chapter 26).

Thyroid hormones and calcium antagonists (verapamil, nimodipine)

There is weak or limited evidence for the use of calcium channel antagonists and thyroid hormones in the treatment of bipolar disorder. High doses of levothyroxine have been used, however, in refractory cases of bipolar disorder, particularly with rapid cycling, but are not licensed for this purpose. Particular caution is required due to cardiovascular side-effects.

Drug choice in bipolar affective disorder

The acute (manic) phase of bipolar affective disorder is often associated with psychosis and therefore treated with antipsychotics such as haloperidol and/or benzodiazepines such as lorazepam for severe cases. These drugs are used for a few days until the effects of lithium are achieved. Recently, the licence for the atypical antipsychotic olanzapine has been extended to include the treatment of moderate to severe manic episode. However, lithium remains the treatment of choice for both acute and long-term prophylaxis; olanzapine may be added to lithium for patients with residual symptoms. Maintenance treatment is given under specialist supervision according to the risk of withdrawing the drug compared to its benefit. The need for continued treatment is assessed regularly and maintenance is only recommended beyond 3–5 years when the benefit of continuing the drug is apparent, for example, the presence of symptoms during a trial of gradual dose reduction.

Other agents such as the anticonvulsants valproate and carbamazepine may be considered when treatment with lithium has failed. Carbamazepine is indicated for the prophylaxis of manic-depressive psychoses for patients unresponsive to lithium therapy. Valproic acid in the form semisodium valproate is licensed for acute mania whereas sodium valproate remains unlicensed for this use. Carbamazepine may particularly benefit patients with rapid cycling between mania and depression (four or more episodes per year). Both carbamazepine and valproate are currently considered to be second choice for prophylaxis due to an inferior efficacy compared to lithium. The anticonvulsants lamotrigine and gabapentin are unlicensed for bipolar disorder and should only be initiated by specialists. Lamotrigine may be considered for the treatment of the depressive phase of bipolar depression when TCA- or SSRI-induced 'switching' to the manic phase is problematic (Calabrese et al., 1999). Recent guidelines published by the World Federation of Societies of Biological Psychiatry suggest that combining SSRIs (or bupropion) with a mood stabiliser (lithium or lamotrigine) reduces the risk of switching, to a level observed when mood stabilisers are used alone (Grunze et al., 2002). It was noted that lithium might also possess antisuicide properties.

Concurrent conditions: additional considerations when prescribing in affective disorders

Some considerations for choosing a suitable antidepressant are summarised in Table 23.1.

Diabetes mellitus

MAOIs should be used with caution due to an increased risk of hypoglycaemia. Lithium ions may impair glucose tolerance and may cause diabetes mellitus. There is no evidence, however, for loss of glycaemic control of existing diabetes but careful monitoring is recommended. Olanzapine has been associated with hyperglycaemia or exacerbation of pre-existing diabetes mellitus and should be used with caution in these patients. Monitoring of patients with risk factors for type 2 diabetes, particularly obesity, is important when prescribing olanzapine, which may also cause weight gain.

Renal impairment

- Lithium should be avoided in renal impairment. For patients with mild renal impairment, a dose reduction and close monitoring are advised.
- SSRIs should be generally avoided in severe renal impairment. In moderate impairment, dose reduction may be needed.
- The dose of venlafaxine also requires reduction in moderate renal impairment.
- Small doses of antipsychotics are used in severe renal impairment. Lower doses of risperidone or olanzapine may be required.

Liver function

TCAs and MAOIs are contraindicated in severe liver disease. TCAs are preferable to MAOIs but sedative effects are increased. Lofepramine is associated with hepatic toxicity. MAOIs are implicated in the development of idiosyncratic hepatotoxicity. Reduced doses of SSRIs are advised with avoidance in severe liver disease. Antipsychotics can precipitate coma and phenothiazines are hepatotoxic. Atypical antipsychotics such as risperidone and olanzapine may be used at reduced doses (*British National Formulary*, appendix 2).

Pregnancy and breast-feeding

TCAs are preferred if necessary for the treatment of unipolar depression during pregnancy and breast-feeding. This is due to greater experience of their use in pregnancy compared to SSRIs. Fluoxetine is the SSRI of choice in pregnancy if the benefit is judged to exceed risk, although fluoxetine, sertraline and paroxetine may all be associated with withdrawal effects in the infant if prescribed close to the delivery date. Sertraline or paroxetine may be preferred during breast-feeding since lower levels of these drugs are found in breast milk compared with fluoxetine.

Drugs used for bipolar disorders are often associated with abnormalities of the fetus and therefore preconception counselling is important. In view of the teratogenic risk associated with lithium in the first trimester, it is recommended that pregnancy be excluded prior to the initiation of lithium therapy. Ideally, all treatment is withdrawn for at least the first trimester. Alternatively, reducing the dose, particularly of lithium, is considered. For patients taking carbamazepine, folic acid 5 mg supplements are recommended before conception and up to the 12th week of pregnancy (Chapters 3 and 22).

Miscellaneous

Lithium is not recommended for patients with Addison's disease, as disturbances in sodium homeostasis may result. Blood pressure monitoring is recommended if doses of venlafaxine exceed 200 mg/day.

Drug interactions

Drug interactions involving antidepressants may result from: altered drug levels due to effects on drug absorption, metabolism or excretion;

overstimulation of monoamine neurotransmission; an increased risk of cardiac arrhythmias due to prolongation of the QT interval and the risk of convulsions due to a lowering of the convulsive threshold. The following section highlights some examples.

Antidepressant combinations

Coprescribing two or more antidepressants is not recommended due to the risk of toxicity. For example, coprescribing MAOIs, particularly irreversible MAOIs, increases the risk of hypertensive crisis and stroke (see above). Despite this, the combinations of some antidepressants such as MAOIs or SSRIs with TCAs or atypical agents may be beneficial but only under expert supervision. Monitoring for adverse drug reactions is advised with all combinations. Examples of problems requiring particular awareness are given in Table 23.2.

Serotonin syndrome

The Sternbach diagnostic criteria indicate that three or more of the following symptoms should be present before differentiating serotonin syndrome from neuroleptic malignant syndrome (Chapter 5): confusion, hypomania, incoordination, tremor, agitation, diaphoresis (sweating), shivering, fever, myoclonus (muscle spasms) and hyperreflexia (Sternbach, 1991).

Lithium and olanzapine

It should be noted that there is no evidence for an interaction between lithium and olanzapine.

Table 23.3 provides examples of drug interactions involving antidepressants.

Monitoring

Renal function and electrolytes (creatinine and sodium)

Hyponatraemia may occur with high doses of TCAs or SSRIs or in elderly patients, and particularly with coprescribed diuretics, laxatives or with concurrent illness leading to dehydration. The

Table 23.2   Problems associated with the coprescribing of antidepressants

Interacting antidepressants	Consequences	Comments
Fluoxetine with TCAs (amitriptyline, clomipramine, imipramine and nortriptyline) or trazodone	• Increased levels of TCAs • Increased risk of sedation due to trazodone	• Dose adjustment is required during concurrent use • Trazodone and fluoxetine are effective when coprescribed but patients may develop increased side-effects such as sedation • The long half-life of fluoxetine means that this interaction may persist after the drug is stopped
Fluvoxamine with TCAs (amitriptyline, clomipramine, imipramine and trimipramine) or maprotiline	Increased serum levels of the TCA or maprotiline	• Dose adjustment is required to prevent toxicity • There is no evidence for the same interaction with desipramine
Lithium with TCAs or SSRIs	An unpredictable risk of serious effects such as serotonin or neuroleptic malignant syndromes (see text)	Lithium is occasionally used successfully with TCAs or SSRIs but monitoring for ADRs is important
Paroxetine with TCAs (desipramine, imipramine and trimipramine)	Increased serum levels of the TCA	Patients should therefore be monitored closely for ADRs and the dose reduced if necessary

TCAs, tricyclic antidepressants; SSRIs, selective serotonin reuptake inhibitors; ADRs, adverse drug reactions.

CSM warns that hyponatraemia should be considered in patients developing confusion, drowsiness or convulsions whilst taking antidepressants.

Lithium (see Chapter 6)

Urea and electrolytes and full blood count

Baseline measurements of blood urea and electrolytes, serum creatinine, thyroid function, a full blood count and the exclusion of pregnancy are required prior to the initiation of lithium therapy. Concurrent diseases such as cardiac disease are also considered (Table 23.1).

During maintenance therapy, the following monitoring is recommended:

• serum creatinine every 6 months
• thyroid function tests every 6–12 months with counselling to report warning symptoms (4–6 weeks if TSH is elevated)
• a full blood count annually
• serum lithium levels at least 3-monthly (Chapter 6)
• urea and electrolytes every 6 months

Ischaemic heart disease
An electrocardiogram is recommended prior to the initiation of lithium treatment for patients with a history of cardiac problems.

Liver function
Liver function should be assessed before and during the first 6 months of treatment with sodium valproate or valproic acid (Chapter 22). Raised liver enzymes may be transient and a clinical assessment of clinical features and liver function tests (Chapter 2), including prothrombin time, should be continued until the levels return to normal. Risk factors include children less than 3 years of age, metabolic or degenerative disease, organic brain disease or severe seizures with mental retardation.

Blood counts
Patients taking mianserin should have blood counts checked every 4 weeks for the first 3 months of treatment. Blood monitoring should be performed for patients taking mianserin or carbamazepine who develop fever, sore throat,

Table 23.3 Examples of drug interactions involving antidepressants

Drug	Consequences	Comments
Antidepressants with alcohol	• Increased side-effects such as drowsiness and reduced alertness • Increased risk of accidents when driving or operating machinery	• Possible antagonism of antidepressant effect with chronic alcohol intake • Temporary mood-enhancing effect may contribute to a vicious cycle of alcohol abuse
Induction of hepatic enzymes: carbamazepine with haloperidol, oral contraceptives or phenytoin	Reduced effects of the latter	• Increased doses may be required
SSRI-mediated inhibition of hepatic enzymes: fluvoxamine with theophylline	• Risk of a rapid and potentially toxic increase in theophylline levels	• The CSM warns that this should be avoided (CSM/MCA, 1994) • Alternatively, the theophylline dose should be reduced to about half • Limited evidence suggests that a similar interaction does not occur between fluoxetine and theophylline
Fluoxetine, fluvoxamine, sertraline and paroxetine **with** anticoagulants, MAOIs, alcohol, selegiline, antipsychotics, lithium, phenytoin, carbamazepine and omeprazole	• Increased effects	• Evidence suggests that the SSRI citalopram does not interact with warfarin • Note that SSRIs differ in their profile of cytochrome P450 inhibition
Lithium levels increased: ACE inhibitors, diuretics (particularly thiazides) and analgesics	• Reduced excretion of lithium	• Consider impairment of renal function as a risk factor • Monitoring is required with a possible reduction in lithium dose • Aspirin and paracetamol are considered safe to use with lithium
Lithium with theophylline or metronidazole	• Increased plasma concentrations of lithium	• Close monitoring is required
Lithium levels reduced: Lithium with ispaghula husk	Serum levels of lithium may be reduced	• Monitoring with appropriate dose adjustment is recommended • The mechanism involved may be due in part to the sodium content of effervescent granules
Lithium with methyldopa or clonazepam	Enhanced neurotoxicity	Avoid concurrent use
Lithium with haloperidol	Risk of rare but serious neurotoxic reaction, particularly in patients with a history of extrapyramidal effects with antipsychotics or if high doses of haloperidol are used	• Symptoms include fever, tremor, confusion, and extrapyramidal effects • Patients should be monitored closely for ADRs, with prompt withdrawal due to a risk of brain damage • The coprescribing of haloperidol with lithium in acute mania is extremely beneficial

Continued

Table 23.3   Continued

Drug	Consequences	Comments
Lithium with baclofen	Increased risk of baclofen-induced hyperkinetic activity	Patients should be monitored closely
MAOIs with pethidine	Risk of a potentially life-threatening reaction	Pethidine should not be given with MAOIs unless a lack of sensitivity is confirmed
Paroxetine or sertraline with tramadol	The combination of two or more serotonergic drugs may lead to a potentially fatal condition resulting from overstimulation of 5-HT receptors	Monitoring for symptoms of serotonin syndrome is advised (see text)
SSRIs or MAOIs with 5-HT agonists (sumatriptan)	Risk of serotonin syndrome (see text)	Avoid concurrent use
SSRIs with NSAIDs	Increased risk of GI bleed	Consider additional risk factors and possible GI protection, for example using a proton pump inhibitor (Chapter 7)
TCAs and some atypical antidepressants (venlafaxine) **with** other drugs known to prolong the QT interval (Table 5.4)	QT interval prolongation and risk of potentially fatal arrhythmias	• The CSM warns against the use of more than one drug known to prolong the QT interval • If concurrent use is unavoidable, patients should report irregular heart beat, palpitations and dizziness immediately
TCAs or SSRIs with other drugs which lower the convulsive threshold (Table 5.9)	Increased risk of convulsions	The CSM advises caution with drugs known to lower the convulsive threshold

SSRI, selective serotonin reuptake inhibitor; CSM, Committee on Safety of Medicines; MCA, Medicines Control Agency; MAOIs, monoamine oxidase inhibitors; ACE, angiotensin-converting enzyme; 5-HT, 5-hydroxytryptamine; ADRs, adverse drug reactions; NSAIDs, non-steroidal anti-inflammatory drugs; GI, gastrointestinal; TCAs, tricyclic antidepressants.

stomatitis or other signs of infection. Mirtazapine treatment warrants blood counts and immediate cessation of treatment if blood dyscrasias are suspected.

Withdrawal

Once a patient has been in remission, withdrawal of the antidepressant should be considered after a sufficient period of sustained remission. Withdrawal may precipitate a reaction (e.g. depression, sensory and balance problems, mood changes and gastrointestinal disturbances) in any patient (particularly with paroxetine) and should involve a dose reduction over at least 4 weeks or up to 6 months in patients who have been on long-term maintenance therapy. Abrupt withdrawal of lithium should be avoided as this may increase the frequency of manic episodes and shorten the time to relapse.

Over-the-counter considerations

An important role of the pharmacist is to recognise and refer patients with symptoms of depression, advise patients about drug interactions associated with antidepressant medication and provide advice and reassurance relating to side-effects and the need for prolonged treatment. Table 23.4 highlights important issues and drug interactions associated with antidepressants and over-the-counter (OTC) prescribing.

Alcohol

TCAs, fluvoxamine, isoniazid, maprotiline, mianserin and trazodone may enhance the effects of alcohol. In patients who are taking MAOIs, the hypotensive effects may be enhanced by alcohol and the tyramine content of certain beers and red wines should also be considered. It should also be noted that alcohol misuse may be related to depression. The central nervous system (CNS)-depressant effect of alcohol may cause or exacerbate depression, with the temporary mood-enhancing properties contributing to a 'vicious circle'.

Caffeine

Lithium levels may be reduced by excess caffeine intake. Levels may increase following abrupt withdrawal of caffeine intake (e.g. Pro Plus and some analgesic preparations). The effects of caffeine may also be deleterious in depression associated with anxiety (Chapter 24).

Dietary supplements

Requests for advice regarding dietary supplements should as always be used as an opportunity to recommend a healthy diet (Chapter 3), particularly including oily fish and foods rich in folic acid. Patients may request supplements such as dehydroepiandrosterone (DHEA), fish oils (particularly rich in the omega-3 fatty acids eicosapentaenoic acid (EPA) and docosahexanoic acid (DHA)), folic acid, phosphatidylserine or *S*-adenosylmethionine. Preliminary observations are interesting. For example, patients with depression have been shown to have low levels of fish

Table 23.4 Antidepressants and over-the-counter (OTC) prescribing

OTC medicines	Comments
Sedative antihistamines such as diphenhydramine, promethazine are licensed for the treatment of insomnia	• Use is limited to 2 weeks. Repeated requests may point to depression • They should not be used concomitantly with TCAs due to enhanced antimuscarinic effects and sedation
Indirectly acting sympathomimetic decongestants (phenylpropanolamine, pseudoephedrine, ephedrine)	• The action of indirectly acting sympathomimetics is likely to be blocked by TCAs • There is, however, limited evidence for this interaction (Chapter 18) • Avoid with MAOIs (Chapter 18)
Directly acting sympathomimetic decongestants (phenylephrine)	These should not be taken by patients prescribed MAOIs or within 14 days of cessation of MAOIs as there is a substantial risk of enhanced pressor activity (i.e. increased blood pressure) (Chapter 18)
Antacids and sodium-containing preparations (cystitis and effervescent products)	These should be avoided with lithium
Cough preparations containing dextromethorphan	A rare but serious interaction (serotonin syndrome) with paroxetine contraindicates concurrent use
Fybogel	May reduce lithium levels
Cimetidine	This inhibits the metabolism of amitriptyline, doxepin, imipramine, moclobemide, nortriptyline, sertraline Use ranitidine as an alternative
NSAIDs	Ibuprofen increases plasma concentrations of lithium. Aspirin or paracetamol are appropriate alternatives

TCAs, tricyclic antidepressants; MAOIs, monoamine oxidase inhibitors; NSAIDs, non-steroidal anti-inflammatory drugs.

oils and folic acid but it is not clear if this is a cause or effect of depression.

Preliminary finding of pharmacological activity associated with the supplements phosphatidyl-serine and S-adenosylmethionine may also warrant further investigation. For example, phosphatidylserine, the most abundant phospholipid in the brain, may interfere with the hypothalamic–pituitary–adrenal axis (HPA), a potential target for the development of new treatments (see below). S-adenosylmethionine may increase dopamine in the brain and preliminary evidence demonstrates antidepressant activity. The supplement choline has been suggested to improve symptoms of mania by increasing the production of acetylcholine, for which it is a precursor, in the brain. There is insufficient evidence to recommend these products to patients, particularly in combination with conventional antidepressants, but healthcare professionals should be aware that patients may be taking them.

Herbal medicines

Herbal medicines should be used with caution due to the lack of safety data available regarding combinations with conventional medicines. St John's wort has been shown to be better than placebo as an antidepressant for the short-term treatment of mild to moderate depression but is associated with significant side-effects and interactions (Chapters 4 and 5). It has been shown to be ineffective in major depression (Shelton *et al.*, 2001). In the context of depression, it inhibits the reuptake of 5-HT, and may potentiate the action of SSRIs, and so should not be used with conventional antidepressants. A Cochrane systematic review concluded that there is insufficient evidence that St John's wort is more effective than other antidepressants (Linde and Mulrow, 2002).

Herbal drugs with sympathomimetic activity (Chapter 4) should not be used with MAOIs and possibly TCAs. Many herbs possess sedative properties (Chapter 4) and may therefore increase side-effects, particularly with TCAs and benzodiazepines. The CNS-depressant effect of these herbs may also oppose the effect of antidepressants. Herbs containing tryptophan (alfalfa, chaparral, fenugreek, ginkgo and plantain) should also be avoided.

General counselling

General counselling points might include:

- To ensure continued treatment, according to the advice of the prescriber, for 6–12 months after recovery to prevent relapse. The analogy between a broken bone healing while in plaster is a useful explanation for the need to continue treatment even when well.
- Not to stop taking medication suddenly or without the advice of the prescriber, but reassure that antidepressants are not addictive.
- Be prepared for a delayed effect of 2–4 weeks and a possible worsening of symptoms in the first week. Sleep improvement may be an early beneficial effect in those receiving sedative TCAs for this purpose.
- The side-effects of antidepressants, particularly nausea, should subside after the first week.
- Patients taking any antidepressant should be cautious when driving due to the risk of drowsiness and impaired reaction times.
- The return of insomnia may provide the first signs of relapse, particularly in bipolar disorder. Patients should be taught to recognise and report early-warning symptoms. Short-term treatment with hypnotics may be appropriate. The maximum benefit of antidepressants is obtained when symptoms are recognised early.
- Women should be advised about adequate contraception and to discuss the issues of antidepressant treatment before planning a pregnancy. This enables the prescriber and patient to discuss the risk versus benefit of antidepressant treatment during pregnancy, the possibility of a trial without treatment or changing to an alternative drug associated with lower risk. This is particularly important for women taking lithium salts.
- In view of the stigma still associated with depression, it may help to reassure patients that depression is common.
- Lifestyle changes such as increasing exercise and reducing alcohol and/or caffeine intake may be beneficial.

- Counselling may help the patient to make appropriate lifestyle changes when possible to prevent recurrence. It may also be useful to explain the importance of the duration of symptoms, comparing depression to normal 'low mood'. It may help to eliminate fear of relapse if the patient is reminded that experiencing occasional low mood is normal.

SSRIs

- Side-effects include gastrointestinal disturbances (nausea, abdominal pain, diarrhoea, constipation, indigestion), postural hypotension, palpitations, increased sweating and sexual dysfunction (impotence, delay or failure of orgasm). There is an increased risk of extrapyramidal effects with paroxetine.
- Sexual dysfunction is a common cause of non-compliance with SSRIs, affecting up to 60% of patients. Sensitive counselling is therefore important when treatment is initiated.
- Reaction times may be impaired and patients should therefore be cautious, particularly when driving.
- Report any rash, particularly with fluoxetine, as treatment may need to be stopped.
- Treatment should not usually be stopped abruptly, particularly paroxetine, as withdrawal symptoms may occur. Patients should be advised to continue their treatment according to the advice of the prescriber, even when feeling better. This prevents the risk of relapse on cessation of treatment, which is withdrawn gradually over at least 4 weeks, or slower if withdrawal symptoms occur.

Tricyclic antidepressants

- TCAs may cause drowsiness and therefore advise caution if driving (less with imipramine and lofepramine). Drowsiness may be enhanced by alcohol.
- The dose should be taken at night if sedation is required and also to limit daytime sedation.
- Side-effects of TCAs include dry mouth, blurred vision and constipation. Initial sedation, confusion and motor incoordination should improve after 1–2 weeks of treatment.
- Patients presenting with signs of infection, such as a sore throat, whilst taking imipramine should be referred for a full blood count.

Newer antidepressants

- Trazodone, nefazodone, reboxetine and venlafaxine may cause drowsiness and therefore patients should be advised to exercise caution if driving. Drowsiness may be increased by alcohol.
- Patients taking venlafaxine should report any rashes, urticaria or related allergic reactions.

MAOIs

- These may cause drowsiness and therefore advise caution if driving. Drowsiness may be increased by alcohol.
- Patients should avoid tyramine-containing food such as cheese, red wine, yeast extracts (e.g. Marmite), chicken and beef liver, salami, soy sauce and avocado. Only fresh food should be eaten and stale food avoided.
- A warning card should be given.
- Side-effects of MAOIs include overexcitement, insomnia, weight gain, dry mouth, blurred vision, constipation and postural hypotension (increased by alcohol). An early warning of food interactions may be a throbbing headache indicating a rapid increase in blood pressure.

Others (mianserin, mirtazapine, flupentixol)

- Patients taking mianserin or mirtazapine should report signs of infection such as fever or sore throat.
- Flupentixol may cause drowsiness but can also be alerting and therefore should not be taken in the evening.

Lithium

- Patients should maintain adequate fluid intake and avoid dietary changes leading to a change in sodium intake (including use of salt substitute) or the sudden introduction or discontinuation of caffeine (Table 23.3).
- Alcohol intake should not exceed the recommended limits (Chapter 3 and Table 23.3).

- A treatment card is available for patients from the National Pharmaceutical Association (www.npa.co.uk).
- Preparations may vary widely in bioavailability. Monitoring may be required if patients change brand.
- Symptoms of drowsiness are usually transient.
- Signs of toxicity, including nausea, vomiting, tremor, lack of coordination, extreme thirst, diarrhoea and excessive urination, should be reported urgently.
- Symptoms of hypothyroidism should prompt referral. These include lethargy, feeling cold and weight gain.
- Fluid loss due to diarrhoea, vomiting and intercurrent infection (particularly with profuse sweating) may necessitate discontinuation of treatment. The prescriber should be contacted.
- Patients should not take ibuprofen.
- Inform patients of the importance of regular blood tests and the need to leave 12 h after the last dose (Chapter 6).
- Patients should inform health professionals that they take lithium.

Antipsychotics

- See Chapter 26.

Anticonvulsants

- See Chapter 22.

Benzodiazepines

- For short-term use only (see also Chapter 25)

Future developments

The search continues for agents with a more rapid onset of action, fewer adverse effects and efficacy in all patients, including those with resistant depression. Products in current development target various permutations of SSRI activity, 5-HT_{1A} receptors, subtypes of 5-HT_{2A} receptors, noradrenaline receptors, neuronal sodium channels, the excitatory amino acid glutamate and/or the inhibitory neurotransmitter GABA, including anticonvulsants such as lamotrigine and gabapentin.

The targeting of three receptor types by single molecules – so-called 'triple action' agents – are also being investigated, for example, combined 5-HT, noradrenaline and dopamine activity. The neuropeptide substance P and at least 40 related peptides are also under investigation since these peptides act at specific receptors in areas of the brain associated with the stress response and containing serotonin- and noradrenaline-containing neurons. For example, neurokinin (NK_1) receptor antagonists are currently being developed. Hormone-based approaches may target the HPA and activity at receptors for corticotrophin-releasing factor (CRF). The role of brain-derived growth factors and the immune system are additional targets for the future.

Practice points

- Be alert for signs of depression in patients as stigma may still prevent patients from volunteering symptoms. Depression remains underdiagnosed in primary care, and undiagnosed or undertreated depression is a significant cause of suicide. Pharmacists may identify patients requesting OTC hypnotics or herbal preparations for stress.
- Close monitoring for signs of suicide is important during early treatment with all antidepressants. Consider also the danger of TCAs when taken in overdose.
- In patients who are at risk of suicide, only small quantities of drugs should be supplied.
- Compliance with treatment may be improved by warning patients of side-effects and worsening of symptoms in the first week of treatment, together with the delayed onset of action.
- In treatment failure, consider compliance and encourage the patient to report troublesome side-effects.
- Avoid abrupt withdrawal of antidepressant treatment.

→

Practice points (continued)

- The majority of MAOIs inhibit MAO irreversibly, and therefore the potential for drug interactions may persist for 2–3 weeks after the cessation of treatment. The SSRI fluoxetine also possesses a long half-life.
- Adequate doses, particularly of older TCAs, should be used to obtain a therapeutic effect.
- The National Service Framework currently advises that TCAs should not be prescribed to people aged over 70 years because of the increased risk of adverse drug reactions in this age group.
- CBT has been shown to be as effective as antidepressants in mild depression and in combination with antidepressants for moderate depression. Beneficial effects include improved compliance and reduced exposure to stress.
- Regular use of propranolol for anxiety associated with depression may worsen depression. SSRIs should be considered (Chapter 24).
- Be alert for the use of alcohol for temporary mood elevation, leading to a worsening of symptoms and risk of alcohol misuse.
- The CSM warns that hyponatraemia should be considered in patients developing confusion, drowsiness or convulsions whilst taking antidepressants.
- Prescriptions for lithium should be written using the brand name.
- It may be useful to repeat patient counselling at least annually during long-term treatment, particularly with lithium, and check that the patient retains the appropriate warning card.

 CASE STUDIES

Case 1
A female patient complains to her pharmacist of anxiety, dizziness, tremor and headache and asks to sit down. She asks if it could be due to stopping her antidepressant treatment. She has been prescribed paroxetine 20 mg daily.

How do you reply?

- Patients taking all antidepressants, but particularly paroxetine, may experience a withdrawal syndrome if treatment is stopped suddenly. The patient should be advised to take a paroxetine tablet as soon as possible and return to her general practitioner (GP) for a discussion about her treatment. You could enquire about the duration of treatment and, if appropriate, reinforce the importance of continuing to take the tablets following remission. Antidepressants should be withdrawn gradually over at least 4 weeks and up to 6 months after long-term maintenance therapy.

Case 2
A female patient requests Nytol tablets for insomnia. Her patient medication record reveals she takes diazepam 2 mg p.r.n. She admits to feeling awful due to a hangover and has been feeling depressed for the last few weeks.

Do you sell the Nytol?

- No! She may be suffering from depression and should be referred to her GP for assessment as she may require an antidepressant. Depression may be exacerbated by benzodiazepine treatment. If appropriate, you could educate her regarding the risk of dependence with benzodiazepines.

continued

CASE STUDIES (continued)

- You could advise her that alcohol causes insomnia and depression and recommend that she should discuss this with her GP.
- She may have depression associated with anxiety, for which an SSRI may be appropriate (Chapter 24).
- An additive effect of Nytol with benzodiazepines (and alcohol) may cause increased drowsiness.

Case 3
A 24-year-old male patient presents a prescription for fluoxetine 20 mg daily and trazodone capsules 100 mg per day.

Are you happy to dispense this prescription?

- Yes. An interaction between the two drugs may result in elevated plasma concentrations of the trazodone, but concurrent use may be beneficial.
- Coprescribing antidepressants is not recommended, but in this case a specialist had prescribed the combination. Advise the patient to report side-effects and particularly excessive sedation.

Case 4
A National Health Service FP10 prescription is presented for fluoxetine liquid 20 mg/5 mL 20 mL/day for postnatal depression. The drug was originally prescribed by the hospital.

Are you happy to dispense the prescription?

- No. The dose is greater than the maximum daily dose for fluoxetine. This prescription should have been for paroxetine 10 mg/5 mL.

Case 5
A patient presents with a prescription for Epipen (adrenaline (epinephrine) injection). You see from his PMR that he is also prescribed lofepramine.

Do you dispense the prescription?

- Interaction between adrenaline and lofepramine may lead to a life-threatening hypertensive crisis.
- If adrenaline is required then an SSRI would be a more appropriate antidepressant.

Case 6
A 55-year-old man known to you for poor compliance with lithium for his bipolar affective disorder complains of tremor. He has difficulty signing his name. He is also taking amitriptyline and tells you he only needs this. He's going to stop his lithium because of the tremor.

What advice should this patient receive?

- Poor compliance is common in patients with bipolar affective disorder as they may fail to recognise their symptoms as abnormal. It is imperative that the patient is encouraged to continue with his lithium.

What is the most likely cause of his tremor?

- Lithium and amitriptyline may interact, causing tremor. The patient should be referred to his GP. The combination of lithium and TCAs can be beneficial but also produces serious and unpredictable problems such as convulsions, serotonin syndrome and neuroleptic malignant syndrome. Patients should be monitored closely. Tremor is a side-effect of lithium and severe tremor may also be a sign of lithium toxicity.

References

American Psychiatric Association (1995). *Diagnostic and Statistical Manual of Mental Disorders* (DSM-IV), 4th edn. Washington, DC: American Psychiatric Press.

Anderson I M, Nutt D J, Deakin J F W (2000). Evidence-based guidelines for treating depressive disorders with antidepressants. *J Psychopharmacol* 14: 3–20.

Barbui C, Hotopf M (2001). Amitriptyline v. the rest: still the leading antidepressant after 40 years of randomised controlled trials. *Br J Psychiatry* 178: 129–144.

Buckley N A, McManus P R (2002). Fatal toxicity of serotoninergic and other antidepressant drugs: analysis of United Kingdom mortality data. *BMJ* 325: 1332–1333.

Calabrese J R, Bowden C L, Sachs G S *et al.* (1999) A double-blind placebo-controlled study of lamotrigine monotherapy in outpatients with bipolar I depression. Lamitcal 602 Study Group. *J Clin Psychiatry* 60: 79–88.

Committee on Safety of Medicines/Medicines Control Agency (1994). *Curr Probl Pharmacovigilance* 20: 12.

Glassman A H, O'Connor C M, Califf R M *et al.* (2002). Sertraline treatment of major depression in patients with acute MI or unstable angina. *JAMA* 288: 701–709.

Greenberger D, Padesky C A (1995). *Mind Over Mood.* New York: Guilford Press.

Grunze H, Kasper S, Goodwin G *et al.* (2002). World Federation of Societies of Biological Psychiatry (WFSBP) guidelines for biological treatment of bipolar disorders, part 1: Treatment of bipolar depression. *World J Biol Psychiatry* 3: 115–124.

Knodel L C, Ley E, Wanke L A *et al.* (1998). Comparative incidence of seizures from antidepressants. *Drug Consults* from Micromedex Healthcare series 12/98.

Kupfer D J, Frank E, Perel J M *et al.* (1992). Five-year outcome for maintenance therapies in recurrent depression. *Arch Gen Psychiatry* 49: 769–773.

Levitt A J, Lam R W, Levitan R (2002). A comparison of open treatment of seasonal major and minor depression with light therapy. *J Affective Disord* 71: 243–248.

Linde K, Mulrow C D (2002). St. John's wort for depression. *Cochrane Systematic Reviews* issue 3. Oxford: Update Software.

Mehta D K (ed.) *British National Formulary*, latest edition. London: British Medical Association and Royal Pharmaceutical Society of Great Britain.

Scott C, Tacchi M, Jones R *et al.* (1997). Acute and one-year outcome of a randomised controlled trial of brief cognitive therapy for major depressive disorder in primary care. *Br J Psychiatry* 171: 289–292.

Shelton R C, Keller M B, Gelenberg A *et al.* (2001). Effectiveness of St John's wort in major depression. *JAMA* 285: 1978–1986.

Sternbach H (1991). The serotonin syndrome. *Am J Psychiatry* 148: 705–713.

Williams R S B, Harwood A J (2000). Lithium therapy and signal transduction. *Trends Pharmacol Sci* 21: 61–64.

World Health Organization (1992). *The International Statistical Classification of Diseases and Related Health Problems* (ICD-10), 10th revision. Geneva: WHO.

Further reading

Anderson I M (2000). Selective serotonin reuptake inhibitors versus tricyclic antidepressants: a meta-analysis of efficacy and tolerability. *J Affect Disord* 58: 19–36.

Anon (2000). The drug treatment of depression in primary care. *MeReC Bull* 11: 33–36.

Anon (2002). Specific issues in depression. *MeReC Briefing* 17: 1–5.

Fraser K, Martin M, Hunter R, Hudson S (2001a). Mood disorders: drug treatment of depression. *Pharm J* 266: 433–442.

Fraser K, Martin M, Hunter R, Hudson S (2001b). Mood disorders: implications for primary care. *Pharm J* 266: 259–262.

Fraser K, Martin M, Hunter R, Hudson S (2001c). Mood disorders: bipolar conditions. *Pharm J* 266: 824–832.

Gaster B, Holroyd J (2000). St. John's wort for depression. A systematic review. *Arch Intern Med* 160: 152–156.

Hazell P (2002). Depression in children. *BMJ* 325: 229–230.

Hirschfield R M, Keller M B, Panico S *et al.* (1997). The National Depressive and Manic-Depressive Association consensus statement on the undertreatment of depression. *JAMA* 277: 333–340.

Lawlor D A, Hopker S W (2001). The effectiveness of exercise as an intervention in the management of depression: systematic review and meta-regression analysis of randomised controlled trials. *BMJ* 322: 763.

Macritchie K A N, Geddes J R, Scott J *et al.* (2002). Valproic acid, valproate and divalproex in the maintenance treatment of bipolar disorder. *Cochrane Systematic Review* issue 3: Oxford: Update Software.

Müller-Oerlinghausen B, Berghöfer A, Bauer M (2002). Bipolar disorder. *Lancet* 359: 241–247.

Perry A, Tarrier N, Morriss R *et al.* (1999). Randomised controlled trial of efficacy of teaching patients with bipolar disorder to identify early symptoms of relapse and obtain treatment. *BMJ* 318: 149–153.

Van Walraven C, Mamdani M M, Wells P S *et al.* (2001). Inhibition of serotonin re-uptake by antidepressants and upper gastrointestinal bleeding in elderly patients: retrospective cohort study. *BMJ* 323: 655–661.

Online resources

www.apni.org is the website for the Association for Post Natal Illness (accessed 4 December 2002).

www.doh.gov.uk/nsf/ is the website containing the National Service Frameworks (accessed 4 December 2002).

www.mind.org.uk is the website for the mental health charity, MIND (accessed 4 December 2002).

www.rcpsych.ac.uk is the website of the Royal College of Psychiatrists (accessed 4 December 2002)

www.sada.org.uk is the website for the Seasonal Affective Disorders Association (accessed 4 December 2002).

www.sane.org.uk is the website of the mental health charity, SANE (accessed 4 December 2002).

www.torsades.org is the website providing an updated list of drugs causing QT interval prolongation (accessed 4 December 2002).

24

Anxiety disorders

Anxiety is a disabling condition, often associated with depression. It is more common in women and displays a peak onset in the early 20s. The term 'anxiety' is applied to a disproportionate response to fearful triggers such as flying and many social situations and encompasses panic, phobic, obsessive-compulsive and general anxiety disorders. There is a significant impact on quality of life and personal achievement and, in extreme cases, patients are unable to leave their home. There is a hereditary component of vulnerability to anxiety, which may be triggered by adverse life events. There is also a link to certain personality traits and anxiety experienced in childhood. Drug-induced causes include:

- caffeine
- initial treatment with selective serotonin re-uptake inhibitors (SSRIs)
- sympathomimetics
- nicotine
- overuse of beta-adrenoceptor agonists, alcohol, amphetamines, cocaine

- withdrawal from alcohol, amphetamines, cocaine, benzodiazepines or antidepressants

Disease characteristics

Before considering the characteristics of anxiety, terms in common use are defined:

- Fear – an emotional reaction to danger accompanied by physiological (mainly autonomic) and behavioural changes such as avoidance of fear-producing situations. Short-term fear such as fear of flying may be managed by single doses of benzodiazepines such as diazepam.
- Anxiety – generalised and often pathological fear, which may be unpredictable and often uncontrollable. It differs from fear in that there is not always an identifiable trigger.
- Phobia – a disabling or pathological fear of an object or situation such as social phobia or arachnophobia (a fear of spiders or arachnids).

Underlying pathology

Anxiety is considered to be pathological when a persistent or distressing response is triggered by non-threatening events and causes significant impairment of normal social or occupational functioning. The underlying pathology remains to be elucidated fully but is thought to involve disrupted serotonergic, glutamatergic, GABAergic and noradrenergic systems together with the involvement of corticotrophin-releasing factor, particularly in the complex interactions of the limbic system, a group of brain regions involved in the physiology of emotion.

Clinical features

Patients present with heightened autonomic symptoms including palpitations, tachycardia, difficulty breathing, dizziness, sweating, tremor, facial flushing and general feelings of panic. Patients may occasionally appear pale. There may also be profound fear of experiencing a heart attack or severe asthma attack. These symptoms may be caused or exacerbated by a number of other medical conditions. The diagnosis may therefore involve ruling out conditions such as asthma, heart disease, hyperthyroidism, vestibular disorders, menopause, hypoglycaemia, epilepsy and phaeochromocytoma (vascular tumour of the adrenal gland). Questioning patients about the frequency and nature of attacks, together with the presence of any fear or phobias, may point to a diagnosis of anxiety. Symptoms of depression may also be present and may form the primary diagnosis (Chapter 23).

Classification

The classification of anxiety disorders is defined in the *Diagnostic and Statistical Manual of Mental Disorders* (DSM-IV: American Psychiatric Association, 1995) and the *International Statistical Classification of Diseases and Related Health Problems* (ICD-10: World Health Organization, 1992). The following section considers the DSM-IV criteria of more common disorders presented to health professionals. These include panic attacks, phobias, obsessive-compulsive disorder (OCD) and general anxiety disorder (GAD). When considering the symptoms suggestive of these disorders, additional causes such as drug abuse, medication or medical conditions including hyperthyroidism are investigated and first excluded. In addition, since the symptoms of mental disorders often overlap, the criteria for similar disorders are considered before confirming a diagnosis. For example, patients presenting with anxiety may fulfil the criteria for major depression, with the latter being diagnosed and treated. For further detail and discussion, the reader is referred to the DSM-IV manual.

General anxiety disorder

GAD differs from panic disorder, phobias and OCD in that it is persistent rather than short-lived and tends not to demonstrate situation-specific triggers. It may occasionally remain following unsuccessful treatment of panic or depressive disorders. Symptoms include a more general description of feeling 'on edge', irritable and tense most of the time. Diagnosis of GAD is made in the presence of the following symptoms:

- excessive anxiety and worry for more than 6 months and occurring on most days
- the patient cannot easily control the worry
- three or more of the following are present for more than 6 months and occur most days:
  - restless or 'on edge'
  - easily fatigued
  - difficult concentrating
  - irritability
  - muscle tension
  - sleep disturbance

Panic disorder

Panic attacks

Panic attacks commonly develop from phobic or hypochondriac symptoms and may progress to agoraphobia. A panic attack is defined by an intense period of fear with four or more of the following symptoms present, having developed abruptly and reaching a peak within 10 min:

- palpitations and/or increased heart rate
- sweating

- tremor
- shortness of breath or sensation of smothering
- choking feeling
- chest pain or discomfort
- nausea or abdominal symptoms
- dizzy or faint feeling
- feeling of depersonalisation or unreality
- fear of losing control
- fear of dying
- paraesthesia ('pins and needles')
- chills or hot flushes

A diagnosis of panic disorder is made when patients suffer recurrent panic attacks according to the following DSM-IV classification:

1. recurrent panic attacks, some of which may occur spontaneously. These may be unpredictable and often unrelated to specific situations
2. at least one of the attacks has been followed by 1 month or more of at least one of the following:
   - worry about future attacks
   - worry about the consequences of an attack such as losing control, suffering an asthmatic or heart attack
   - a significant change in behaviour due to the attack such as avoidance behaviour

Agoraphobia

Agoraphobia is indicated by anxiety associated with places or situations and a fear of embarrassment or that it is difficult to escape or that help is not available. These include being alone outside the home, in a crowd, standing in a line, on a bridge and travelling by bus, train or car. Avoidance behaviour or severe distress occurs in relation to these triggers. Social or specific phobias are considered if avoidance behaviour relates to a limited number of situations such as social situations.

Specific phobias

The sufferer describes excessive fear occurring in response to an object or situation such as flying, animals, heights or the sight of blood. Exposure to the trigger often produces anxiety symptoms and may fulfil the criteria for a panic attack.

Avoidance behaviour may be present. Normal social and occupational functioning is adversely affected as a result of the phobia. Again, diagnosis is made following the exclusion of other mental disorders, disease- or drug-related causes.

Children

Symptoms in children may present as tantrums, crying, freezing or clinging, particularly described as a variant of normal behaviour. The duration of specific phobias is at least 6 months for those aged under 18 years.

Social phobia

Social phobia is diagnosed in the presence of symptoms described for specific phobias. However, the trigger relates to social situations or performance, during which sufferers worry that they will be humiliated or embarrassed.

Children

Social phobia is identified following an assessment of age-related social relationships with familiar people and the anxiety must occur during interaction with peers and not just with adults. Symptoms are the same as for specific phobias but with a social trigger.

Obsessive-compulsive disorder

OCD comprises a continuous and difficult-to-control preoccupation with an object, activity or recurrent thoughts. With the exception of children, the patient tends to be aware that the behaviour is unnecessary or unreasonable. Again, a diagnosis is also dependent on the duration (e.g. more than 1 h/day) and/or the impact on the patient's quality of life. The diagnosis of OCD is made in the presence of obsessions or compulsions as follows:

Obsessions
- the presence of inappropriate recurrent and persistent thoughts, impulses or images causing distress or anxiety
- the above cannot be explained as excessive worries triggered by adverse life events
- patients attempt to ignore or substitute the thoughts, impulses or images and recognise them as produced by their own mind

Compulsions

- The patient feels driven to repetitive behaviour such as hand washing, checking that a door is locked, counting or praying. This occurs in response to an obsession or strict rules, for example, not stepping on the cracks in the pavement.
- The behaviour is intended to prevent the occurrence of an adverse situation such as injury but is not a realistic method of avoiding such occurrences, for example, believing that avoiding the cracks in the pavement will prevent a serious illness.

Posttraumatic stress disorder

This involves a reaction to a traumatic event which carries the threat of death or serious injury to the patient or other. There is also a significant level of continued experience in dreams, as 'flashbacks' or feelings associated with the incident are triggered by stimuli reminiscent of the scene. For example, getting into a car may trigger the distress of a previous car accident. Avoidance behaviour may also be present. Additional symptoms not present prior to the event and with a duration of at least 1 month include two or more of:

- insomnia
- irritability or outbursts of anger
- poor concentration
- increased vigilance
- exaggerated response to non-threatening stimuli

Children

The effect of posttraumatic stress in children may present as agitated or disorganised behaviour. The event may be revisited through play or in dreams.

Acute stress disorder

The presentation of acute stress disorder is similar to that for posttraumatic stress disorder but with the exception that the duration is at least 2 days but not more than 4 weeks. Acute stress disorder occurs within 4 weeks of the traumatic event and three or more symptoms of dissociation are present in a positive diagnosis:

- numbness, detachment or lack of an emotional response
- reduced awareness of surroundings or being 'in a daze'
- the situation does not feel real to the patient (derealisation)
- the patient feels 'unreal', as in depersonalisation
- the patient has incomplete recollection of important aspects of the event (dissociative amnesia)

Goals of treatment

Treatment is initiated when symptoms meet the criteria detailed above together with a significant impairment of social and/or occupational functioning and relationships with others. The goals of treatment are to alleviate the symptoms of panic and anxiety, improve the quality of life and prevent relapse and recurrence. Initially, this may include identifying and dealing with causes such as associated depression and substance abuse.

Pharmacological management

Drugs such as benzodiazepines or beta-blockers may offer symptomatic relief though the use of the former is limited due to the risk of tolerance and dependence (Chapter 25). The use of antidepressants with behavioural therapy combined with lifestyle advice, including the importance of regular exercise and the avoidance of drugs causing anxiety such as caffeine, may improve the long-term outcome.

It should be noted that anxiolytics and particularly benzodiazepines were previously described as 'minor tranquillisers', in an attempt to differentiate these drugs from antipsychotics or 'major tranquillisers'. These terms are inaccurate and therefore no longer used.

Beta-adrenoceptor antagonists (propranolol)

Propranolol is the most commonly used beta-blocker for treating the physical symptoms of anxiety associated with the affects of adrenaline (epinephrine)-mediated activation of beta-adrenoceptors. These include palpitations, tremor and tachycardia.

Benzodiazepines

See Chapter 25.

Antidepressants

Many antidepressants have been shown to be effective anxiolytics and, unlike buspirone, are also effective for panic attacks. See also Chapter 23.

Buspirone

Buspirone is rarely used, as antidepressants or occasional use of benzodiazepines are preferred. Buspirone activates 5-HT_{1A} receptors, binds to dopamine receptors and may also target noradrenergic and dopaminergic transmission in the brain. The effects on 5-HT are thought to be the main mechanism by which buspirone exerts its anxiolytic effects. Side-effects include dizziness, nausea and headache, as occur with SSRI antidepressants. There is also a delay of 2–3 weeks prior to an anxiolytic effect. Buspirone differs from the benzodiazepines in that it does not cause sedation.

Drug choice in anxiety

The treatment of anxiety involves a combination of short-term symptomatic relief and long-term use of drugs such as SSRI antidepressants with or without behavioural therapy.

Symptomatic treatment

For rapid resolution of symptoms, a short course of a benzodiazepine may be indicated if symptoms are severe and disabling. Low doses of the longer-acting benzodiazepines diazepam, alprazolam or chlordiazepoxide are used. Short-acting alternatives such as lorazepam or oxazepam are administered to patients with hepatic impairment

but these are more likely to produce withdrawal symptoms.

For patients with significant autonomic symptoms, beta-adrenoceptor antagonists such as propranolol are effective and often prescribed for intermittent use. These drugs exhibit a rapid onset of action. Buspirone is also used but a response may be delayed for 2–3 weeks. Symptomatic treatment may help to break the cycle of conditioned anxiety, as occurs when anxiety is experienced in a situation which may have evoked an attack in the past. This short-term treatment, combined with counselling and lifestyle advice, may be sufficient to control anxiety.

Long-term pharmacological intervention

According to severity, SSRIs may be used, particularly if the anxiety is associated with underlying depression (Chapter 23) or chronic symptoms of more than 4 weeks, or when benzodiazepine treatment has failed (Table 24.1). A delay of 2–4 weeks may precede the onset of efficacy of antidepressants in anxiety disorders. However, symptoms may persist for 4–8 weeks in panic disorder and up to 10 weeks in OCD. Treatment is continued for at least 6 months on cessation of symptoms, as for depression, and maintenance treatment may be indicated for recurrent episodes. The treatment of OCD may be continued for a year or more.

It is important to note that antidepressants and particularly paroxetine are associated with an initial worsening of panic symptoms when used to treat panic disorder. Starting with low doses and coprescribing a benzodiazepine in the short term prevents this. The most common adverse effects reported by patients taking SSRIs long-term include tiredness, weight gain and sexual dysfunction.

Non-pharmacological intervention

Counselling such as cognitive behaviour therapy (CBT) may be used to help the patient overcome fear and phobias, thereby aiding recovery and reducing the risk of relapse since many anxiety disorders follow a chronic course. Patients may also benefit from relaxation techniques such as progressive muscle relaxation. Behavioural therapy may include a gradual exposure to feared situations.

Table 24.1   The use of antidepressants in anxiety disorders

Anxiety disorder	Drugs indicated
General anxiety disorder	SSRIs (particularly paroxetine), imipramine (unlicensed), venlafaxine or trazodone
Obsessive-compulsive disorder	Fluoxetine, fluvoxamine, paroxetine, sertraline or clomipramine
Panic disorder	Antidepressants, particularly citalopram or paroxetine, imipramine (unlicensed) or clomipramine (unlicensed)
Panic disorder resistant to antidepressants	Lorazepam or clonazepam (unlicensed indications)
Phobias	Antidepressants generally, particularly clomipramine
Social phobia	Paroxetine or moclobemide
Posttraumatic stress disorder	Paroxetine

SSRIs, selective serotonin reuptake inhibitors.

General anxiety disorder

The use of benzodiazepines should be particularly restricted when treating GAD since this tends to be lifelong and therefore represents a high risk for long-term dependence of these agents. The risk of depression resulting from regular use of benzodiazepines and beta-blockers should also be considered (Chapter 5).

Buspirone may be effective in GAD, although it exhibits a slower onset of action compared with benzodiazepines. Beta-blockers do not appear to be effective in GAD. CBT may particularly benefit GAD due to the chronic nature of this disorder. This may be combined with drug treatment, which may produce a more rapid reduction in symptoms. Patients are assisted in identifying and changing negative, worrying and anxious thoughts. Relaxation techniques are also important.

Table 24.1 summarises the use of antidepressants for anxiety disorders.

Concurrent disease

Prescribing decisions in treating anxiety in the presence of concurrent diseases include:

Beta-blockers (propranolol)

Beta-blockers are a compelling choice for anxious patients with ischaemic heart disease, hypertension or migraine but should be avoided in asthma and chronic obstructive pulmonary disease

(COPD). It should be noted that long-term use may cause or exacerbate depression (see also Chapter 5).

Benzodiazepines

See Chapter 25.

Antidepressants

See Chapter 23.

Buspirone

Buspirone is contraindicated in epilepsy, severe hepatic or renal impairment, pregnancy and breast-feeding.

Drug interactions

These are largely dealt with elsewhere (beta-adrenoceptor antagonists, Chapter 11; benzodiazepines, Chapter 25; antidepressants, SSRIs, Chapter 23).

Buspirone

- contraindicated with monoamine oxidase inhibitors
- increased drowsiness and weakness when combined with alcohol
- risk of serotonin syndrome with citalopram and possibly fluoxetine and other SSRIs. Fluvoxamine may reduce the effects of buspirone

- cytochrome P450 enzyme inhibitors such as erythromycin and itraconazole increase buspirone levels, requiring a dose reduction. Diltiazem, verapamil and possibly ketoconazole may interact by the same mechanism
- rifampicin induces cytochrome P450 and may therefore reduce levels of buspirone and necessitate an increased dose

Herbal medicines

Patients may request or take damiana, cowslip, hops, lady's slipper and St John's wort for anxiety (Chapter 4). These products cannot be recommended by healthcare professionals on the basis of a lack of clinical evidence for safe and efficacious use and should be avoided with conventional treatment for anxiety. Of particular note is kava, a herbal preparation for anxiety which has been withdrawn for investigation into safety following reports of hepatotoxicity. There was also a case reported in which a patient developed a semicomatosed state following concurrent ingestion of kava with alprazolam.

Patients with anxiety should particularly avoid herbs with sympathomimetic activity (Chapter 4) and stimulants such as ginseng. Herbs with sedative properties include valerian, St John's wort and possibly ginseng and should not be taken with benzodiazepines (Chapters 4 and 25). Other herbs associated with causing anxiety include cola and maté.

Counselling

Patients benefit from an empathic approach together with education to increase their understanding of their symptoms. General counselling may include lifestyle advice, as outlined in Chapter 3. Particular emphasis should be placed on smoking cessation and the avoidance of excessive caffeine intake. Motivation for regular exercise may be gained by an explanation of the 'fright or flight' response as occurs when faced with threatening situations. Anxiety is a magnified reaction to situations that may not actually be threatening but invoke a 'fright or flight' response in the patient. A summary of counselling regarding non-pharmacological interventions includes:

- Avoid excess intake of caffeine, alcohol, nicotine and decongestants. It should be noted that caffeine is present in many over-the-counter (OTC) products, including analgesics, tonics and some products marketed to increase energy.
- Patients may be at risk of abusing alcohol due to a temporary relief of symptoms. A vicious circle may result, as described in Chapter 23, and therefore it is useful to highlight this to patients considered at risk.
- Relaxation tapes may help to alleviate anxiety symptoms.
- Practise relaxation techniques, including:
  - progressive muscle relaxation, involving progressive tensing and relaxing of major muscle groups
  - yoga, a Hindu tradition consisting of a series of exercises encompassing stretching, balance and muscle toning, with a focus on controlled breathing throughout
  - meditation, a method of relaxation of the mind involving repetitive internal or vocal chanting of a word, phrase or sound.
- A diary of symptoms together with situations which provoke or alleviate symptoms may help the patient to feel in control and serves to highlight progress. It also helps health professionals to determine the severity of the disorder.

Specific counselling

Specific counselling for SSRIs, tricyclic antidepressants, beta-adrenoceptor antagonists and benzodiazepines is given in Chapters 23, 11 and 25. Points particularly relevant in the treatment of anxiety include the following.

Antidepressants

Patients may be confused by the use of antidepressants for anxiety. It may therefore be helpful to inform patients that antidepressants are used to treat anxiety disorders even in the absence of depression.

SSRIs

- In the treatment of panic disorder with paroxetine, panic symptoms may worsen during initial treatment. Patients should be reassured that this is normal and not a reason to stop treatment.

- The treatment should not be stopped abruptly and should be continued for at least 6 months or up to 12 months or longer.

Benzodiazepines

- These are only recommended for short-term (2–4 weeks) symptomatic relief, for example when SSRIs are initiated. Use is restricted due to the risk of tolerance and dependence.

Beta-blockers (propranolol)

- Beta-blockers treat the symptoms of anxiety and tend to be used on a 'when required' basis. If they are taken regularly, they should not be stopped suddenly as rebound anxiety will occur, with the risk of developing a 'vicious circle' and subsequent psychological dependence on beta-blockers.

Buspirone

- A response may not be observed for up to 2 weeks.
- This is indicated for short-term use, although the risk of dependence and abuse is low.
- Side-effects include dizziness, headache, nervousness, light-headedness, excitement and nausea. These tend to be transient, occurring at the start of treatment.
- Buspirone rarely causes sedation but patients should be advised not to drive until they have established that they do not suffer any sedative effects with buspirone.

Future treatment

Future treatment may include additional selective targets such as subtypes of 5-HT receptors and antagonists of the neuropeptide cholecystokinin (CCK).

Practice points

- Benzodiazepines are reserved for the short-term treatment of severe anxiety.
- Lifestyle advice is important to prevent long-term psychological dependence on drugs.
- Underlying depression should be identified and treated.
- Some antidepressants are indicated for anxiety disorders.
- Beta-blockers are associated with a rare but unpredictable life-threatening bronchospasm and should therefore be avoided by patients with asthma or COPD. This includes low doses.
- Patients often present with physical symptoms, thereby delaying a diagnosis.

 CASE STUDY

A 26-year-old male reports sporadic difficulty with breathing, which usually occurs when he is sitting in an office full of people at work. He is concerned that he may have asthma but has no history of asthma, although he does suffer from hayfever. He is not taking any medication at the moment.

Should this patient receive a salbutamol inhaler?

- This is an interesting case, with vague symptoms that may point to asthma, particularly as he has a history of hayfever. On further questioning, however, the patient also reported an increase in heart rate, sweating, facial flushing and feelings of panic about his breathing. Salbutamol was therefore not appropriate and could have exacerbated his symptoms. He admitted to regular consumption of alcohol and caffeine, although he regularly visited a gym. A diagnosis of panic attacks was made; the patient was advised to cut down on alcohol and particularly caffeine, and continue with his exercise. He was given a prescription for 60 propranolol 10 mg tablets t.d.s. p.r.n.

→

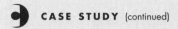

CASE STUDY (continued)

What are possible alternative causes of these symptoms?

- Underlying conditions such as hyperthyroidism and asthma may produce the above symptoms and these should be excluded. The exclusion of asthma is particularly important when prescribing propranolol, which would otherwise be contraindicated. The measurement of lung function may be considered (Chapter 20). Cardiac causes are perhaps unlikely in view of his age. Substance abuse should also be excluded.

What advice should be given regarding propranolol?

- Propranolol may help with the symptoms of anxiety but regular use may lead to rebound anxiety on withdrawal, and without appropriate advice this may progress to chronic use of propranolol. The patient should be advised to use the propranolol occasionally for the temporary relief of symptoms. For example, propranolol may be taken prior to difficult situations known to trigger an attack with a view to breaking the association between the situation and an attack (conditioned anxiety). The importance of lifestyle changes with or without CBT should be stressed.
- The patient should be advised to report symptoms of wheeze and return if his symptoms do not improve. He could also be warned that propranolol will decrease exercise tolerance. Anxiety may be associated with depression, therefore chronic use of propranolol may not be appropriate as it may cause or exacerbate depression. An SSRI and/or CBT may be indicated. This case was resolved with lifestyle changes and intermittent use of propranolol. The patient identified an association with drinking caffeine and excess alcohol.

References

American Psychiatric Association (1995). *Diagnostic and Statistical Manual of Mental Disorders* (DSM-IV), 4th edn. Washington, DC: American Psychiatric Association.

World Health Organization (1992). *The International Statistical Classification of Diseases and Related Health Problems* (ICD-10), 10th revision. Geneva: WHO.

Further reading

Kapczinski F, Schmitt R, Lima M S (2002). The use of antidepressants for generalised anxiety disorder. *Cochrane Systematic Review* 2. Oxford: Update Software.

Livingston M, Jarvie S (2002). Treatment of generalised anxiety disorder. *Prescriber* 13: 17–28.

Nash J, Nutt D (2002). Primary-care treatment of panic disorder. *Prescriber* 13: 29–41.

Online resources

www.adaa.org The Anxiety Disorders Association of America, a comprehensive educational site, provides up-to-date information for patients and healthcare professionals on the nature and treatment of anxiety disorders (accessed 4 December 2002).

www.alcoholics-anonymous.org.uk Alcoholics Anonymous (AA) services, including nationwide support groups (accessed 4 December 2002).

www.crusebereavementcare.org.uk Cruse Bereavement Care is a charity providing information about bereavement (accessed 4 December 2002).

www.phobics-society.org.uk The Anxiety Disorders Charity providing help and advice for patients and carers of phobics, including access to literature, counselling and support groups (accessed 4 December 2002).

www.rcpsych.ac.uk is the website for the Royal College of Psychiatrists (accessed 4 December 2002).

25

Insomnia

Characteristics

Insomnia is an extremely common complaint, affecting one in 10 people, particularly elderly patients, and may have multiple causes such as stress, chronic illness, pain and depression. The effects on quality of life are extensive and insomnia and its treatment are also risk factors for accidents.

Causes of insomnia

There are numerous causes of insomnia, which if addressed may resolve the problem without the requirement for treatment with hypnotic drugs. Causes of insomnia include:

- environmental factors: noise, extremes of temperature, poor ventilation
- lifestyle factors: stress, shift work, jet lag
- disease: poorly controlled asthma or chronic

obstructive pulmonary disease, heart failure, chronic pain, hyperthyroidism, dementia, schizophrenia, anxiety and depression or menopausal symptoms
- drugs, including sympathomimetics, selective serotonin reuptake inhibitors, beta-blockers, thyroid hormones, corticosteroids, caffeine, theophylline and alcohol
- indirect drug causes: diuretics if taken at night, hypoglycaemia following insulin administration or a persistent cough due to angiotensin-converting enzyme inhibitors
- withdrawal from drugs including nicotine, alcohol, antidepressants, hypnotics, opioids, cannabis, amphetamines, and MDMA (3, 4-methylenedioxymethamfetamine) or ecstasy.

Clinical features

Symptoms of insomnia include a delay in falling asleep, failure to maintain sleep or early-morning wakening. The result is often permanent tiredness. The most common presentation is a delay in falling asleep and this is particularly associated with stress, shift work, noise or drugs. Insomnia is classified according to the duration of the problem, as shown in Table 25.1.

Goals of treatment

Initially, potential causes of insomnia should be identified and any underlying problems such as pain or depression treated. There is an important role for patient education and non-pharmacological methods such as counselling and relaxation techniques. The aim is to establish a normal sleep pattern without the use of long-term hypnotics. Patients dependent on hypnotics, including over-the-counter (OTC) preparations, should be supported during gradual withdrawal from these drugs. Referral for cognitive behavioural therapy or specific abuse counselling may be required for chronic insomnia. Sleep clinic referrals are reserved for sleep apnoea, epilepsy during sleep, long-standing insomnia resistant to treatment, or following suspicion of exaggeration by the patient.

Pharmacological basis of management

Benzodiazepines

Flunitrazepam, flurazepam, loprazolam, lormetazepam, nitrazepam, temazepam

Benzodiazepines reduce anxiety and aggression, induce sleep, reduce muscle tone and coordination and produce an anticonvulsant effect. The main mechanism of action involves increased activity of the inhibitory neurotransmitter, gamma-aminobutyric acid (GABA), in the brain. This occurs following binding of the drug to a regulatory site, the benzodiazepine receptor, on $GABA_A$-receptor complexes. Differences in the sensitivity of numerous subtypes of $GABA_A$-receptors to benzodiazepines account for some of

their different clinical uses. For example, clonazepam and diazepam exhibit greater anticonvulsant activity. Short-acting benzodiazepines such as temazepam, lormetazepam or loprazolam are reserved for the treatment of insomnia to reduce the risk of a hangover effect persisting the following day. Tolerance and dependence are also problematic with benzodiazepines.

Related hypnotics

'Z-drugs': zaleplon, zolpidem, zopiclone

These newer agents which have a non-benzodiazepine structure have been developed with the aim of reducing adverse effects such as hangover and dependence. These drugs exhibit a shorter duration of action and are thought to be selective for subtypes of benzodiazepine receptor and/or selectively target individual sub-units of these receptors. In practice, however, the adverse effects appear to be similar to conventional benzodiazepines.

Sedating antihistamines

Diphenhydramine, promethazine

Sedating antihistamines are histamine H_1-receptor antagonists (Chapter 19). They also exhibit antimuscarinic effects, resulting in side-effects, including dry mouth, blurred vision, constipation and urinary retention. They are available in OTC preparations for the short-term relief of insomnia.

Barbiturates

Amobarbital, butobarbital, secobarbital

Traditionally, barbiturates were used as hypnotics and tranquillisers. These are non-selective central nervous system (CNS)-depressants acting to increase GABA transmission in a less selective manner compared with benzodiazepines. Side-effects are therefore even more troublesome than those associated with benzodiazepines, and barbiturates are seldom used, with the exception

Table 25.1 Classification of insomnia according to the duration of symptoms

Description of insomnia	Duration	Common causes
Transient	2–3 days	Noise, shift work, jet lag
Short-term	3–4 weeks	Stress, depression, drugs such as caffeine or decongestants
Chronic	Most nights for 3 weeks or longer	Severe disease, drug abuse, including alcohol and mild hypnotic dependence

of anaesthesia and occasionally epilepsy. They exhibit numerous drug interactions due to the induction of hepatic cytochrome P450 enzymes, produce tolerance and dependence and are toxic in overdose.

Drug choice

Treatment may often require non-pharmacological intervention such as lifestyle changes or reviewing drug-related causes or treating underlying illness. Occasionally, pharmacological intervention with benzodiazepines is required but this should be short-term due to the following problems:

- an increased risk of falls in the elderly
- a hangover effect the next morning
- confusion, amnesia, cognitive impairment and impaired coordination
- a risk of road traffic accidents associated with benzodiazepines with long half-lives and the short-acting hypnotic zopiclone
- the disruption of normal sleep patterns
- chronic use is associated with anxiety and depression
- tolerance and therefore the requirement for higher doses
- the risk of dependence and abuse
- withdrawal effects, including rebound insomnia
- a risk of life-threatening respiratory depression if an overdose of benzodiazepines is taken with alcohol, although they are relatively safe if taken without alcohol or other substances of abuse

Summary

Hypnotics are licensed for the short-term treatment of insomnia for no more than 3 weeks and ideally for only 1 week and using intermittent doses such as every third night. Agents with a short half-life should be given. These include temazepam, loprazolam and lormetazepam.

Short-acting benzodiazepines (temazepam, loprazolam, lormetazepam)
These agents are preferred due to a reduced risk of hangover effect in the short-term treatment of insomnia. Loprazolam exhibits erratic absorption, which may increase its duration of action.

Long-acting benzodiazepines (diazepam, flurazepam, flunitrazepam, nitrazepam)
The longer-acting benzodiazepines are rarely used to treat insomnia due to residual side-effects, particularly affecting elderly patients. The exception is diazepam used for insomnia associated with anxiety. It is also the preferred agent for withdrawal from chronic use of benzodiazepines as withdrawal effects are less pronounced.

Other hypnotics
'Z-drugs' are associated with withdrawal symptoms, tolerance and dependence. Current evidence suggests they offer little advantage over benzodiazepines. Chloral hydrate is no longer recommended as there is no evidence of real benefit for elderly patients and the treatment of children is rarely justified. Clomethiazole is occasionally used for elderly patients due to reduced confusion and hangover effects. Short-term use is again indicated due to the risk of dependence.

Concurrent disease

Table 25.2 indicates disease states that may preclude the use of certain hypnotics.

Hepatic impairment

Hypnotics should be avoided in severe liver disease as they may precipitate coma. Reduced doses of some hypnotics may be used in milder hepatic disease and the *British National Formulary* and/or summary of product characteristics should be consulted.

Renal impairment

Small doses of hypnotics are recommended due to increased cerebral sensitivity associated with severe renal impairment.

Special groups

Pregnancy and breast-feeding
Non-pharmacological treatment is preferred during pregnancy and breast-feeding.

The elderly
The requirement for sleep is reduced in the elderly and this group is likely to expect to sleep for longer than is actually required. Hypnotic use in this group should be avoided due to an increased risk of side-effects, particularly drowsiness and confusion, which may increase the risk of falls. The enhanced effects are mainly due to an age-related reduction in hepatic metabolism. Reduced doses are indicated if treatment is necessary.

Children
Hypnotics should not be used in children, with the possible exception of night terrors and

Table 25.2 Concurrent disease states to be considered when prescribing hypnotics

Disease	Comments
Cardiac disease	Chloral hydrate is contraindicated.
COPD	Hypnotics should be used with caution, particularly in patients with hypoxia, due to reduced respiratory drive
Dementia	• Benzodiazepines may cause or worsen dementia. Avoid if possible, or use low doses of short-acting agents • Zolpidem has also been associated with memory impairment and vigilance is required for these effects with all 'Z-drugs'
Depression	• Hypnotics should not be used alone as long-term use may exacerbate depression • Sedating TCAs (e.g. amitriptyline, dosulepin), maprotiline, mianserin or trazodone may be appropriate • SSRIs may cause insomnia
Gastritis	Chloral hydrate is contraindicated
Glaucoma, prostatic hypertrophy and urinary retention	Antimuscarinic side-effects of sedative antihistamines mean that they should be used with caution in these conditions
Muscle weakness	Benzodiazepines should be used with caution.
Osteoporosis	The risk of fractures may be increased in elderly patients due to falls associated with hypnotics
Porphyria	Some antihistamines, benzodiazepines and chloral hydrate may be unsuitable (see *British National Formulary* section 9.8.2)
Respiratory depression	All hypnotics should be avoided
Sleep apnoea	Benzodiazepines, zaleplon, zolpidem and zopiclone should be avoided

COPD, chronic obstructive pulmonary disease; TCAs, tricyclic antidepressants; SSRIs, selective serotonin reuptake inhibitors.

somnambulism (sleep walking). Alternatives for treating night terrors include waking the child 15 min before the time a night terror usually occurs and then allowing him or her to go back to sleep. A bedtime routine is particularly important for children.

Drug interactions

Drug interactions with hypnotics generally result from an additive effect with other drugs with sedative properties such as alcohol, antihistamines, antidepressants and opioids. Barbiturates are rarely used as they exhibit numerous interactions due to activation of hepatic cytochrome P450 enzymes.

Plasma levels of benzodiazepines may be elevated in patients taking cimetidine, due to cytochrome P450 inhibition. However this interaction appears not to be very important clinically. Possible increases in side-effects may occur.

Over-the-counter considerations

Sedating antihistamines are available for the short-term relief of insomnia but patients should be advised to consult their general practitioner (GP) if symptoms persist after 2 weeks. However these drugs are associated with a hangover effect and may also lead to tolerance, headaches, psychomotor impairment (including impaired reaction times) and antimuscarinic effects.

Herbal medicines

Patients with insomnia may commonly take or request products containing valerian, camomile, hops, valerian, gentian, passionflower (*Passiflora*), wild lettuce and pulsatilla. For example, combinations of these herbs are present in Kalms, HRI night and Nytol herbal. Until more information regarding the pharmacological activity, efficacy and safety of these products is known, the same precautions observed with conventional hypnotics may be appropriate. For example, the potential for drug interactions and concurrent disease as outlined above should be considered. Advice about non-pharmacological intervention is also relevant. For a discussion on the recommendation of herbal preparations, the reader is referred to Chapter 4.

Patients who take herbal preparations for insomnia should avoid herbs with sympathomimetic activity (Chapter 4) and stimulants such as ginseng. Herbs with sedative properties (Chapter 4) should not be taken with hypnotics. Camomile and pulsatilla have been associated with hypersensitivity reactions and should be avoided by susceptible individuals such as asthmatics.

Dietary supplements

Melatonin is a hormone involved in the sleep–wake cycle, being secreted during the night. This is taken as a dietary supplement for jet lag and by shift workers but reliable evidence for efficacy and long-term safety is lacking. People with depression, prescribed CNS-depressants or women trying to conceive should avoid it.

Withdrawal from chronic benzodiazepine treatment

See Chapter 5.

Counselling

General counselling should focus on non-pharmacological options:

- Try to establish a routine of retiring to bed and rising at the same time each day.
- Avoid lying in bed worrying about being awake, as this may also contribute to conditioned insomnia and is more tiring than being awake and not worrying.
- Regular exercise may benefit insomnia but should be avoided a few hours before going to bed. A short walk in the evening may help.
- Alcohol should not be used to aid sleep as it is a diuretic, disturbing sleep in the latter part of the night and also produces 'unrestful' sleep. Chronic use may itself cause insomnia.

- Avoid caffeine, nicotine (including 24-h patches), thyroid hormones and decongestants, particularly after 4 p.m.
- Do not work, eat or watch television in the bedroom as conditioned insomnia may result whereby the bedroom is associated with being awake.
- Avoid napping during the day.
- Avoid intellectual activity before going to bed.
- Establish a routine each night such as reading, drinking warm milk or having a warm bath with lavender oil before retiring to bed.
- Eliminate environmental causes such as noise, light, extremes of temperature or poor air quality.
- Listen to relaxation tapes.
- Relaxation techniques are particularly useful for patients with stress-related insomnia who have difficulty in falling asleep. These include:
  - progressive muscle relaxation, involving progressive tensing and relaxing of major muscle groups
  - yoga, a Hindu tradition consisting of a series of exercises encompassing stretching, balance and muscle toning, with a focus on controlled breathing throughout
  - meditation, a method of relaxation of the mind involving repetitive internal or vocal chanting of a word, phrase or sound.
- A sleep diary may be useful for identifying the cause, pattern and severity of insomnia. Patients may benefit from feeling more in control of the problem and from observing their progress. This method may also reveal patients with an unrealistic expectation of the duration and depth of sleep required. The following points may be recorded:
  - the time of retiring to bed and approximate time taken to fall asleep
  - the duration of sleep
  - the number of times of waking during the night and the duration
  - a score out of 10 of the feeling of tiredness each day
  - a score out of 10 of the feeling of tension and irritability

  - general comments such as alcohol or caffeine intake and other potential causes.

Counselling and the use of hypnotics

Generally, patients should be warned that hypnotics only help the symptoms and not the causes of insomnia. They are only recommended for short-term intermittent use. Informing patients that withdrawal from regular use of hypnotics causes rebound insomnia leading to the desire to continue taking the treatment may help prevent this road to dependence.

- Intermittent use, preferably every third night, is recommended to avoid tolerance. It may be useful to explain that this means that the sedative effect is lost if hypnotics are taken every night.
- Treatment is ideally restricted to no more than 1 week to prevent the development of dependence.
- Hypnotics may cause drowsiness, which may persist to the next day. Patients should therefore be cautious if driving or performing other skilled tasks. Alcohol adds to these effects and should be avoided.
- Following withdrawal from hypnotics, sleep may be disturbed for a few days and may feature vivid dreams due to increased rapid eye movement (REM) sleep for many weeks.

Practice points

- Reinforce non-pharmacological options for treating insomnia.
- Patients should be asked about the use of over-the-counter hypnotics and frequent requests should lead to a referral to the GP.
- Long-term users of benzodiazepines should be changed to the equivalent dose of diazepam prior to gradual withdrawal, with regular review and encouragement.
- Patient education relating to the risks and benefits of withdrawing from hypnotics may improve the outcome.

CASE STUDIES

Case 1
A 45-year-old male with a history of bipolar affective disorder requests a sedative antihistamine from his pharmacist. He currently takes lithium and is away from home for a business meeting.

Should a supply be made?

- Insomnia may be an early sign of relapse in patients with bipolar affective disorder and therefore referral to the GP is warranted. This patient was away from home and therefore could not see his GP until the following week and did not want to see a GP not familiar with his case. He was driving and therefore a sedating antihistamine was not the best choice due to the possibility of hangover effect the next morning. However, due to the risk of relapse of bipolar disorder, the problem of driving when tired and the absence of other symptoms, a supply was made with the recommendation that the patient only take a tablet every third night until he returned home. He was advised not to take them too late at night to prevent the residual effects next morning and to consult his GP if his symptoms did not improve within a week. He was also given advice and an information leaflet about non-pharmacological treatment of sleep problems, particularly the importance of avoiding alcohol and caffeine. He telephoned to thank the pharmacist on his return, saying that the advice and treatment helped him through a difficult week and he was now feeling much better.

Case 2
A 25-year-old female with Crohn's disease presented to her GP complaining of insomnia mainly due to her painful condition. She was taking venlafaxine 75 mg b.d. in addition to her immunosuppressant therapy. She felt that her prednisolone treatment was aggravating her low mood and her Crohn's symptoms were still not controlled.

What course of action could the GP take?

- The patient should be referred back to her specialist to review her Crohn's medication, as this is likely to be the main cause of her insomnia. However, the GP may consider changing the antidepressant to a more sedating agent such as trazodone and reviewing her medication for pain. General counselling about sleep may also be beneficial, as outlined above.

Case 3
A 20-year-old female student presents with insomnia before her exams and asks for a prescription for sleeping tablets. She says she 'has a few drinks' every night to help her unwind but wakes up in the night and cannot get back to sleep.

Would a short-term hypnotic help this patient?

- A short-term hypnotic may help depending on the amount of distress to the patient and the nature and duration of the exams. However, non-pharmacological intervention could be considered first, for example, advising that alcohol is not an effective sedative due to disturbed sleep later in the night. She should be advised not to revise late in the evening and to try to revise somewhere other than where she sleeps. Further questioning of this patient revealed that she was taking Pro Plus, a caffeine-containing product, during the day. She was advised to reduce this gradually and was given a leaflet outlining general counselling for people with insomnia and to return if her problem did not improve.

Reference

Mehta D K (ed.) *British National Formulary*, latest edition. London: British Medical Association and Royal Pharmaceutical Society of Great Britain.

Further reading

Anon (2002). An update on benzodiazepines and non-benzodiazepine hypnotics. *MeReC Briefing* 17: 6–8.

Hallström C (2002). A primary-care guide to insomnia management. *Prescriber* 13: 65–74.

Online resource

www.rcpsych.ac.uk The Royal College of Psychiatrists provides up-to-date information and informative patient information leaflets (accessed 4 December 2002).

26

Schizophrenia

Characteristics

Schizophrenia presents with psychotic symptoms similar to the manic phase of bipolar affective disorder but differs in that deterioration of cognitive function is often observed over time. Many patients suffering from schizophrenia are unable to continue with their normal daily life. Approximately 1% of the population is affected: onset tends to be in the early 20s and has both genetic and environmental components. Patients may be reassured that one in five patients may only suffer a single acute episode, although seven in 10 suffer at least two acute episodes. Drugs such as amphetamines may induce psychotic symptoms or worsen schizophrenia, mainly as a result of dopamine release.

Clinical presentation

The symptoms of schizophrenia are grouped as positive or negative. Patients may describe positive symptoms as 'dreaming while awake':

Positive symptoms

- Hallucinations – false perceptions of sounds, images, taste, smells or other sensory images that do not have a real stimulus.
- Delusions – these are irrational beliefs, which cannot be altered by logical reasoning. For example, being controlled by others.
- Thought disorder and disorganised communication. For example:
  - thought broadcasting – thoughts are 'expressed freely' to others
  - thought insertion – thoughts are inserted by another person
  - thought withdrawal – thoughts are stolen by another person

Negative symptoms

- reduced activity with emotional flattening (psychomotor retardation, Chapter 23)
- withdrawal from society
- cognitive deficit and therefore unemployment

Other

Catatonic

A catatonic state encompasses motor (movement) abnormalities, including overactivity and violence or standing in strange positions.

Classification

The term 'schizophrenia' literally translates as 'split mind' and is often misinterpreted as a split personality. According to the *Diagnostic and Statistical Manual of Mental Disorders* (DSM-IV: American Psychiatric Association, 1995), a diagnosis of schizophrenia is made if two or more of the following symptoms are present for most of the time during a period of 1 month. The required time period is shorter if the symptoms are treated successfully with medication. Symptoms include:

• delusions
• hallucinations
• disorganised speech
• disorganised or catatonic behaviour
• negative symptoms: affective (emotional) flattening

Schizophrenia results in considerable impairment of social and occupational functioning, including interpersonal relationships and self-care. A diagnosis may also be made on the basis of the presence of hallucinations alone if these comprise a voice giving a running commentary on the patient's behaviour or thoughts, or two or more voices communicating with each other. A longer period, 6 months or more, of milder symptoms may also result in a diagnosis of schizophrenia and may include milder manifestations of at least two of the above symptoms (such as strange beliefs) or only negative symptoms. Finally, substance abuse and concurrent disease are excluded as the cause before a positive diagnosis of schizophrenia can be made.

Pathophysiology

Schizophrenia is considered a neurodevelopmental rather than neurodegenerative disease, mainly affecting the cerebral cortex, as predicted from the cognitive symptoms. The pathophysiology of schizophrenia remains elusive, although new and interesting theories are beginning to emerge. Historically, schizophrenia has been associated with overactivity of dopaminergic neurotransmission and conventional treatment has been with dopamine receptor antagonists such as chlorpromazine. This theory, however, does not provide a complete explanation. For example, the efficacy of antipsychotics (chlorpromazine, clozapine, sulpiride, trifluoperazine) is delayed for 7–10 days or more, suggesting an additional mechanism to simple antagonism of receptors. Alternative mechanisms may include a change in the number of receptors expressed in cells or perhaps an effect on signal transduction within cells. Current theories (Glen, 2001) involve the modulation of neurotransmission at the cellular level and particularly arachidonic acid derived from membrane phospholipids and leading to the production of prostanoids (Chapter 20). The importance of the intake of polyunsaturated fat from the diets is therefore under investigation.

The modulation of dopaminergic neurotransmission remains important in newer, atypical antipsychotics but the role of 5-hydroxytryptamine (5-HT) is also recognised and effective treatment such as with clozapine is thought to be due to a greater effect on serotonergic transmission compared with dopaminergic systems. This may partly explain the beneficial effect of clozapine on negative symptoms. Other systems targeted include glutamatergic, GABAergic and noradrenergic, which are involved in the modulation of dopaminergic neurotransmission. For example, antagonism of the glutamate N-methyl-D-aspartate receptor by drugs such as phencyclidine and ketamine produce symptoms similar to those observed in schizophrenia.

Pharmacological basis of management

All antipsychotics are dopamine D_2-receptor antagonists, thereby inhibiting dopaminergic neurotransmission, and this remains an important target for effective antipsychotic activity. Extra-pyramidal and endocrine symptoms are often troublesome, particularly at higher doses. For example, hyperprolactinaemia may also follow the inhibition of dopamine transmission, resulting in increased prolactin secretion. The reverse occurs when the dopamine receptor agonist bromocriptine is used to suppress lactation. Most antipsychotics also act as antagonists at receptors for other monoamines, including alpha-adrenoceptors, muscarinic and 5-HT receptors (mainly 5-HT$_2$). The affinity for these receptors determines the side-effect profile. Histamine receptors may also be modulated by antipsychotics, but this is not thought to result in antipsychotic activity.

Conventional antipsychotics

The conventional antipsychotics were previously termed 'major tranquillisers' but this term is no longer used since this is not the main effect exploited in the treatment of schizophrenia. The term 'antischizophrenic' is also inaccurate since these drugs are 'antipsychotic' and are also used to treat psychotic symptoms associated with major depression and bipolar disorder (Chapter 23) and delusional disorders. The main groups of these typical antipsychotics include:

- phenothiazines comprising three further groups (see *British National Formulary*):
  - group 1 (aliphatic), e.g. chlorpromazine
  - group 2 (piperidine), e.g. thioridazine (restricted to second-line treatment of schizophrenia under specialist supervision)
  - group 3 (piperazine), e.g. prochlorperazine and trifluoperazine

The following groups resemble the structure of the group 3 phenothiazines:

- butyrophenones, e.g. haloperidol, droperidol
- diphenylbutylpiperidines, e.g. pimozide
- thioxanthines, e.g. flupentixol
- substituted benzamides: sulpiride (often grouped with 'atypical' antipsychotics due to its reduced extrapyramidal effects)

Atypical antipsychotics

e.g. Clozapine, olanzapine, risperidone, sertindole

Atypical antipsychotics have vastly improved the treatment of schizophrenia, mainly as a result of reduced extrapyramidal effects. In addition, clozapine is one of the only antipsychotics to benefit negative symptoms and has a central role in treatment-resistant schizophrenia. These drugs are now considered for first-line treatment and are also used in the treatment of bipolar affective disorder (Chapter 23). They are not, however, devoid of adverse effects. For example, weight gain and metabolic effects are common and sexual dysfunction is a major factor in reduced compliance. Clozapine is associated with agranulocytosis and is therefore restricted to patients who have failed to respond to at least two antipsychotics (see below). Sertindole is currently restricted to named patients due to its association with arrhythmias and sudden death.

Adverse effects of antipsychotics

With the introduction of atypical antipsychotics, frightening extrapyramidal effects are less common, being associated with conventional antipsychotics and particularly the group 3 phenothiazines, the butyrophenones and particularly depot preparations of these groups. Common adverse effects with atypical antipsychotics include weight gain, sexual dysfunction and the risk of diabetes mellitus.

Weight gain

Weight gain is common with antipsychotics and may be a factor in the cause or exacerbation of type 2 diabetes mellitus.

Sexual dysfunction

Sexual dysfunction often has a significant effect on personal relationships and quality of life but is not discussed due to embarrassment. Symptoms range from altered libido to impotence in men or reduced lubrication in women and failure of orgasm. Fertility may therefore be an important issue. Sexual dysfunction is an important cause of non-compliance with both conventional and atypical antipsychotics.

Galactorrhoea and amenorrhoea

Endocrine effects such as galactorrhoea occur due to increased prolactin secretion. This includes an enlargement of the breasts and milk production. Other effects include missed periods (amenorrhoea), reduced libido and therefore reduced fertility.

Movement disorders

As described above, many of the adverse effects of antipsychotics result from the blockade of dopamine receptors and therefore include disorders of movement or endocrine disorders. These include parkinsonian symptoms such as tremor and rigidity. This is not surprising considering the use of levodopa to replenish dopamine levels, thereby improving the symptoms of Parkinson's disease. Antimuscarinic drugs such as procyclidine are prescribed 'when required' to counteract these effects but should be used with caution due to the risk of irreversible tardive dyskinesia. The following terms are used to describe movement disorders.

Extrapyramidal effects

Extrapyramidal neurons comprise a system of nerves connecting the cerebral cortex, basal ganglia, thalamus, cerebellum, reticular formation and spinal neurons in complex systems not included in the pyramidal system. Extrapyramidal motor disorders are those affecting movement, which is regulated by dopamine in the extrapyramidal system. These include:

- akinesia: literally 'lacking movement', a loss of normal muscular tone or responsiveness
- parkinsonism: symptoms associated with Parkinson's disease, including tremor, rigidity, salivation (drooling) and akinesia of the face. These effects are reversible when they are drug-induced

- acute dystonia: abnormal or impaired posture or muscle spasms due to altered muscle tone. This often involves sustained contractions of neck and facial muscles and is reversible
- akathisia: an unwanted effect of antipsychotics (phenothiazines) involving involuntary movements or restless overactivity of the legs and/or body, for example, pacing up and down, constantly changing leg position or foot tapping. This may easily be confused with the agitation for which the drug was prescribed. There is currently no reliable evidence for or against the use of antimuscarinic agents to treat acute akathisia induced by antipsychotics (Lima *et al.*, 2002)
- tardive dyskinesia: a chronic condition characterised by repetitive involuntary movements, usually of the tongue, face, fingers, hands, legs and trunk and resulting in drooling and lip smacking. The concurrent use of drugs with antimuscarinic activity may aggravate the condition, which may be irreversible, and therefore careful monitoring is important

Cardiovascular effects

Cardiac arrhythmias are a particular problem with sertindole but may also occur with phenothiazines and particularly thioridazine and chlorpromazine. The prescribing of thioridazine was recently limited to the second-line treatment of schizophrenia in adults under specialist supervision. Sertindole was withdrawn in 1998 but has recently been reintroduced for named patients, only for those stabilised on sertindole and when other antipsychotics are not appropriate.

Severe postural hypotension may occur with chlorpromazine and other phenothiazines due to the antagonism of alpha-adrenoceptors (Chapter 11).

Antimuscarinic effects

The antimuscarinic affects of drugs may be peripheral or central. Peripheral effects such as dry mouth, blurred vision, urinary retention and constipation are summarised in Chapter 5. This pharmacological activity also accounts in part for the use of phenothiazines as antiemetics

(Chapter 8). The following central effects may occur with antipsychotics as a result of antimuscarinic activity:

- confusion
- disorientation
- visual hallucinations
- agitation
- irritability
- delirium
- memory impairment
- aggression and possibly violent behaviour
- sedation

Caution is required in identifying drug-related central antimuscarinic effects to prevent the coprescribing of antipsychotics with additional antimuscarinic effects. The subsequent occurrence of extrapyramidal effects such as dystonia, akathisia, tremor or rigidity then becomes apparent, with a risk of further antimuscarinic drugs such as procyclidine being added to control these effects. The iatrogenic problem is then worsened, with the risk of causing serious adverse drug reactions such as irreversible tardive dyskinesia, heat stroke or paralytic ileus (Chapter 5).

Idiosyncratic and hypersensitivity reactions

Type B adverse drug reactions are less predictable from the pharmacological activity of antipsychotics and include photosensitivity, particularly with chlorpromazine (and also contact sensitivity), agranulocytosis, jaundice and neuroleptic malignant syndrome (Chapter 5).

Tables 26.1 and 26.2 include a comparison of side-effects between different groups of phenothiazines and a consideration of the most prominent side-effects, considering both conventional and atypical agents.

Drug choice

The aims of treatment are to manage the initial psychotic symptoms, improve the quality of life and reduce the risk of relapse but with minimum adverse effects (particularly frightening extrapyramidal effects). The most difficult symptoms to treat are negative symptoms, for which clozapine may be required. Atypical antipsychotics have been associated with fewer extrapyramidal side-effects and have been recommended by the National Institute of Clinical Excellence (NICE, 2002) as first-line treatment for newly diagnosed schizophrenia. Specified agents include amisulpiride, olanzapine, quetiapine, risperidone and zotepine and low doses should be used for the first episode. This recommendation excludes clozapine due to the risk of agranulocytosis. Additional recommendations by NICE for the appropriate use of atypical antipsychotics include the following:

- Patients taking conventional antipsychotics and experiencing intolerable side-effects (usually extrapyramidal) may be switched to an atypical antipsychotic.
- Patients suffering relapse and symptoms who

Table 26.1   A comparison of severity of common side-effects of phenothiazines

Adverse effect	Phenothiazines		
	Group 1	Group 2	Group 3
Extrapyramidal effects	++	+	+++
Antimuscarinic effects	++	+++	+
Drowsiness	+++	++	+

+++ severe, ++ moderate and + fewer in comparison to the other phenothiazines.
Information derived from *British National Formulary*, vol. 44.

Table 26.2 Examples of common side-effects produced by antipsychotics

Side-effect	Drugs implicated	Drugs least likely to cause the ADR
Extrapyramidal effects	Haloperidol, phenothiazines (see Table 26.1 for comparison), depot preparations	Atypical antipsychotics, including amisulpiride, sulpiride and particularly clozapine, olanzapine, quetiapine and risperidone
Antimuscarinic effects	Phenothiazines (see Table 26.1), clozapine	Haloperidol, amisulpiride, olanzapine, quetiapine, risperidone, sulpiride
Cardiac arrhythmias	Sertindole, phenothiazines (particularly thioridazine), pimozide, clozapine	Amisulpiride, flupentixol, sulpiride, olanzapine, risperidone
Galactorrhoea	Sulpiride	Atypical antipsychotics
Parkinsonism	Fluphenazine, perphenazine, trifluoperazine, prochlorperazine	Atypical antipsychotics
Photosensitivity	Chlorpromazine	
Jaundice	Conventional antipsychotics, particularly phenothiazines (Chapter 5)	
Hypotension	Haloperidol, phenothiazines, sertindole, seroquel	Amisulpiride, sulpiride, clozapine, risperidone, flupentixol, olanzapine, quetiapine
Drowsiness	Chlorpromazine (Table 26.1)	Amisulpiride, haloperidol, flupentixol, pimozide, quetiapine, sulpiride or zotepine
Sexual dysfunction (Chapter 5)	Phenothiazines, pimozide and sulpiride	
Weight gain	Chlorpromazine, sertindole, risperidone, olanzapine, clozapine	Pimozide
Agranulocytosis	Clozapine	All antipsychotics, except clozapine

ADR, adverse drug reaction.

were previously poorly controlled by conventional agents may benefit from an atypical antipsychotic.

• Symptoms of schizophrenia poorly controlled following trials with two or more antipsychotics (including at least one atypical) for 6–8 weeks may benefit from clozapine but only initiated in a hospital inpatient setting. Patients are required to register with a centralised monitoring service for early detection of agranulocytosis. A second antipsychotic may be added if there is a poor response with clozapine.

• There is convincing evidence that clozapine is more effective than conventional antipsychotics for the treatment of schizophrenia and that agranulocytosis is more likely to occur in children, adolescents and the elderly (Wahlbeck et al., 2002).

• Changing to an atypical antipsychotic is not appropriate if symptoms are controlled and side-effects are mild and acceptable.

Aggressive symptoms

Haloperidol is the common choice for violent or aggressive patients and often first choice for acute treatment of psychosis, prescribed 'when required' alongside other antipsychotics. Drugs such as lorazepam or haloperidol may be administered by intramuscular injection. It should be noted that haloperidol is often the choice for elderly patients as it has a lower incidence of hypotension. For further information regarding the management of acute schizophrenia, including rapid tranquillisation, the reader is referred to guidelines issued by NICE (2002).

Depot preparations

Depot preparations may be used for maintenance therapy, given every 1–4 weeks, particularly when compliance is a problem, and may benefit people who exhibit considerable first pass metabolism. A test dose may be given initially (see *British National Formulary* or summary of product characteristics). There may however be an increased risk of extrapyramidal side-effects compared with oral agents. Problems include difficulty in titrating doses, pain on injection and variable pharmacokinetics according to muscle mass and rate of metabolism. Side-effects may take weeks to dissipate following the last dose. A depot preparation of the atypical antipsychotic, risperidone, is now licensed and available and may be associated with fewer side-effects, as discussed above.

Duration of maintenance treatment

Treatment with antipsychotics is often long-term. However, patients who appear to be in remission may withdraw gradually from treatment with regular monitoring for signs of relapse for at least 2 years following the last acute episode (NICE, 2002). These patients include those who have suffered only one acute psychotic episode during 1–2 years of treatment and have responded well to treatment. Patients who have suffered two or more psychotic episodes are continued on medication for at least 5 years.

Non-pharmacological interventions

Cognitive behavioural therapy (CBT) is recommended alongside drug treatment, to help patients to understand their symptoms and develop coping mechanisms in order to control them. It is particularly beneficial for persistent psychotic symptoms: longer courses of more than 6 months and at least 10 sessions are recommended (NICE, 2002). Shorter courses may only benefit depressive symptoms. Carers may

also benefit from support in the form of CBT or counselling and supportive psychotherapy. These interventions are beneficial for the patient and aim to prevent relapse, reduce symptoms, increase insight and improve compliance with medication (NICE, 2002). It should therefore be possible for patients to live a fairly normal life and this should be emphasised at the start of treatment.

The effect of environmental factors on patients with schizophrenia is recognised and benefit may be gained from moving patients to a low-stress environment. Social, group and physical activities are also beneficial.

Concurrent disease

Table 26.3 summarises possible influences on the choice of antipsychotic drugs.

Drug interactions

Some of the older antipsychotic agents may cause QT prolongation and increase the risk of torsade de pointes arrhythmias. Accordingly, these drugs should be used with caution in the elderly, those with pre-existing arrhythmias and with other drugs which may prolong the QT interval. Atypical antipsychotics do not normally alter the QT interval but should be used with caution with drugs that do. Additional interactions are summarised in Table 26.4.

Monitoring

General

Monitoring for patients prescribed antipsychotics may include blood pressure due to the risk of hypotension, electrocardiogram (ECG), weight, urinary glucose and temperature. Temperature monitoring is useful for the early diagnosis of neuroleptic malignant syndrome, although this is rare.

Cardiovascular

An ECG should be performed for patients at risk of cardiotoxicity such as those with pre-existing

Table 26.3   Concurrent disease and the prescribing of antipsychotics

Disease	Comment
Cardiovascular disease (e.g. angina, arrhythmias, chronic heart failure)	• Increased risk of arrhythmias, particularly with thioridazine (contraindicated), sertindole and pimozide • Increased risk of hypotension in susceptible patients, e.g. the elderly or those prescribed antihypertensives. Reduced doses of antipsychotics may be recommended
Closed-angle glaucoma	• Antimuscarinic drugs reduce drainage, therefore worsening this condition. Prochlorperazine and chlorpromazine use should be avoided • Patients at increased risk include those with diabetes mellitus and/or a family history of glaucoma
Prostatic hypertrophy	Antimuscarinic effects may lead to urinary retention
Depression	• There is currently no evidence for the benefit of antidepressants in patients with schizophrenia (Whitehead et al., 2002). The appropriateness of electroconvulsive therapy for patients with severe major depression (Chapter 23) and schizophrenia is currently under review by NICE • See also drug interactions (Table 26.4)
Diabetes mellitus	• Risk of type 2 diabetes due to weight gain with antipsychotics and particularly chlorpromazine, sertindole, risperidone, clozapine and olanzapine • Risk of exacerbation or ketoacidosis (olanzapine)
Dementia and the elderly	• Drugs with antimuscarinic effects may cause or worsen dementia (Chapter 5) • Atypical antipsychotics such as risperidone are preferred for elderly patients
Epilepsy	• The convulsive threshold is lowered by antipsychotics. Reduced doses may be indicated (e.g. clozapine) • Additional risk factors for convulsions are listed in Chapters 5 and 22
Parkinson's disease	Antipsychotics may exacerbate symptoms, mainly as a result of dopamine receptor antagonism
Severe respiratory disease	Use with caution, particularly in combination with other CNS-depressants such as alcohol

NICE, National Institute of Clinical Excellence; CNS, central nervous system.

cardiovascular disease, elderly patients and those taking medication associated with prolongation of the QT interval and those prescribed high doses of antipsychotics. For patients prescribed thioridazine, ECG and electrolytes are measured prior to starting treatment and then following every dose increase and then every 6 months.

Elderly

Drugs used in the treatment of schizophrenia may increase the risk of falls due to postural hypotension. Accordingly, lower doses are indicated. Note that thioridazine is no longer appropriate for the treatment of agitation. This was previously a

Pharmacological basis of management **327**

Table 26.4 Examples of drug interactions involving antipsychotics

Drugs	Consequences	Comments
Clozapine with anticonvulsants (carbamazepine, phenytoin)	• Clozapine levels are reduced • Risk of additive bone marrow suppression (carbamazepine) • Risk of neuroleptic malignant syndrome (Chapter 5)	• Dose of clozapine may need to be doubled when used with carbamazepine or phenytoin • Monitor for signs of infection or neuroleptic malignant syndrome
Haloperidol and anticonvulsants (phenobarbital, carbamazepine, phenytoin) or rifampicin	Reduced levels of haloperidol	• Note that haloperidol may also increase carbamazepine levels • Sodium valproate appears not to interact • Isoniazid may increase haloperidol levels
Clozapine with benzodiazepines	Risk of severe hypotension and respiratory depression	• Monitor closely for signs of these adverse effects • Lorazepam may be prescribed 'when required' during acute schizophrenia
Clozapine with SSRIs (fluoxetine, fluvoxamine, paroxetine, sertraline)	Increased levels of clozapine and also increased risk of serotonin syndrome as both drugs increase serotonergic neurotransmission	• Dose of clozapine may require adjustment • This combination may be beneficial and is used commonly • Citalopram does not appear to interact
Haloperidol with fluvoxamine or quinidine	Risk of increased haloperidol levels	The dose of haloperidol may require adjustment
Haloperidol with indometacin	Severe drowsiness and confusion	Avoid combination or monitor closely
Haloperidol or phenothiazines with tobacco or cannabis smoke	Reduced levels	Smokers may require an increased dose of haloperidol and chlorpromazine or a reduced dose on cessation of smoking
Conventional antipsychotics (butyrophenones, phenothiazines and thioxanthenes) with antimuscarinics	Additive antimuscarinic effects (Chapter 5) with the risk of rare but serious effects including: • heat stroke • severe constipation • paralytic ileus • psychosis • reduced efficacy of antipsychotic treatment due to reduced plasma levels	• Concurrent use may be beneficial • Monitor for signs of antimuscarinic effects (see text) and consider risk factors such as exposure to hot and humid conditions, polypharmacy, high doses and/or impaired renal or hepatic function
Chlorpromazine and other antipsychotics with lithium	• Reduced levels of chlorpromazine • Risk of severe extrapyramidal effects and neurotoxicity	• Dose adjustment of chlorpromazine may be required • Severe side-effects are rare but monitoring for these is important
Phenothiazines with trazodone	Severe hypotension	Additive hypotensive effects. Consider patients at increased risk such as those taking antihypertensive medication

Continued

Table 26.4   Continued

Drugs	Consequences	Comments
Phenothiazines with TCAs	• Increased TCA levels and possibly phenothiazine levels • Increased risk of tardive dyskinesia, which may be caused and masked by elevated levels of either or both drugs	• This combination is often used but the safety of coprescribing is not certain • For a discussion of effects on the QT interval, see text • Additional risk factors include high doses and polypharmacy
Pimozide with clarithromycin	Increased levels of pimozide	Increased risk of cardiotoxicity. Consider also use with other drugs known to prolong the QT interval (Chapter 5)
Sertindole interactions (e.g. cimetidine, fluoxetine, paroxetine or QT-prolonging drugs: see text)	Risk of cardiotoxicity with increased levels and/or those that prolong the QT interval	Sertindole was withdrawn in 1998 as a result of cardiotoxicity but has recently been reintroduced for restricted indications (see text)
Sertindole with carbamazepine or phenytoin	Reduced levels of sertindole	Increased dose may be required.
Thioridazine with phenylpropanolamine	Risk of fatal cardiac arrhythmia	Pseudoephedrine may produce an adrenaline (epinephrine)-like mechanism leading to ventricular tachycardia and should therefore be avoided with thioridazine and other drugs which prolong the QT interval (Chapter 5)

SSRIs, selective serotonin reuptake inhibitors; TCAs, tricyclic antidepressants.

popular choice due to reduced extrapyramidal effects compared with other phenothiazines and prior to the introduction of the atypical antipsychotics. Low doses of chlorpromazine or haloperidol are occasionally prescribed for short-term treatment. Alternatively, olanzapine or risperidone are used but these are unlicensed indications. The underlying cause of these symptoms must be investigated.

Renal impairment

Lower doses of antipsychotics may be required in severe renal impairment, due to increased cerebral sensitivity. Lower doses of clozapine, quetiapine, risperidone or olanzapine are required in mild to moderate renal impairment

with avoidance of clozapine in severe impairment. Sulpiride should be avoided in moderate renal impairment or lower doses used if essential.

Hepatic impairment

All antipsychotics have the potential to precipitate coma in patients with hepatic disease (Chapter 10). Phenothiazines are hepatotoxic. Lower doses of clozapine, risperidone, quetiapine or olanzapine may be appropriate with regular monitoring of liver function.

Pregnancy and breast-feeding

Phenothiazines and butyrophenones tend to be preferred and in particular chlorpromazine, trifluoperazine or haloperidol, due to greater experience of use during pregnancy. Depot preparations are avoided unless compliance is a significant problem. Treatment is assessed according to risk versus benefit. There is evidence of neonatal toxicity during the third trimester. Symptoms observed in the fetus include tremor, increased muscle tone, abnormal movements and feeding difficulties. Antipsychotics such as chlorpromazine, trifluoperazine or haloperidol or possibly flupentixol may be continued with caution during breast-feeding as necessary but the infant should be monitored for adverse effects such as oversedation.

Over-the-counter considerations

Patients may request supplements of polyunsaturated fatty acids such as evening primrose oil for symptoms of schizophrenia. Preliminary evidence supports the use of evening primrose oil, which may improve symptoms and does not appear to cause adverse effects (Joy *et al.*, 2002). Drug interactions with decongestant preparations containing phenylpropanolamine are given in Table 26.4.

Counselling

Recent guidance issued by NICE (2002) emphasises the importance of providing 'an atmosphere of hope and optimism' for patients and carers and forming 'a supportive and empathic relationship' with them. Reassurance should be given that drug treatment is effective and, with adequate support, the patient should be given the opportunity to return to employment if desired. Pharmacists have key roles in empathic support and the provision of information relating to treatment as necessary.

General lifestyle advice (Chapter 3) should be given due to the risk of weight gain, diabetes mellitus and cardiac effects with antipsychotics. Alcohol or drug misuse may exacerbate schizophrenia and should therefore be avoided and patients referred for additional support if necessary.

Compliance with antipsychotic medication is a common problem due to side-effects as described above and there may initially be a lack of insight, resulting in patients not recognising that they are ill. The importance of maintenance treatment in preventing relapse should be emphasised and patients or carers informed that intermittent therapy is not recommended. The side-effects and particularly movement disorders should also be explained when treatment is initiated. Patients should be advised that treatment requires gradual withdrawal and should therefore not be stopped without the advice of their doctor.

Changing treatment

Patients should be warned about the risk of relapse and a transient worsening of side-effects when changing to an alternative antipsychotic. It is important to reinforce that adherence to treatment should improve symptoms with fewer side-effects over time. However, if symptoms persist, an alternative antipsychotic may be tried.

Blood dyscrasias

Patients should be advised to report symptoms of infection such as sore throat and pyrexia, particularly when prescribed clozapine.

Weight gain

Weight gain and the onset of type 2 diabetes should be monitored, particularly in patients prescribed chlorpromazine, sertindole, risperidone, olanzapine or clozapine and also in patients at risk, such as those with obesity. When initiating treatment, it is useful to reinforce a healthy diet and exercise (Chapter 3). Urinary glucose should be monitored.

Sexual effects

Counselling at the onset of treatment may help reduce the effect on relationships and quality of life. The importance of compliance should be stressed due to the risk of relapse, and the patient encouraged to discuss problematic effects as they occur. Patients should also be advised to discuss a planned pregnancy.

Antimuscarinic effects

Patients should be warned of antimuscarinic effects, including dry mouth and eyes, blurred vision and constipation. Artificial saliva (e.g. Luborant) or sugar-free boiled sweets, artificial tears or laxatives should be prescribed as necessary. Coprescribing with other drugs having antimuscarinic activity may increase the risk of these effects and particularly severe constipation (risk of paralytic ileus and obstruction, particularly with clozapine), heat stroke (Chapter 5) and psychosis. Patients should be advised of the importance of maintaining regular fluid intake, particularly in hot or humid conditions, due to the increased risk of heat stroke. There is also a risk of hypothermia during cold weather, due to poor temperature regulation.

Cardiac effects

Symptoms suggestive of arrhythmias should be explained and reporting encouraged. For example, patients may become aware of palpitations and/or an altered pulse rate. Prescribers should monitor patients for these symptoms and particularly those at risk (discussed above). Blood pressure should be monitored as hypotension may occur, particularly when treatment is initiated.

Drowsiness (all antipsychotics and particularly chlorpromazine)

General counselling should be to warn the patient about drowsiness and the effect on driving and operating machinery. This may be particularly prevalent when treatment is initiated.

Photosensitivity

Photosensitivity may occur, particularly with chlorpromazine and therefore exposure to the sun or sunlamps should be avoided. High-factor sunscreen should be applied when exposure to ultraviolet light is unavoidable.

Extrapyramidal symptoms

Patients should be advised about the risk of extrapyramidal symptoms, as these can be frightening (see above).

Tardive dyskinesia

Patients should be advised to consult their doctor urgently if they develop fine involuntary movements of the tongue, as this adverse effect is often irreversible.

Visual disturbances

Monitoring for visual defects is recommended with long-term thioridazine treatment.

Future developments

In addition to more selective receptor targets, longer-acting injectable atypical antipsychotics continue to be developed, with the aim of improving compliance and increasing treatment in the community and reducing the need to section patients under the Mental Health Act.

Practice points

General

- Prompt diagnosis of patients with psychosis may improve the clinical outcome.
- Lifestyle changes are important in the management of schizophrenia (see sections on Monitoring and Counselling).
- Regular screening for side-effects and particularly weight gain, sexual dysfunction, drowsiness and extrapyramidal effects (e.g. tardive dyskinesia) is important.

→

Practice points (continued)

Antipsychotics

- Starting treatment at a low dose and increasing gradually (ideally once a week or longer) reduces side-effects.
- Patients should be maintained on the lowest effective dose.
- Concurrent use of antipsychotics should only be used in the short term, for example, when changing to an alternative antipsychotic.
- The dose for intramuscular injection is lower than the oral dose, due to the absence of first-pass metabolism by hepatic enzymes.
- Withdrawal should be gradual following long-term treatment with antipsychotics, because of the risk of withdrawal symptoms and possible relapse.
- Treatment should be withdrawn in the presence of early symptoms suggestive of tardive dyskinesia, as this is usually irreversible.
- When the patient is stabilised on an antipsychotic, the dosage interval may be reduced to once-daily administration as these drugs have a long half-life.
- Suspensions of thioridazine should not be diluted but some may be mixed together to provide an intermediate strength.
- It should be noted that the use of antipsychotic doses greater than the recommended limit constitutes use outside the product licence and increases the risk of side-effects without any improvement in symptom control. Alternatives include switching to another antipsychotic. The duration of use of high doses should be limited and reviewed regularly. It is recommended that the dose be reduced if no improvement is observed after 3 months (advice from the Royal College of Psychiatrists reported in the *British National Formulary*, vol. 44).

 CASE STUDIES

Case 1
40-year-old male patient presents with worsening auditory hallucinations associated with messages he feels are being given to him by characters in a television soap opera. He recognises these symptoms and consults his general practitioner (GP) urgently according to previous advice. He is currently taking trifluoperazine 5 mg daily. He has been stable on this treatment for 20 years.

What action do you take?

- A short-term increase in his dose to 15 mg daily may control his symptoms until the period of stress has passed. Further increases (consider divided dosing) can be made at intervals of 3 days according to response. The dose can then be reviewed, particularly if side-effects become troublesome. It may be useful to remind him about possible side-effects and to discuss these if they become problematic. This case represents the benefits of education as the patient has control of his condition, helped by the support of his GP.

Case 2
The police arrest a 22-year old male due to his involvement in a fight. He becomes uncommunicative and fails to cooperate. A friend at the scene comments that he has been concerned about his

continued

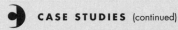

CASE STUDIES (continued)

friend for some time as he recently lost his job and became uninterested in his appearance. He mentioned that aliens were laughing at him and told him that a group of men were planning to attack him before he started the fight. He was not provoked.

Which symptoms are typical of schizophrenia?

- This patient has negative symptoms, including lack of communication and loss of interest in his appearance. These may be the first symptoms to occur in schizophrenia and may also include a loss of interest in previous activities and relationships. Positive symptoms include hallucinations, paranoia and thought disorder.

What is the likely treatment for this patient?

- If the patient continues to be aggressive, he may be given haloperidol in the short term, possibly with an antimuscarinic agent 'when required' for the short-term prevention of extrapyramidal effects. He is likely to be prescribed an atypical antipsychotic. The misuse of drugs such as cocaine should be investigated as this may trigger schizophrenia.

References

American Psychiatric Association (1995). *Diagnostic and Statistical Manual of Mental Disorders* (DSM-IV), 4th edn. Washington, DC: American Psychiatric Press.

Glen I (2001). Schizophrenia. Aetiology and pathophysiology. *Hosp Pharm* 8: 187–191.

Joy C B, Mumby-Croft R, Joy L A (2002). Polyunsaturated fatty acid (fish or evening primrose oil) for schizophrenia. *Cochrane Systematic Review* issue 3. Oxford: Update Software.

Lima A R, Weiser K V, Bacaltchuk J *et al.* (2002). Anticholinergics for neuroleptic-induced acute akathisia. *Cochrane Systematic Review* issue 3. Oxford: Update Software.

Mehta D K (ed.) *British National Formulary*, latest edition. London: British Medical Association and Royal Pharmaceutical Society of Great Britain.

NICE (2002). *Core Interventions in the Treatment and Management of Schizophrenia in Primary and Secondary Care*. Clinical guideline 1. London: National Institute for Clinical Excellence.

Wahlbeck K, Cheine M, Essali M A (2002). Clozapine versus typical neuroleptic medication for schizophrenia. *Cochrane Systematic Review* issue 3. Oxford: Update Software.

Whitehead C, Moss S, Cardno A *et al.* (2002). Antidepressants for people with both schizophrenia and depression. *Cochrane Systematic Review* issue 3. Oxford: Update Software.

Further reading

Bazire S (2001). *Psychotropic Drug Directory 2001*. Wiltshire: Quay Books.

Glen I (2001). Schizophrenia. Review of antipsychotics. *Hosp Pharm* 8: 192–194.

Maclean F, Lee A (1999). Drug-induced sexual dysfunction and infertility. *Pharm J* 262: 780–784.

McGrath J, Emmerson W B (1999). Treatment of schizophrenia (clinical review). *BMJ* 319: 1045–1048.

Part G

Pain and palliation

27

Pain management

Pain is one of the most common complaints and impacts greatly on patients' quality of life, possibly leading to reduced mobility, insomnia and depression. Management of pain is complicated, particularly in the elderly, due to side-effects such as constipation; drowsiness with opioids and gastrointestinal bleeding with non-steroidal anti-inflammatory drugs (NSAIDs) with numerous drug interactions add to this prescribing challenge.

Acute pain is an important protective mechanism preventing or reducing injury by enabling rapid removal from harm. Chronic pain, lasting 6 months or longer, is not beneficial and is widely considered to be a disease.

Physiology of pain

The detection of pain occurs via nociceptive afferent neurons, mechanoreceptors and thermoreceptors, which transmit sensory information to the brain or dorsal horn of the spinal cord. Fast, reflex actions involve direct transmission to the dorsal horn of the spinal cord without involving the brain, prior to the defence or motor response. A detailed description of pain physiology is beyond the scope of this book but terminology in common usage is defined as follows:

- noci: a prefix denoting pain or injury
- nociceptive: describes nerve fibres, endings or pathways concerned with pain
- nociceptors: any receptor which responds to stimuli resulting in the sensation of pain
- thermoreceptors: receptors activated by heat
- mechanoreceptors: receptors activated by light touch
- afferent (sensory) neurons transmit impulses from the sense organs and receptors to the brain or spinal cord
- efferent (motor) neurons transmit impulses from the brain or spinal cord (dorsal horn) to various tissues in response to stimulation by the sensory fibres, leading to defence responses

335

such as muscle contraction to move away from the pain source

- nociceptive afferent (sensory) neurons: afferent fibres directly involved in the detection of pain. These are neurons with sensory endings in peripheral tissues. They are essentially bare nerve endings and are activated by mechanical, thermal or chemical stimuli. They may also set up local reflexes, such that stimulation may elicit a local response, for example, vasodilatation
- Aδ, Aβ and C-fibres describe different types of nerve fibre involved in pain transmission

Other transmitters of pain (inflammatory mediators, neurotransmitters and neuropeptides)

As described above, physical or chemical insults activate nociceptors resulting in neurotransmission to the brain and/or spinal cord. Inflammatory mediators, including bradykinin, histamine and 5-hydroxytryptamine (5-HT) produced by injured tissues, may modify the transmission of pain impulses. In addition, prostanoids, which do not produce pain directly, sensitise nociceptors.

Neuropeptides involved in pain transmission include the tachykinins: substance P (neurokinin-1), neurokinin A and calcitonin gene-related peptide (CGRP). These are released from sensory neurons and release inflammatory mediators such as histamine, 5-HT, leukotrienes and prostaglandins from mast cells. This is known as neurogenic inflammation. These inflammatory mediators sensitise nociceptive nerve endings, lowering the trigger threshold of the nerve to produce hyperalgesia.

Ultimately, the perception of pain occurs in the cerebral cortex. An emotional component from the limbic system is also thought to contribute and explains the subjective response according to psychological characteristics such as anxiety and depression.

Excitatory and inhibitory neurotransmitters

Pharmacological targets include receptors for neurotransmitters involved in complex spinal neural activity. These include N-methyl-D-aspartate (NMDA) receptors for the endogenous excitatory amino acid, glutamate. Anaesthetic agents such as dizocilipine, and the less potent ketamine, are NMDA channel antagonists. The neurotransmitters gamma-aminobutyric acid (GABA) and noradrenaline (norepinephrine) produce inhibitory effects. Adenosine is also thought to be involved, indicating a potential target for caffeine, a methylxanthine and adenosine receptor antagonist.

Opioids

Opioid receptors for the endogenous opioids (endorphins, enkephalins and dynorphins) are also involved in pain transmission and perception affecting both the brain and spinal cord. Activation of these receptors in the spinal cord leads to presynaptic inhibition and blockade of pain transmission.

Gate theory

The gate theory describes the modulation of pain signals either to prevent or enhance the signal received by the brain. Noxious stimuli activate afferent neurons, invoking a neuronal impulse to the spinal cord. This signal may then be inhibited or enhanced prior to its transmission to the brain. The pathways involved in the transmission of pain, together with pharmacological targets of analgesics, are summarised in Figure 27.1.

Types of pain

Pain is described as somatic, visceral or neuropathic according to its origin:

Somatic

Somatic pain is pain relating to the body wall but excluding the viscera. Pain tends to be localised and follows stimulation of peripheral pain receptors (nociceptors) in the skin and musculoskeletal system. Examples include osteo- or rheumatoid arthritis and myalgia.

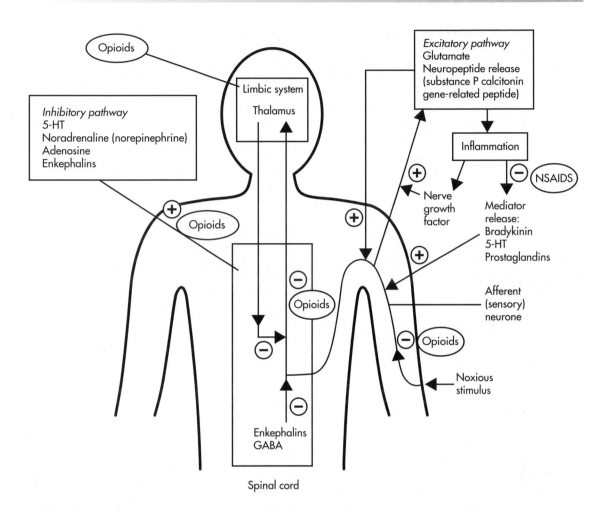

Figure 27.1   Pharmacological targets for analgesics in the pain pathway. Noxious stimuli trigger a neuronal response along sensory neurons to the spinal cord and brain. 5-HT, 5-hydoxytryptamine; GABA, gamma-aminobutyric acid; NSAIDs, non-steroidal anti-inflammatory drugs. Based on a figure in Rang *et al.* (1999).

Visceral

Visceral pain originates in the viscera, that is, the internal organs of the body, particularly the abdominal and thorax organs. Visceral pain is usually poorly localised and often referred to peripheral sites, for example, the pain associated with gallstones, myocardial infarction or appendicitis.

Neuropathic pain

As the name suggests, neuropathic pain results from nerve damage arising in the central or peripheral nerves. Neuropathic pain occurs as a result of disease affecting the sensory pathway and is independent of damage to peripheral tissue. This usually results from damage to neural tissue. Examples include postherpetic neuralgia, phantom limb, peripheral neuropathies (e.g. associated with diabetes), rheumatoid arthritis, trauma, central pain (following a stroke or in multiple sclerosis) and cancer pain due to the tumour impinging on nerves. Neuropathic pain occurs due to a lack of sensory input following sensory nerve damage and is often accompanied by allodynia, that is, pain caused by non-noxious stimuli (e.g. touch).

The pathophysiology of neuropathic pain is not yet fully elucidated but is thought to involve spontaneous activity in the damaged sensory neurons. The pain is described as burning, shooting or scalding. Sensitivity to noradrenaline due to the expression of alpha-adrenoceptors may develop, resulting in sympathetically mediated pain.

Clinical features

See Chapter 1.

Goals of treatment

The goals of treatment are to improve the quality of life and to delay disease progress by good pain control but with minimal side-effects.

Pharmacological basis of management

e.g. Aspirin, diclofenac, diflusinal, flurbiprofen, ibuprofen, naproxen, piroxicam

NSAIDs are amongst the most widely used drugs for a number of conditions associated with inflammation. In addition to their anti-inflammatory effects, most NSAIDs possess analgesic and anti-pyretic effects.

Anti-inflammatory effects

When considering anti-inflammatory effects, it is useful to consider the process of inflammation. Important physiological mechanisms combine to produce vasodilatation, increased vascular permeability and cell accumulation. A number of mediators produce these effects to different extents depending on the nature of the inflammation. These mediators include nitric oxide, leukotrienes, prostaglandins, and thromboxane. For example, the prostaglandins PGE_2 and PGI_2 produce vasodilatation and oedema, in addition to sensitisation of nociceptors, as described

above. Those mediators produced by cyclo-oxygenase (COX) activity, prostaglandins and thromboxane are the targets for NSAIDs. Production of the inflammatory mediators from membrane phospholipid and COX activity is detailed in Figure 27.2.

The inhibition of cyclooxygenase

The predominant mode of action of NSAIDs is inhibition of the COX enzyme, resulting in subsequent inhibition of prostaglandin and thromboxane production. Most NSAIDs are competitive inhibitors of COX, whilst aspirin irreversibly inactivates COX by acetylation. This action of aspirin is exploited for antiplatelet effects (Chapter 13).

The anti-inflammatory effects vary between NSAIDs, with ibuprofen being the weakest and indometacin and piroxicam the most potent. Ibuprofen is therefore not considered suitable for the treatment of acute gout. Most NSAIDs are antipyretic due to inhibition of prostaglandin effects, which disrupt the hypothalamic regulation of temperature.

The difference in anti-inflammatory activity of NSAIDs is small compared to tolerability by patients. In the treatment of rheumatoid arthritis, therefore, larger doses of 1.6–2.4 g daily of ibuprofen, which possesses only weak anti-inflammatory activity, are required. Longer-acting NSAIDs with more potent anti-inflammatory activity such as naproxen and piroxicam are useful in the treatment of chronic pain.

Analgesic effect
As described above, prostaglandins produced by inflamed tissue sensitise nociceptors to inflammatory mediators such as bradykinin and 5-HT. NSAIDs therefore produce an analgesic effect in conditions associated with prostaglandin production. The beneficial effect in headache may result from inhibiting prostaglandin-mediated vasodilatation of the cerebral vasculature. Actions in the spinal cord may also contribute to the central effect.

Adverse effects
NSAIDs are associated with many adverse drug reactions (ADRs: Chapter 5) but predominantly

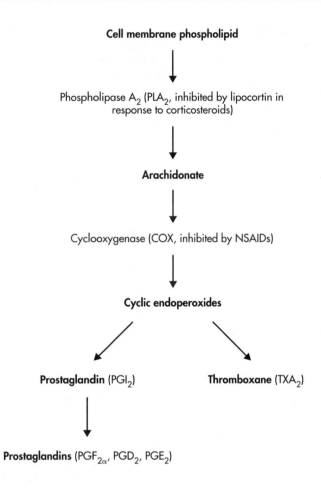

Figure 27.2   Production of the inflammatory mediators from membrane phospholipid and cyclooxygenase (COX) activity. NSAIDs, non-steroidal anti-inflammatory drugs.

gastric toxicity with a risk of haemorrhage (Chapter 7). Other ADRs include diarrhoea, nausea, rashes, urticaria, photosensitivity, sodium and water retention (with worsening of hypertension and congestive heart failure) and renal impairment. Renal toxicity may be due to inhibition of the effects of prostaglandins on renal blood flow, or due to nephropathy. Some NSAIDs may precipitate asthma in certain individuals (Chapter 20).

Adverse effects due to salicylates
In addition to the adverse effects caused by other NSAIDs, salicylates may also cause 'salicylism'

including tinnitus, impaired hearing and vertigo. This usually occurs only after chronic use of larger doses, which may also lead to compensated respiratory alkalosis due to increased respiration. Aspirin may also cause encephalitis and liver problems, known as Reye's syndrome, in children aged under 12 years and those under 15 years with fever and/or viral illness. This advice is regarded as too complex in view of the wide availability of aspirin through general sale and the Medicines Control Agency (www.mca.gov.uk/) has therefore recommended that aspirin should not be taken by any child under 16 years of age.

COX-2 inhibitors (e.g. coxibs (celecoxib and rofecoxib), etodolac, meloxicam)

There are two subtypes of COX, COX-1 and COX-2, which show some variation in distribution and roles. COX-1 is the constitutive or 'physiological' isoform, found in most tissues and in blood platelets. COX-2 is inducible and is produced in activated inflammatory cells and is, therefore, the COX subtype involved in the production of prostaglandins and thromboxanes involved in inflammation. The main anti-inflammatory activity of NSAIDs is therefore due to COX-2 inhibition. COX-1 inhibition is thought to produce toxic effects, including gastric irritation (Chapter 7). Drugs selective for COX-2 have therefore been developed and are thought to be more selective for inhibition of prostanoids associated with inflammation, rather than those involved in physiological regulation. It is becoming apparent, however, that COX-2 inhibitors may not be as free from gastric toxicity as first thought (Jüni *et al.*, 2002). A recent systematic review of the efficacy and safety of celecoxib compared with traditional NSAIDs for the treatment of osteoarthritis and rheumatoid arthritis reported similar efficacy for both treatments and an improvement in gastrointestinal safety and tolerability with celecoxib (Deeks *et al.*, 2002).

Paracetamol

Paracetamol is the first-choice analgesic for conditions not associated with inflammation. It possesses analgesic and antipyretic activity with similar efficacy to aspirin, but is not thought to exhibit significant anti-inflammatory effects. Its mechanism of action is yet to be fully elucidated but recent research has suggested that paracetamol inhibits COX-3, a novel COX variant, which is located in the brain (Chandraeskharen *et al.*, 2002). Inhibition of COX-3 may therefore explain the analgesic and antipyretic actions of paracetamol.

In normal doses, paracetamol is well tolerated; however, hepatotoxicity occurs with doses only two to three times the maximum recommended dose due to saturation of metabolism involving conjugation with glutathione. Toxic metabolites are produced, causing liver necrosis and damage to renal tubules. Early administration of acetylcysteine or methionine increases glutathione formation and therefore prevents liver damage. As few as 20 tablets can produce severe hepatocellular necrosis in the absence of symptoms in the first few days. Nausea and vomiting subside within 24 h but patients should be admitted to hospital urgently. Additional signs of liver toxicity include jaundice, abdominal tenderness (right upper quadrant) and hypoglycaemia. Patients at increased risk of liver damage include those taking concurrent enzyme-inducers (carbamazepine, alcohol, phenytoin, rifampicin) and malnourished patients.

Nefopam

Nefopam is used for moderate pain resistant to treatment with non-opioid analgesics. Adverse sympathomimetic and antimuscarinic effects limit its use. These include nervousness, tachycardia, urinary retention, dry mouth and blurred vision.

Opioids

The term 'opioid' applies to morphine-like synthetic and endogenous compounds. Synthetic opioids are used to treat moderate to severe pain, often visceral in origin. They are reserved for more severe pain due to their unwanted effects of drowsiness, constipation, nausea and vomiting, tolerance and dependence. High doses may produce respiratory depression and hypotension.

Opioid receptors

The effects of opioids are mediated by opioid receptors. To date, three subtypes have been identified and termed μ, κ, and δ receptors. The main pharmacological effects are mediated by μ-receptors and include analgesia, respiratory depression, euphoria, miosis (pupil constriction), physical dependence, constipation and sedation. The κ-receptors are thought to produce dysphoria.

Most morphine-like drugs have a high affinity for μ-receptors with lower affinities for κ- and δ-receptors. The potency of agents such as codeine, methadone and dextropropoxyphene is lower than that of morphine, resulting in reduced pharmacological effects even at maximum doses.

Opioid receptors are distributed throughout the brain and spinal cord. The administration of morphine inhibits nociceptive pathways in the brain and dorsal horn of the spinal cord and from the peripheral terminals of nociceptive afferent neurons. Effects on the brain also contribute to the euphoric effect and subsequent reduction in the psychological component of pain.

Weak opioids (e.g. codeine, dextropropoxyphene, dihydrocodeine)
Dihydrocodeine and codeine have similar moderate potencies, followed by dextropropoxyphene, which is a very mild opioid with a lower potency than codeine. Weak opioids are available in combination with paracetamol (co-proxamol, co-codamol, co-dydramol) but are no more effective than aspirin or paracetamol alone when given as single doses.

Strong opioids (e.g. buprenorphine, diamorphine, fentanyl, morphine)
Strong opioids form step 3 of the analgesic ladder (described below) and are prescribed for chronic non-malignant pain or in palliative care (Chapter 29). It should be noted that the risk of psychological dependence is minimal when opioids are used for severe pain and this is not a reason to withhold treatment.

Adverse effects of opioids
The most common adverse effects of opioids are constipation, nausea and vomiting and drowsiness. Respiratory depression is thought to result from reduced sensitivity of the respiratory centre (in the brain) to carbon dioxide, when higher doses of opioids are administered.

Nausea and vomiting Nausea and vomiting occur due to the effects of opioids on the chemoreceptor trigger zone in the brain. This is fairly common but usually transient. Antiemetics (Chapter 8) such as metoclopramide or prochlorperazine are often required when more potent opioids such as morphine are first prescribed. Dystonic (abnormal muscle tone, e.g. muscle spasms) reactions may occur, particularly in the young and elderly.

Constipation Constipation is common with opioids (Chapter 9) and coprescribing of laxatives is required. Bulk-forming laxatives may not be appropriate due to the reduced motility of the colon and, therefore, the reduced reflex effect of increased bulk produced by these agents. Stool softeners combined with stimulants are often used (Chapter 9). It should be noted that constipation occurs with low doses of codeine, including those used for cough suppression (Chapter 18).

Tolerance and dependence Chronic opioid use may result in tolerance requiring an increase in dosage. Alternatively, another opioid may be administered. Tolerance to analgesia, emetic, euphoria and respiratory effects of opioids occurs but that to constipation and pupil constriction is much less marked. Dependence may be physical, involving a withdrawal syndrome, or psychological.

Other
Other adverse effects of opioids include bronchoconstriction (induced by morphine due to histamine release from mast cells), hypotension, bradycardia, pruritus and immunosuppression (following long-term opioid misuse). Table 27.1 summarises some important properties of opioids.

Tramadol

Tramadol exhibits opioid effects and also enhances the effects of 5-HT and adrenergic pathways. The use of this drug for moderate to severe pain has increased due to reduced opioid side-effects. Psychiatric reactions may however occur. The response of patients to tramadol varies considerably and the dose is therefore adjusted accordingly.

Local anaesthetics (e.g. lidocaine (lignocaine), bupivacaine, levobupivacaine and prilocaine)

Local anaesthetics inhibit reversibly the transmission of nerve impulses via blockade of voltage-sensitive sodium channels. Side-effects include agitation, confusion, tremors, convulsions and respiratory depression. Cardiovascular side-effects include myocardial depression, vasodilatation and subsequent hypotension.

Table 27.1 A summary of some important properties of opioid analgesics

	Comments
Opioids for mild to moderate pain	
Codeine	• Constipating when used long-term • Laxatives should be prescribed for all patients prescribed regular codeine
Dextropropoxyphene	• Less potent than codeine • Combination products with paracetamol (co-proxamol) increase the danger of overdose due to respiratory depression added to hepatotoxicity of paracetamol • Combination products with paracetamol or aspirin are not proven to be more effective than single doses of these agents used alone
Dihydrocodeine	Nausea and vomiting increase with higher doses
Opioids for moderate to severe pain	
Alfentanil, fentanyl and remifentanil	• Injections used for intraoperative analgesia • Fentanyl patch used in palliative care (Chapter 29)
Buprenorphine	• Partial agonist at opioid receptors and therefore precipitates withdrawal symptoms in patients dependent on other opioids. This may result in breakthrough pain in patients changing from other opioids during treatment for pain • Longer duration of action, with the sublingual preparation producing analgesia for 6–8 h
Dextromoramide (Palfium)	Shorter duration of action than morphine and less sedating
Diamorphine (heroin)	Less nausea and hypotension than with morphine
Dipipanone (Diconal)	• Contains cyclizine and therefore not recommended in palliative care (see Cyclimorph, Chapter 29) • Less sedating than morphine
Meptazinol (Meptid)	• Lower incidence of respiratory depression • Rapid onset of action, 15 min
Methadone	• Less sedating than morphine • Long half-life and may therefore accumulate with repeated doses
Oxycodone	• Similar to morphine • Used in palliative care (Chapter 29)
Pethidine	• Rapid onset of action but short-acting and therefore not recommended for chronic pain • Less constipating than morphine but less potent analgesic
Tramadol	• Fewer opioid side-effects, including reduced potential for addiction • May cause adverse psychiatric effects such as hallucinations and confusion

Tricyclic antidepressants – see Chapter 23

The pyschotropic effects of antidepressants may be of benefit for pain in patients with anxiety and depression. Tricyclic antidepressants (TCAs) also possess analgesic activity independent of these pyschotropic effects. Indeed, the analgesic effect tends to occur at lower doses than used for depression. The mechanism is largely unclear but may involve inhibition of spinal neurons in pain pathways by increasing noradrenaline and 5-HT concentrations in inhibitory pathways. TCAs may also block sodium channels and they are also NMDA-receptor antagonists.

Anticonvulsants – see Chapter 22

Anticonvulsants such as carbamazepine, sodium valproate or phenytoin stabilise neuronal membranes. They are particularly useful, therefore, to relieve neuropathic pain.

Carbamazepine is widely used for neuropathic pain, including diabetic neuropathy. Its use may be limited by dose-related side-effects (Chapter 22). Phenytoin may be used as an alternative but consideration should be given to zero-order pharmacokinetics (Chapter 6). It may take 3–4 weeks to reach steady state if loading doses are not used. Lamotrigine is also increasingly being used for neuropathic pain. Although the mechanism of action is unclear, the anticonvulsants are believed to block sodium channels, suppressing neuronal discharge at sites of injury. The anticonvulsant gabapentin also has a role in the management of neuropathic pain but its mechanism of action is less clear and may involve altering GABAergic or calcium channel function.

Caffeine

Caffeine is added to a number of over-the-counter (OTC) preparations with the claim that it increases the analgesic effect of drugs such as paracetamol and aspirin. There is little evidence to support this and the regular use of these preparations may lead to chronic daily headache (see below) and be mildly habit-forming. The alerting effect of caffeine may also be a disadvantage.

Counterirritants

Aδ and C-fibres transmit pain signals to the dorsal horn of the spinal cord. These signals may be modulated by Aβ-fibres, thereby preventing transmission to the brain. This explains the effect of counterirritants such as menthol and capsaicin and/or rubbing, which activate Aβ-fibres and provide relief from pain caused by activation of C-fibres.

Cannabinoids

Although not licensed for pain management, there is good evidence that cannabinoids may exert analgesic effects both through inhibition of synaptic transmission at the spinal level and also at higher centres. Analogous to the opioid story, endogenous cannabinoids such as anandamide have been identified and may play a role in endogenous pain relief. Patients with certain chronic conditions such as multiple sclerosis appear to gain effective pain relief from canna-

binoids. Current aims are to produce routes of administration which do not involve smoking and to identify cannabinoids with analgesic but without psychoactive properties.

Chronic pain and central sensitisation

Dosing 'when required' is not appropriate in the treatment of chronic pain due to the principle of central sensitisation. This phenomenon also explains the benefit of administration of opioids prior to surgery. Following damage to peripheral tissue, spinal neurons exhibit hyperresponsiveness to impulses from afferent neurons. This results in an increased perception of a similar intensity of pain. Therefore, if chronic pain recurs, it may be difficult to regain pain control due to the reduced threshold of the spinal neurons. Higher doses may be required to regain pain control. Maintenance treatment also removes the psychological component of fear and a dose reduction may then be possible.

Medication overuse headache

Medication overuse headache (MOH) is a common subtype of chronic daily headache (CDH). It may be caused by a withdrawal effect following the chronic use of analgesic preparations and results in a vicious circle whereby analgesic administration is continued. It is becoming increasingly recognised as a problem associated with the overuse of analgesics in the treatment of headache. Inappropriate use of OTC analgesia is a particular problem due to the widespread availability of analgesics such as paracetamol, aspirin and ibuprofen from supermarkets and pharmacies.

MOH may follow the regular daily use of simple analgesics such as paracetamol, NSAIDs (more than four times per week), opioids or ergotamine more often than twice a week (Silberstein and Young, 1995). Compound preparations containing caffeine or sympathomimetics may also contribute to MOH. Health professionals should be aware of the problem in patients presenting with chronic headache. The suspected causative drug should be withdrawn gradually and the patient monitored for improvement.

A recent study reported the occurrence of MOH due to excessive use of triptans. A critical number of dosages was reported as 10 single doses per month, above which MOH included a migraine-like daily headache or an increase in frequency of migraine attacks. It was recommended that, on suspicion of triptan-induced MOH, the drug should be withdrawn temporarily (Limmroth *et al.*, 2002).

Drug choice

The World Health Organization (1996) recommends that effective analgesia is given 'by the mouth, by the clock and by the ladder'. That is, the oral route is preferred for drug administration if possible and analgesia should be given regularly rather than 'when required'. The analgesic ladder starts with simple analgesics such as paracetamol or ibuprofen and progresses to mild and then strong opioids. Adjuncts including simple analgesics or pyschotropic agents may be added at any stage. Patients are then reviewed regularly and treatment stepped up or down as appropriate. In summary, the steps comprising the analgesic ladder are as follows:

Step 1: (Mild): simple non-opioid analgesics such as paracetamol or NSAIDs

Step 2: (Moderate): opioids for mild to moderate pain, such as codeine or dihydrocodeine, with or without a non-opioid

Step 3: (Severe): opioids such as morphine for moderate to severe pain, with or without a non-opioid

Adjunct analgesics such as TCAs or anticonvulsants may be added at any step.

Paracetamol

Paracetamol is a common first-line agent, particularly for elderly patients, due to the reduced side-effect profile and fewer drug interactions. The main problem of paracetamol use is life-threatening hepatotoxicity in overdose.

NSAIDs

Aspirin is indicated for the treatment of headache, transient muscle pain, dysmenorrhoea and pyrexia. For inflammatory conditions, safer alternatives include ibuprofen (Chapter 7).

NSAIDs are indicated for inflammatory conditions such as back pain, soft-tissue inflammation and rheumatoid arthritis. High doses are required to achieve a full anti-inflammatory effect. NSAIDs may also be useful in the treatment of advanced osteoarthritis (Chapter 28).

It is important to note that it may take up to a week to achieve the full analgesic effect of NSAIDs, while the full anti-inflammatory effect may take up to 3 weeks. A poor response after this time should be followed by an alternative NSAID since their responses vary.

Topical NSAID preparations are widely available but their efficacy is uncertain and the benefit of topical agents over oral preparations has not yet been demonstrated.

Opioids

Mild opioids include codeine, dextropropoxyphene and dihydrocodeine and may be prescribed in addition to simple analgesics when these have failed to control pain when used alone. If this fails, more potent opioids may be introduced at step 3. This includes the treatment of chronic pain, which may not always be due to malignancy. For the use of opioids in palliative care see Chapter 29.

Compound preparations

The use of compound preparations containing paracetamol or aspirin with a low dose of opioid (8 mg codeine or 10 mg dihydrocodeine) is discouraged due to the lack of evidence, from single-dose studies, of efficacy compared with paracetamol or aspirin alone (Anon, 2000). Coupled to this is the difficulty of titrating individual drug doses and the risk of opioid side-effects such as drowsiness and constipation, particularly in elderly patients. Initial prescribing of more than one agent should be for individual drugs and then fixed doses of combination products used once control is achieved if compliance is a problem. If regular use of higher doses is required, patients may be advised that tolerance to most side-effects will develop, with the exception of constipation and pupillary effects. Elderly patients may require a lower dose of codeine such as 15–30 mg daily. The use of combination analgesics for chronic pain may be appropriate for these patients and may improve compliance.

An alternative regimen includes the use of regular paracetamol at 500 mg up to four times a day, with a single dose of up to 60 mg of codeine when required for more severe pain as a beneficial second step, although opioid side-effects may be problematic. This type of regimen limits the development of tolerance and dependence to opioids (Anon, 2000).

Topical preparations

Capsaicin is licensed for neuropathic pain but its use is limited due to an intense burning sensation, occurring when treatment is initiated. Capsaicin is the constituent of chilli powder and acts on vanilloid receptors to release and deplete neurotransmitters from sensory nerves, leading to counterirritation.

Nerve block

This involves the injection of local anaesthetics such as lidocaine close to a sensory nerve or plexus.

Steroids

Corticosteroids are used to treat pain associated with nerve compression, tissue swelling or raised intracranial pressure (Chapter 29).

Non-pharmacological treatment

Non-pharmacological treatments used in pain management include simple measures such as rest, cooling, compression and elevation, the use of transcutaneous electrical stimulation, warmth, physiotherapy and/or psychological support. Following a soft-tissue injury, rest, ice, compression and elevation (RICE) are recommended to reduce swelling and inflammation. Subsequent treatment may include the application of warmth, which aims to improve circulation of the affected area.

Transcutaneous electrical nerve stimulation (TENS)

Current is applied to the painful area via two electrodes placed approximately 2 cm apart, until paraesthesia is experienced. Aβ-fibres are stimulated, closing the gating mechanism in the spinal cord and therefore inhibiting the transmission of A- and C-fibres. The release of endogenous opioids may also be stimulated. TENS machines are battery-operated and portable, though not suitable for use while driving. They are particularly useful for chronic pain, postoperative pain and labour pain. Acupuncture is thought to work by a similar mechanism.

Physiotherapy

Physiotherapy may also include the use of warmth or electrical currents. This physical technique also encompasses massage, exercises, infrared and ultraviolet rays and manipulation of the affected joints or muscles.

Psychological support

Depression, insomnia, anxiety, fear, anger, boredom and social isolation all reduce the pain threshold. Conversely, sleep, rest, antidepressants, sympathy, diversion and understanding all raise the pain threshold. Consideration of psychological and lifestyle factors is an important part of pain management.

Specific conditions

The choice of analgesic is determined according to the cause and nature of the pain. The following section deals with specific conditions associated with pain.

Fever

Paracetamol is used first-line due to its tolerability. Alternatively, ibuprofen may be used for pyrexia and is often added to paracetamol treatment when pyrexia is difficult to control.

Headache

Treatment should follow the analgesic ladder, with paracetamol being a suitable first-line choice. Diagnosis may include tension, cluster headaches, raised intracranial pressure, CDH, arteritis in patients aged over 60 years or sinusitis. For a discussion of signs and symptoms and appropriate referral, see Chapters 1 and 21.

Migraine

See Chapter 21.

Dysmenorrhoea

Dysmenorrhoea or painful periods may be relieved by oral contraceptives and may resolve following a pregnancy. First-line analgesia is paracetamol and/or NSAIDs. Treatment is started a few days before a period to improve pain control of severe dysmenorrhoea (see Chronic pain and central sensitisation, above). More severe or secondary dysmenorrhoea, often associated with endometriosis, may also lead to vomiting and require treatment with an antiemetic.

Neuropathic pain

Neuropathic pain, including trigeminal neuralgia, postherpetic neuralgia and phantom limb pain, often responds poorly to conventional analgesics. Adjuvant analgesics such as TCAs or anticonvulsants are used. Dextropropoxyphene (60 mg every 6–8 h), methadone, tramadol and oxycodone are the most effective opioids and are administered after alternatives have failed. Nerve block or TENS and physiotherapy may be of benefit.

Amitriptyline is commonly the first-choice drug (unlicensed indication), at lower doses compared with those used for the treatment of depression, ranging from 10–25 mg at night and increasing to a maximum dose of 75 mg if required. Doses rarely need to exceed 75 mg daily and an effect should be observed in 3–7 days. Once again, the sedating properties of amitriptyline would be beneficial if sleep is disturbed. In the absence of a response, other TCAs such as clomipramine or maprotiline may be used. Gabapentin and topical capsaicin are also licensed for neuropathic pain and specialists may prescribe sodium valproate, phenytoin, ketamine or lidocaine. Corticosteroids may help pain associated with compression neuropathy.

Trigeminal neuralgia

Again, only a partial response is observed following treatment with opioids. Carbamazepine is used in acute trigeminal neuralgia and in extreme cases surgery may be required. Plasma levels of carbamazepine should be monitored at higher doses. Alternatives include oxcarbazepine, gabapentin, lamotrigine or phenytoin.

Postherpetic neuralgia

This results from acute herpes zoster (shingles) and is treated with amitriptyline or gabapentin (Chapter 32). Capsaicin or topical local anaesthetic may be used.

Concurrent disease

The following section summarises the effect of concurrent disease on the prescribing of analgesics.

Gastrointestinal irritation and ulceration

(Chapter 7)

Cardiovascular disease

As discussed in Chapter 13, low-dose aspirin has a major role in the prevention of myocardial infarction and stroke. However, other COX inhibitors may not be used in place of aspirin for this role. Furthermore, COX-2 inhibitors exhibit adverse effects on cardiovascular disease and are therefore contraindicated in chronic heart failure. COX-2 inhibitors have also been associated with an apparent increase in thrombosis, possibly as they may, unlike NSAIDs, inhibit the production of prostacylin but not thromboxane, favouring platelet aggregation (Cheng et al., 2002). The VIGOR trial (Bombardier et al., 2000) reported an increased risk of myocardial infarction in patients taking rofecoxib compared with those prescribed naproxen.

Table 27.2 summarises these and other considerations, including hypersensitivity reactions to NSAIDs. It should be noted that the cautions highlighted for opioids become less important in palliative care.

Drug interactions

Table 27.3 highlights some important drug interactions involving analgesics.

Pregnancy and breast-feeding

If possible, as with all drugs, analgesics should be avoided in the first trimester. If required for headache, pyrexia, musculoskeletal or dental pain, paracetamol is used first-line. The use of analgesics during pregnancy and breast-feeding is summarised in Tables 27.4 and 27.5.

Over-the-counter considerations

Many analgesic preparations are available OTC and pharmacists are ideally placed to monitor pain control, identify drug interactions (see above) and refer conditions such as suspected rheumatoid arthritis for prompt assessment and prescribing of higher doses of anti-inflammatory agents. Misuse and the risk of MOH may also be identified. The provision of lifestyle advice may benefit conditions such as gout, migraine and general painful conditions.

Simple analgesics such as ibuprofen and paracetamol are widely available from many outlets, including supermarkets. Accordingly, health professionals should always enquire about self-medication to ensure the correct use of medicines and avoidance of ADRs, for example, worsening asthma associated with overuse of NSAIDs (and possibly paracetamol) or the risk of gastro-intestinal toxicity with chronic NSAID use.

Counselling

General counselling should encourage patients to take analgesics if they are in pain. This may sound obvious but many patients are reluctant to take these drugs due to extensive publicity about side-effects. Conversely, patients who take chronic analgesia, including OTC preparations, require regular review of treatment and the underlying cause of their pain. For example, chronic use of co-codamol preparations for headache may be investigated for analgesia-induced headache or migraine.

Elderly patients may often report 'aches and pains' deemed to be an inevitable consequence of old age. Chronic pain is common in the elderly and may coexist with depression. Health professionals have an important role in identifying these patients and advising on appropriate treatment to enable pain control. Education, reassurance, support and patient counselling are particularly important in achieving good pain control. A pain diary outlining the influence of activity and analgesics may be useful in attaining good pain control. Pharmacists or carers may prepare monitored dosage systems as a memory aid for taking medication. These usually include four compartments per day so that all tablets are taken at the appropriate times.

Drug-specific counselling points are detailed below.

Paracetamol

- Paracetamol is one of the safest drugs at normal doses.
- Liver damage may occur after exceeding recommended doses and may take a few days or more to develop – help should be sought immediately.
- Take care not to exceed the maximum recommended dose by combining with other paracetamol-containing products such as OTC preparations for colds.
- Do not take more than two 500 mg tablets at a time.
- 4–6 h should be left between doses.
- Do not take more than eight 500 mg tablets in 24 h.

NSAIDs

- Patients should report symptoms of indigestion, wheezing or rashes immediately.

Table 27.2   Effects of concurrent conditions on drug choice

Condition	Drug implicated	Comments
Chronic heart failure	NSAIDs, including COX-2 inhibitors	• May cause worsening CHF and fluid overload, due to sodium and water retention (Chapter 14) • An alternative such as paracetamol should be used if possible
Hypertension, oedema, renal failure, ischaemic heart disease and chronic heart failure	Effervescent preparations	• The sodium salt content of six effervescent co-codamol tablets is approximately equal to the recommended daily maximum intake of 6 g (2.4 g sodium). These preparations should be avoided, particularly by patients with renal failure or taking diuretics, as increased sodium intake may reduce the efficacy of these drugs • COX-2 inhibitors should not be used with low-dose aspirin, as any benefit of the former will be reduced • The combination of an NSAID added to low-dose aspirin should be avoided if possible due to the increased risk of gastrointestinal toxicity
Hypotension	Opioids	• Worsening of hypotension
Asthma	NSAIDs (chronic paracetamol), opioids	• NSAIDs are contraindicated if there is a history of asthma, angioedema, urticaria or rhinitis induced by previous exposure (Chapter 20) • Preliminary evidence indicates that long-term, high-dose paracetamol use may worsen asthma (Shaheen et al., 2000). However, Levy and Volans (2001) concluded that any deterioration of asthma was short-lived but that practitioners should be alert to the possibility of worsening asthma • Opioids should not be used during an acute asthma attack, due to the risk of respiratory depression
Colitis	NSAIDs	• May cause or exacerbate inflammatory bowel disease
Female infertility	NSAIDs	• Female fertility may be reduced by long-term treatment
Hepatic impairment	Paracetamol, opioids, NSAIDs	• Dose-related toxicity, therefore larger doses of paracetamol should be avoided • Avoid or reduce doses of opioids, due to the risk of precipitating coma • Risk of fluid retention with NSAIDs, and increased gastrointestinal bleeding (secondary to impaired clotting). Avoid in severe liver disease
Prostatic hypertrophy	Opioids, nefopam	• Increased risk of urinary retention

Continued

Table 27.2   Continued

Condition	Drug implicated	Comments
Renal impairment	NSAIDs (including topical preparations), opioids	• Use with caution, due to the risk of deterioration in renal function as a result of reduced renal perfusion, particularly in elderly patients and those with heart failure and cirrhosis. Additional risk factors include hypertension, diabetes and coprescribing of drugs excreted renally, such as ACE inhibitors, digoxin and lithium • Use the lowest effective dose and monitor renal function (Chapter 2) • Avoid NSAIDs in moderate to severe renal failure • The effects of opioids may be increased and prolonged in moderate to severe renal failure and so they should be avoided or their doses reduced
Thyroid dysfunction	Opioids	• Use with caution in hypothyroidism due to worsening of symptoms such as bradycardia and hypotension
Epilepsy	Tramadol, nefopam	• The CSM recommends the avoidance of tramadol in patients with a history of epilepsy • Nefopam should not be used in patients with a history of convulsions

NSAIDs, non-steroidal anti-inflammatory drugs, COX-2, cyclooxygenase 2; CHF, chronic heart failure; ACE, angiotensin converting enzyme.

• NSAIDs are best taken with or after food and not on an empty stomach.
• Diclofenac and indometacin have a tendency to cause dizziness and patients should be warned that caution is advised when driving.
• Enteric-coated and slow-release preparations should be swallowed whole and not chewed.
• Enteric-coated tablets should not be taken at the same time of day as indigestion preparations.

Tiaprofenic acid
• Report urinary symptoms, including increased frequency, nocturia, urgency, pain on urinating or blood in the urine and stop taking medication immediately.

Indometacin
• There is a high incidence of side-effects with indometacin, including headache, dizziness and gastrointestinal disturbance.

Topical NSAIDs
• Avoid contact with the eyes, mucous membranes, inflamed or broken skin.
• Discontinue taking if a rash develops.
• Wash hands immediately after application.
• Do not use with occlusive dressings.
• Avoid excess exposure of the treated area to sunlight as photosensitivity may increase.
• As absorption occurs, the same precautions with hypersensitivity to oral preparations should be observed, particularly when applying large amounts of topical NSAIDs.

Nefopam
• Urine may appear pink.
• Side-effects include nervousness, palpitations, dry mouth, blurred vision and other sympathomimetic or antimuscarinic effects.

Table 27.3   Some important interactions with analgesics

Interaction	Consequences	Comments
NSAIDs with ACE inhibitors	Reduced antihypertensive effect due to effects on renal prostaglandins. Increased risk of renal damage	Monitor blood pressure and renal function
NSAIDs (except aspirin) with lithium	Increased levels of lithium and possible intoxication	Avoid unless lithium levels are closely monitored and the dose adjusted as necessary
NSAIDs with warfarin	Risk of bleeding due to increased anticoagulant effects and/or stomach irritation	Normal doses of ibuprofen interact only rarely. Careful monitoring, particularly in elderly patients. Azapropazone is contraindicated
NSAIDs with alcohol	Possible increase in gastric irritation	
Paracetamol with warfarin		Paracetamol is the analgesic of choice for patients taking warfarin. However, long-term use of larger doses may increase the anticoagulant effect
Dextropropoxythene with warfarin	Rare increases in the effects of warfarin	Monitor, particularly at the start of treatment
NSAIDs with alendronate	Risk of severe oesophagitis	Avoid concurrent use
NSAIDs with corticosteroids	Increased risk of gastrointestinal bleeding and ulceration	'Steroid-sparing effect' of indometacin and naproxen may allow dose reduction of corticosteroids
NSAIDs with SSRIs	Increased risk of gastrointestinal bleeding and ulceration	
NSAIDs with loop diuretics	Antihypertensive and diuretic effects reduced or abolished	Ibuprofen, meloxicam and ketoprofen may not interact but monitoring is advised with all NSAIDs. Increased doses of diuretics may be required
NSAIDs with ciclosporin	Renal function may be reduced by some NSAIDs, resulting in nephrotoxicity and/or increased ciclosporin levels	Renal function should be monitored. Low doses of diclofenac should be used when newly prescribed
NSAIDs with methotrexate	Excretion of methotrexate may be reduced	Dose of methotrexate should be monitored closely
Colestyramine with diclofenac, ibuprofen, meloxicam, naproxen, piroxicam	• Reduced absorption of diclofenac and ibuprofen • Delayed absorption of naproxen (limited importance) • Increased clearance of meloxicam and piroxicam	• Doses should be separated by at least 2 h • The separation of doses may reduce but not abolish the interaction involving piroxicam and meloxicam
Tramadol with SSRIs/TCAs	• Small risk of serotonin syndrome • The CSM advises caution due to risk of convulsions (CSM/MCA, 1996)	Monitor
Opioids with alcohol	Enhanced sedation	

Continued

Table 27.3   Continued

Interaction	Consequences	Comments
Opioids with antibacterials	Rifampicin may reduce the plasma concentrations of methadone and possibly morphine	The dose of methadone or morphine may need to be increased
Opioids with antidepressants	The analgesic effects of morphine may be increased by clomipramine and possibly amitriptyline	This may be an advantageous interaction
Opioids with antiepilepetic drugs	Enzyme inducers may reduce the concentration of methadone	The dose of methadone may need to be increased
Pethidine with cimetidine	Reduced elimination of pethidine	Proton pump inhibitors or ranitidine are not known to interact
Morphine with metoclopramide	Increased absorption and enhanced effects of morphine	
Nefopam with anticonvulsants, TCAs and MAOIs	Nefopam may cause convulsions in susceptible patients. TCAs may reduce seizure threshold	Nefopam should not be used in patients with a history of convulsions. Nefopam may have sympathomimetic activity and should not be given with MAOIs
Pethidine with phenothiazines	Increased analgesia and side-effects	This may be used to advantage

NSAIDs, non-steroidal anti-inflammatory drugs; ACE, angiotensin-converting enzyme; SSRIs, selective serotonin reuptake inhibitors; TCAs, tricyclic antidepressants; CSM, Committee on Safety of Medicines; MCA, Medicines Control Agency; MAOIs, monoamine oxidase inhibitors.

Gabapentin (Chapter 22)

- Do not stop taking this medicine without the doctor's advice. Withdrawal should be gradual, over at least 1 week.
- Do not take indigestion remedies at the same time of day as this medicine.

Phenytoin and carbamazepine

See Chapter 22.

Opioids

- Opioids may cause drowsiness, therefore caution is required when driving or operating machinery.
- Patients should avoid alcohol.
- Opioids may cause constipation. Laxatives may be required with long-term treatment, preferably softeners and stimulants rather than bulk-forming agents.
- They may cause tolerance, requiring increasing doses during chronic treatment.
- Patients should avoid taking opioids regularly unless advised by a doctor or pharmacist, due to the risk of side-effects, tolerance and dependence.

Future

New drugs being investigated in the search for anti-inflammatory drugs with reduced gastric toxicity include nitric oxide-donating NSAIDs and dual inhibitors of COX and 5-lipoxygenase. These drugs target gastric and duodenal protective mechanisms by increasing nitric oxide levels and inhibiting 5-lipoxygenase activity.

Table 27.4 The use of analgesic drugs in pregnancy

Drug	Trimester of risk	Comment
Paracetamol		• Not known to be harmful • Used first-line, avoiding high doses and chronic use as a precaution
Aspirin	3	• May delay or prolong labour due to COX inhibition • Impaired platelet function and risk of haemorrhage
NSAIDs	3	• Ketorolac is contraindicated • Avoid during pregnancy unless benefit outweighs risk • If necessary, use lowest effective dose (usually ibuprofen first-line) and avoid high-potency NSAIDs such as indometacin • Use in late pregnancy associated with risk of closure of the fetal ductus arteriosus whilst *in utero* and possibly pulmonary hypertension of the newborn • Delayed onset and increased duration of labour • NSAID use has been associated with increased risk of miscarriage (Nielsen *et al.*, 2001) • Possible increased incidence and duration of bleeding in fetus and mother during delivery • No NSAID should be used after 32 weeks' gestation
Codeine, dihydrocodeine	3, particularly last few weeks	• Opioids may be used for moderate to severe pain • Long-term *in utero* exposure may result in neonatal withdrawal symptoms
Tramadol		Caution, as there is limited experience

Information derived from the *British National Formulary and Therapeutics in Pregnancy and Lactation* by Lee *et al.* (2000).
COX, cyclooxygenase; NSAIDs, non-steroidal anti-inflammatory drugs.

Table 27.5 Analgesic use during lactation

Drug	Comment
Paracetamol, codeine	Small quantities excreted into breast milk but they appear to be safe. Paracetamol is used first-line. Codeine may cause constipation in the mother or baby and colic in the baby
NSAIDs (ibuprofen, naproxen, diclofenac)	Excreted into breast milk in small quantities but appear to be safe
Aspirin	Avoid, due to risk of Reye's syndrome

Information derived from the *British National Formulary and Therapeutics in Pregnancy and Lactation* by Lee *et al.* (2000).
NSAIDs, non-steroidal anti-inflammatory drugs.

Practice points

General

- Try paracetamol or ibuprofen first for mild to moderate pain. Patient counselling regarding the correct dose and effectiveness of paracetamol may help compliance.
- Analgesic combination products are not recommended as these products prevent the titration of individual drug doses. In addition, many combination products containing milder opioids with paracetamol or aspirin are no more effective than either drug alone when given as a single dose. Combination products may however be appropriate for the treatment of chronic pain and/or for patients with compliance problems.
- Chronic pain management should be managed 'by the mouth, by the clock and by the ladder', according to World Health Organization (1996) guidelines.

NSAIDs

- The use of two or more NSAIDs is not recommended and this includes low-dose aspirin (Committee on Safety of Medicines/Medicines Control Agency, 2002). Low-dose aspirin should only be combined with another NSAID if absolutely necessary. Gastrointestinal protection with a proton pump inhibitor should be considered, particularly for elderly patients and when prescribing NSAIDs long-term.
- The benefits of COX-2 inhibitors are negated in combination with other NSAIDs, including low-dose aspirin.
- Allow up to a week to achieve the full analgesic effect of NSAIDs. The full anti-inflammatory effect may take up to 3 weeks at full doses.
- Aspirin should not be prescribed for children under 16 years due to the risk of Reye's syndrome.
- The use of NSAIDs to treat postoperative pain may reduce the requirement for high doses of opioid analgesics.

Opioids

- Avoid regular use of opioids due to tolerance, dependence, constipation and the risk of falls in the elderly. For severe pain, however, there is little risk of psychological dependence and the use of strong opioids is indicated (Chapter 29).
- Regular opioid treatment should be accompanied by laxatives.

 CASE STUDIES

Case 1

A patient complains that he is not having much pain relief with the co-proxamol you dispensed for him a week earlier for his osteoarthritis. He has been taking 2 tablets in the morning, as he doesn't like to take too many. He has not tried paracetamol as he says 'it's not strong enough for this condition'.

- A common misconception exists that paracetamol is effective to treat a headache or fever but little else. In fact, patients can be reassured that paracetamol is an extremely effective analgesic and relatively free from side-effects. This is a suitable first choice in osteoarthritis and should be tried for at least a week of regular dosing. As this patient has not been taking regular co-proxamol, it may be appropriate to try paracetamol 1 g q.d.s. alone for at least a week. He should be advised that he may need to take them regularly to control the pain.

continued

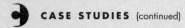 **CASE STUDIES** (continued)

- Co-proxamol is generally not recommended due to the difficulty in titrating the individual doses, the low dose of paracetamol (325 mg) and the risk of side-effects of dextropropoxyphene.

Case 2
Whilst performing a medication review, you come across the following record for an 80-year-old hypertensive female patient with 'painful knees':

Dosulepin 75 mg b.d.
Co-codamol 8/500 mg 2 up to q.d.s.
Bendroflumethiazide 5 mg o.d.

How do you respond?

- The first consideration relates to the high risk of constipation with all three drugs. It is very likely that this patient will require treatment with laxatives such as a combination of lactulose solution (up to 15 mL b.d.) and senna tablets (1–2 o.n. p.r.n.). The dose of bendroflumethiazide is high for hypertension and may increase dehydration and subsequent electrolyte disturbances without a further reduction in blood pressure. Perhaps the addition of atenolol could be considered? The TCA may not be appropriate for this age group and a selective serotonin reuptake inhibitor (SSRI) may be more appropriate (see Chapter 23). Successful treatment of her depression is an important component of her pain management.

    Her analgesia should be reviewed. For example, has she tried paracetamol alone at adequate doses? If so, this patient may be a candidate for a COX-2 inhibitor due to her age and particularly if prescribed an SSRI. Her blood pressure should be monitored for any worsening due to regular use of NSAIDs or COX-2 inhibitors. A COX-2 inhibitor can be added to paracetamol, avoiding the side-effects of the low codeine dose.

Case 3
The following repeat prescription is for a 46-year-old female.

Diclofenac gel 1.16% apply t.d.s. 100 g
Diclofenac sodium E/C tablets 50 mg take 1 t.d.s. 84
Fluoxetine 20 mg caps 84 take 1 o.m.

What should be the course of action?

- This patient is at risk of gastrotoxicity from the above prescription. SSRIs are associated with increased risk of bleeding events and using two NSAID preparations further increases this risk.
- The nature of her pain should be determined and pain control reviewed. Has paracetamol and/or ibuprofen been used? A proton pump inhibitor should be considered if the diclofenac and fluoxetine are continued. Review the need for both diclofenac tablets and gel due to increased risk of side-effects. Check for a history of peptic ulcer disease. Question the patient about signs and symptoms such as dyspepsia, gastric pain, dark stools and symptoms of anaemia.

References

Anon (2000). The use of oral analgesics in primary care. *MeReC Bull* 11: 1–4.

Bombardier C, Laine L, Reicin A *et al.* (2000). Comparison of upper gastrointestinal toxicity of rofecoxib and naproxen in patients with rheumatoid arthritis. VIGOR Study Group. *N Engl J Med* 343: 1520–1528.

Chandraeskharen N V, Dai H, Roos K L T *et al.* (2002). COX-3, cyclo-oxygenase variant inhibited by acetaminophen and other analgesic/antipyretic drugs: cloning, structure and expression. *Proc Natl Acad Sci USA* 99: 13926–13931.

Cheng Y, Austin S C, Rocca B *et al.* (2002). Role of prostacyclin in the cardiovascular response to thromboxane A. *Science* 296: 539–541.

Committee on Safety of Medicines/Medicines Control Agency (1996). *Curr Probl Pharmacovigilance* 22: 11.

Committee on Safety of Medicines/Medicines Control Agency (2002). *Curr Probl Pharmacovigilance* 28: 1–2.

Deeks J J, Smith L A, Bradley M D (2002). Efficacy, tolerability, and upper gastrointestinal safety of celecoxib for treatment of osteoarthritis and rheumatoid arthritis: systematic review of randomised controlled trials. *BMJ* 325: 619–623.

Jüni P, Rutjes A W S, Dieppe P A (2002). Are selective COX 2 inhibitors superior to traditional non steroidal anti-inflammatory drugs? *BMJ* 324: 1287–1288.

Lee A, Inch S, Finnigan D (2000). *Therapeutics in Pregnancy and Lactation*. Oxon: Radcliffe Medical Press.

Levy S, Volans G (2001). The use of analgesics in patients with asthma. *Drug Safety* 24: 829–841.

Limmroth V, Katsarava Z, Fritsche G *et al.* (2002). Features of medication overuse headache following overuse of different headache drugs. *Neurology* 59: 1011–1014.

Mehta D K (ed.) *British National Formulary*, latest edition. London: British Medical Association and Royal Pharmaceutical Society of Great Britain.

Nielsen G L, Sorensen H T, Larsen H *et al.* (2001). Risk of adverse birth outcome and miscarriage in pregnant users of non-steroidal anti-inflammatory drugs: population based observational study and case–control study. *BMJ* 322: 266–270.

Rang H P, Dale M, Ritter J M (1999). *Pharmacology*, 4th edn. Edinburgh: Churchill Livingstone.

Shaheen S O, Sterne J A C, Songhurst C E *et al.* (2000). Frequent paracetamol use and asthma in adults. *Thorax* 55: 266–270.

Silberstein S D, Young W B (1995). Analgesic rebound headache. How great is the problem and what can be done? *Drug Safety* 13: 133–144.

World Health Organization (1996). *Cancer Pain Relief, With A Guide To Opioid Availability*, 2nd edn. Geneva: WHO.

Further reading

Anon (1997). Topical non-steroidal anti-inflammatory drugs: an update. *MeReC Bull* 8: 29–32.

Blenkinsopp J (2002). Over-the-counter analgesics and the treatment of pain. *Pharm J* 268: 252–256.

Chapman V (2000). *Future Pain Drugs*. London: Smi.

Loeser J D, Melzack R (1999). Pain: an overview. *Lancet* 353: 1607–1609.

Skelly M M, Hawkey C J (2002). Potential alternatives to COX 2 inhibitors. *BMJ* 324: 1289–1290.

Silverstein F E, Faich G, Goldstein J L *et al.* (2000). Gastrointestinal toxicity with celecoxib vs non-steroidal anti-inflammatory drugs for osteoarthritis and rheumatoid arthritis: the CLASS study: a randomized controlled trial. Celecoxib Long-term Arthritis Safety Study. *JAMA* 284: 1247–1255.

Van Walraven C, Mamdani M M, Wells P S *et al.* (2001). Inhibition of serotonin reuptake by antidepressants and upper gastrointestinal bleeding in elderly patients: retrospective cohort study. *BMJ* 323: 1–6.

28

Musculoskeletal pain

Disorders of the muscles, joints and bones are a common cause of chronic illness and inability to work and have a considerable impact on quality of life. Musculoskeletal conditions include rheumatoid arthritis (RA), osteoarthritis, gout, muscle cramps and osteoporosis.

Disease characteristics and clinical features

Arthritis

Arthritis, literally inflammation of the joints, includes osteo- or rheumatoid types.

Osteoarthritis

Osteoarthritis is the most common form and is a degenerative disease of the joints due to wearing of articular cartilage with subsequent changes in the underlying bone. This may be secondary to obesity, fractures, dislocation, sports injuries, hyperparathyroidism, haemophilia, RA, gout and Paget's disease.

The pain of osteoarthritis differs from RA in that it usually occurs following exercise and at night. Any stiffness occurring in the morning tends to be transient. The pain may be present at rest and there is often tenderness. Joints of the feet (particularly the big toe), knees, hips, cervical and lumbar spine are often affected. Diagnosis is usually by X-ray of painful joints, revealing a narrowing of the joint space due to loss of cartilage and the presence of osteosclerosis (increased bone density), osteocytes and cysts in the bone. There are no systemic (extra-articular) features.

Rheumatoid arthritis

RA is a chronic inflammatory condition affecting the synovial lining of the joints. Disease progression leads to ligament damage and erosion of bone: joints become deformed and tendons may rupture. RA tends to follow a relapsing, remitting course and is progressive.

The assessment of presenting symptoms of pain (Chapter 27) includes the location of affected joints and timing of the pain, which is often worse in the morning and persists for an hour or more. The principal features include inflammation and swelling predominantly affecting the hands, wrists and knees. Symptoms progress to muscle wasting due to joint disuse, joint deformity and joint erosion. Extra-articular symptoms may also be present and include (Greene and Harris, 2000):

- Non-specific: tiredness, depression and fever
- Dermatological: nodules, palmar erythema (red palms), sweaty palms
- Circulatory: Raynaud's syndrome, pericarditis, myocarditis, vasculitis, anaemia
- Opthalmic: keratoconjunctivitis sicca (dryness of the cornea and conjunctiva due to reduced production of tears), episcleritis (inflammation of the episclera resulting in painful red eyes sensitive to light) or scleritis (inflammation of the white of the eye)
- Neurological: trapped nerves, peripheral neuropathy
- Pulmonary: lung nodules, pleurisy and pulmonary fibrosis

RA is an autoimmune disease with rheumatoid factors (autoantibodies against immunoglobulin G (IgG)) detected in serum. X-ray changes are also observed. The erythrocyte sedimentation rate (ESR) is elevated (Chapter 2).

Gout

Gout occurs due to the overproduction of purines, resulting in acute arthritis. The metabolism of purines leads to the production of uric acid, which forms urate crystals in joints, particularly affecting the big toe (podagra). This triggers an inflammatory response. Gout may also occur as an adverse drug reaction (ADR) (Chapter 5), particularly due to thiazides, which impair the excretion of uric acid. Disorders such as heart failure, hypercalcaemia and hypertensive nephropathy are also associated with gout.

Gout presents with inflammation and joint pain affecting the big toe and may also affect the ankles, knees, elbows, wrists and fingers. The skin

of the affected joint may flake after the initial onset of pain. The attack may resolve spontaneously after a few days or weeks. Laboratory tests reveal hyperuricaemia, although this is occasionally present with arthritic conditions.

Osteoporosis

Osteoporosis is a disorder of bone structure with a characteristic reduction of bone mass resulting in brittle bones at increased risk of fracture. Bone is constantly being absorbed by osteoclasts and new bone formed by osteoblasts. In osteoporosis, absorption exceeds formation, with reductions in bone matrix and therefore strength. Causes include oestrogen deficiency, particularly following an early menopause, and age-related degeneration of bone, declining from a peak in the 20s. There are hereditary and lifestyle components and the most common drug cause is corticosteroids.

Osteoporosis may be asymptomatic, being diagnosed following fracture. Patients presenting with a fracture resulting from minimal trauma, also known as 'low trauma' fracture, are treated for osteoporosis and further investigations may not be necessary, as management is the same. Bone-density scans (commonly dual-energy X-ray absorptiometry or DEXA scans) are useful for early diagnosis and are increasingly performed for patients with risk factors for osteoporosis as follows:

- early menopause (under 45 years of age, also prolonged secondary amenorrhoea)
- aged over 65 years
- family history of osteoporosis or low trauma fractures
- poor diet (lacking in calcium and vitamin D)
- low exposure to sunlight (reduced vitamin D)
- low body weight (body mass index less than 20)
- smoking
- excess alcohol intake
- low level of physical activity
- concurrent disease should be considered and treated (hyperthyroidism, hyperparathyroidism, osteomalacia or hypogonadism)
- drugs (corticosteroids more than 7.5 mg equivalent of prednisolone daily for 3 months or more)

Pharmacological basis of management

The management of musculoskeletal conditions predominantly involves the relief of pain and the reduction of inflammation. In treating osteoporosis, lifestyle factors are also important and treatment may include the correction of calcium and vitamin D intake. Additional treatments target the mineralisation of bone using bisphosphonates, antioestrogens and oestrogens. Bisphosphonates reduce bone turnover and oestrogens and antioestrogens target and reduce the resorption of bone.

The pharmacology of analgesics, including non-steroidal anti-inflammatory drugs (NSAIDs), cyclooxygenase-2 (COX-2) inhibitors and topical counterirritants, together with non-pharmacological options, is discussed in Chapter 27.

Osteoarthritis

Osteoarthritis involves joint degeneration and may be improved by lifestyle measures such as weight reduction and increased exercise. Paracetamol is used first-line, particularly in the elderly, followed by an NSAID with or without paracetamol. Topical capsaicin may provide relief. Advanced osteoarthritis may require full doses of NSAIDs. It should be noted, however, that NSAIDs do not alter the disease process and are mainly used for their analgesic effects. The benefits of NSAIDs are therefore compared to the risks, such as gastrointestinal toxicity (Chapter 7), and alternative interventions such as lifestyle measures may be preferred (Chapter 27).

Rheumatoid arthritis

NSAIDs are used for symptomatic treatment of pain associated with inflammation in RA and corticosteroids are occasionally injected locally into the affected joints, providing temporary relief. Disease-modifying antirheumatoid drugs (DMARDs) such as penicillamine, gold salt or antimalarials are used to suppress the disease process. These drugs are given for 4–6 months before a full response is observed. This may allow a subsequent reduction in the dose of NSAID. Sulfasalazine or methotrexate may be tolerated better than alternative DMARDs. It is also interesting to note that minocycline has been used to treat RA (American College of Rheumatology, 2002).

Disease-modifying anti-rheumatoid drugs

NSAIDs control the symptoms associated with RA but do not alter the disease progression and may even make it worse due to the increased availability of arachidonic acid as a substrate for lipoxygenase-mediated production of leukotrienes. DMARDs are therefore used to slow disease progression and include:

- gold compounds
- penicillamine
- sulfasalazine
- methotrexate
- chloroquine
- hydroxychloroquine

Their mechanisms of action are complex and are yet to be fully elucidated. Immunosuppressants such as azathioprine, ciclosporin and corticosteroids are also used as DMARDs.

Corticosteroids

These drugs are used in the treatment of RA, for example, when treatment with other anti-inflammatory drugs is unsuccessful. If long-term treatment is required, prophylaxis for the prevention of osteoporosis is required (see below). Courses of corticosteroids should use the lowest effective dose, for example 7.5 mg of prednisolone. This is sufficient to reduce the rate of joint destruction in patients with moderate to severe disease which has been present for less than 2 years. Prednisolone treatment is required for 2–4 years for beneficial effects on joint destruction, prior to gradual dose reduction to prevent long-term adverse effect. It should also be noted that the effects of reduced joint destruction persist despite a possible reduction in symptom control, which may occur after 6–12 months, and this does not necessarily indicate a higher dose of prednisolone.

Osteoporosis

Agents used for the prevention or treatment of osteoporosis include bisphosphonates, vitamin D derivatives, hormone replacement therapy (HRT), calcitonin and selective oestrogen receptor modulators (SERMs). It is also important that concurrent medication and other risk factors for falls are assessed in these patients and that preventive counselling includes advice regarding diet and exercise (see Counselling, below). For example, concurrent diseases that may increase the risk of falls include hypothyroidism, epilepsy, diabetes mellitus, Ménière's disease or cardiovascular disease (particularly with a history of transient ischaemic attacks or arrhythmias). Drugs associated with an increased risk of falls, particularly in elderly patients include:

- diuretics
- other antihypertensives, particularly alpha-blockers, and the concurrent use of angiotensin-converting enzyme (ACE) inhibitors with diuretics
- antipsychotics
- benzodiazepines, sedating antihistamines and other drugs with sedative properties (Chapter 5)
- alcohol

Bisphosphonates (alendronate, etidronate, risedronate)

Bisphosphonates reduce the risk of vertebral fracture (alendronate and risedronate have been shown to reduce the risk of non-vertebral fractures) by reducing the turnover of bone. These drugs are enzyme-resistant analogues of pyrophosphate and, by binding to hydroxyapatite crystals, slow dissolution. They also inhibit osteoblast-mediated resorption.

Vitamin D and its derivatives

Vitamin D and derivatives, together with parathyroid hormone, cytokines and calcitonin, are involved in the metabolism and mineralisation of bone. Vitamin D requirements are met through diet, metabolism in the liver and kidney and from reactions in the skin occurring in the presence of sunlight. The supplementation of vitamin D is partly dependent on the cause of deficiency, as follows:

1. Poor diet or malabsorption is treated with supplements of vitamin D_2 (ergocalciferol) which is formed in plants or vitamin D_3 (colecalciferol), formed in the skin in the presence of ultraviolet radiation. High doses (up to 1 mg or 40 000 units daily) of ergocalciferol are required by patients with intestinal malabsorption or chronic liver disease.
2. In renal failure, 1,25-hydroxyvitamin D_3 (calcitriol) or 1α-hydroxycholecalciferol (alfacalcidol) are given. Deficiency would otherwise result as these hydroxylated compounds are usually formed in the kidney.

Hormone replacement therapy

Both HRT and bisphosphonates are indicated for the treatment of osteoporosis. Oestrogens have a protective effect on bone by preventing bone resorption. Postmenopausal women may benefit from HRT prophylaxis for osteoporosis, particularly following an early menopause.

Tibolone

Tibolone possesses mixed oestrogenic, progestogenic and androgenic effects and is used for the prevention of hot flushes and bone loss. This is only given at least 1 year following the menopause because of problems with irregular bleeding. If the patient is to be changed from cyclical HRT, a withdrawal bleed is induced using progestogens, given until the withdrawal bleed has stopped. This minimises the risk of irregular bleeding during tibolone therapy.

Calcitonin

Calcitonin may be a useful alternative for the prophylaxis or treatment of postmenopausal osteoporosis when HRT and bisphosphonates are not appropriate. Following vertebral fracture, breakthrough pain resistant to analgesics may respond to calcitonin, given for up to 3 months. Calcitonin is a hormone secreted by the thyroid gland.

It acts to inhibit calcium resorption into bone and reduces reabsorption of calcium and phosphate in the kidney. An increased plasma calcium level stimulates endogenous calcitonin secretion.

Raloxifene

Raloxifene is an SERM used to treat osteoporosis. This is an analogue of tamoxifen, developed following the observation that, despite possessing antioestrogen activity, tamoxifen produces agonist-like oestrogenic activity in bone, as it is a partial agonist.

Prevention of osteoporosis

The first step in the prevention of osteoporosis is to identify patients who are at risk, as outlined above. Interventions such as lifestyle changes may then be addressed and the need for drug treatment considered. For example, calcium and vitamin D intake are corrected by supplementation and HRT

initiated for female patients particularly after premature menopause. Treatment is continued for 5–10 years for full benefit. This is a highly effective intervention for the prevention or treatment of osteoporosis. It should also be noted when prescribing HRT that:

- Women with an intact uterus should be given HRT containing a progestogen to reduce the risk of endometrial cancer.
- Following hysterectomy, a progestogen is not required.
- Oestrogens are contraindicated for patients with previous oestrogen-receptor-positive breast cancer.

When HRT is not appropriate (Table 28.1), bisphosphonates may be prescribed. It should be noted that disodium etidronate administration is alternated with calcium carbonate (Didronel PMO) as it can increase the risk of fractures due to reduced calcification of bone. Raloxifene is also being investigated for its role in the prevention of

Table 28.1 Some considerations of the effects of concurrent conditions on drug choice in musculoskeletal conditions

Disease	Drug(s)	Comments
Ischaemic heart disease (IHD)	Colchicine, sulfinpyrazone, HRT	• Sulfinpyrazone may cause salt and water retention and should therefore be used with caution • The CSM warns that HRT is not indicated for the prevention of IHD (Chapter 13: MCA/CSM, 2002)
Upper gastrointestinal disorders: dysphagia, oesophagitis, gastritis, duodenitis or ulcers	Alendronic acid and risedronate sodium	May cause or exacerbate these disorders (Chapter 7)
Delayed gastric emptying	Alendronic acid and risedronate sodium	Contraindicated
Peptic ulcer disease	Sulfinpyrazone	Use with caution
Gastrointestinal disease	Colchicine	Use with caution since colchicine may exacerbate all gastrointestinal disease
Hypocalcaemia	Alendronic acid, risedronate sodium	Contraindicated
Venous thromboembolism (VTE)	HRT, raloxifene	• HRT is contraindicated in patients with a history of confirmed VTE, active or recent arterial thromboembolic disease • Raloxifene also increases the risk of thromboembolism

HRT, hormone replacement therapy; MCA, Medicines Control Agency; CSM, Committee on Safety of Medicines.

osteoporosis. Further lifestyle interventions are outlined below (see Counselling).

Prevention of corticosteroid-induced osteoporosis

It is recognised that treatment with cortico-steroids equivalent to more than 7.5 mg of pred-nisolone daily for 3 months or more constitutes a risk factor for the development of osteoporosis. Such patients may benefit from a DEXA scan and may require treatment as indicated above, particularly in the presence of additional risk factors. Drugs with the best evidence to support their use for preventing corticosteroid-induced osteoporosis appear to be the bisphosphonates (Adachi and Papaioannou, 2001). The American College of Rheumatism (2001) recommendations include the use of calcium and vitamin D supplements for all patients taking corticosteroids.

Current recommendations by the British Society for Rheumatology (see Online resources, below) are that patients prescribed a 6-month course (or longer) of the equivalent of 7.5 mg of prednisolone daily should be offered treatment for the prevention of osteoporosis following the results of a DEXA scan. It is suggested that a DEXA scan revealing a T-score (number of standard deviations from the value of peak bone density of a 25–30-year-old woman) of –1.5 or less would indicate preventive treatment. American guidelines recommend scanning patients prescribed a course of corticosteroids equivalent to 5 mg of prednisolone per day for 3 months or longer and prophylactic treatment following a T-score of –1 or less (American College of Rheumatism, 2001).

Gout

The treatment of gout involves the use of NSAIDs, with the exception of aspirin, which reduces urate excretion and ibuprofen due to its weak anti-inflammatory activity. Additional treatment may include allopurinol, colchicine, sulfinpyrazone and probenecid.

Acute gout

Acute gout is treated with high doses of NSAIDs including diclofenac, indometacin, ketoprofen, naproxen, piroxicam or sulindac. Allopurinol should not be initiated during or within 1 month of an acute attack as it may prolong the attack. The manufacturers recommend that prophylaxis with an NSAID or colchicine be given for the first month of treatment as allopurinol may precipitate a further attack. Patients already taking allopurinol when suffering an exacerbation should continue treatment. Weight loss and dietary measures are also important (see Counselling, below).

Chronic gout

The long-term management of gout includes prophylaxis with allopurinol or colchicine (short-term only during initial treatment with allopurinol) and the reduction of inflammation by NSAIDs during an acute exacerbation.

Allopurinol Allopurinol is a xanthine oxidase inhibitor and reduces the synthesis of uric acid.

Colchicine The mechanism of action of colchicine in the treatment of gout involves inhibition of leukocyte migration into the joint by reducing the production of chemotaxins.

Sulfinpyrazone and probenecid Sulfinpyrazone and probenecid inhibit uric acid reabsorption by the kidneys, thereby increasing excretion.

Nocturnal leg cramps

Quinine salts are used for nocturnal leg cramps but are only effective in a small proportion of patients. For example, quinine sulfate or quinine bisulfate is given. It should be noted that quinine bisulfate 300 mg contains less quinine than 300 mg of quinine sulfate.

Concurrent disease

Some considerations are summarised in Table 28.1.

Drug interactions

Table 28.2 highlights some important drug interactions involving drugs used to treat musculoskeletal disorders. For interactions associated with NSAIDs, see Chapter 27.

Table 28.2 Some drug interactions involving drugs used in musculoskeletal conditions

Drugs	Consequences	Comments
Absorption interactions		
Alendronate with antacids and calcium supplements	Reduced absorption	• Separate the administration of alendronate from calcium supplements and antacids by at least 30 min
Penicillamine with aluminium or magnesium-containing antacids and iron salts		• Separate the administration of penicillamine by 2 h • Caution if iron is withdrawn when patients are stabilised on penicillamine, due to risk of toxicity
Allopurinol with theophylline	Increased levels of theophylline	There is limited evidence for this interaction but monitoring for signs of theophylline toxicity is recommended
Alendronate with NSAIDs	Risk of severe oesophagitis	Avoid concurrent use
Allopurinol with warfarin	Increased bleeding	This interaction is reported to be uncommon but monitoring is prudent
Calcium and vitamin D supplements or corticosteroids with thiazide diuretics	Increased risk of hypercalcaemia or hypokalaemia	• Thiazides retain calcium and therefore monitoring of plasma calcium may be required (Chapter 2) • Increased risk of hypokalaemia if thiazides are given with corticosteroids (Chapter 2)
Quinine with digoxin	Small risk of increased levels of digoxin	Monitor for signs of digoxin toxicity
Methotrexate with NSAIDs	Reduced excretion and therefore increased risk of methotrexate toxicity	• Increased risk with higher doses of methotrexate and/or impaired renal function • Careful monitoring is recommended
Methotrexate with corticosteroids	• Increased risk of methotrexate toxicity • Possible steroid-sparing effect	Monitor for signs of methotrexate toxicity or reduced efficacy of corticosteroids
Methotrexate with co-trimoxazole or trimethoprim	Risk of severe bone marrow depression	Avoid concurrent use or monitor full blood count closely
Penicillamine with digoxin	Limited reports of reduced levels of digoxin	Monitor for signs of reduced efficacy (Chapter 14)

NSAIDs, non-steroidal anti-inflammatory drugs.

Monitoring requirements

More detailed monitoring information is produced by the British Society for Rheumatology (see Online resources, below).

Penicillamine

A full blood count and urine (protein) should be monitored before the start of treatment, every 1–2 weeks for 2 months, every 4 weeks, and the week following a dose increase. In the presence of proteinuria, urea and electrolytes and 24-h urine are tested (Chapter 2).

Sulfasalazine

• Monitor differential white cell, red cell and platelet counts initially and at monthly intervals for the first 3 months.

- Liver function tests should be monitored monthly for the first 3 months.
- Renal function should be monitored at regular intervals.

Methotrexate (Committee on Safety of Medicines advice)

- Carry out a full blood count, renal and liver function tests before starting treatment and repeat weekly until therapy is stabilised, then every 2–3 months. See also Counselling, below.
- Treatment should not be started or should be discontinued if any abnormality of liver function tests or liver biopsy is present or develops during treatment. Abnormalities return to normal after 2 weeks and treatment may be restarted if appropriate.
- Risk factors for haematopoietic suppression include advanced age, renal impairment and concomitant treatment with a second anti-folate drug.

Gold

- Urine tests and full blood counts (including total and differential white cell and platelet counts) should be performed before treatment is started and before each intramuscular injection.
- During oral treatment, urine and blood tests are carried out monthly.
- The occurrence of blood disorders or protein-uria (repeatedly above 300 mg/L and without urinary tract infection) necessitates withdrawal of treatment.

Antimalarials

- Measure renal and liver function before starting treatment.
- Monitor visual changes.

Corticosteroids

Monitoring during treatment with corticosteroids may include blood pressure, urinary glucose, weight gain, bone density, visual changes and lung function.

Sulfinpyrazone

Regular blood counts are recommended.

Vitamin D supplements (e.g. ergocalciferol, calcitriol)

All patients receiving vitamin D supplements for the prevention and treatment of osteoporosis should have their plasma calcium levels monitored weekly when treatment is initiated and then at regular intervals and when presenting with nausea and vomiting, which may suggest hypercalcaemia. Breast milk from mothers taking vitamin D supplements may also cause hyper-calcaemia in the infant.

Disodium etidronate

Serum phosphate and alkaline phosphatase (and urinary hydroxyproline) should be measured before starting treatment and then every 3 months.

Alendronic acid and risedronate sodium

Hypocalcaemia and vitamin D deficiency should be corrected prior to initiating treatment.

Renal function

The following points are intended to highlight drugs to be used with caution in renal impairment:

- Allopurinol: dose adjustment is required in moderate to severe renal failure. There may be increased toxicity and rashes.
- Methotrexate: dose adjustment is required.
- Penicillamine is nephrotoxic and should be avoided if possible, or the dose reduced.
- Sulfasalazine should be avoided in severe renal failure. In moderate failure, there is an increased risk of toxicity, including crystalluria. A high fluid intake is therefore required.
- Antimalarials: use with caution.
- Alendronic acid or risedronate sodium is not recommended if creatinine clearance is less than 35 or 30 mL/min, respectively.
- Disodium etidronate should be avoided in moderate to severe renal impairment or administered at a reduced dosage in mild impairment.

Hepatic function

The following points are intended to highlight drugs to be used with caution in hepatic disease:

- Methotrexate: dose-related toxicity, avoid in non-malignant conditions.
- Allopurinol: reduce dose.
- Gold: avoid in severe liver disease.
- Antimalarials: use with caution.

Pregnancy

Table 28.3 summarises examples of issues associated with drug use for musculoskeletal conditions during pregnancy. For information regarding NSAIDs, the reader is referred to Chapter 27.

Over-the-counter considerations

The availability of analgesic preparations over the counter is discussed in Chapter 27. In relation to musculoskeletal disorders, pharmacists are ideally placed to refer conditions such as suspected RA for prompt assessment and prescribing of higher doses of anti-inflammatory agents and/or DMARDs. The provision of lifestyle advice may benefit conditions such as gout, migraine and general painful conditions. Pharmacists may also provide a screening service for osteoporosis as part of the multidisciplinary healthcare team.

Counselling

Patient counselling should comprise a combination of lifestyle factors, including advice regarding diet and exercise, together with information relating to drug treatment. Careful exercise is important to improve joint mobility, muscle strength, aerobic fitness and function, with the aim of promoting both physical and psychological health without worsening any fatigue or joint symptoms. This is also important in the elderly to prevent falls.

Osteoporosis

- Patients with risk factors for developing osteoporosis should maintain a high intake of calcium and vitamin D (milk, Cheddar cheese, Edam, yogurt, canned sardines and whitebait). For example, half a litre (1 pint) of semi-skimmed milk or 100 g (4 oz) of Cheddar cheese contains 700–800 mg of calcium. Supplements of calcium should be considered when a risk of deficiency is recognised, such as in strict vegetarians. Vitamin D should be included for the housebound and others with low exposure to sunlight.

Table 28.3 Some considerations of drug use in pregnancy

Drug	Trimester of risk	Comment
DMARDs	3	Sulfasalazine is the DMARD of choice in pregnancy
Bisphosphonates	All	Contraindicated
Colchicine	All	Contraindicated
Corticosteroids		• Assess risk of not treating. Commonly used in asthma and inflammatory bowel disease during pregnancy • Risk of neonatal adrenal suppression with long-term high-dose treatment
Antimalarials	All	Hydroxychloroquine and chloroquine (except in malaria prophylaxis) should be avoided in pregnancy and breast-feeding

DMARDs, disease-modifying antirheumatic drugs.

- Recommended intakes of calcium and vitamin D are as follows:
  - Calcium
    males 11–18   1000 mg daily
    females 11–18   800 mg daily
    adults 19+ years 700 mg daily
  - Vitamin D   400 IU daily
- Weight-bearing exercise should be emphasised, particularly to women in their 20s, and immobility should be avoided. Exercise programmes are useful for patients with osteoporosis in building muscle strength, general well-being and improving posture, thereby reducing the risk of further fractures.
- Patients should stop smoking and avoid excess alcohol intake.
- Excess dieting and vigorous exercise routines, which result in amenorrhoea, should also be avoided by women of all ages.
- Hip protectors may help prevent hip fractures in elderly patients.

Bisphosphonates

- Bisphosphonates may cause gastrointestinal disturbance, oesophagitis (particularly alendronic acid) and occasionally bone pain.
- Premenopausal women initiated on bisphosphonates should be counselled about the appropriate use of contraception.

Alendronic acid

- Alendronic acid may be administered as a weekly dose.
- Patients should stop taking alendronate if they develop symptoms of oesophageal ulceration, e.g. dysphagia, dyspepsia, pain on swallowing or retrosternal pain.
- Tablets should be swallowed whole with a tumbler full of water while standing and not immediately before rising or retiring to bed.
- Tablets should be taken 30 min before breakfast (and other medication) and patients advised to remain standing or to sit upright for at least 30 min. Patients should not lie down until after breakfast.

Risedronate

- Food, particularly calcium-containing food (milk), iron and mineral supplements and antacids should be avoided for at least 2 h before and after tablets are taken.
- Tablets are usually taken 30 min before breakfast (and other medication).
- Patient should remain standing or sit upright for at least 30 min. Patients should not take the tablets before rising or at bedtime.

Disodium etidronate

- Food, particularly calcium-containing food (milk), iron and mineral supplements and antacids should be avoided for at least 2 h before and after tablets are taken.

Vitamin D

- Excess intake may lead to hypercalcaemia, including symptoms of constipation, depression, nausea and vomiting, polyuria and polydipsia, weakness and fatigue. These symptoms should be reported to the prescriber.

NSAIDs

See Chapter 27.

Topical counterirritants (capsaicin)

See Chapter 27.

Quinine salts for nocturnal leg cramps

- Stretching the affected muscle regularly may reduce leg cramps.
- Take quinine salts for up to 4 weeks before improvement is observed.
- Reassess every 3 months.
- Caution is required as quinine is extremely toxic and has caused fatalities in children.

Allopurinol

- The affected joint should be rested.
- Avoid purine-rich food, including offal, anchovies, sardines, herring, mackerel, shrimps, crab, fish roes and meat extract.
- Reduce intake of protein.
- Maintain an adequate fluid intake of 2–3 L/day. This reduces plasma urate levels and prevents the formation of renal urate stones.

- Try to limit alcohol intake to 1 unit per day. Alcohol reduces the solubility of urate and beer contains high levels of purines.
- Gradual weight loss may improve symptoms. Avoid overeating.
- Take with or after food with plenty of water.
- Do not stop taking allopurinol unless advised by the prescriber.

Colchicine

- Dietary advice is as for allopurinol.
- Take until either pain is relieved or vomiting and diarrhoea occur, or a maximum dose of 6 mg has been reached (12 tablets of 500 µg).

Sulfinpyrazone

- Maintain an adequate fluid intake of 2–3 L/day.
- Take with or after food.
- Do not take with aspirin.

Penicillamine

- Penicillamine may cause nausea, therefore take 30–60 min before food or on retiring to bed.
- Do not take indigestion remedies or medicines containing iron or zinc at the same time of day as this medicine.
- The dose will be increased gradually.
- Penicillamine may cause loss of taste after 6 weeks' treatment, but taste will then return.
- Mineral supplements are not recommended during penicillamine treatment.
- Report sore throat, fever, infection, unexplained bleeding and bruising, purpura, mouth ulcers, metallic taste or rash to the doctor immediately.
- Penicillamine may cause rashes in the first few months of treatment. These should disappear when the drug is stopped, allowing reintroduction at a lower dose and gradually increasing. Later rashes may require cessation of treatment.
- Patients who are allergic to penicillin may also be hypersensitive to penicillamine, although this is rare.

Sulfasalazine

- Report unexplained bleeding, bruising or purpura, sore throat, fever or malaise. These symptoms are most likely to occur in the first 3–6 months of treatment.
- Sulfasalazine may cause rashes and gastrointestinal intolerance. Upper gastrointestinal intolerance is common at doses greater than 4 g/day.
- Contact lenses may be stained.
- Urine may be coloured orange.

Methotrexate

- Treatment is taken weekly. This is an important safety issue and all prescriptions for methotrexate that are not for a weekly dose should be queried.
- Folic acid supplement 5 mg weekly will reduce side-effects resulting from folic acid deficiency.
- Contact the doctor immediately with breathlessness or cough.
- Do not take over-the-counter aspirin or ibuprofen without the prescriber's advice.
- Pregnancy: avoid conception (this applies to males and females) for at least 6 months after stopping treatment.

Gold

- Report sore throat, fever, infection, unexplained bleeding and bruising, purpura, mouth ulcers, metallic taste or rash to the doctor immediately.
- Also report breathlessness or cough immediately.
- Rashes with pruritus often occur after 2–6 months of intramuscular treatment and may require cessation of treatment.
- The most common side-effect of oral therapy, diarrhoea, with or without nausea or abdominal pain, may respond to bulking agents or temporary dose reduction.
- Stop treatment at least 6 months before conception.

Antimalarials

- Report any visual disturbances.
- Do not take indigestion remedies at the same time of day.

Corticosteroids

See Chapter 20.

Practice points

- For NSAIDs, see Chapter 27.
- Methotrexate is given as a *weekly* dose.
- To reduce the risk of corticosteroid-induced osteoporosis, doses should be low and the course duration as short as possible. Long-term use of inhaled steroids may also reduce bone mineral density.
- Early intervention to prevent osteoporosis is important for patients prescribed corticosteroids since the greatest loss of bone occurs in the first 6–12 months.
- Prophylaxis for the prevention of osteoporosis should be considered alongside additional risk factors in patients prescribed the equivalent of 7.5 mg prednisolone or more daily for 3 months or more and particularly in patients aged over 65 years. Otherwise, a bone scan should be offered if treatment is likely to be continued for 6 months or longer.
- Patients suffering a fracture following relatively low trauma should be treated as for osteoporosis.
- Patients aged over 65 years and those with low exposure to sunlight may be advised to take supplements of vitamin D (400 IU daily). Calcium supplements are indicated if requirements are not met by the diet. Calcium and vitamin D supplements are recommended for all frail elderly people, including those at home, in hospital or in nursing or residential homes.
- The effects of calcium are less than HRT or other agents in the prevention and treatment of osteoporosis.
- Exclude vitamin D deficiency and secondary hyperparathyroidism in elderly patients with osteoporosis or osteomalacia.

 CASE STUDY

Case study
A 70-year-old woman with RA comes to ask you if you sell sulfur tablets for arthritis. She has just heard a radio programme talking about the benefits of sulfur for arthritis. She asks what you think and if you know of anything that might be better. You check her patient medication record which shows regular supplies of ibuprofen 200 mg t.d.s. p.r.n. and co-proxamol 2 tablets q.d.s. p.r.n.

What is the first issue you should consider?

- The fact that this patient is requesting additional treatment demonstrates poor pain control and this should be reviewed. The dose of ibuprofen is low for arthritis and may not be providing sufficient anti-inflammatory activity (Chapter 27). Co-proxamol may not be appropriate and the patient should be asked about any side-effects such as constipation and how often she has been taking her p.r.n. analgesics (Chapter 27).

Do you recommend sulfur tablets?

- This patient was particularly interested in alternative remedies but, as she is seeking advice from her health professional, information should be evidence-based. If she insists on taking alternative products such as sulfur tablets, you could offer to check the literature and/or the manufacturer for any known interactions or problems with her current medication. The opportunity should be taken to recommend a healthy diet as before (Chapter 3), and particularly a high intake of fish oils. You could recommend a fish oil supplement to help her joint pain and any morning stiffness (providing 1–2 g eicosapentaenoic acid/docosahexanoic acid per dose). This intervention would also benefit patients with concurrent cardiovascular disease (Chapters 12 and 13).

References

Adachi J D, Papaioannou A (2001). Corticosteroid-induced osteoporosis – detection and management. *Drug Safety* 24: 607–624.

American College of Rheumatology (2001). Recommendations for the prevention and treatment of glucocorticoid-induced osteoporosis. *Arthritis Rheum* 44: 1496–1503.

American College of Rheumatology (2002). Guidelines for the management of rheumatoid arthritis. *Arthritis Rheum* 46: 328–346.

Greene R J, Harris N D (2000). *Pathology and Therapeutics for Pharmacists*. London: Pharmaceutical Press.

Further reading

Anon (1997). Topical non-steroidal anti-inflammatory drugs: an update. *MeReC Bull* 8: 29–32.

Anon (1999). Prevention and treatment of osteoporosis. *MeReC Bull* 10: 25–28.

Cummings S R, Meltin L J (2002). Epidemiology and outcomes of osteoporotic fractures. *Lancet* 359: 1761–1767.

Delmas P D (2002). Treatment of postmenopausal osteoporosis. *Lancet* 359: 2018–2026.

Kanis J A (2002). Diagnosis of osteoporosis and assessment of fracture risk. *Lancet* 359: 1929–1936.

MCA/CSM (2002). *Curr Probl Pharmacovigilance* 28: 1–6.

National Institutes of Health (2001). Osteoporosis prevention, diagnosis, and therapy. *JAMA* 285: 785–795.

Seeman E (2002). Pathogenesis of bone fragility in women and men. *Lancet* 359: 1841–1850.

Solomon C G (2002). Bisphosphonates and osteoporosis. *N Engl J Med* 346: 642.

Online resources

www.nos.org.uk National Osteoporosis Society is a charity providing information for both patients and healthcare professionals. The main aims are to improve the diagnosis, prevention and treatment of osteoporosis (accessed 11 December 2002).

www.rheumatology.org.uk. is the website of the British Society for Rheumatology with access to latest guidelines, including recommendations for monitoring requirements (accessed 11 December 2002).

29

The cancer patient: cancer and palliative care

After cardiovascular disease, neoplastic disease or cancer represents the next largest cause of mortality, with more than one in three people developing cancer in their lifetime and one in four people dying as a result of it. The treatment of cancers is a highly specialised area and as such is beyond the scope of this book. This chapter describes the main pharmaceutical care issues involved in palliative care such as limiting the side-effects associated with treatment and optimising pain relief. In addition, the importance of prevention, screening, diagnosis, treatment and care as outlined in the *NHS Cancer Plan* (Department of Health, 2000) is discussed. This plan aims to lower the cancer death rate and improve survival rates and quality of life for both patients and carers.

Prevention, detection and screening

The primary aim is to reduce the risk of cancer by lifestyle changes such as smoking cessation and a healthy diet (Chapter 3) and improved screening. Cancers may affect many organs and tissues within the body: cancers of the lungs, skin, breast and gastrointestinal tract are the most common. The outcome of cancer treatment varies between the sites affected and the stage at presentation. For example, lung cancer has a very poor 5-year survival rate as it often presents at a late stage when it has spread via metastases (in general this means spread to distant sites, including the liver, brain, lungs and bone). By contrast, treatment of testicular cancer often has a high cure rate if detected early. Healthcare professionals therefore have an important role in the education of patients to recognise and report serious symptoms early (Chapter 1). This is particularly important for patients with additional risk factors such as a family history of breast or bowel cancer and these patients should be encouraged to undertake regular screening. Interventions include:

- the provision of information relating to the importance of self-examination for lumps of the breast, testicles, neck or arm pits
- to alleviate fear and encourage early referral to improve outcome

- to encourage patients to attend screening such as cervical smears and mammograms and to discuss concerns with healthcare professionals
- to educate patients about the risk of skin cancer and the importance of protecting skin from the sun, particularly for those with fair skin (Chapter 32). Vigilance of changes to moles suggestive of melanoma is also important
- to educate patients to recognise other warning symptoms such as sudden unexplained weight loss, rectal bleeding or haemoptysis (Chapter 1)
- future screening may include screening for colorectal and ovarian cancers

Treatment

Treatment of cancer is usually by hospital specialists and is divided into surgery, chemotherapy and radiotherapy. The aim of surgery is to remove the tumour and, if the tumour is localised, this may be curative. Surgery may also be used palliatively, for example to remove obstructions, or even preventively, such as the removal of a second breast in women at very high risk of the recurrence of breast cancer.

Chemotherapy is the use of cytotoxic drugs to kill fast-growing cells. Drugs used in anticancer chemotherapy generally target the synthesis of nucleotides (antimetabolites such as methotrexate and mercaptopurine), may chemically modify the DNA by alkylation (e.g. busulfan, chlorambucil, cyclophosphamide), cause fragmentation (e.g. bleomycin) or interchelation (e.g. dactinomycin) or may destroy mitotic spindle fibres (vinca alkaloids) involved in cell division. Corticosteroids also have a role, although this is poorly understood. In targeting these processes, the agents kill rapidly dividing cells in the tumour but also suppress growth of 'normal' cells with high rates of division, such as bone marrow cells producing blood cells and epithelial cells. Accordingly, the lack of selectivity gives rise to a wide range of side-effects, including myelosuppression leading to pancytopenia, which is associated with anaemia, increased susceptibility to infections due to neutropenia and increased bleeding due to thrombocytopenia. Myelosuppression is a common occurrence with many agents and is a reason to carry out chemotherapy in cycles, as this allows the bone marrow to recover between cycles. Colony-stimulating factors may be used under some circumstances to increase the white cell count and reduce the time between cycles. Prophylactic antimicrobial agents may also be required. Because of the toxic nature of cytotoxic agents they may exhibit a range of side-effects which, depending on the agent, may include:

- alopecia
- nausea and vomiting
- mouth ulcers
- renal damage
- bladder damage
- infertility
- lung damage
- cardiotoxicity
- carcinogenic effects

In the treatment of cancers, chemotherapy may be curative, for example in the treatment of testicular cancer, or may be used to kill leukaemia cells prior to bone marrow transplantation leading to a cure. Chemotherapy may be used in addition to surgery. For example, following the removal of a solid tumour, courses of anticancer chemotherapy may be used to prevent recurrence or suppress the growth of any metastases. It may also be used in palliation to reduce tumour size or growth and to prolong life. There are a number of chemotherapeutic agents and these are often used in specific combinations, generally involving three agents. The purpose of using combinations is to attack different pharmacological targets and so limit the development of resistance. Aside from the conventional agents mentioned above, newer approaches include the use of monoclonal antibodies which selectively target certain cell types. For example, rituximab targets B-lymphocytes and is used in non-Hodgkin lymphomas.

Hormonal-based therapy plays a significant role in certain tumours. For example, the oestrogen receptor antagonist tamoxifen is widely used in oestrogen receptor-positive breast cancer. It is given after surgery, with or without chemotherapy, and is effective at suppressing the growth of oestrogen-sensitive cells, including residual cells and metastases. Other approaches include the use of aromatase inhibitors, such as aminoglutethimide, which prevent the metabolism of androgens to oestrogens.

Radiotherapy also plays a role, whether by radiation from isotopes or from X-rays. By targeting the radiation on the tumour, cancerous cells may be killed. Certain tumours are especially sensitive to irradiation (such as bladder cancers) and radiotherapy may play an important role in localised disease. Radiotherapy is also used when surgery is not possible in vital organs such as in the head and neck. Additionally, radiotherapy may be used after surgery, in palliation to reduce the size of tumours, to reduce obstruction of the vena cava and for relief from bony metastases. This may allow a reduction in doses of analgesics and/or stepping down the analgesic ladder.

Palliative care

The following section is intended as an introduction to some of the issues encountered during palliative care, particularly relating to common symptoms, the importance of regular monitoring to optimise treatment and the education of patients and carers. Specialist information should be sought from references given at the end of the chapter and local palliative care teams.

What is palliative care?

The term 'palliative' is used to describe treatment that addresses and alleviates symptoms associated with an incurable disease. Palliative care is therefore applied commonly to the treatment of terminal malignancy but may also include conditions such as the end-stages of chronic heart failure, respiratory diseases, acquired immune deficiency syndrome (AIDS) and motor neuron disease. The aim of treatment is to improve the quality of life of both patients and carers and includes the control of physical symptoms and attention to spiritual, emotional and social needs. A multidisciplinary palliative care team therefore comprises specialist nurses, doctors, pharmacists, counsellors, dieticians, physiotherapists, social workers and ministers of religion. The

World Health Organization (WHO, 1990) also includes the following recommendations as to the role of palliative care:

- Consider dying as a normal process (see Nuland, 1997).
- Death should not be hastened or postponed.
- Patients should be offered the support required enabling them to live as actively as possible until death.
- The quality of life should be enhanced and care may also provide a positive influence throughout the course of illness.

Types of cancer pain

Pain is one of the most common and feared symptoms of cancer. However, this is not inevitable and approximately a third of patients do not suffer severe pain at any stage of their illness. When treating pain, the first step is to determine the location and likely source as this will determine the choice of treatment. For example, pain resulting from compression by a tumour may be reduced by chemotherapy or radiotherapy to remove or reduce the size of the tumour. Some types of pain (Chapter 27) respond to treatment with opioids, but neuropathic or bone pain may be more resistant to opioids. Bone pain is a somatic pain produced by nociceptors in the bone and tends to be localised, described as gnawing or aching, and often results from secondary tumours in the bone. Visceral pain is triggered by infiltration, compression, distension or stretching of the viscera due to the presence of a tumour and tends to be diffuse and constant.

WHO analgesic ladder

Once the nature and likely cause of pain are assessed, the recommendation of analgesia follows the analgesic ladder, as recommended by the WHO (Chapter 27). Analgesia is prescribed continually and not 'when required' for optimum pain management and therefore improved quality of life. Additional analgesia is prescribed for pain occurring despite continuous treatment. This is commonly described as breakthrough pain, for which 'when required' analgesia is appropriate.

Adjuvants may be added to treatment at any stage and include tricyclic antidepressants, anticonvulsants and corticosteroids (Chapter 27). Choice is dependent on the nature of the pain, risk of drug interactions and the side-effect profile.

Other symptoms

Other common symptoms of advanced cancer may include fatigue, weakness, anorexia, weight loss, lack of energy, dry mouth, constipation, dyspnoea and early satiety. Symptoms may be drug-related and may vary according to the nature of the tumour. For example, cancer of the head and neck often causes dysphagia whereas dyspnoea is associated with lung, breast or other cancers affecting the thorax. The cause and treatment of common symptoms are summarised in Table 29.1.

Pharmacology

The pharmacology of analgesics is described in Chapter 27. The pharmacology of corticosteroids is summarised in Chapter 20.

Drug choice

Treatment is given according to the analgesic ladder, as described in Chapter 27. The following section outlines analgesic choice according to the analgesic ladder, as applied to palliative care.

Step 1

Regular paracetamol is an effective first choice and is often an adequate analgesic used alone for mild pain, with or without a non-steroidal anti-inflammatory drug (NSAID). This should be used regularly and may be continued at all stages of the ladder.

Step 2

Mild opioids such as codeine, dihydrocodeine or dextropropoxyphene may be added (see Chapter 27).

Tramadol

Tramadol is considered suitable for use at the second step of the analgesic ladder, as it has fewer opioid side-effects such as constipation and respiratory depression compared with strong opioids. It should however be used with caution in patients with epilepsy or those prone to seizures, for example patients with cerebral tumours or uraemia. It should be avoided with other drugs known to lower the convulsive threshold, such as antidepressants (Chapter 5).

Step 3

Strong opioids

The properties of the strong opioids such as fentanyl, morphine, pethidine, oxycodone and buprenorphine are summarised in Tables 27.1 and 29.2. The latest *British National Formulary* (BNF) should be consulted for equivalent doses of opioids when calculating doses of strong opioids following treatment with milder agents. For example, codeine, dihydrocodeine and dextro-propoxyphene are approximately one-tenth the potency of morphine and the use of these opioids is considered when calculating the morphine dose. Despite the introduction of agents such as oxycodone, morphine remains the strong opioid in common use regardless of the frequent occurrence of nausea and vomiting when treatment is initiated. Morphine causes euphoria and mental detachment, which may be beneficial, as well as reducing respiratory symptoms. Exceptions are bone pain and neuropathic pain, which are often resistant to even strong opioids.

Where possible, it is reasonable to give drugs orally, even in advanced cancer. For patients with vomiting or difficulty swallowing, oral suspensions, patches or suppositories may be used. Alternatively syringe drivers provide a useful and continuous method of drug administration (see below).

Syringe drivers

For patients in the final stages of a terminal illness, syringe drivers can provide an extremely useful way of delivering medication. Syringe drivers provide a continuous subcutaneous

Table 29.1   Examples of the causes and treatment of common symptoms encountered in palliative care

Symptom	Treatment	Comments/common causes
Anorexia	Identify and treat the cause. A short course of corticosteroids may be given or high doses of a progestogen such as megestrol acetate or medroxyprogesterone	• Possible causes include dry mouth, nausea, constipation, anxiety, dyspepsia, pain, gastric stasis, hypercalcaemia, uraemia, depression and malodorous tumours • Dietary supplements may be added but do not replace normal meals. The intake of calorific food such as cheese and full-fat milk should be encouraged • The effects of progestogens may be delayed for a few weeks and side-effects such as oedema and the risk of thromboembolic disease may prevent their use. They tend only to be used if the prognosis is greater than 3 months
Anxiety	SSRIs, beta-blockers, benzodiazepines, e.g. lorazepam sublingually	• May be associated with depression and this may worsen pain (Chapter 23) • Benzodiazepines may be appropriate and the risk of dependence may not be relevant
Breathlessness	• Identify cause and treat as appropriate. Breathing techniques may be beneficial, particularly when dyspnoea is worsened by anxiety • Opioids may be of symptomatic benefit due to reduction of the central respiratory drive • Oxygen is required if the patient is hypoxic	Causes include anaemia, bronchospasm, fluid retention, respiratory infection, COPD, pulmonary embolism, congestive heart failure or drugs such as beta-blockers or aspirin (Chapter 14)
Confusion	Identify cause. Treatment may include haloperidol or chlorpromazine if the patient is agitated or distressed	• Hyponatraemia, hypercalcaemia, uraemia, pain, constipation, infection, urine retention • Drug causes include opioids, hypnotics and antimuscarinics (Chapter 5)
Constipation	A softener and stimulant are required. For example, regular lactulose and senna or co-danthrusate (Chapter 9). Suppositories or enemas may be required if severe	• Opioids, reduced mobility, dehydration • Laxatives should be given to all patients prescribed regular opioids
Dehydration	Small amounts of fluids may be administered regularly. Causes should be identified and treated	• Causes include diuretics, laxatives, sweating or difficulty swallowing • Dehydration may lead to deterioration of renal function and should therefore be avoided or identified and corrected promptly

Continued

Table 29.1   Continued

Symptom	Treatment	Comments/common causes
Depression	Tricyclic or SSRI antidepressants (Chapter 23)	• Consider the prognosis and delayed efficacy before initiating antidepressants • Monitor for hyponatraemia as a cause of confusion and drowsiness • Antimuscarinic effects of tricyclics may be a disadvantage. Review other medications for risk of additive effects and consider problems such as dry mouth and constipation
Diarrhoea	Loperamide (Chapter 9), other opioids, rehydration	Causes include impacted faeces, bowel obstruction or infections. Drug causes include opioid withdrawal, antibiotics, iron salts, laxatives, NSAIDs and magnesium salts (Chapter 5)
Dry mouth and oral candidiasis	• Sugar-free chewing gum or sweets may help to stimulate saliva production (consider sorbitol as a cause of diarrhoea), artificial saliva, ice or unsweetened pineapple chunks and regular sips of water • Candidiasis may be present and is treated with nystatin or miconazole oral gel • Antiseptic mouth washes (e.g. chlorhexidine) may be used if patients are unable to brush their teeth	• Drug causes include opioids, drugs with antimuscarinic effects (sedating antihistamines, TCAs, hyoscine: see Chapter 5) • Reduce the prescribing of antimuscarinic drugs if possible • Glycerine-based mouthwashes are best avoided as they cause drying • Broad-spectrum antibiotics and steroids (particularly inhaled) and general debilitation may cause candidiasis • Asthmatic patients treated with inhaled steroids are at increased risk of developing oral candidiasis and may benefit from using a spacer device and should be advised to rinse their mouth after inhaler use
Hiccup	Antacid with antiflatulent (dimeticone) e.g. Asilone suspension or Maalox Plus, metoclopramide or chlorpromazine	• May be caused by gastric distension • Avoid antacids containing aluminium salts alone, which may cause constipation • Avoid bicarbonate salts, which may increase flatulence from carbon dioxide production
Insomnia	Benzodiazepines, e.g. temazepam	• Causes include anxiety, depression, cramps, pain, night sweats, joint stiffness, fear or discomfort • Drug causes include corticosteroids (administer dexamethasone before 6 p.m.), caffeine, alcohol, sympathomimetics (Chapter 25) or withdrawal from benzodiazepines

Continued

Table 29.1 Continued

Symptom	Treatment	Comments/common causes
Intractable cough	Consider changing posture, particularly at night or opioids, e.g. morphine	Gastric distension
Muscle spasm	Diazepam, baclofen or dantrolene	• Pressure or nerve irritation • The efficacy of dantrolene may be delayed by a few weeks
Nausea and vomiting	The cause should be determined and treated if appropriate. Antiemetics include domperidone, metoclopramide, haloperidol, cyclizine, levomepromazine, prochlorperazine when required (Chapter 8). Ondansetron may be used for chemotherapy-induced nausea and vomiting	• For example, gastric stasis, constipation, bowel obstruction, hypercalcaemia (stop drugs such as thiazides, which retain calcium), renal failure, raised intracranial pressure, motion sickness, severe pain, cough, severe anxiety, infection, uraemia or chemotherapy • Antimuscarinic drugs may oppose prokinetic drugs (Chapter 5) • Common cause is initial treatment with opioids but this is usually transient, resolving after a few days • Review every 24 h • Many drugs cause nausea and vomiting (Chapter 5) • Note that extrapyramidal effects of metoclopramide are more common in children
Pruritus	Emollients (cool in the fridge) and/or oral antihistamines. Avoid heat and try cotton clothing. Obstructive jaundice may require treatment with colestyramine	Jaundice or drugs such as opioids (Chapter 32). Note that itching due to opioids is more common in children
Sedation	Reduction of opioid dose if pain is controlled. Also review other drugs causing sedation such as antihistamines (chlorphenamine), antidepressants (amitriptyline, dosulepin (dothiepin), trazodone) or benzodiazepines	• Tends to occur when opioid dose is increased and should be transient, resolving after a few days • Patient should not perform skilled tasks such as driving • If sedation persists, consider toxicity and review dose and factors such as deteriorating renal function
Sweating	Paracetamol or NSAIDs, or hyoscine (opioid-induced sweating)	• Malignancy, infection, anxiety, hyperthyroidism, menopause. Drug causes include antidepressants • Monitor for dehydration, e.g. diuretic doses may need to be withheld

SSRIs, selective serotonin reuptake inhibitors; COPD, chronic obstructive pulmonary disease; NSAIDs, non-steroidal anti-inflammatory drugs; TCAs, tricyclic antidepressants.

infusion and therefore allow effective control of symptoms. When converting from oral morphine to a syringe driver, the more soluble opioid diamorphine is used and the equivalent doses of these opioids are tabulated in the BNF. The dose may however need to be increased because of worsening pain and/or increased tolerance by patients at the time a syringe driver is initiated. It should be noted that a misconception exists whereby patients and carers view the administration of opioids via the parenteral route to be more effective than the oral route, and an inevitable part of the treatment of advanced disease. The BNF indications for the parenteral route include patients unable to take medication by mouth, e.g. due to dysphagia or nausea and vomiting and, importantly, when patients request that they receive their medication by this route.

Important roles for pharmacists include the calculation of diamorphine dose required when converting from oral morphine and assessing the compatibility of drugs to be added to diamorphine infusions, thereby maintaining the stability of the infusion and preventing adverse effects in the patient. The infusion solution should be checked regularly for discolouration or precipitation. Examples from the BNF of drugs which may be added to diamorphine infusions include:

- cyclizine
- dexamethasone
- haloperidol
- hysoscine butylbromide
- hyoscine hydrobromide
- metoclopramide
- midazolam

Drugs contraindicated for use in syringe drivers include chlorpromazine, prochlorperazine and diazepam due to irritation at the injection site. The latest BNF and *The Syringe Driver* (Dickman *et al.*, 2002) should be consulted for further information.

Adjuncts used in the treatment of pain

Adjuncts may be added at any step of the analgesic ladder and include corticosteroids, antidepressants and anticonvulsants. Other treatment includes nerve block, relaxation therapy and the use of transcutaneous electrical nerve stimulation (TENS) machines (Chapter 27).

Corticosteroids

Corticosteroids such as dexamethasone are particularly useful for treating pain due to nerve compression, tissue swelling or raised intracranial pressure.

Dexamethasone (doses up to 16 mg/day) is used for raised intracranial pressure, severe bone pain, nerve or soft-tissue infiltration by the tumour or oedema, and hepatic capsular pain. The last dose should be given before 6 p.m. to avoid causing insomnia. Additional benefits include increased appetite, energy and general well-being. To avoid side-effects, the lowest effective dose is prescribed and the course duration is as short as possible. For patients taking corticosteroids and NSAIDs, gastric protection in the form of a proton pump inhibitor is appropriate.

Neuropathic pain

Neuropathic pain (Chapter 27) results from treatment such as radiotherapy, or from infiltration of a tumour into peripheral nerves or the central nervous system, causing compression or damage. It may be described as burning, stabbing, tingling, a constricting sensation or shooting pains. The skin may feel numb or oversensitive. Neuropathic pain is often unresponsive to opioids and is managed by a combination of corticosteroids, tricyclic antidepressants and anticonvulsants (Chapters 22 and 23). Specialists may also consider the use of ketamine or antiarrhythmics such as flecainide, mexiletine or lidocaine.

Bone pain

Bone pain often arises from secondary tumours, which result in either increased or reduced bone density and the release of prostaglandins. NSAIDs are therefore the analgesics of choice. If an NSAID remains ineffective after 1 week, an alternative NSAID is selected (Chapter 27). The addition of a weak opioid may be considered but is not often beneficial. Bisphosphonates or calcitonin may

Table 29.2   A summary of some important characteristics of strong opioids in relation to palliative care

Opioid	Comments
Buprenorphine	• Vomiting may be a problem and withdrawal effects may occur if added to high-dose opioid treatment, resulting from its partial agonist activity. It is therefore not often suitable for cancer pain • Patches have recently been introduced
Cyclimorph	• Cyclimorph is a combination product containing both morphine and cyclizine. This is not appropriate for chronic pain since nausea is a transient effect of opioid treatment and therefore ongoing treatment with cyclizine is not necessary. In addition, dose increases lead to excessive sedation due to cyclizine • Diconal is a combination product of cyclizine and dipipanone and is therefore also unsuitable in palliative care
Dextromoramide	• A short duration of action makes dextromoramide unsuitable for control of continuous pain and this is rarely used • Available as a sublingual tablet
Diamorphine	• More soluble than morphine and therefore used for infusion due to reduced volume • Activity one-quarter to one-third that of oral morphine • Injection is given by the subcutaneous route, which is easier to administer and less painful than other routes
Fentanyl	• The efficacy of fentanyl is comparable with morphine and this is therefore not a suitable alternative when pain is not controlled by morphine (suspect opioid-resistant pain). The time taken for transdermal fentanyl to reach steady state also makes this preparation unsuitable for unstable pain • Patches changed at the same time every 3 days are useful for patients with dysphagia, malabsorption or poor compliance • Less constipating than morphine and more suitable in renal impairment as there are no active metabolites, although dose reduction may be required • Oral transmucosal fentanyl citrate lozenges are now available for breakthrough pain • New preparations should be started 12 h after the last patch is removed. It should also be noted that fentanyl effects remain for up to 72 h following removal of the patch • When starting fentanyl treatment, apply patch at the same time as the last dose of slow-release morphine. The full effect may take 36–48 h and therefore breakthrough pain may occur and should be treated as required • When changing from morphine, withdrawal symptoms such as colic, diarrhoea, nausea, sweating and restlessness may persist for a few days, although pain may be controlled. Doses of short-acting oral morphine may be given • Adjuncts or alternative analgesia should be considered if pain is not controlled by doses above 300 µg/h
Hydromorphone	• To date, hydromorphine appears to demonstrate efficacy and tolerability comparable to morphine and is reserved for patients with confusion, loss of concentration, vivid dreams or hallucinations occurring with even low doses of morphine • The contents of controlled-release capsules may be sprinkled on cold soft food
Methadone	Useful in renal failure
Morphine	• Remains the first choice for the treatment of chronic cancer pain • Oral slow-release and quick-acting preparations available for good pain control, including breakthrough pain • Suppositories offer alternative routes of administration
Oxycodone	• Role in relation to morphine remains to be established as side-effect profile and efficacy appear similar but may provide an alternative if symptoms such as hallucinations become problematic with morphine
Pentazocine	• Avoided due to high risk of confusion and hallucinations
Pethidine	• Pethidine is avoided in palliative care due to the short half-life, reduced potency compared with morphine and the accumulation of toxic metabolites during regular use

be used to reduce bone turnover or inhibit calcium resorption into bone, respectively. Corticosteroids are also useful for treating bone pain due to anti-inflammatory properties and also by reducing oedema surrounding the tumour. Regular use of paracetamol is also useful at each step of the analgesic ladder.

Colicky pain

Pain associated with the gastrointestinal tract and reported as 'colicky' pain may respond to antimuscarinic agents, such as hyoscine, which reduce intestinal transit.

Common symptoms

Table 29.1 summarises the causes of some common symptoms associated with cancer and their management.

Concurrent disease

Analgesic prescribing decisions complicated by concurrent diseases are outlined in Chapter 27. Key considerations include gastrointestinal toxicity due to NSAIDs and worsening renal function. For patients with effective pain control with NSAIDs, a proton pump inhibitor may be added for gastric protection. Misoprostol may not be suitable due to colic and diarrhoea. It should be noted, however, that respiratory depression in terminal care does not preclude the use of strong opioids and careful dose titration prevents this effect. Signs of opioid overdose include drowsiness, reduced respiratory rate and the presence of hallucinations and pain tends to be well controlled. Opioid toxicity may be precipitated by renal impairment.

In general, the risks of initiating further treatment are compared to the likely benefits. Unnecessary treatment is withheld to prevent further complications of drug regimens. For example, the treatment of hyperlipidaemia may not be appropriate in terminal care. Palliative care is one of the exceptions when polypharmacy is often necessary and adverse drug reactions (ADRs) are treated as they arise. Patients and carers should be as involved as possible in treatment choices and

the impact on quality of life considered. For example, the use of drugs with sedative properties may be avoided for as long as possible in patients wishing to retain the independence gained from driving.

Terminal symptoms

Terminal symptoms occur when death is likely to be within days. These include noisy breathing (death rattle), confusion, fever and severe fatigue. Symptoms should be monitored regularly and those considered to be causing distress, such as urinary retention, constipation, pain and dyspepsia, should be identified and treated. It should be noted that restlessness and agitation may occur in the presence of worsening pain but this is not always the case and care should be taken to avoid misinterpretation. Increasing doses of opioids may worsen such symptoms and dose reduction or an alternative opioid should be considered when other causes, including pain, have been excluded. Any unnecessary treatment such as antihypertensives, diuretics, antiarrhythmics and hypoglycaemics may be stopped. Artificial feeding such as via a nasogastric tube is not appropriate as it may cause distress to both the patient and carers.

Drug interactions

See Chapter 27.

Monitoring

The impairment of renal or hepatic function may increase side-effects, particularly to opioids, and requires dose reduction or less frequent dosing (Chapter 27).

The role of the community pharmacist

The community pharmacist is an important source of support and information, particularly for carers of cancer patients who are often involved in collecting and administering medication. Pharmacists are an essential part of the palliative care team, being experts on the use and availability of medicines. For example, pharmacists can advise on alternative preparations such as suspensions, suppositories and patches available for patients with dysphagia.

Perhaps the most important role of the pharmacist is in the education of patients and carers on the best use of medicines since this improves compliance. The needs of the patient and carers should be considered, for example a complicated medication regimen is of no benefit if it causes anxiety and poor compliance. Verbal and written information should be provided; an up-to-date list of medication, dosing information and indications for use of each product may help both patients and carers. Advice may need to be repeated. Regular supply of medication should be ensured and patients and carers encouraged to report new or altered symptoms for early recognition of ADRs or new symptoms. Providing a list of contacts and sources of further information is also helpful, particularly in the early stages of the disease. Pharmacist input to medication assessment and review as part of a multidisciplinary palliative care team staffing palliative care clinics is also to be encouraged as this improves pharmaceutical care for patients (Needham and Wong, 1999; Austwick *et al.*, 2002).

General advice for patients and carers

- Key words to consider when providing advice include *education, empathy, reassurance, approachability* and *resourcefulness.*
- Good mouth care should be encouraged to prevent problems such as infection.
- Take care not to run out of medicines.
- Pharmacists may consider producing specific information leaflets to cover the use of medicines outside the product licence.

Pain

- Patients and carers may fear the use of morphine, as it is wrongly associated with 'imminent death'. Reassurance should be given that morphine is an extremely safe and useful analgesic, which may be used for years and with little risk of psychological dependence when used for severe pain.

- Drowsiness caused by strong opioids is often transient. Skilled tasks such as driving should be avoided and prolonged drowsiness should be reported to the prescriber.
- Advice should be given as to the timing of morphine doses. For example, regular administration of a long-acting preparation twice a day means as close to 12 h as practical between doses, with additional doses of an immediate-release preparation (usually morphine solution) given up to every 4 h as required for breakthrough pain. The total amount of oral solution taken during a 24-h period allows the prescriber to calculate the 12-hourly dose required.
- Reassurance should be given that the effectiveness of morphine will persist even if started early in the disease. It is a common misconception by patients that starting morphine treatment too early may leave them without adequate pain control when the pain worsens.
- The control of neuropathic pain may take a week or more but if the pain worsens the prescriber should be contacted. If agents such as antidepressants or anticonvulsants are used, the use of these drugs for neuropathic pain should be explained.

Opioids, NSAIDs and adjuvant counselling

See Chapter 27.

Fentanyl patches

- Patches should be changed at the same time every 3 days.
- A new patch should be applied to a different area of skin, and not applied to inflamed skin, scar tissue, swollen or broken skin.
- Direct contact of heat such as from hot-water bottles should be avoided.
- There should be good contact between the skin and the patch and porous adhesive tape (e.g. Micropore) may be used if necessary.
- Used patches should be folded inwards, protecting the side which contained the drug, and disposed of carefully.

Co-danthramer

- This may colour urine red.

Practice points

- Psychosocial and spiritual support for both patient and family are important components of palliative care and may impact on the severity of symptoms.
- The progressive nature of cancer means that the symptoms and patients' needs are constantly changing. Regular review of medication is therefore essential and should identify ADRs and new symptoms and assess the continued benefit from treatment. Palliative care medicine is a balance between symptom control and avoidance of unacceptable ADRs.

General pain control

- Pain control should follow the stepped approach recommended by the WHO (Chapter 27).
- The WHO also recommends that analgesia be provided continually and not 'when required', although additional analgesia is prescribed for use when required for breakthrough pain.
- Frequent review is required for optimum pain control.
- Consider the timing of doses, for example prior to painful changing of dressings.
- It may be useful to ask the patient to indicate the severity of each symptom on a scale of one to 10 to assess treatment outcome and the need for dose changes or further intervention. A list of drugs, including those found to be ineffective, is useful to prevent omissions and unnecessary treatment.

Opioids

- The total daily dose of morphine should be reviewed daily and the regular dose adjusted according to the number of rescue doses required. In practice, a doubling of the rescue dose may be given at night (50% increase for elderly patients) to ensure a pain-free night and prevent the patient waking for a further dose.
- There is no maximum dose for morphine and therefore the dose is titrated according to increased pain relief compared to side-effects. A poor response may necessitate the introduction of adjuncts. For example, the cause of pain should be reassessed if more than 200 mg/day of morphine is required.
- There are now many brands of morphine which are designed for either daily or twice-daily administration. When prescribing, it is good practice to indicate both the generic and brand name to avoid over- or underdosing.
- Patients sensitive to the adverse effects of one strong opioid can be changed to a similar opioid so long as toxicity has been excluded, but note that frequent changes result in poor pain management.
- Softener and stimulant laxatives (Chapter 9) should be started when any opioid is initiated and the dose increased according to response rather than the opioid dose. When changing from high doses of morphine, however, laxative doses should be halved as severe diarrhoea may occur.
- Note that, unlike stronger opioids, opioids for mild to moderate pain produce a maximum analgesic effect, which is not exceeded by further dose increases. At this stage, stronger opioids are substituted according to step 3 of the WHO analgesic ladder. Substituting for an alternative weak opioid is of no benefit.

Syringe drivers

- Check infusion solutions regularly for discoloration or precipitation and ensure the correct rate of infusion.
- Infusion solutions should not be used for longer than 24 h to reduce the risk of infection.
- Breakthrough pain may be treated with subcutaneous (or intramuscular) injections of diamorphine (a sixth of the total 24-h dose being given by subcutaneous infusion).
- Monitor the injection site and consider changing to an alternative site if there is pain or prominent inflammation.

References

Austwick E A, Brown L C, Goddyear K H *et al.* (2002). Pharmacist's input into a palliative care clinic. *Pharm J* 268: 404–406.

Dickman D, Littlewood C, Varga J (2002). *The Syringe Driver. Continuous Infusions in Palliative Care*. Oxford: Oxford University Press.

Mehta D K (ed.) *British National Formulary*, latest edition. London: British Medical Association and Royal Pharmaceutical Society of Great Britain.

Needham D, Wong I (1999). An expert panel review to evaluate the effectiveness of community pharmacist's interventions in the palliative care setting. *Pharm J* 263 (Suppl): R32–R33.

Nuland S B (1997). *How we Die.* Berkshire: Vintage.

World Health Organization (1990). *Cancer Pain Relief and Palliative Care: Report of a WHO Expert Committee.* Geneva: WHO.

Further reading

Allen M, Taylor R (1999). Pain control in palliative care. *Pharm J* 262: 620–624.

Costello P (2001). Palliative care – an introduction. *Hosp Pharm* 8: 211–214.

Department of Health (2000). *NHS Cancer Plan.* London: Department of Health.

Montgomery F (2001). Palliative care. Managing chronic cancer pain. *Hosp Pharm* 8: 215–218.

Montgomery F (2002). Pain management in palliative care. *Pharm J* 268: 254–256.

Quigley C (2002). Hydromorphone for acute and chronic pain (Cochrane review). In: *The Cochrane Library,* issue 4. Oxford: Update Software.

Twycross R, Wilcock A (2001). *Symptom Management in Advanced Cancer,* 3rd edn. Oxford: Radcliffe Medical Press.

Twycross R, Wilcock A, Charlesworth S *et al.* (2002). *PCF2 – Palliative Care Formulary*, 2nd edn. Oxford: Radcliffe Medical Press.

Urie J, Fielding H, McArthur D *et al.* (2000). Palliative care. *Pharm J* 265: 603–614.

Williams J (2001). *Palliative Care Prescribing.* Drug information letter no. 117. North West Medicines Information Service and Aintree Hospitals NHS Trust. Available in PDF format from: www.nwrocancer.org.uk/PallCare.htm#Pathways (accessed 4 November 2002).

Online resources

http://www.palliativedrugs.com Provides access to drug information on the use of drugs in palliative care, access to books such as the *Palliative Care Formulary* and a monthly newsletter (accessed 4 November 2002).

http://www5.who.int/cancer for WHO cancer information and publications, including the International Agency for Research on Cancer (IARC) (accessed 4 November 2002).

www.cancerbacup.org.uk Cancer BACUP provides information for health professionals, patients and carers, a telephone helpline and access to information centres throughout the UK (accessed 4 November 2002).

www.doh.gov.uk/cancer/index.htm for the National Health Service (NHS) cancer plan, current information and research, recommendations for good practice and links to cancer services within the NHS (accessed 4 November 2002).

www.macmillan.org.uk For Macmillan Cancer Relief, a charity providing information and support to patients with cancer and their carers, including information on access to Macmillan nurses and a telephone helpline (accessed 4 November 2002).

www.mariecurie.org.uk. For access to Marie Curie Cancer Care, providing access to ongoing research, education and Marie Curie Hospices across the UK (accessed 4 November 2002).

www.nice.org.uk for access to National Institute of Clinical Excellence (NICE) recommendations for cancer treatment (accessed 4 November 2002).

Part H

Infections

30

Bacterial infections

Bacterial infections comprise a wide range of diseases from simple, troublesome conditions to life-threatening events. The purpose of this chapter is to give a brief overview of common infections and antibacterial agents. In some cases infections such as respiratory tract and skin infections are dealt with elsewhere (Chapters 18, 20 and 32). The aim is to illustrate common examples and principles: more detailed sources and guidelines should be consulted for specific information relating to bacterial sensitivity to antibiotics.

Disease characteristics

Infection or invasion by foreign, pathogenic organisms may result from those living as commensals on the body or from gut flora, in addition to those present in soil, food or on other animal hosts. Pathophysiological changes may result from bacterial infection of any part of the body, often entering by a wound or mucous membranes, by contact, by ingestion or opportunistic infection, for example, of immunocompromised patients.

Risk factors for infection include reduced immunity in the young, elderly, immunocompromised, malnourished, those with diabetes mellitus, those with prosthetic valves or joints, or following surgery or as a result of burns. Foreign travel may also result in infection due to exposure to organisms for which immunity has not developed previously.

Clinical features of common infections (Table 30.1)

Signs and symptoms of infection may include pyrexia, sweating, tachycardia, hypotension, nausea and vomiting, pallor, local pain and inflammation or purulence. A full blood count may indicate elevated white cells to more than 12×10^9/L, with neutrophilia but may be reduced due to depletion in chronic infections (such as

tuberculosis (TB), although monocytes may be elevated) or in septicaemia. There may also be a raised erythrocyte sedimentation rate (ESR, Chapter 2).

Table 30.1   Some common examples of bacteria and their related conditions

	Associated disease
Gram-positive cocci	
Staphylococcus aureus	Associated with styes, impetigo, conjunctivitis, sinusitis, food poisoning, endocarditis, meningitis, pneumonia, UTI and osteomyelitis
Streptococcus pyogenes	Causes scarlet fever, acute tonsillitis, erysipelas; dangerous if it affects wounds as it may cause sepsis
Streptococcus pneumoniae	Pneumonia, bronchitis, infections of the ears and sinuses, meningitis
Streptococcus viridans	Endocarditis
Gram-negative cocci	
Neisseria gonorrhoeae	Purulent ophthalmia or gonorrhoea
Neisseria meningitidis	Cerebrospinal fever or meningococcal meningitis
Gram-positive rods	
Bacillus spp. (B. anthracis, B. cereus)	Anthrax, food poisoning
Clostridium spp. (C. botulinum, C. tetani, C. difficile)	Dangerous anaerobes causing tissue damage affecting wounds and leading to gangrene, food poisoning (botulism), tetanus, pseudomembranous colitis (often secondary to use of broad-spectrum antibiotics such as clindamycin)
Gram-negative rods	
Pseudomonas aeruginosa	Dangerous secondary infection of wounds, pneumonia, eye infections, UTI
Helicobacter pylori	Associated with peptic ulcer
Haemophilus influenzae	Infantile meningitis, conjunctivitis, chronic bronchitis, infections of ear and sinuses
Escherichia coli	Enterobacteria (inhabitants of intestines) causing enteritis in young infants, also pyelitis, pyelonephritis and UTIs
Salmonella spp.	Enteric bacteria causing typhoid, food poisoning
Shigella spp.	Enteric bacteria causing dysentery
Proteus spp.	Enteric bacteria infecting the urinary tract and wounds
Klebsiella pneumoniae	Enteric bacteria and cause of acute bronchopneumonia
Campylobacter jejunum	Enteritis due to food poisoning. Anaerobe
Bacteroides fragilis	Oropharyngeal or gastrointestinal infection. Anaerobe
Chlamydia trachomatis	Trachoma, conjunctivitis and non-gonococcal urethritis
Legionella pneumophila	Legionnaires' disease transmitted in water, pneumonia
Acid-fast organisms	
Mycobacterium tuberculosis	Tuberculosis (Mycobacterium spp. also cause leprosy)
Spirochaetes	
Leptospira icterohaemorrhagiae	Weils' disease (jaundice) carried by rats
Borrelia vincenti	Vincent's angina

UTI, urinary tract infection.

Gastrointestinal infections

Infections of the gastrointestinal tract include gastroenteritis, *Campylobacter* enteritis, invasive salmonellosis, shigellosis, typhoid fever, antibiotic-associated pseudomembranous colitis, biliary tract infection (cholangitis) and peritonitis. Specific symptoms include diarrhoea, vomiting and abdominal pain. Cholangitis presents as pain in the right upper quadrant of the abdomen and may be associated with jaundice and high fever. Chronic infection of the stomach or duodenum with *Helicobacter pylori* is associated with ulceration and is dealt with in Chapter 7.

Cardiovascular infections

Endocarditis, inflammation of the lining of the heart cavity (endocardium) and valves, may result from rheumatic fever or bacterial infection by species of streptococci, enterococci and staphylococci. Patients with existing abnormalities of the heart such as valvular disease are at an increased risk. Specific clinical features are chest pain, murmur, tachycardia and palpitations. Patients may be frightened that they are suffering a heart attack, as symptoms are severe and rapid in onset.

Respiratory infections

Respiratory infections include bronchitis and pneumonia, which are discussed in Chapters 18 and 20.

The incidence of TB is increasing, mainly due to the spread of acquired immune deficiency syndrome (AIDS), increased homelessness and the emergence of resistant strains. An initial latent phase may be asymptomatic. Progressive pulmonary TB produces symptoms of fatigue, night sweats, weight loss, cough with haemoptysis and chest pain. Chest radiology reveals abnormalities such as pulmonary infiltration, visible cavities and fibrosis. These abnormalities may occur before the clinical symptoms. The causative organisms are *Mycobacterium tuberculosis* and *M. avium*, of which multidrug-resistant strains are common.

Central nervous system

The most common infection of the central nervous system is meningitis, or infection with inflammation of the membrane (meninges) surrounding the brain. *Neisseria meningitidis* (meningococci), *Streptococcus pneumoniae* (pneumococci), *Haemophilus influenzae* and *Listeria monocytogenes* are important causative agents of bacterial meningitis. Clinical features include photophobia, neck stiffness, headache, rash which does not blanch under pressure (the glass test), general malaise and fever. A rash is not always present. Suspected meningitis is treated with 'blind' antibiotic therapy.

Urinary tract

Bacturia may indicate genitourinary infection affecting the kidney (pyelonephritis), bladder (cystitis) or prostate in men (prostatitis) or urethra (urethritis), collectively known as urinary tract infections (UTIs). Acute pyelonephritis is an acute kidney infection presenting with fever, chills, rigors and pains and tenderness. Lower UTIs are more common in women due to a shorter urethra and produce symptoms of urgency, frequency and dysuria (painful urination). More serious symptoms indicating renal involvement include haematuria, lower back or loin pain and fever with diarrhoea and vomiting.

Risk factors for developing UTI include diabetes mellitus, pregnancy, impaired voiding and catheters. *Escherichia coli* causes most UTIs occurring in the community. UTIs acquired during a stay in hospital may include infection by staphylococci, streptococci, *Pseudomonas* or *Proteus* species. UTIs are also commonly associated with long-term urinary catheters.

Genital infections

Genital infections include gonorrhoea, uncomplicated genital chlamydial infection, non-gonococcal urethritis and non-specific genital infections, pelvic inflammatory disease and, rarely, syphilis. *N. gonorrhoeae* can infect the urethra, cervix, rectum, pharynx and conjunctiva. Infection is associated with a purulent discharge and may be otherwise asymptomatic and a cause of infertility. Non-gonococcal infection may produce a thinner discharge but also requires further investigation. Pyrexia and pelvic pain require urgent referral.

Genital infections are often transmitted sexually and partners should be referred for screening even in the absence of symptoms. Recurrent requests for cystitis or thrush treatment, particularly when previous treatment has been unsuccessful, should be referred to the general practitioner (GP) or genitourinary clinic for further investigation. This is particularly important due to the risk of complications such as infertility.

Blood

Septicaemia (blood poisoning) often results from an existing infection and in susceptible patients such as the elderly or immunocompromised. It may be caused by any of a number of pathogens. Treatment is therefore dependent on the nature of the initial infection. Symptoms include chills, diarrhoea, fever and vomiting. Urgent treatment is required to prevent spread, leading to secondary infection of organs and ultimately life-threatening septic shock, which involves severe hypotension and may lead to multiorgan failure.

Musculoskeletal system

Prompt treatment of osteomyelitis (infection and inflammation of bone marrow) and septic arthritis is imperative to prevent bone or joint damage. Alerting symptoms of infection include red, hot and painful swelling of the affected site with difficult movement. Septic arthritis most often involves *Staphylococcus aureus* and occasionally *H. influenzae* or *N. gonorrhoeae* (gonococci). Patients with existing damage to joints, such as those with rheumatoid arthritis and patients taking corticosteroids, are at increased risk of developing septic arthritis. This may also follow osteomyelitis affecting a nearby bone. Osteomyelitis may follow a fracture or bone surgery. Treatment includes high doses of antibiotics, aspiration, analgesia and support of the affected joint or limb.

Eye

Purulent conjunctivitis may indicate bacterial infection requiring antibiotic eye drops such as chloramphenicol or gentamicin. Fusidic acid is used to treat suspected staphylococcal infections. Gonococcal conjunctivitis requires both topical and systemic antibiotics.

Ear, nose and throat

Infections affecting the ear, nose and throat include dental infections, sinusitis, otitis externa, otitis media and throat infections, which are covered in Chapter 18.

Acute otitis media

Acute otitis media is dealt with in Chapter 18.

Skin

Infections of the skin produce the conditions impetigo, erysipelas (*Streptococcus pyogenes* infection of the skin and underlying tissue of the face and scalp), cellulitis or acne. See Chapter 32.

Goals of treatment

The aims of antibacterial treatment are to:

- eradicate the infection
- prevent spread
- prevent complications such as septicaemia or secondary infection

The appropriate antibiotic is chosen with the spectrum of activity to cover the specific infection whilst avoiding the development of resistance. Symptomatic treatment may include the use of analgesics such as paracetamol and/or ibuprofen.

Prophylaxis

The use of antimicrobial agents to prevent infection plays an important role in patients at risk due to concurrent disease, surgery or contact with infection. Important examples where prophylaxis is appropriate include:

- patients with rheumatic fever who receive antibiotic prophylaxis until the age of 25 years

of age and for subsequent surgery and dental surgery
- patients with a history of endocarditis and/or those with prosthetic heart valves who require antibiotic prophylaxis prior to dental surgery
- patients in contact with meningitis or tuberculosis
- patients undergoing surgery

Pharmacological basis of management

The aim of pharmacological treatment is the selective destruction of pathogens without harming human cells. Possible targets are mechanisms unique to pathogens and include protein synthesis and disruption of the unique construction and presence of a cell wall.

Beta-lactam antibiotics (penicillins, cephalosporins)

Penicillins

Amoxicillin, ampicillin, benzylpenicillin (penicllin G), flucloxacillin, phenoxymethylpenicillin (penicillin V)
Penicillins target bacterial cell wall synthesis, by inhibiting cross-linking of peptide side chains, and so are only effective against dividing organisms. Penicillins are thus bactericidal, causing lysis of the bacteria. Some penicillins are inactivated by beta-lactamases secreted by resistant bacteria (see below). Benzylpenicillin is only active following parenteral administration.

Cephalosporins

e.g. Cefaclor, cefalexin, cefotaxime, cefradine, cefuroxime
Cephalosporins exhibit similar pharmacology to penicillins, binding to beta-lactam-binding sites and inhibiting cell wall synthesis. They show cross-reactivity with penicillins and approximately 10% of penicillin-allergic patients will also be allergic to cephalosporins.

Glycopeptides

Teicoplanin, vancomycin
These also inhibit bacterial cell wall synthesis by inhibiting the growth of the peptidoglycan chain.

Antibiotics which target bacterial protein synthesis

Tetracyclines

e.g. Doxycycline, minocycline, oxytetracycline, tetracycline
Tetracyclines are bacteriostatic following inhibition of protein synthesis, through interfering with tRNA binding. They are broad-spectrum antibiotics taken up into bacteria by active transport. Resistance has reduced the clinical indications for tetracyclines (Table 30.2).

Aminoglycosides

Amikacin, gentamicin, neomycin, tobramycin
Aminoglycosides bind irreversibly to the bacterial ribosomes leading to an inhibition of protein synthesis. They enter the bacterial cells via an oxygen-dependent active transport process and are therefore less effective against anaerobes. The bactericidal activity of aminoglycosides is enhanced when they are used with agents that target cell wall synthesis such as penicillins and vancomycin.

Macrolides

e.g. Azithromycin, clarithromycin, erythromycin
Macrolides prevent the translocation movement of the bacterial ribosome along the mRNA and so prevent protein synthesis, resulting in bacteriostatic actions. In some organisms they are bactericidal.

Quinolones

e.g. Ciprofloxacin, norfloxacin, ofloxacin
These are bacterial DNA gyrase inhibitors, which inhibit the supercoiling of the bacterial DNA, which is essential for DNA repair and replication. This group of agents is bactericidal.

Table 30.2   Some antibiotic sensitivities

Antibiotic	Sensitivities	Comments and indications
Penicillins (phenoxymethylpenicillin)	Streptococcal (including *Streptococcus pneumoniae*), *Neisseria gonorrhoea* and *N. meningitidis* infection	• Phenoxymethylpenicillin is less active than benzylpenicillin but may be given orally for respiratory tract infections in children, streptococcal tonsillitis and as prophylaxis against streptococcal infections following rheumatic fever and against pneumococcal infections following splenectomy or in sickle cell disease • Benzylpenicillin may be given intravenously for bacterial meningitis • See text for note on resistance • Co-amoxiclav is used for animal bites
Penicillinase-resistant penicillin (flucloxacillin)	Penicillin-resistant *Staphylococcus* spp.	Otitis externa, adjunct in pneumonia, impetigo, cellulitis, wound infections, osteomyelitis and endocarditis if infection is known or likely to be caused by *Staphylococcus* spp. producing penicillinases
Broad-spectrum penicillins (ampicillin, amoxicillin)	Gram-positive and Gram-negative bacteria but inactivated by penicillinases secreted by common Gram-negative bacilli and *Staphylococcus aureus*	• Indicated for exacerbation of chronic bronchitis, otitis media and UTIs • See text for note on resistance
Cephalosporins	Varying sensitivities to Gram-positive and Gram-negative bacteria depending on generation of the cephalosporin	Septicaemia, pneumonia, meningitis, biliary tract infections, peritonitis and UTIs
Glycopeptides	Only Gram-positive bacteria	• Vancomycin and teicoplanin are used against MRSA infections • Vancomycin is effective against *Clostridium difficile*
Macrolides	Similar spectrum to penicillins. Also active against *Chlamydia*, *Mycoplasma*, *Campylobacter*, *Legionella*	• Suitable alternative in patients who are allergic to penicillin • Respiratory infections, whooping cough, Legionnaires' disease, *Campylobacter* enteritis • Poor activity against *Haemophilus influenzae*
Chloramphenicol	Broad-spectrum against mainly Gram-positive cocci and Gram-negative bacteria	• It is associated with aplastic anaemia and systemic use is reserved for life-threatening infections such as *Haemophilus influenzae* • It is widely used for bacterial conjunctivitis
Tetracyclines	Gram-positive and Gram-negative bacteria	• Resistance is a problem • *Chlamydia*, exacerbation of chronic bronchitis (*Haemophilus influenzae*), periodontal disease, acne, respiratory and genital *Mycoplasma* infections

Continued

Table 30.2   Continued

Antibiotic	Sensitivities	Comments and indications
Quinolones	Aerobic Gram-negative bacilli, particularly *Pseudomonas aeruginosa*, *Haemophilus influenzae*, *Campylobacter*	• Nalidixic acid and norfloxacin used to treat UTIs • Ciprofloxacin for respiratory infection (except pneumococcal pneumonia), UTIs, gastrointestinal infections (including typhoid), gonorrhoea and septicaemia • Ofloxacin for UTIs, lower respiratory tract infections, gonorrhoea, non-gonococcal urethritis and cervicitis • Many staphylococci are resistant to quinolones, which are therefore avoided for MRSA infections
Metronidazole	Anaerobes and protozoa	• Trichomonal vaginosis (*Gardnerella vaginalis*), giardiasis (*Giardia lamblia*), surgical and gynaecological sepsis (*Bacteroides fragilis*), pseudomembranous colitis, fungating tumours and rosacea • Resistance is common
Sulphonamides and trimethoprim	*Pneumocystis carinii*, methicillin-resistant *Staphylococcus* spp., some Gram-negative rods	• Decreased use due to resistance and availability of less toxic alternatives • Trimethoprim is now often used alone in place of sulfamethoxazole plus trimethoprim (co-trimoxazole) • Pneumonia in AIDS patients, toxoplasmosis and nocardosis. Acute exacerbation of chronic bronchitis, acute otitis media in children and UTI if good bacteriological evidence
Aminoglycosides	Some Gram-positive and many Gram-negative	• Gentamicin is administered systemically (thus hospital use) and plays an important role in serious infections such as septicaemia, meningitis, acute pyelonephritis and endocarditis • Inactive against anaerobes and poor activity against haemolytic streptococci and *Streptococcus pneumoniae* • Synergism with agents that target cell wall synthesis such as penicillins and vancomycin • Requires therapeutic drug monitoring (Chapter 6)
Clindamycin	Gram-positive cocci, including penicillin-resistant staphylococci, many anaerobes	• Staphylococcal joint and bone infections, e.g. osteomyelitis and intra-abdominal sepsis • Limited use due to toxic side-effects

UTIs, urinary tract infections; MRSA, methicillin-resistant *Staphylococcus aureus*; AIDS, acquired immune deficiency syndrome.

Others

- Clindamycin inhibits protein synthesis by a similar mechanism to the macrolide antibiotics (see above).
- Chloramphenicol inhibits protein synthesis by binding to the bacterial ribosome and inhibiting the formation of peptide bonds.
- Fusidic acid is a narrow-spectrum antibiotic inhibiting predominantly protein synthesis by Gram-positive bacteria.

Sulphonamides and trimethoprim

Sulphonamides inhibit the growth of bacteria (bacteriostatic) by inhibiting the enzyme dihydropteroate synthase involved in the synthesis of folate from *para*-amino benzoic acid. The availability of DNA and RNA precursors is therefore reduced. Human folate synthesis is also reduced, though it may be obtained from the diet. The presence of thymidine and purines from pus and tissue breakdown bypass the need for folic acid, thereby reducing the effectiveness of these agents in such situations.

Trimethoprim is structurally related to folate, thereby acting as a folate antagonist and inhibiting dihydrofolate reductase, which converts folate to tetrahydrofolate. Previously, trimethoprim was widely used in combination with sulfamethoxazole (co-trimoxazole), but the side-effects of sulfamethoxazole are pronounced and therefore trimethoprim tends to be used alone.

Metronidazole

Metronidazole was originally developed to treat amoebiasis (protozoan infection). The mechanism of action is thought to be via DNA damage due to toxic oxygen products generated from the drug by these parasites. It is also active against anaerobic bacteria, containing nitroreductases, which activate metronidazole. It is useful for the treatment of dental abscesses, fungating tumours, pseudomembranous colitis and sepsis secondary to bowel disease when anaerobic infection is suspected.

Antituberculous drugs

Ethambutol, isoniazid, pyrazinamide, rifampicin

First-line agents include a combination of isoniazid, rifampicin, ethambutol (if resistance to isoniazid is likely) and pyrazinamide. Combination therapy is given in two phases to prevent resistance. The initial phase includes the use of at least three drugs for 2 months. A combination of two drugs is then given for the continuation phase lasting 4 months or longer in drug-resistant infection, meningitis or bone/joint involvement. Intermittent regimens are recommended when compliance is a problem.

Isoniazid

Isoniazid possesses selective bacteriostatic activity against mycobacteria species with some bactericidal activity against the actively dividing mycobacteria. It is actively taken up: possible inhibition of *Mycobacterium*-specific mycolic acid constituents of the cell wall is the suggested mechanism. Disruption of cell metabolism may also be involved.

Resistance occurs due to reduced penetration of the drug. Side-effects include allergic skin eruptions, fever, hepatotoxicity, haematological changes, arthritis and vasculitis (Chapter 5).

Rifampicin

Rifampicin binds to and inhibits DNA-dependent RNA polymerase in prokaryotic cells but not eukaryotic cells. It is also active against some Gram-positive and Gram-negative species. Resistance occurs rapidly due to a mutation in the chromosome encoding the DNA-dependent RNA polymerase. Adverse drug reactions (ADRs) include skin eruptions, jaundice, hepatotoxicity, fever and gastrointestinal disturbances.

Ethambutol

Ethambutol inhibits the growth of mycobacteria, though resistance is common if used alone. The development of optic neuritis is dose-related, with an increased risk in renal impairment. Colour blindness and reduced visual acuity may occur and therefore monitoring of visual symptoms is required. Additional ADRs include gastrointestinal disturbance, arthralgia, headache, dizziness and mental disturbances.

Pyrazinamide

This agent becomes tuberculostatic at acidic pH. It is effective against intracellular mycobacteria found in macrophages following phagocytosis. Pyrazinamide is most effective against rapidly dividing intracellular organisms and is most effective in the first 2 months. Unwanted effects include gout, gastrointestinal disturbances and hepatotoxicity.

Drug choice

Current guidelines can be found at the beginning of section 5 of the *British National Formulary*. Local guidelines may be available from health authorities or primary care trusts or the local infectious diseases centre. Table 30.2 summarises examples of the main sensitivities of some antibiotics in regular use. Factors for consideration when prescribing antibiotics include:

- the likely causative organism
- risk of pathogen resistance
- age and sex of patient
- history of drug allergy
- tolerance of gastrointestinal side-effects
- renal and hepatic function
- concurrent illnesses, e.g. epilepsy (Table 30.3)
- concurrent drug treatment (Table 30.4)
- route of elimination (renal excretion of active drugs resulting in therapeutic concentrations in the urinary tract, a distinct advantage in UTIs)
- is the patient pregnant or breast-feeding?
- risk factors, e.g. immunocompromised
- is the patient taking oral contraceptives?

Common organisms causing disease in humans

Bacteria are classified according to a staining method developed by Christian Gram in the 19th century. Gram-positive bacteria retain a solution of dye, which can be washed away from Gram-negative bacteria due to differing cell wall structures. Further nomenclature results from additional properties including morphology, the formation of spores and movement. Acid-fast bacteria are also named according to a staining reaction. For examples of disease-causing bacteria see Table 30.1; some sensitivities of antibacterial agents are indicated in Table 30.2.

Resistance

Antibiotic resistance is an increasing problem. It occurs as a result of evolution of the rapidly dividing populations of bacteria. The spread of resistance occurs by the transfer of bacteria between people and the transfer of genetic material encoding resistance properties between bacteria. Mechanisms of resistance include:

- development of pumps to exclude the drug from the bacteria, e.g. resistance to quinolones
- impermeability of bacteria to drugs, e.g. resistance to streptomycin
- inactivation of the drug, e.g. production of the enzyme beta-lactamase by *Staphylococcus* spp. results in the breakdown of both penicillin V and penicillin G. Flucloxacillin is penicillinase-resistant and is therefore used for treating infections caused by penicillin-resistant *Staphylococcus* spp. Alternatively, the combination of the broad-spectrum penicillin amoxicillin with clavulanic acid may be given. Clavulanic acid inhibits beta-lactamase
- some Gram-negative bacteria have reduced permeability of the cell wall, thereby impeding penetration of hydrophilic antibiotics to the target site
- alternative metabolic pathways to bypass blockade, e.g in resistance to trimethoprim
- alteration in the drug target so that it is no longer recognised by the drug, e.g. in resistance to erythromycin, aminoglycosides

Methicillin-resistant *Staphylococcus aureus*

Resistance of *Staphylococcus aureus* bacteria to the discontinued drug methicillin is known as methicillin-resistant *Staphylococcus aureus* (MRSA).

Table 30.3 Concurrent disease and antibiotic prescribing

Concurrent disease	Drugs to avoid or use with caution	Comments
Arrhythmias	Macrolides	Prolongation of QT interval
History of allergy	Penicillins (phenoxymethylpenicillin, flucloxacillin, amoxicillin, pivmecillinam)	Increased risk of penicillin hypersensitivity including urticaria, fever, joint pains, rashes, angioedema
Penicillin allergy	Penicillins and cephalosporins	• If possible, penicillin side-effects should be differentiated from true penicillin allergy (see text) • Usually occurs within 72 h of starting treatment • Penicillin allergy is a contraindication to using penicillins and a reason not to use cephalosporins
Asthma (see also above)	Co-trimoxazole	May cause shortness of breath or pulmonary infiltrates
Epilepsy	Quinolones	May induce convulsions
Immunocompromised	All antibiotics	Higher doses are often required, as infections may be severe
Porphyria (hereditary disorder of haem biosynthesis)	Flucloxacillin, cephalosporins, erythromycin, isoniazid, sulphonamides, chloramphenicol, co-trimoxazole, trimethoprim, nitrofurantoin, nalidixic acid, tinidazole, oxytetracyline	For complete list see *British National Formulary* section 9.8.2
Sore throat	Broad-spectrum penicillins (ampicillin, amoxicillin)	Due to a rash with glandular fever
Psychiatric disorders	Quinolones	Discontinue if there is a psychotic reaction
Diabetes mellitus	Cephalosporins, nitrofurantoin	False-positive urinary glucose (test for reducing substances)
Myasthenia gravis	Aminoglycosides	Impairment of neuromuscular transmission
Diarrhoea	Clindamycin	Contraindicated
History of deafness	Vancomycin, gentamicin	Ototoxic

Resistance to flucloxacillin has also been reported. The mechanism includes the modification of bacterial penicillin-binding sites. Treatment is indicated according to the infecting strain and currently includes vancomycin and teicoplanin. New antibiotics effective against MRSA are reserved for strains resistant to conventional antibiotics and as such are currently beyond the scope of this book. These agents include linezolid (an oxazolidinone) and a combination of the streptogramin antibiotics quinupristin and dalfopristin.

Measures to limit resistance include:

• the use of short courses of antibiotics such as a 3-day course to treat uncomplicated UTI
• a reduction in unnecessary use of antibiotics in the treatment of viral infections and other self-limiting infections
• the avoidance of antibiotics on repeat prescriptions
• the avoidance of inappropriate prescribing of broad-spectrum agents (Table 30.2)
• ensuring that patients complete courses of

antibiotics, so that more resilient strains do not survive

- in the case of TB, the use of combination therapy

Penicillin allergy

Reports of penicillin allergy are common and it is often difficult to distinguish between true penicillin allergy (Chapter 19) and less serious ADRs. A high proportion of patients reporting penicillin allergy may lack immunoglobulin E (IgE) antibodies specific for penicillin. It has been suggested that the unnecessary use of broad-spectrum antibiotics may be avoided by performing penicillin skin tests (Solensky *et al.*, 2002). This study revealed that patients with a previous history of true penicillin allergy might safely receive subsequent courses of penicillin following a negative skin test result.

Concurrent conditions

Although bacterial sensitivity of the causative organisms is a prime factor in the choice of appropriate antibacterial agents, concurrent conditions should also be taken into account. Some considerations are detailed in Table 30.3.

Children less than 12 years of age should not receive tetracyclines due to deposition in the teeth, leading to discoloration.

Pregnancy

The safest antibiotics for use during pregnancy are considered to be the penicillins, erythromycin and cephalosporins. The following drugs should be avoided or used with caution:

- Ciprofloxacin and other quinolones: adverse effects on developing cartilage have been reported in animal studies, even though there is no evidence of teratogenicity in humans.
- Co-trimoxazole: this is a folate antagonist, so there is a possible teratogenic risk.
- Fusidic acid: not known to be harmful; consider risk versus benefit.
- Gentamicin: there is a risk of auditory damage to the fetus.

- Metronidazole: avoid high doses if possible but this is an important treatment of trichomoniasis and giardiasis infections.
- Nitrofurantoin may cause nausea.
- Tetracycline: there is a risk of deposition in growing bones and teeth and the resultant risk of fetal abnormalities if given during pregnancy.

Breast-feeding

Amoxicillin, erythromycin or cephalosporins are appropriate for use during breast-feeding. Penicillins may in theory produce hypersensitivity in the infant and therefore mothers should be vigilant for signs of allergy such as a rash. Tetracyclines are not recommended, although calcium should prevent the infant from absorbing the small amounts present in breast milk.

Drug interactions

Antibacterial agents comprise a diverse group of drugs and can be expected to exhibit a range of interactions. In particular, the macrolides are inhibitors and rifampacin an inducer of cytochrome P450 with the ability to alter the metabolism of a range of other drugs. An important consideration is the interaction with oral contraceptives and broad-spectrum antibiotics which, although rare, should always be borne in mind. Some important interactions are detailed in Table 30.4.

General counselling

- Antimicrobials should be taken regularly, at evenly spaced intervals, and the prescribed course should be completed to prevent recurrence and resistance. Explaining that more resistant bacteria may survive if the course is not completed, creating an increased risk of resistance to subsequent treatment, may aid compliance.
- Women of child-bearing age should be counselled regarding the possible interaction between antibiotics and oral contraceptives (Table 30.4).

Table 30.4   Examples of drug interactions involving antibiotics

Drugs	Consequences	Comments
Aminoglycosides with furosemide (frusemide)	Increased risk of aminoglycoside toxicity	• Monitor carefully for signs of nephrotoxicity and/or ototoxicity • Bumetanide does not appear to interact
Aminoglycosides with vancomycin	Increased risk of nephrotoxicity due to both drugs	Monitor for signs of nephrotoxicity
Broad-spectrum antibacterials (penicillins, trimethoprim and co-trimoxazole, tetracyclines, erythromycin, metronidazole) with oral contraceptives	Rarely, contraceptive failure and pregnancy	• Additional precautions should be taken during treatment and for at least 7 days thereafter • During long-term antibiotic treatment, additional precautions are recommended for the first 3 weeks of treatment • This rare interaction is thought to be due to alterations in gut bacteria, which are involved in the enterohepatic cycling of oestrogens
Quinolones with oral contraceptives	No reports of an interaction	This combination is included in view of confusion regarding the interaction of antibiotics with oral contraceptives
Rifampicin with oral contraceptives	Risk of contraceptive failure and pregnancy	Additional precautions are required during treatment and for 4–8 weeks after withdrawal due to enzyme induction and accelerated metabolism of oestrogens
Quinolones (ciprofloxacin, ofloxacin) with NSAIDs and drugs lowering seizure threshold (Chapter 5)	Increased risk of seizures	• Rare and limited evidence • These drugs should not be used in combination in patients with epilepsy
Quinolones with antacids	Reduced absorption of quinolones	• Aluminium and magnesium antacids particularly may reduce serum levels to below therapeutic concentrations • Separate administration by 2–6 h
Ciprofloxacin with theophylline	Increased serum levels of theophylline	• Dose reduction (by half) is required with ciprofloxacin, enoxacin, and possibly norfloxacin • Monitor for signs of theophylline toxicity (Chapter 6)
Metronidazole, tinidazole, the cephalosporin cefamandole with alcohol	Risk of disulfiram-like reaction	• Most antibiotics do not interact with alcohol • Avoid alcohol with the drugs listed, as reaction may be frightening, although not serious
Erythromycin with alcohol	Erythromycin may increase the plasma concentrations of alcohol	• Some reports have also shown that alcohol reduces the absorption of erythromycin ethyl succinate • Drivers should be advised of this potential interaction

Continued

Table 30.4   Continued

Drugs	Consequences	Comments
Antibiotics with warfarin	Effects of warfarin may be increased	See Chapter 15
Isoniazid with phenytoin, carbamazepine	Increased levels of anticonvulsants	Isoniazid inhibits cytochrome P450
Rifampicin with corticosteroids, oestrogens, phenytoin, carbamazepine, sulphonylureas, anticoagulants	Reduced levels	Rifampicin induces cytochrome P450, therefore increasing metabolism
Macrolides with ciclosporin	Increased levels	• Reduced ciclosporin dosage is usually required (approximately 60% with erythromycin). Monitor levels • Azithromycin appears not to interact
Erythromycin, clarithromycin, with other drugs which prolong the QT interval (Chapter 5)	Risk of potentially life-threatening cardiac arrhythmias	The CSM advises that the concurrent use of two or more drugs that prolong the QT interval should be avoided because of the risk of additive effects (CSM/MCA, 1996)
Erythromycin with various drugs: (alfentanil, theophylline, warfarin, atorvastatin, some benzodiazepines, nadolol, carbamazepine (may become toxic), ciclosporin, digoxin (occasionally), felodipine, omeprazole	Inhibition of metabolism and therefore increased levels	Erythromycin inhibits cytochrome P450 enzymes
Erythromycin with zafirlukast	Reduced plasma concentrations	Monitor treatment outcome with zafirlukast

NSAIDs, non-steroidal anti-inflammatory drugs; CSM, Committee on Safety of Medicines; MCA, Medicines Control Agency.

- Patients should be advised that antibacterial agents will take several days for an effect but if the condition does not resolve by the end of the course patients should visit their GP.
- Patients should be advised not to hoard antibacterials or allow them to be used by others.
- A key point to reinforce is that colds and most sore throats are viral in origin and will not respond to antibacterial agents (Chapter 18).
- An important point is that taking broad-spectrum antibiotics is associated with super-infection, which may lead to candidiasis and diarrhoea. If the diarrhoea is severe (possibly accompanied by pain and pyrexia), this may indicate pseudomembranous colitis and patients should contact their GP urgently. This is particularly associated with clindamycin treatment (Chapters 5 and 9).
- Many antibacterial agents are associated with rashes and this is particularly true of penicillin allergy. In the case of penicillin allergy, antihistamines may relieve the rash. However, as with any drug, if there is itching, angioedema or breathing difficulties, then medical attention should be sought immediately as this may be due to anaphylaxis (Chapter 19).
- A prominent record of penicillin allergy should be made on all medical records and patients should also be advised to inform GPs, dentists, pharmacists and nurses.

Penicillins

- Penicillins should be taken an hour before food or on an empty stomach for improved absorption, with the exception of amoxicillin.
- Penicillins should not be taken by patients with a history of penicillin allergy.
- Side-effects are mild and may include diarrhoea or indigestion.
- Flucloxacillin may rarely cause jaundice.

Cephalosporins

- Report increased bruising or signs of bleeding, due to possible interference with blood-clotting factors.

Quinolones

- Separate administration of antacids, particularly aluminium and magnesium-containing preparations, by 2–6 h as these antacids may reduce serum levels to below therapeutic concentrations.
- Quinolones may impair performance of skilled tasks such as driving. Advice given in the *British National Formulary* suggests that these effects are enhanced by alcohol, but evidence presented in *Drug Interactions* by Stockley (2002) suggests that quinolones do not interact with alcohol.
- Due to risk of tendon damage, the Committee on Safety of Medicines (CSM) warns that treatment should be withdrawn at the first sign of pain or inflammation (CSM/Medicines Control Agency, 1995). The affected limb should be rested until tendon symptoms have resolved. Contact the GP immediately.

Macrolides

- Macrolides may cause nausea, so should be taken with or after food.
- Macrolides and erythromycin in particular are associated with a high incidence of nausea and vomiting.

Tetracyclines

- Do not take at the same time as milk, iron or zinc supplements, calcium supplements or indigestion remedies that may hinder absorption. Separate doses by at least 2 h.
- Swallow whole with plenty of water while sitting or standing.
- Doxycycline may cause photosensitivity, therefore avoid exposure to the sun or use high-factor sun cream. Avoid using sun beds and sun showers.

Metronidazole and tinidazole

- Do not take these with alcohol due to very unpleasant effects such as flushing.
- Take with or after food.
- Swallow whole, and do not chew.
- Take with plenty of water.
- For treatment exceeding 10 days, consider providing advice about the increased risk of adverse effects such as peripheral neuropathy (see Monitoring, below).

Trimethoprim

- Contact the GP if a rash and/or itching develop.
- If taking trimethoprim long-term, report signs of bruising, bleeding, mouth ulcers or sore throat due to rare effects of this antibiotic on the blood.

Clindamycin

- Capsules should be swallowed whole with plenty of water.
- See comments above regarding diarrhoea.

Antituberculous drugs

- Soft contact lenses should not be worn during treatment with rifampicin. Gas-permeable or hard lenses are appropriate.
- The patient should report any signs of liver disease such as persistent nausea, vomiting, malaise or jaundice immediately.
- Rifampicin may colour the patient's urine orange-red.
- Isoniazid should be taken 30–60 min before food.
- The patient should report visual deterioration with ethambutol immediately. This may be irreversible if treatment is continued.
- The importance of compliance should be explained.

- Pyridoxine (vitamin B_6) should be taken with isoniazid to prevent peripheral neuropathy. Increased risk factors include diabetes mellitus, alcohol misuse, renal failure and malnutrition.

Eye drops and ointments

- Eye drops should be applied at least every 2 h and then the frequency reduced as the infection is controlled.
- Treatment should be continued for 48 h after symptoms have cleared.
- Eye ointment may be used at night or three to four times a day if used alone.
- Remaining drops or ointment should be discarded.
- Sterile saline solution may help soothe the eyes and remove discharge.

Monitoring

Metronidazole

Laboratory and clinical monitoring is advised if treatment with metronidazole exceeds 10 days. This is due to an increased risk of adverse effects, particularly peripheral neuropathy, and possibly transient seizures, cholestatic hepatitis, jaundice and leucopenia. Full blood counts and liver function tests may be required (Chapter 2).

Renal impairment

Many drugs require dose reduction, particularly in severe renal impairment. Some general considerations are:

- Piperacillin: dose adjustment is required.
- Aminoglycosides: dose reduction and monitoring are required with even mild renal impairment. Plasma concentrations should be monitored due to renal and ototoxicity.
- Ethambutol: dose reduction and monitoring are required.
- Isoniazid: maximum dose recommended in severe impairment is 200 mg/day.
- Sulphonamides: maintain a high fluid intake with moderate impairment due to the risk of crystalluria.
- Tetracyclines: other than doxycycline and minocycline, may exacerbate renal failure and should not be given to patients with renal disease.
- Trimethoprim: dose reduction is required in moderate renal failure. Avoid if creatinine clearance is less than 10 mL/min unless plasma trimethoprim levels are monitored.

Hepatic function

Many antibiotics may cause hepatic disease (Chapter 5) and therefore monitoring for suspected ADRs is important.

- Clindamycin: dose reduction is required.
- Co-amoxiclav: CSM warns of risk of cholestatic jaundice. Treatment should not normally exceed 14 days.
- Erythromycin may cause idiosyncratic hepatotoxicity.
- Flucloxacillin: CSM warns of a risk of cholestatic jaundice.
- Fusidic acid: impaired biliary excretion and increased risk of hepatotoxicity. A reduced dose is used if treatment is necessary.
- Isoniazid: monitor liver function tests regularly and particularly during the first 2 months of treatment.
- Metronidazole: in severe hepatic disease, the dose of metronidazole is reduced by a third and given once a day.
- Minocycline: monitor liver function tests if treatment exceeds 6 months.
- Pyrazinamide: avoid in liver disease.
- Rifampicin: monitor for toxicity.
- Tetracyclines should be avoided or used with caution in liver disease.

Over-the-counter considerations

Pharmacists are ideally placed to reassure patients and recommend symptomatic relief of infections which do not require antibiotics. Consultations regarding infections are particularly important in the identification of underlying disease. Patient counselling on the appropriate use of anti-infective agents and preventive measures is important, particularly in preventing drug resistance and treatment failure. General lifestyle advice (Chapter 3) may also be appropriate.

Genitourinary infection

Recurrent UTIs or *Candida* infections may indicate diabetes mellitus, recent antibiotic treatment or undiagnosed sexually transmitted disease. Appropriate referral including the first UTI in men, pregnant women, abdominal or lower back pain, resistance to treatment and haematuria is warranted.

The following advice is important in the prevention of recurrent infection:

- the avoidance of nylon underwear (cotton is preferred)
- the importance of sexual hygiene, including urination after sexual intercourse
- drink plenty of water
- urinate frequently with double voiding (go again after 5 min)
- cranberry juice has been shown to be effective at preventing bacteria adhering to bladder epithelial cells and may be helpful in the treatment of UTIs
- consider treating partners

ADRs

Requests for antidiarrhoeal agents should be dealt with carefully to exclude possible antibiotic-associated colitis. For example, the severity and duration of diarrhoea should be determined.

Throat preparations containing local anaesthetics may cause hypersensitivity.

Drug interactions

For interactions between non-steroidal anti-inflammatory drugs or antacids with antibiotics, see Table 30.4.

Products for cystitis containing sodium are inappropriate for patients with hypertension or those prescribed lithium. Alternative products containing potassium salts should not be given to patients taking angiotensin-converting enzyme inhibitors or potassium-sparing diuretics such as spironolactone or amiloride.

Practice points

- Broad-spectrum antibiotics are more likely to result in fungal infections (vaginitis or pruritus ani) or ADRs such as pseudomembranous colitis.
- Viral infections such as simple coughs and colds and viral sore throats should not be treated with antibacterials.
- Whenever possible, an accurate diagnosis and clear documentation of penicillin hypersensitivity should be made.

 CASE STUDIES

Case 1
A 60-year-old female requests loperamide for acute diarrhoea. On further questioning you discover she is taking clindamycin.

Do you give loperamide?

- No! Clindamycin is associated with antibiotic-associated colitis, which is potentially fatal. This is most common in middle-aged and elderly women and particularly postoperatively. The antibiotic should be stopped immediately.

Case 2
A 65-year-old male presents at Accident and Emergency complaining of a persistent productive cough with haemoptysis and general ill health. A chest X-ray reveals a lesion.

→

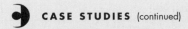

CASE STUDIES (continued)

How would TB be confirmed?

- TB is becoming more prevalent. A positive Mantoux (tuberculin test) confirms TB together with the above symptoms and possibly a sputum sample culture, though the former is the quickest means of diagnosis.

What tests would be carried out before starting drug treatment?

- Liver function tests are required, as isoniazid, rifampicin and pyrazinamide are all associated with liver toxicity. Renal function would be determined as doses of ethambutol and isoniazid may need to be adjusted. Visual acuity is monitored with ethambutol as this can cause loss of acuity, colour blindness or restriction of visual fields.

Is it necessary to treat contacts?

- Yes. Chemoprophylaxis with isoniazid for 6 months is the current recommendation.

What are the possible causes of treatment failure?

- Treatment failure may result from incorrect prescribing, poor compliance or drug resistance. Taking a sample of urine, which is orange-red when taking rifampicin, may be a useful method to monitor compliance.

Case 3
A 55-year-old male patient presents with an acute exacerbation of chronic bronchitis. He has seen adverts about overuse of antibiotics and is reluctant to take them. He reports purulent green sputum.

What is the appropriate treatment?

- Amoxicillin is an appropriate first-line treatment, assuming this patient is not allergic to penicillin. His symptoms and history indicate the use of antibiotics and he should be advised accordingly. Amoxicillin is a broad-spectrum antibiotic covering the main organisms causing community-acquired infection, such as *Streptococcus, Pneumonia, Haemophilus influenzae* or *Staphylococcus aureus*. Erythromycin is a suitable alternative in penicillin allergy, though drug interactions should be considered. Smoking cessation advice should be reinforced if necessary.

References

Committee on Safety of Medicines/Medicines Control Agency (1995). *Curr Probl Pharmacovigilance* 21: 8.

Committee on Safety of Medicines/Medicines Control Agency (1996). *Curr Probl Pharmacovigilance* 22: 1–2.

Mehta D K (ed.) *British National Formulary*, latest edition. London: British Medical Association and Royal Pharmaceutical Society of Great Britain.

Solensky R, Earl H S, Gruchala R S (2002). Lack of penicillin resensitization in patients with a history of penicillin allergy after receiving repeated penicillin courses. *Arch Intern Med* 162: 822–826.

Stockley I H (2002). *Drug Interactions*, 6th edn. London: Pharmaceutical Press.

Further reading

Hugo W B, Russell A D (eds) (1987). *Pharmaceutical Microbiology*, 4th edn. Oxford: Blackwell Scientific Publications.

Standing Medical Advisory Committee, subgroup on antimicrobial resistance (SMAC 1998). *The Path of Least Resistance*. London: HMSO.

Online resource

www.phls.co.uk The Public Health Laboratory Service for the latest information relating to infectious diseases (accessed 4 December 2002).

31

Non-bacterial infections

The term 'parasite' describes organisms which rely on another organism or host for food and shelter without providing a positive contribution to the host. Parasitic infections therefore include bacteria, fungi, worms, viruses and protozoa. Non-bacterial infections comprise:

- fungal: *Candida albicans* and tinea (Chapter 32)
- viral: herpes simplex and varicella-zoster (Chapter 32), influenza (Chapter 18)
- protozoan: *Plasmodium* spp. (malaria)
- helminthic: roundworms (ascariasis), thread worms (enterobiasis)
- ectoparasitic infections: head lice (*Pediculus humanus capitis*), crab lice (*Pthirus pubis*) and scabies (*Sarcoptes scabiei*)

Goals of treatment

The main aims of treatment are to:

- prevent infection such as malaria
- prevent spread of lice or scabies

- prevent reinfection by implementing hygiene measures and contact tracing

Malaria

Malaria is a potentially fatal mosquito-borne infection of red blood cells (erythrocytes) caused by the protozoan parasites *Plasmodium falciparum, P. vivax, P. ovale* and *P. malariae.* Red blood cells are destroyed by the parasites, resulting in haemolytic anaemia. Other symptoms include shivering, fever and sweating.

Drug treatment for prophylaxis of malaria

The choice of antimalarial agent depends largely on the destination of travel and the presence of resistance. Recommendations for effective prophylaxis are reviewed regularly and therefore the latest guidelines should be sought from the National Pharmaceutical Association (NPA),

405

Schools of Tropical Medicine (contact details are in the *British National Formulary* (BNF) section 5.4), the Department of Health or World Health Organization.

4-aminoquinolines (chloroquine)

Chloroquine is a disease-modifying antirheumatoid drug (DMARD, Chapter 28). In protozoal infections, chloroquine becomes concentrated in infected erythrocytes as it binds to a breakdown product of haemoglobin. It then inhibits haem polymerase, an enzyme produced by *Plasmodium* spp., which prevents the parasite from digesting haemoglobin. It is therefore effective against the erythrocytic forms *P. malariae*, *P. ovale* and *P. vivax*. It is not however effective against latent forms of *P. ovale* and *P. vivax*, which reside in the liver. The resistance of *P. falciparum* to chloroquine tends to result from increased efflux of the drug and/or reduced uptake.

Quinoline-methanols (quinine, mefloquine)

Quinine is active against all erythrocytic forms of *Plasmodium* spp. but is mainly used to treat *P. falciparum* infections. In view of its adverse effects, it is not appropriate for prophylaxis. Quinine is an alkaloid with negative inotropic effects on the heart, a mild oxytocic effect on the uterus in pregnancy (although use is appropriate for malaria treatment), and has a weak antipyretic effect. Mefloquine has no effect on hepatic forms of the parasites but is often used for prophylaxis or treatment of *P. falciparum* infection and particularly against chloroquine-resistant forms. Quinine resistance occurs following increased expression of an efflux transporter.

Drugs affecting the synthesis or utilisation of folate (pyrimethamine, proguanil)

These agents exhibit activity similar to that of sulphonamides (Chapter 30) in that they inhibit the utilisation of folate by inhibiting dihydrofolate reductase. Combinations of folate antagonists with drugs targeting folate synthesis are used to produce a synergistic action resulting from blockade of different parts of the synthetic pathway.

8-aminoquinolones (primaquine)

Primaquine is active against the latent phase of *P. ovale* and *P. vivax* and may be used in combination with other drugs such as chloroquine. It enters the parasites in the liver and is thought to inhibit mitochondrial respiration. Active metabolites may also bind to parasitic DNA. Resistance is currently rare.

Doxycycline

Doxycycline may be used as an alternative when antimalarials are contraindicated (Chapter 30).

Drug choice

Local guidelines may be available from health authorities, primary care trusts or on the advice of the local infectious disease centre. Factors for consideration when prescribing include:

- risk of pathogen resistance
- age and sex of patient
- history of drug allergy
- concurrent disease (Table 31.1)
- is the patient pregnant or breast-feeding?
- time and destination of travel

Patient counselling

Patients should be encouraged to consult healthcare professionals at least 2 months before foreign travel to ensure time for vaccinations.

Antimalarials

- Preventive measures are important, even during prophylaxis with antimalarials.
- The application of repellents containing diethyltoluamide (DEET, now called diethylmethylbenzamide), with increasing concentration (up to 50%) or frequency of applications, offers greatest protection (Fradin and Day, 2002).
- Mosquito nets should be used at night. Nets impregnated with permethrin and vaporised insecticides are also effective.

Table 31.1 The effects of concurrent disease on drug choice

Concurrent disease	Drugs to avoid or use with caution	Comments
Arrhythmias	Mefloquine, quinine	Prolongation of QT interval (Chapter 5)
Asthma and/or eczema	Pesticides containing alcohol	Some pesticide preparations may trigger an allergic response. All pesticides should be applied in a well-ventilated room
Epilepsy	Chloroquine, mefloquine, piperazine	May induce convulsions and should therefore be avoided
Gastrointestinal disease (severe)	Chloroquine	Use with caution
Glucose-6-phosphate dehydrogenase (G6PD) deficiency	Primaquine	• G6PD activity should be assessed prior to initiating treatment • Patients with G6PD deficiency may suffer haemolysis if given standard doses • Reduced doses are appropriate
Hepatic disease	Mefloquine, pyrazinamide	Avoid
Psychiatric disorders	Mefloquine	Contraindicated for patients with a history of psychiatric disorders including depression
Psoriasis	Chloroquine	May exacerbate psoriasis
Renal impairment	Proguanil (avoid or reduce dose), piperazine	• Chloroquine, mefloquine or doxycycline are appropriate for malaria prophylaxis • The dose of chloroquine may require reduction in severe impairment • Piperazine should be avoided in severe renal impairment

- Protective clothing should be worn in the evening, after dusk.
- Patients may be concerned about side-effects from antimalarials and should be advised of the importance of taking these drugs since malaria is life-threatening. For example, many people are worried about the psychiatric effects of mefloquine (Chapter 5).
- Prophylaxis is recommended for 1 week before travel (2–3 weeks for mefloquine to identify psychiatric adverse drug reactions prior to travel), during the stay and for 4 weeks after return.
- Any illness within 1 year of travel to an area associated with risk of malaria should be reported, particularly within the first 3 months.

Helminthic and ectoparasitic infections

Pruritus is the most common feature of the presence of worms, head lice, crabs or scabies. These parasites may then be observed, for example, head lice on the hair or worms in the faeces. Scabies are more difficult to diagnose as they burrow under the skin but close examination will reveal 'tracks' along the skin and a magnifying glass may be used to view the mites. Suspicion of scabies is aroused if more than one patient living in the same house is affected and often the wrists are the first sites of infection.

Pharmacological basis of management

Anthelminthics

Mebendazole, piperazine

Anthelminthics target the formation of intracellular microtubules in helminths (parasitic worms). They must penetrate the cuticle of the worm or be eaten by the worm. The resultant effects are paralysis, partial digestion or an immune response to the damaged cuticle. Alternatively, helminth metabolism may be targeted. This is a species-dependent effect, explaining the varied activity of some anthelminthics.

Mebendazole is a broad-spectrum agent and may take several days to expel worms by targeting intracellular organelle function such as microtubules.

Piperazine is used to treat common roundworm (*Ascaris lumbricoides*) and threadworm (*Enterobius vermicularis*). It inhibits neuromuscular transmission in the worm, possibly by activation of gamma-aminobutyric acid (GABA)-gated chloride channels in nematode muscle leading to muscle relaxation. The paralysed worms are passed alive. Side-effects include gastrointestinal disturbance and urticaria.

Drug choice

Anthelminthics

These are combined with hygiene measures to prevent reinfection. Mebendazole is used to treat threadworms in patients over 2 years of age. This is available over-the-counter (OTC) but not for use during pregnancy. A fatty meal aids the absorption of mebendazole, which is given as a single dose for threadworm infection, or twice a day for 3 days to treat hookworms or roundworms and repeated after 2–3 weeks. Mebendazole is the most commonly used benzimidazole: gastrointestinal disturbances are the main side-effect.

Piperazine is an alternative, for example given to children aged from 3 months by a general practitioner (GP), given as a single dose and repeated after 14 days for threadworm infections or monthly for up to 3 months for roundworms.

Head lice preparations

The choice of preparation depends upon previous treatment and the presence of asthma or skin sensitivity such as eczema (Table 31.1). If a previous treatment has failed, then an alternative agent should be used. It should be noted that the presence of live head lice 7–9 days following treatment indicates the survival of eggs and therefore not treatment failure. The same treatment should be repeated. Evidence suggests the following order of efficacy: Suleo M > Prioderm > Derbac M > Lyclear rinse. This is based on the increased efficacy of products with a high alcohol content. Products with an aqueous base, such as Derbac M, are preferred for asthmatics and sensitive skin. Lotions, liquids or creme rinse formulations are recommended rather than shampoos, as the latter may be too dilute.

Carbaryl

It should be noted that carbaryl preparations have been restricted to prescription-only use due to the observation that carbaryl is potentially carcinogenic. The risk is reported to be theoretical, especially if use is intermittent.

Crab lice

Permethrin, phenothrin and malathion are licensed for the eradication of crab lice. Aqueous preparations are applied to all parts of the body for 12 h.

Patient counselling

Head lice preparations

Prevention

- Parents should be reassured that head lice have no preference for dirty or clean hair. Long hair may however be more accessible since head lice 'walk' from head to head. They do not hop, jump or fly. Long hair should therefore be braided close to the head if possible. Head lice are not harmful but may cause an itchy scalp.
- Regular checking for lice is advisable using a fine nit comb when the hair is wet, going

through a small section at a time. This will help to remove lice, aid early diagnosis and prevent the spread of head lice. The excessive use of pesticides may then be prevented. The use of conditioner may help the manual removal of lice. The eggs may appear similar to dandruff but are differentiated as they stick to the hair.

- Motivation is important when using wet combing as a treatment method as this process may take 30 min. The BNF recommends an interval of 4 days and a minimum of 2 weeks. Pesticides are considered to be a more effective treatment.
- The presence of lice should be confirmed before treating, as infection is not prevented by treatment. The hair may be combed over white paper to identify live lice.
- Contact tracing is important to prevent spread of the infection. This includes all close contacts such as grandparents who should be treated if infected.

Treatment

- Most products require a 12-h application and should be applied to dry hair at night, in a well-ventilated room. The hair and scalp should be soaked in the product and then allowed to dry naturally. The hair may then be washed the following morning.
- A second application may be required after 7–9 days, after which time any eggs not eradicated by the initial treatment may begin to hatch. This should not be confused with treatment failure or reinfestation.
- The manufacturers of Lyclear recommend that overuse of hair conditioners may reduce the efficacy of the product. Hair should be washed with a non-medicated shampoo without conditioner before using the product.
- Repeat applications should be avoided within a week and for more than 3 consecutive weeks. The manufacturers suggest that not more than five applications of head lice preparations are used per year. The likelihood of eradication is not increased.
- It should be noted that Full Marks mousse contains alcohol and may not be suitable for patients with asthma or eczema.

Crab lice

- Apply lotion to all parts of the body for 12 h. A second treatment is recommended after 7 days to kill lice hatching from eggs which may have survived the initial treatment (BNF).

Anthelminthics

- Combine with hygiene measures to break the cycle of reinfection. Hands should be washed and nails scrubbed before each meal and after each visit to the toilet. A bath immediately after rising will remove ova laid during the night. Fingernails should be kept short.
- A second dose may be required to prevent reinfection.
- Infected patients should use separate towels.
- Avoid using dirty towels in public toilets.
- All members of the same household should be treated, even if asymptomatic.

Concurrent conditions

Table 31.1 provides examples of the influence of concurrent disease on the choice of non-antibiotic anti-infective drugs.

Pregnancy

Antimalarials

Ideally, travel to areas with malaria should be avoided during pregnancy but proguanil or chloroquine may be used. Folic acid 5 mg supplementation is required with proguanil. Mefloquine is considered for areas of chloroquine resistance but the manufacturer recommends that it should be avoided. Doxycycline is contraindicated.

Anthelminthics

Mebendazole should be avoided during the first trimester. The BNF reports a lack of evidence of harm with piperazine.

Drug interactions

Table 31.2 summarises examples of drug interactions with antimalarial and anthelminthic drugs.

Table 31.2 Examples of drug interactions with antiparasitic agents

Drugs	Consequences	Comments
Antimalarials with antacids or antidiarrhoeals	Reduced absorption of chloroquine and proguanil	Doses of antimalarials and antacids (particularly magnesium trisilicate or kaolin) should be separated by at least 2–3 h
Mefloquine or quinine with drugs which prolong the QT interval (Chapter 5)	Increased risk of arrhythmias	• Mefloquine and quinine prolong the QT interval • The WHO has warned that mefloquine should be used with caution with concurrent antiarrhythmics, beta-blockers, calcium channel blockers, antihistamines or phenothiazines
Chloroquine with cimetidine	Increased effects of chloroquine due to reduced hepatic metabolism	• Risk of increased adverse effects of chloroquine • Ranitidine may be a suitable alternative
Mebendazole with cimetidine	Increased levels of mebendazole	Monitor for adverse effects of mebendazole
Mebendazole with phenytoin or carbamazepine	Reduced levels of mebendazole	Increased doses of mebendazole may be required but not when treating infections of the gut
Mefloquine with beta-adrenoceptor antagonists, calcium channel blockers, digoxin or antidepressants	Increased risk of bradycardia	Concurrent use should be avoided if possible, particularly for patients considered to be at increased risk of developing bradycardia, until more is known about these interactions
Quinine with cimetidine	Increased levels of quinine	• Monitor for adverse effects of quinine • Ranitidine is a suitable alternative

WHO, World Health Organization.

Practice points

Malaria

• The latest guidelines should always be consulted when recommending malaria prophylaxis due to increased resistance and the potentially fatal nature of this disease.

→

Practice points (continued)

Helminthic and ectoparasitic infections

- Contact tracing should be encouraged when eliminating head lice.
- Hygiene measures are important when recommending treatment for worms and head lice.
- Repeat applications of pesticides are generally recommended after 7–9 days for head lice.
- The mosaic approach to head lice treatment is no longer used. Current recommendations consist of using a different insecticide for a second application following treatment failure.
- Pharmacists should refer treatment failure and infants less than 6 months for assessment of scabies. Pharmacists may wish to refer to a GP patients exceeding five applications of pesticide per year and when counselling has failed.

References

Fradin M S, Day J F (2002). Comparative efficacy of insect repellents against mosquito bites. *N Engl J Med* 347(1): 13–18.

Mehta D K (ed.) *British National Formulary*, latest edition. London: British Medical Association and Royal Pharmaceutical Society of Great Britain.

Further reading

Anon (1998). Treating head louse infections. *Drug Ther Bull* 36(6): 45–46.

Online resources

www.doh.gov.uk/traveladvice/tables.htm tables of immunisation and malaria prophylaxis requirements for each country (accessed 13 December 2002).

www.fitfortravel.scot.nhs.uk is the website for National Health Service travel and health information (accessed 13 December 2002).

www.who.int/ith/ is the website for World Health Organization travel and health information (accessed 13 December 2002).

Part I

Dermatology

32

Dermatology

Dermatology is a relatively specialised area but the pharmacist has important roles, which include:

- identifying and treating common skin diseases or advising appropriate referral
- dispensing and monitoring treatment in more complicated cases
- identifying and referring serious skin diseases or serious diseases presenting with skin changes

Dermatology encompasses common conditions such as eczema and skin infections to serious conditions (such as skin cancers) and rare conditions, which are only likely to be dealt with by hospital specialists. In addition, adverse drug reactions may manifest as dermatological changes, which are considered in Chapter 5. This chapter will concentrate on common skin conditions including eczema, psoriasis, acne, fungal infections and some cancers. In order to aid recognition of dermatological conditions the reader is referred to the many textbooks and atlases of dermatology, such as *Colour Guide – Dermatology* by Wilkinson and Shaw (1998).

Eczema

Disease characteristics

This is a common inflammatory skin condition, which has many forms. Within dermatology, the terms 'eczema' and 'dermatitis' are both used but eczema should be used for the endogenous inflammatory conditions and dermatitis for reactive changes, for example to allergens. Examples of eczema/dermatitis include:

- atopic or infantile eczema
- irritant contact dermatitis
- allergic contact dermatitis
- seborrhoeic eczema – cradle cap in infants and a dry and itchy scalp in older children and adults

In addition, rarer forms include pompholyx (vesicles on hands or feet, which may be related to heat, stress, a reaction to fungal foot infections or may be cryptogenic); hyperkeratotic palmar eczema (typically occurring in middle age, and presenting with fissured eczema on hands); asteatotic eczema (reduced lipids in the skin, drying and cracking, which give rise to a 'crazy paving' appearance); discoid eczema (rare, discoid lesions, perhaps related to alcohol abuse).

Atopic eczema

Atopic or infantile eczema is the most common form of eczema and is associated with an inherited tendency for asthma and hayfever. It often appears in babies at around 3 months of age and by the age of 5 almost a third of children will have been diagnosed as having atopic eczema at some stage. Fortunately, most children grow out of the condition. It is characterised by:

- prominent pruritus – this is a central feature and its absence may suggest another condition
- itchy papules on the cheeks
- the skin is often dry or inflamed and lichenified, especially around the flexures of the elbows and knees
- there may be sensitivity to allergens. The dry and inflamed skin may be aggravated by cold, heat, hard water, infections and clothes (especially wool)
- the affected area is often scratched and may become infected, particularly with staphylococci or streptococci, and this may lead to a flare of eczema and, sometimes, impetigo. Viral infection with herpes simplex (eczema herpeticum) leads to painful vesicles and is

a serious complication requiring immediate antiviral treatment.

Management

Guidelines for the management of eczema have been produced on behalf of the British Association of Dermatologists (McHenry *et al.*, 1995) and these should be consulted.

The initial treatment is regular use of emollients, which hydrate the skin and prevent drying. Emollients have a range of constituents which may include liquid and soft paraffins and cetomacrogol. The most effective are the oily emollients but these may be cosmetically less acceptable. To prevent dehydration of the skin, soap and bubble bath should be avoided and bathing should be with emollient bath oils and using emollient creams as a soap substitute. Other lifestyle measures include keeping the house cool (to reduce itchiness), limiting allergens such as house dust mite (Chapter 19), as this may reduce severity (although this is not recommended by McHenry *et al.* (1995), on the grounds of a lack of proven effect) and cutting the child's nails to reduce scratching. Children may also benefit from an oral sedating antihistamine (e.g. alimemazine, chlorphenamine) to aid sleep and to prevent nocturnal scratching.

Pharmacological management

Topical steroids
When emollients are not sufficient, then topical steroids should be considered for treatment, especially in inflamed eczema. Topical 1% hydrocortisone is the first-line agent and is the only agent suitable for infants under 1 year of age. It is very effective at reducing the inflammatory response and should be used for short bursts of aggressive treatment rather than occasional 'dabbing'. Ointments give better skin penetration for the steroid than creams, although creams are less greasy and may be more acceptable to patients. Topical 1% hydrocortisone is a mild corticosteroid and is rarely associated with side-effects. However, failure of treatment may lead to the short-term use of more potent corticosteroids such as hydrocortisone butyrate, betamethasone and clobetasol propionate to bring the condition under control. These are, however, more likely to

be associated with side-effects, especially if used for prolonged periods or excessively, and these include:

- secondary infections due to immunosuppression
- thinning of the skin
- telangiectasia (appearance of dilated arterioles in the skin due to thinning)
- acneiform lesions
- they may cause glaucoma if applied near to the eyes or on the eyelids and so should be used with caution
- mild depigmentation
- pituitary–adrenal axis suppression
- Cushing's syndrome

Eczema which is severe may require oral steroids (e.g. prednisolone), in which case height suppression is an important side-effect in children and this should be monitored.

The steroid creams may also be combined with topical antibacterial agents or antifungal agents to prevent infection. Oral antibacterial agents may also be required occasionally to bring any infections under control.

Additional treatments
Ultraviolet phototherapy is used by hospital dermatologists in some patients. In severe disease dermatologists are now increasingly using systemic azathioprine and ciclosporin in children to suppress the immune response. These agents may be preferable to oral steroids. Although not licensed for the treatment of eczema, leukotriene receptor antagonists (Chapter 20) may lead to an improvement in some patients.

Evening primrose oil
This has been advocated for use in eczema but there is no convincing evidence to support its effectiveness.

Counselling

Lifestyle measures are the first step and are detailed earlier.

Emollients
- These are best applied after bathing when the skin is hydrated.

- They may sting on application.
- They should be applied liberally at least twice daily.
- They should be used even after the condition has improved.

Topical steroids
The use of topical steroids requires clear counselling:

- They are very effective and safe in the treatment of eczema if they are used correctly.
- Steroids have different potencies and mildly potent agents such as topical hydrocortisone have few side-effects. More potent steroids may be used to bring the eczema under control.
- Apply the cream or ointment thinly.
- The steroid should be applied once or twice daily as directed.
- Avoid application to the face (unless specifically prescribed). This is to limit systemic absorption, facial telangiectasia and acne.
- Avoid application to the anogenital region (unless specifically prescribed) to limit systemic absorption.
- Over-the-counter (OTC) use is only appropriate for children over 10 years of age and for 7 days. Longer treatment or application to the face or anogenital region requires referral to the general practitioner (GP).
- Avoid application to infected areas including cold sores, acne and fungal infections (in the absence of a concomitant antifungal agent).
- The preparation is applied in 'fingertip units' in adults:

  hand: 1 unit
  face: 2.5 units
  arm: 3 units
  leg: 6 units
  foot: 2 units
  front of trunk: 7 units
  back of trunk: 7 units

Contact dermatitis

This is also a common form of eczema, which is either an irritant reaction to chemicals such as detergents, or an allergic reaction to chemicals such as nickel, cosmetics and creams (e.g. some constituents such as lanolin, sodium stearate). It is characterised by inflammation with dryness and chapping following exposure to the irritant or allergen. The initial management is to remove or avoid the cause, coupled with emollients, barrier creams, topical steroids or oral antihistamines as appropriate. Occupational causes should be referred for patch testing to identify the irritant.

Napkin dermatitis

This form of contact dermatitis is due to the irritant effects of ammonia from faeces and urine in the nappy region and may often coexist with fungal infection. In napkin rash which is solely due to irritation, the skin folds are relatively spared, as there is less contact in these areas. Treatment should include improved hygiene, such as frequent nappy changes, leaving the nappy off for a time and washing, with the application of barrier creams (e.g. dimethicone) to prevent contact and emollients to hydrate the skin. In more severe dermatitis not responding to these measures 1% hydrocortisone cream may be prescribed for up to a week. Fungal infection should be suspected if the skin folds are affected or there are small red dots, as the fungi may spread. Accordingly, antifungal treatment with a topical imidazole, clotrimazole (see later), is appropriate, often with hydrocortisone to reduce the inflammation. Bacterial infections may present as pustules.

Seborrhoeic eczema

In infants this manifests on the scalp as cradle cap, for which there are a number of preparations, some of which include oils to soften the skin and facilitate removal.

In children and adults seborrhoeic eczema may present as a dry and flaky scalp for which corticosteroid lotions are effective. The condition may be related to a hypersensitivity to yeast infection due to *Pityrosporum* and ketoconazole shampoo is effective.

Other forms

In relation to the rarer forms of eczema, pompholyx may be managed by potent topical steroids and potassium permanganate. Oral antihistamines may provide symptomatic relief and if the condition is a reaction to a fungal infection, then this should be treated with antifungal agents (see later). Hyperkeratotic palmar eczema is treated with emollients, topical steroids, keratolytics and, in severe disease, immunosuppressants. Asteatotic eczema is treated with emollients, emollient bath oils and weak topical steroids. Discoid eczema is treated with emollients and steroids.

Psoriasis

This is a reasonably common inflammatory skin condition which affects 2–3% of the population and is due to rapid epidermal transit caused by increased cell division and increased passage of keratinocytes through the epidermis. As part of the inflammatory response, there is infiltration of the dermis with lymphocytes and the epidermis with neutrophils. The release of cytokines and lymphokines stimulates keratinocyte proliferation and alters their maturation.

The most common form is plaque psoriasis, which presents as a well-demarcated, erythematous region with thick silvery scales and is associated with pruritus. The plaques may be localised to a few areas or are extensively distributed. Less common forms include guttate psoriasis ('raindrop' lesions which may follow a streptococcal throat infection in younger patients), pustular psoriasis (a rare and serious condition, which presents as sterile pustules) and flexural psoriasis (well-demarcated erythematous regions). Decreased levels of cyclic adenosine monophosphate are found in lesions and beta-blockers may exacerbate the condition. In addition, lithium may exacerbate psoriasis.

Pharmacological management

There are a number of pharmacological approaches to psoriasis which may be tried and used according to their response. A central theme of the agents used is to reduce the proliferation of dermal cells and the inflammatory response, which contribute to the condition.

Emollients

As with eczema, emollients play an important role in hydrating the skin and should be used widely.

Topical steroids

Their anti-inflammatory actions may be of benefit but they may become less effective on continued use and there may be rebound effects on withdrawal.

Topical dithranol

This is often used first-line in plaque psoriasis and has antiproliferative properties by inhibiting mitotic activity. It may lead to hypersensitivity and so patch testing is sometimes used prior to treatment. The ability of this agent to stain skin and clothes may limit its acceptability with patients.

Topical vitamin D₃ analogues

Calcipotriol, tacalcitol

Vitamin D_3 analogues act on keratinocyte vitamin D receptors, with antiproliferative actions and reduce epidermal proliferation. They are also anti-inflammatory by interfering with the release of cytokines and suppression of both lymphocyte proliferation and neutrophil accumulation. Calcipotriol has now been formulated with betamethasone (in Dovobet) and appears to give good control of stable plaque psoriasis.

Coal tar

The keratolytic, antipruritic and anti-inflammatory actions of coal tar provide relief.

Phototherapy

Phototherapy with ultraviolet A (UVA) reduces dermal cell proliferation by interfering with DNA synthesis and reduces lymphocyte infiltration of the psoriatic epidermis. In extensive disease, the patients are treated with oral or topical methoxsalen (a psoralen) as a photosensitising agent, to enhance the effects of UVA, and this is known as PUVA (psoralen UVA). Alternatively, the patient may receive narrow-band UVB treatment, which does not require a photosensitising agent.

Oral retinoids

Acitretin

Acitretin (a metabolite of etretinate) binds to nuclear retinoic acid receptors and affects gene transcription, resulting in antiproliferative actions and normal keratinocyte maturation. It should be avoided in pregnancy and in females of child-bearing age; adequate contraception should be used and conception should be delayed for 2 years after stopping treatment. Acitretin may also alter the lipid profile by increasing plasma triglycerides and cholesterol and so this should be monitored along with liver function tests. Tazarotene is available as a topical retinoid.

Other treatments

Low-dose methotrexate is used by dermatologists for its cytotoxic actions, which reduce cellular turnover. Ciclosporin is also used by dermatologists for its immunosuppressant actions.

Counselling

Emollients and steroids

See earlier.

Dithranol

- This should be applied for 30–60 min and then washed off.
- It should only be applied to the lesions.
- It may stain skin and clothes.
- Patients should wash their hands thoroughly after application.

Oral acitretin

- This agent is teratogenic and should not be used during pregnancy. In females, conception should be delayed for at least 2 years after the patient has stopped taking the drug.
- Acitretin may also cause cracked and dried lips, which may be helped by the application of Vaseline.

- It may cause a drying of mucous membranes.
- It may cause thinning of the skin.
- The effects may be delayed for 2–4 weeks.
- The patient should not donate blood for at least 1 year after stopping treatment.
- Excessive exposure to sunlight should be avoided.

Acne

Acne vulgaris is a common condition, typically affecting teenagers, but in a few patients it may persist beyond these years. It is due to excessive sebum production in response to androgens, and results in the formation of comedones and pustules. Closed comedones are white cysts and open comedones are blackheads.

The bacterium *Propionibacterium acnes* is present in the skin and can lead to inflammatory lesions. The lipid-rich sebum favours the growth of *P. acnes,* which produces lipases that act on the sebum to release fatty acids, favouring comedone formation. The *P. acnes* also activates the complement system, leading to the release of proteases, which cause inflammation. Pustules form as part of the inflammatory lesions.

Management

In the mild form of the disease, general cleansing may provide relief. There is no evidence that altering the diet will bring about an improvement. The treatments for acne are directed against the comedones and/or the infected lesions and the following are used.

Topical agents

Topical benzoyl peroxide
Topical benzoyl peroxide is used for its keratolytic and bactericidal properties and is used in all forms of acne.

Azelaic acid
This may be used as an alternative to benzoyl peroxide and is less irritating.

Topical retinoids
If topical benzoyl peroxide fails then topical applications of retinoids (tretinoin and isotretinoin) are used for their keratolytic actions by reducing adhesion between epidermal cells. The main adverse effect is skin irritation. Retinoids are teratogenic and are only used in patients who are not pregnant.

Topical antibiotics
Topical antibiotics erythromycin, tetracycline or clindamycin are prescribed. When used alone they are ineffective against comedones but in pustular disease they are as effective as tretinoin and benzoyl peroxide. However, resistance may develop and this may be partly overcome by combining either zinc (such as Zineryt, which is erythromycin plus zinc acetate) or benzoyl peroxide with the antibiotic. They are often used for a 10–12-week trial.

Systemic treatments

Oral antibiotics
In moderate to severe acne or when there is a poor response to topical treatments, oral antibiotics are used. Tetracycline is used first-line, with oxytetracycline, minocycline, erythromycin, clindamycin or trimethoprim as alternatives. The penetration of the antibiotics into the sebaceous glands is low and so treatment can take up to 3–4 months for an effect: maximal effects may take up to 2 years. Tetracycline and erythromycin may exert additional anti-inflammatory actions, independent of their antibacterial activity.

When minocycline is used for longer than 6 months the *British National Formulary* recommends that hepatotoxicity, skin pigmentation and signs of systemic lupus erythematosus are monitored every 3 months.

Oral retinoids (tretinoin and isotretinoin)
A failure of oral antibiotics or severe acne may lead to referral to a dermatologist, who may prescribe the oral retinoid isotretinoin. This inhibits sebum production by reducing the number and activity of sebaceous glands. It can be highly effective but is associated with depression. It may also alter the lipid profile by increasing plasma triglycerides and

cholesterol and so this should be monitored along with liver function tests. It is teratogenic and is only used in patients who are not pregnant and who should be advised to avoid conception for at least 1 month after stopping treatment.

Hormonal therapy

In females only, Dianette (oral cyproterone, a testosterone receptor antagonist, plus ethinyl-estradiol) may be used as it will alter the hormonal balance away from androgens.

Counselling

General counselling should include hygiene advice and emphasise the importance of not touching lesions, to reduce the spread of infection.

Benzoyl peroxide

- Benzoyl peroxide may bleach hair and clothes.
- Benzoyl peroxide may irritate the skin and cause dryness.
- Apply once daily in the evening to begin with, in case there is redness or peeling.
- If there is irritation, reduce the frequency or stop and consider reintroducing gradually.
- Apply to the affected area, not just the spots.

Topical retinoids

- These are a photoirritant: patients should avoid UV sun beds and may need to wear sunscreen in the sunshine.
- Topical retinoids are teratogenic and females should take adequate contraceptive measures.

Oral antibiotics

- See Chapter 30.
- Broad-spectrum antibiotics may reduce the effectiveness of combined oral contraceptives containing ethinylestradiol (by altering the gastrointestinal flora) and so alternative barrier contraceptive measures should be used. This reduction in effectiveness only lasts for 3 weeks as resistance within the gastrointestinal

flora develops and so additional measures need only be taken for this time.
- Patients developing severe diarrhoea whilst taking antibiotics (especially clindamycin) should stop taking them and consult their GP urgently.
- An improvement may take 3–4 months.

Oral isotretinoin

- This is teratogenic and females must not become pregnant during treatment and for at least 1 month after treatment.
- Patients should not donate blood during treatment and for 1 month afterwards.
- This drug may cause depression.
- Patients should not exceed the daily allowance of vitamin A and should not take supplements containing vitamin A without consulting their pharmacist or GP.
- Patients should not take other products for acne unless advised to by their GP or dermatologist.
- Isotretinoin may cause thinning of the skin: patients should not wax or epilate their skin for 5–6 months after stopping treat-ment. Vaseline may be helpful in preventing dry and cracked lips. Dry eyes may also affect vision and hypromellose eye drops may be helpful.
- Patients should avoid strong sunlight and UV light and wear sunblock if exposed.

Dianette

- As with other oestrogen-containing contraceptives, there is a risk of thromboembolism, which is compounded by other risk factors such as smoking and increased age.
- An improvement may take several months.
- This may be used as a contraceptive for patients with acne.

Rosacea

Rosacea is an inflammatory condition with acneiform lesions, and telangiectasia (prominent and dilated arterioles) but without comedones. It is more common in women with fair skin, especially around the menopause. It may be precipitated by sunshine, alcohol and spicy foods. Hypertrophy of sebaceous glands around the nose may lead to an enlargement, rhinophyma, which is more common in men.

Management

The first active treatment is topical metronidazole gel (0.75%) and this may be followed by oral erythromycin or tetracycline. Beta-blockers or clonidine may be used to help the symptoms of flushing. Sunscreen should be used to reduce the effects of the sun.

Fungal infections

The skin is a common site of fungal infection due to tinea (dermatophyte) or *Candida,* and is commonly encountered in primary care. Common forms are as follows.

Ringworm (tinea infections)

This may occur at different sites on the body, as shown in Table 32.1.

Pityriasis versicolor

This is a relatively common condition, which presents as hypo- or hyperpigmented macules. It is due to infection by the yeast *Pityrosporum* spp.

Candidiasis

This is a common yeast infection due to *Candida albicans* and is known as thrush. It commonly affects the skin and mucous membranes. Skin infections tend to present as moist, inflamed regions, which are less well demarcated than in tinea infection, presenting with pain and itching. The infections are favoured by warm and moist skin folds, such as the groin, breasts, armpits and buttocks, especially in the obese (intertrigo). Mouth infections present as white patches and vaginal infections as pruritus with a creamy discharge, which is sometimes described as being like cottage cheese in appearance but is sometimes watery. Candidiasis is favoured by the use of antibiotics, corticosteroids, in diabetes mellitus, in eczema and in immunocompromised patients. Patients who have recurrent candidiasis should be investigated to exclude diabetes mellitus. It may also present as angular stomatitis at the corner of the mouth. Nails may also be affected and may become discoloured.

Management

In superficial infections, simple hygiene measures should be advocated and these may involve thorough drying after washing, not sharing towels and avoiding occlusive clothing (e.g. nylon). In athlete's foot, more frequent changes of socks and shoes may help.

Topical imidazoles

Clotrimazole, miconazole, tioconazole
These act to inhibit a cytochrome P450-dependent demethylase which converts lanosterol

---

Table 32.1   The different forms, sites and features of tinea infection

Form	Site	Features
Tinea corporis	Trunk and limbs	Discoid, erythematous scaly plaques
Tinea capitis	Scalp	Bald, scaly patches
Tinea pedis (athlete's foot)	Between the toes	May present as scaling or inflammation between the toes
Tinea unguium	Nails	Nails become yellow and crumbly
Tinea cruris	Groin	Reddened and scaly groin.

to ergosterol, a fungal membrane lipid. This results in the accumulation of lanosterol which disrupts the membrane phospholipids. The imidazoles are fungistatic and so must be used for about 2 weeks after healing to prevent a relapse. They are widely used in superficial skin infections and are effective against both tinea and candidial infections.

Oral imidazoles and triazoles ('azoles')

The imidazole ketoconazole and the triazoles itraconazole and fluconazole are orally active and act via inhibition of cytochrome P450-dependent demethylase, as described above. The azoles are associated with hepatotoxicity.

Polyenes

Nystatin
This polyene macrolide binds to fungal ergosterol in the cell membrane. It disrupts the cells and is effective in candidiasis but not tinea.

Allylamines

Terbinafine
Terbinafine inhibits the conversion of squalene to lanosterol, with the accumulation of squalene causing cell death. This fungicidal action has the advantage that shorter treatment courses are required. Terbinafine is available as either a cream for superficial infections or orally for deeper infections, such as those affecting the nails.

Griseofulvin

This interferes with fungal microtubules and nucleic acid synthesis but has largely been replaced by oral terbinafine and azoles. This is suitable for tinea infections but not candidiasis, as it is ineffective against the yeast.

Topical steroids

These may be used in addition to antifungal agents to relieve the symptoms due to irritation and are especially useful in concomitant eczema.

In terms of the use of antifungal agents, then topical agents are used in more superficial infections and oral agents for deeper infections. The agents are chosen according to the spectrum of activity: some recommendations are given in Table 32.2.

Counselling

A long course is often required and should be completed.

Imidazole creams

- For cutaneous infections, these should be applied two to three times daily and for 2 weeks after the infection has healed.
- For vaginal infections, hygiene advice should be given and sexual partners treated if they are symptomatic. Other sources of infection may include fingernails, umbilicus, gastrointestinal tract and bladder.
- Vaginal preparations (excluding nystatin pessaries) may damage latex condoms and diaphragms.
- Vaginal preparations should be administered high into the vagina and may be used during menstruation.
- They may cause a burning sensation on application.

Oral azoles and oral terbinafine

- These may cause gastrointestinal side-effects. Itraconazole capsules (but not liquid) and ketoconazole should be taken with food.
- Patients taking oral antifungal agents should report signs of liver toxicity such as nausea, vomiting, dark urine or jaundice (Chapters 5 and 10).

Nystatin

- The cream may stain clothes yellow.

Griseofulvin

- Avoid during pregnancy.
- Males should avoid fathering children for 6 months after stopping treatment.

Table 32.2   Treatment for fungal infections

Condition	Possible primary treatments
Tinea corporis	• Topical imidazole, continued for 2 weeks after healing • Topical terbinafine: 1–2 weeks. Topical imidazole is first-line while terbinafine is reserved for resistance
Tinea capitis	• Oral griseofulvin: 8 weeks • Oral terbinafine: 4 weeks (unlicenced) • Oral itraconazole (unlicenced)
Tinea pedis (athlete's foot)	• Topical imidazole, continued for 2 weeks after healing • Topical terbinafine: 1 week
Tinea unguium	• Oral terbinafine: 6 weeks to 3 months, sometimes longer in toenail infections • Oral itraconazole: 3 months or 2 pulses (fingernails) or 3 pulses (toenails) • Oral griseofulvin for 6 months (fingernails) or 12 months (toenails) • In mild infection limited to 1–2 nails, local therapy with amorolfine or tioconazole may be used
Tinea cruris	• Topical imidazole, continued for 2 weeks after healing • Topical terbinafine: 1–2 weeks Topical imidazole is first-line while terbinafine is reserved for resistance
Pityriasis versicolor	• Selenium sulfide shampoo daily for 1 week • Topical imidazole for 10 days • Itraconazole for 1 week
Candidiasis – cutaneous	• Topical imidazole for 2 weeks after healing • Topical terbinafine: 2 weeks • Topical nystatin, continued for 7 days after healing
Candidiasis – nail	• Oral itraconazole: 3 months or 2 pulses (fingernails) or 3 pulses (toenails)
Vaginal candidiasis	• Either clotrimazole pessaries (single-dose) or cream (10% clotrimazole is available for single application); oral fluconazole (150 mg as a single dose), it may also be used for candidal balanitis

Failure of topical treatment or extensive infection should be treated with oral agents, such as terbinafine or itraconazole. Pulses of itraconazole are high doses (200 mg b.d. for 7 days followed by subsequent courses after 21 days). The recommended agents and duration of the above therapies are largely derived from the *British National Formulary*.

Other infections affecting the skin

In addition to fungal infections, the skin is also the site of a wide range of bacterial and viral infections, which vary from the benign to potentially serious. Some of the infections may be related to increased susceptibility due to chronic skin conditions, for example impetigo (as a complication of eczema) and due to manifestations of viral infections with both skin and systemic symptoms. A summary of the features and management of a range of common skin infections is given in Table 32.3.

Pruritus

This is a symptom of a range of conditions and presents as itchiness. Possible causes include (Greene and Harris, 2000):

- dermatological inflammatory conditions
  - eczema
  - psoriasis
- skin infections
  - lice/scabies
  - viral infection – chickenpox, herpes
  - fungal infection
- reactions
  - drug reactions
  - urticaria
- psychogenic
- ageing
- manifestations of systemic changes
  - diabetes
  - pregnancy
  - liver failure
  - renal failure
  - malignancy

The treatment should be directed at the cause, but additional symptomatic measures include the use of crotamiton cream or lotion and oral antihistamines. Colestyramine is used in pruritus associated with liver failure, as it will bind bile salts and so reduce plasma bilirubin which causes pruritus (Chapter 10). Anogenital pruritus may be due to fungal infection, haemorrhoids or contact dermatitis due to irritation by poor hygiene. It should be treated with hygiene measures, antifungal agents, emollients if due to dry skin or short-term hydrocortisone as appropriate but topical local anaesthetics are best avoided as they may lead to hypersensitivity.

Manifestations of systemic disease

In addition to pruritus as a symptom, systemic diseases may manifest as changes in the skin. Examples of this include:

- Pigmentation which may be yellow in jaundice (due to increased bilirubin in liver disease), or a lemon tinge in renal failure or vitiligo in Addison's disease.
- Spider naevi are dilated central arterioles with spidery arterioles feeding from them, and are present, especially above the nipple line, in liver cirrhosis, frequently due to alcohol.

- Fungal infections which recur may suggest that the patient has impaired immunity. Frequent candidiasis occurs in diabetes mellitus.

Skin cancers

The incidence of skin cancers is on the increase and they are dealt with by specialists in dermatology. However, recognition of potential skin cancers in primary care is clearly important and the pharmacist should be vigilant for changes in the skin which require referral.

Basal cell carcinoma (rodent ulcer)

This is the most common skin cancer and presents as a colourless lump with pearly edges but may become ulcerated and crusty in the centre and is often on the edge of the ear, temple or side of the nose. It is very slow-growing and may have been present for several years. Although it is a malignant tumour, it has only very limited local invasion and is cured by surgical removal. Extensive invasion may require radiotherapy or cryotherapy. Topical 5-fluorouracil is also used. Prevention of occurrence or recurrence (which is common) should be stressed by advising sun protection measures, such as wearing a hat in the sun and using a high-factor sun block.

Solar keratosis

These are common, premalignant lesions with crusts on an erythematous base. Solar keratosis is associated with exposure to the sun and occurs more often on fair-skinned patients on the forehead, scalp, face or hands. It may be managed by cryotherapy and topical 5-fluorouracil.

Squamous cell carcinoma

This is a relatively common malignancy, often appearing on sun-damaged skin on the hand and face, especially the ear and lip. It is remove surgically but metastases may occur if it is untreated.

Table 32.3   Additional skin infections and their treatment

Condition	Comments	Management
Impetigo	Usually a staphylococcal or occasionally streptococcal infection of the skin. Reddening with a golden crust. Contagious and may complicate eczema	Limited infection may be treated with topical fusidic acid or mupirocin (use limited to 10 days to prevent the emergence of resistance). More extensive infections require oral flucloxacillin (or phenoxymethylpenicillin if there is streptococcal infection) or erythromycin if penicillin-allergic. Antiseptic bath oils may reduce colonisation
Cellulitis	Deep streptococcal or staphylococcal infection, often following trauma. There may be a red, oedematous rash which may be accompanied by pyrexia	Phenoxymethylpenicillin plus flucloxacillin or erythromycin if penicillin-allergic
Erysipelas	Superficial cellulitis of the skin, often due to *Streptococcus pyogenes*. Often affects the face or legs	Phenoxymethylpenicillin in mild infections. Flucloxacillin is added if staphylococcal infection is suspected
Herpes simplex	Painful vesicles on mucous membranes and skin due to herpes simplex virus. Tingling precedes the lesions	Analgesics provide symptomatic relief. Topical aciclovir and penciclovir reduce the length of symptoms if started at the first signs of an attack. Oral aciclovir may be less effective
Chickenpox	• Varicella infection leading to fever and vesicular rash. Usually uncomplicated in children but in adults may be complicated by pneumonia, hepatitis, encephalitis, and myocarditis • Smoking increases the chances of complications of pneumonia • Chickenpox is especially severe in patients taking systemic steroids	• Antihistamines may provide symptomatic relief • Emollients may be soothing • Older remedies such as calamine lotion may be ineffective • Aciclovir is indicated for high-risk patients who develop the infection and should be started in the first 24 h • Immunoglobulin is appropriate for pregnant contacts and those taking steroids who do not have immunity
Shingles	Reactivation of varicella-zoster virus leading to pain, with red papules which become vesicular. Shingles cannot be caught from contact with chickenpox but contact of patients with shingles may lead to chickenpox in patients who are not immune	• Aciclovir is indicated for patients over 60 years of age or immunocompromised. It should be started within 72 h of the appearance of the rash • Neuralgic pain after infection may require low doses of tricyclic antidepressants such as amitriptyline or carbamazepine, which are routinely used in older patients as a preventive measure
Warts and verrucae (plantar warts)	Warts are hyperkeratotic papules and verrucae are deep lesions on the soles. They are caused by the human papillomavirus	• Warts generally resolve but may be treated with salicylic acid, glutaraldehyde or cryotherapy with liquid nitrogen or dry ice • Verrucae may be treated with salicylic acid plasters or podophyllin/salicylic acid ointment or cryotherapy

Continued

Table 32.3 Continued

Condition	Comments	Management
Molluscum contagiosum (water blisters)	Drop-like papules affecting infants and children due to a virus	None indicated and reassurance is all that may be required
Hand, foot and mouth disease	Coxsackie viral infection in children with vesicles around the mouth, palms and soles	None
Scabies	Severe pruritus due to scabies mite infestation	• Malathion or permethrin as aqueous preparations as alcohol may irritate damaged skin (Chapter 31) • All members of the family should be treated • Treatment should be applied to the whole body, particularly to the web of digits and fingernails • Two applications, 1 week apart are recommended • Crotamiton and/or sedating antihistamines may be used for pruritus

Malignant melanoma

This involves evolution and possibly malignant transformation in a large mole. This is more likely in larger moles and in sun-exposed skin. The following features may be seen:

Asymmetry
Border irregular
Colour irregular
Diameter >0.5 cm
Elevation irregular

Any change in a mole requires referral for an expert opinion. In malignant melanoma, surgical excision has a good outlook in small lesions, which are caught early. Chemotherapy is palliative in disease which has spread.

Drug interactions involving drugs widely used in dermatology

In drugs used in dermatology there are a wide range of potential drug interactions, generally affecting the oral azoles, and also ciclosporin and methotrexate which are only initiated by specialists. Table 32.4 (see page 430) contains a summary of some important interactions.

  CASE STUDIES

Case 1
Toddler TR is 2 years old and has scaly inflamed skin on her back and on the back of her knees. A diagnosis of atopic eczema has been made.

1. How might the parents manage this condition using lifestyle changes and OTC treatments?

continued

CASE STUDIES (continued)

- Simple lifestyle measures should involve regular but not excessive washing, and using emollients in place of soap. After bathing, emollient should be applied liberally and reapplied throughout the day. Keeping the house cool may help reduce the discomfort of itching. Limiting allergens in the house is controversial and may or may not help. The child's nails should be kept short to avoid scratching and a sedative oral antihistamine given at night might help her sleep and reduce scratching at night.

2. Might the toddler benefit from topical antihistamines?

- These are of no benefit in eczema and they may actually sensitise the skin.

3. What are the treatment options open to her GP?

- For poorly controlled and inflamed eczema, topical corticosteroids (1% hydrocortisone preferred in infants) may be prescribed (not OTC at this age) for short periods to bring the condition under control.

4. What other conditions will she be susceptible to?

- Atopic individuals are more susceptible to asthma and hayfever.

Toddler TR's skin condition deteriorates and becomes covered with a golden crusty coat over a red and inflamed surface. The GP decides that she has an impetigo-like infection.

5. What is impetigo?

- A staphylococcal or streptococcal infection of the skin leading to reddening with a golden crust which may complicate eczema.

6. How would this be treated?

- In limited infection, topical fusidic acid (2%) is used. If widespread, either oral flucloxacillin (125 mg q.d.s.) or erythromycin (250 mg q.d.s.) is appropriate. If streptococcal infection is suspected then phenoxymethylpenicillin (125 mg q.d.s.) may be prescribed.

Case 2
Ms GS is a 16-year-old (50 kg) female with acne vulgaris.

1. What are the goals of treatment?

- eradication of acne, which is important both cosmetically and psychologically
- reduction in sebum production
- to limit the growth of the bacteria involved
- to prevent recurrence
- to prevent scarring

2. What would the ladder of treatment be in her case?

- Step 1: Mild acne – general cleansing.
- Step 2: Topical benzoyl peroxide for its keratolytic and bactericidal actions.

→

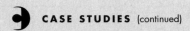

CASE STUDIES (continued)

- Step 3: If there is a poor response to the above, then topical tretinoin or topical antibiotics (not effective against comedones).
- Step 4: If there is a poor response to the above, then oral antibiotics.
- Step 5: If there is a poor response to the above, then oral isotretinoin.
- Any stage: oral cyproterone plus ethinylestradiol (Dianette) may be used. Severe acne should be referred to a dermatologist.

At one stage she is prescribed tetracycline (500 mg b.d.).

3. How would you counsel her?

- Do not take at the same time as milk and antacids: take at least 30 min before food or on an empty stomach. Calcium in milk and antacids will bind tetracycline and prevent it from being absorbed.
- Complete the course.
- Avoid direct sunlight/UV due to photosensitivity.
- An improvement may take 3–4 months.

4. What might be tried if there is no improvement?

- Oral erythromycin or trimethoprim might be tried.

Later her dermatologist prescribes isotretinoin p.o.

5. Suggest an appropriate dosage.

- 500 µg/kg daily, therefore her dose is 25 mg daily.

6. How would she be counselled?

- Isotretinoin is teratogenic and she will require a pregnancy test and must not become pregnant until at least 1 month after stopping treatment. She should use effective contraception.
- Her skin may become thin.
- She should avoid waxing or epilation, as this will strip skin.
- Her lips may become dry and Vaseline may help.

References

Greene R J, Harris N D (2000). *Pathology and Therapeutics for Pharmacists*. London: Pharmaceutical Press.

McHenry P M, Williams H C, Bingham E A (1995). Management of atopic eczema. *BMJ* 310: 843–847.

Mehta D K (ed.) *British National Formulary*, latest edition. London: British Medical Association and Royal Pharmaceutical Society of Great Britain.

Stockley I H (2002). *Drug Interactions*, 6th edn. London: Pharmaceutical Press.

Wilkinson J D, Shaw S (1998). *Colour Guide – Dermatology*. Edinburgh: Churchill Livingstone.

Further reading

Brown S K, Shalita A R (1998). Acne vulgaris. *Lancet* 351: 1871–1876.

Table 32.4   Some important drug interactions for drugs used in dermatology

Interacting drugs	Consequences	Comments
Methoxsalen with phenytoin	Phenytoin may, by enzyme induction, reduce concentrations of methoxsalen	This combination should be avoided
Acitretin with ciclosporin	An increase in ciclosporin concentration may occur	
Acitretin with methotrexate	Increased toxicity of methotrexate	BNF recommends avoiding concomitant use of acitretin and methotrexate
Isotretinoin with carbamazepine	The plasma concentration of carbamazepine may be reduced	Epileptic control should be monitored
Isotretinoin with tetracycline/minocycline	Increased risk of benign intracranial hypertension	Their concomitant use should be avoided
Methotrexate	Toxicity of methotrexate is known to be enhanced by NSAIDs and so extreme caution should be exercised, although this is less likely to occur at the lower doses used for psoriasis	Methotrexate exhibits a wide range of interactions and *Drug Interactions* by Stockley (2002) should be consulted
Ciclosporin		Ciclosporin exhibits a wide range of interactions and *Drug Interactions* by Stockley (2002) should be consulted
Oral cyproterone plus ethinylestradiol (Dianette)	Efficacy may be reduced by broad-spectrum antibiotics and enzyme inducers. When used with minocycline there may be an enhancement of facial pigmentation	
Oral imidazoles and triazoles	• Phenytoin reduces the plasma concentrations of itraconazole and ketoconazole but fluconazole may increase the concentrations of phenytoin • Carbamazepine may reduce the plasma concentrations of itraconazole • Rifampicin reduces the plasma concentrations of itraconazole, fluconazole and ketoconazole Additional interactions include reduced absorption of ketoconazole and itraconazole (but not fluconazole) by antacids and H_2-receptor antagonists	• These are inhibitors of cytochrome P450 and will inhibit the metabolism of a range of drugs, increasing their plasma concentrations (Chapter 5) • Similarly, inducers of cytochrome P450 may accelerate the metabolism of the azoles, reducing their plasma concentrations • Inhibitors of cytochrome P450 may inhibit the metabolism of azoles and increase their concentrations
Antifungals (fluconazole, itraconazole, ketoconazole and miconazole) with warfarin	Increased anticoagulant effect	• Includes oral and vaginal preparations of miconazole
Griseofulvin with warfarin	In some patients, griseofulvin decreases the plasma concentration of warfarin	Monitoring is recommended
Itraconazole with clarithromycin	Itraconazole levels doubled	Monitoring and possible dose reductions are recommended

Continued

Table 32.4 Continued

Interacting drugs	Consequences	Comments
Ketoconazole with omeprazole	Reduced antifungal effects	• Fluconazole is a suitable alternative for patients prescribed omeprazole • Alternative proton pump inhibitors such as lansoprazole may also interact and an alternative such as H_2-antagonists is recommended
Terbinafine with rifampicin	Reduced levels of terbinafine	A doubling of the terbinafine dose may be required
Oral terbinafine	• Plasma concentrations are decreased by concomitant rifampicin and its dose may need to be increased • Terbinafine may increase plasma levels of theophylline but this is unclear	The interaction of terbinafine and oral contraceptives is not believed to be clinically significant
Amphotericin with corticosteroids	• Adverse cardiac effects due to potassium loss and water and sodium retention	Electrolytes should be monitored, particularly in patients at risk (e.g. elderly)
Oral aciclovir	• There is a report of aciclovir reducing plasma concentrations of phenytoin and sodium valproate • Aciclovir can increase plasma concentrations of theophylline, which may lead to toxicity	Monitoring may be appropriate

NSAIDs, non-steroidal anti-inflammatory drugs; BNF, *British National Formulary.*

Cunliffe W (2002). A rational approach to acne management. *Prescriber* 13: 46–67.

Hindle E (2001). Eczema: first- and second-line drug treatments. *Prescriber* 12: 49–71.

Rudikoff D, Lebwohl M (1998). Atopic dermatitis. *Lancet* 351: 1715–1721

Stern R S (1997). Psoriasis. *Lancet* 350: 349–353.

Online resources

www.eczema.org is the website of the UK National Eczema Society (accessed 4 December 2002).

www.bad.org.uk is the website of the British Association of Dermatologists providing professional and patient information. (accessed 11 July 2003).

Part J

Endocrine disorders

33

Diabetes mellitus

Diabetes mellitus is a serious condition associated with a considerable disruption to a patient's life and potentially serious long-term consequences. In particular, diabetes mellitus is a major risk factor for cardiovascular disease, comparable to hypertension and hypercholesterolaemia. Diabetes mellitus is broadly classed as either type 1 (also known as insulin-dependent diabetes mellitus, IDDM), or type 2 (non-insulin dependent diabetes mellitus, NIDDM). Both conditions are characterised by impaired glucose metabolism. In type 1, there is an inability to produce insulin while in type 2 there is reduced production and/or a reduced sensitivity to its actions. Type 1 is generally associated with onset at an early age, whilst type 2, previously termed 'maturity-onset diabetes', presents later in life and is strongly associated with obesity. A small subset of type 2 diabetes is maturity-onset diabetes of the young (MODY), a genetic condition, with onset at an earlier age. It is now recognised that the incidence of type 2 diabetes mellitus is increasing, with many cases remaining undiagnosed, and it

is believed that we are on the edge of a hidden epidemic. Type 2 diabetes represents 90% of patients who have diabetes.

Common clinical features of diabetes are:

- increased thirst (secondary to increased plasma osmolality)
- increased urination (due to osmotic diuresis secondary to glucose in the urine)
- glycosuria
- increased superficial infections such as genital candidiasis due to glucose in the urine
- tiredness
- weight loss in type 1
- ketoacidosis (in the form of dehydration, nausea, vomiting, thirst, weight loss, hyperventilation, ketone breath) in type 1, rarely in type 2

Diagnosis may be secondary to complications of diabetes, such as hypertension, myocardial infarction, retinal damage, peripheral vascular disease and renal damage. Diabetes can be induced in certain conditions such as pregnancy (gestational diabetes), endocrine conditions associated with the increased production of counterregulatory hormones (such as corticosteroids in Cushing's syndrome and growth hormone in acromegaly), diseases of the pancreas such as chronic pancreatitis, and by certain drugs (e.g. thiazides, corticosteroids).

Diagnosis is based on elevated plasma glucose levels of greater than 7.0 mmol/L in the fasting state or 11.1 mmol/L on a random test on two occasions. An oral glucose tolerance test may also be carried out and involves measuring plasma glucose levels before and 2 h after a challenge with a glucose-rich drink (75 g). In this test, a diagnosis is made if the fasting glucose is greater than 7.0 mmol/L or the 2-h glucose is greater than 11.1 mmol/L. A fasting value of 6–7 mmol/L is consistent with impaired glucose tolerance. Diabetes may be suggested by detection of glucose in the urine, but this is a less valuable test as individuals vary in their renal threshold (c. 7–15 mmol/L) for the appearance of glycosuria.

Type 1 diabetes mellitus

This form is generally associated with onset at a young age (<40 years old) but may occur at any age. It may be caused by destruction of beta-cells of the islets of Langerhans following certain viral infections or due to an autoimmune process. It is characterised by an inability of the beta-cells to produce insulin and is fatal if not treated.

Pharmacological management

Treatment is directed towards replacing the insulin in an attempt to return blood glucose to normal and preventing diabetic complications. The insulin used is now generally the human peptide derived from recombinant DNA technology, although insulin derived from porcine and bovine (rarely) pancreases are used. The insulin is given by injection and in the maintenance phase by subcutaneous injection. Insulin acts on insulin receptors on target tissues of the body to enable blood glucose to be controlled. This follows the insertion of glucose transporters to promote glucose uptake into muscle, liver and adipose tissue, and by stimulation of glycogen, triglyceride and fatty acid synthesis.

Insulin preparations

As insulin has a short plasma half-life, it may be complexed with various agents to retard its absorption and so prolong its action.

Human insulin analogues
These are modified insulin peptides (insulin lispro and insulin aspart) which have a rapid onset but short duration of action and may be injected just before a meal or when necessary just after a meal. These preparations increase flexibility and are particularly useful for patients prone to pre-lunch hypoglycaemia and those who tend to eat late in the evening and may therefore be at risk of nocturnal hypoglycaemia.

Short-acting insulins
Soluble insulins have relatively short-lived effects of 6–8 h, with peak effects at 2–5 h. These are given approximately 15–30 min before meals.

Intermediate and long-acting insulins
Combination of insulin with protamine gives rise to intermediate-acting insulin (isophane insulin), binding to zinc gives intermediate to long-acting insulin and combination with protamine plus zinc gives long-acting insulin. Crystalline insulin zinc suspensions are also long-acting. Biphasic preparations contain both an intermediate-acting agent (e.g. isophane insulin) with a shorter-acting form (e.g. soluble insulin).

The aim of insulin therapy is to maintain a plasma glucose level as close to 7.5 mmol/L as possible to prevent future complications but also to avoid hypoglycaemia. The ideal situation is to match the physiological changes in insulin profile in non-diabetic patients. One method of achieving good glycaemic control is by multiple insulin injections of differing durations of action in an attempt to mimic physiological responses. The aim is to give a long-acting agent to achieve a basal level and to add short-acting preparations in relation to a meal; this is termed basal bolus dosing. The disadvantage here can be one of compliance, as patients are required to monitor blood glucose frequently and administer multiple injections per day. This can be difficult to achieve.

There are no fixed rules and regimens can be adopted to suit the individual needs of the patient. Here are some of the regimens which are commonly used:

- Twice-daily regimens: two daily injections, one 30 min before breakfast and one before the evening meal of short- and longer-acting insulins in combination, with two-thirds of the insulin given as the morning dose. This is the most common regimen.
- Multiple dosing regimens: a single dose of medium-acting insulin is given at bedtime and doses of short-acting insulin are given 30 min before each meal. This allows more flexibility with the timing of meals.

  Alternatively, a short-acting insulin mixed with intermediate-acting insulin is given before breakfast; short-acting insulin is given before the evening meal and an intermediate-acting insulin is given at bedtime.
- Single daily regimens: these are rarely used but involve one daily injection before breakfast or at bedtime of intermediate-acting insulin, with or without a short-acting insulin. They are generally for patients with type 2 diabetes who are unable to control their blood glucose with antidiabetic drugs.

Insulin requirement is increased by stress, infection, accidental or surgical trauma, puberty (effects of growth hormone) and during the latter two trimesters of pregnancy. Reduced insulin requirements may occur in coeliac disease, renal or hepatic impairment and endocrine disorders such as untreated Addison's disease.

Insulin administration

Intravenous infusion of soluble insulin is a reliable route of administration and may be used in hospital in an acute setting, to bring the diabetes under control. The amount required to control blood glucose may give an indication of daily requirements for future treatment. In the early stages, patients may encounter what is termed a 'honeymoon period', during which time less insulin is required (due to residual beta-cell function). The most conventional route is via subcutaneous injection using a disposable syringe, in which the different insulins may be mixed to achieve the desired combination. This method has largely been superseded by the introduction of more convenient injection pens and biphasic insulins.

Insulin pumps may be used which allow continuous subcutaneous administration. These are particularly useful in diabetes which is difficult to control. They have the advantage of providing a continuous infusion, which may be increased at meal times. However, they are expensive and are not available on prescription.

Complications of insulin therapy

As the role of insulin is to reduce blood glucose levels, excessive dosing in relation to food intake can lead to hypoglycaemia. Patients may become aware of this through autonomic (anxiety, sweating, trembling, tachycardia and hunger) and neuroglycaemic (confusion, drowsiness, and problems with concentration, speech and coordination) symptoms. Awareness of these symptoms is important so that action may be taken such as intake of 10–20 g of glucose in lumps or in glucose-rich drinks to prevent a hypoglycaemic coma. For example, 10 g glucose is provided by two teaspoons of sugar, three sugar lumps, 200 mL of milk, 50–55 mL of Lucozade, 90 mL of Coca-Cola or 15 mL of Ribena original (to be diluted). If this is not sufficient, the same dose may be repeated in 10–15 min. Hypostop gel may be easier to administer with a reduced risk of choking and it contains 10 g per 23 g ampoule. Glucagon may be given by subcutaneous, intramuscular or intravenous injection for acute insulin-induced hypoglycaemia resulting in unconsciousness.

Strict glycaemic control and the use of human insulin may also impair hypoglycaemic awareness, and it is for this reason that some patients prefer to be maintained on porcine or bovine insulin. Hypoglycaemia is also common at night, as the evening insulin injection may have peak effects at this time, even if the patient has an evening snack (see insulin regimens).

Exercise not only reduces insulin requirements as glucose is used, but also accelerates the absorption of insulin from the subcutaneous sites. Accordingly, patients may need to reduce the dose of insulin before and after exercise and also to take a snack prior to exercise. In highly trained patients, multiple daily insulin injections may be the best approach to attain glycaemic control, and avoid hypoglycaemia.

Subcutaneous injection of insulin may lead to changes in the skin. At a site of repeated injections, there may be lipohypertrophy, leading to unpredictable insulin absorption. It is for this reason that patients should rotate the sites used.

Drug interactions and effects on concurrent diseases

A number of drugs may alter glucose control and hence the effects of insulin (Table 33.1). By altering glucose metabolism they will also affect

control in diabetes and in some cases uncover diabetes.

Intercurrent illnesses and conditions

As commented in Chapter 1, patients with diabetes are a special group who should have a lower threshold for general practitioner (GP) referral during illness. In addition, during an illness there may be a loss of appetite but patients should not reduce their insulin intake. In fact, the illness itself may increase blood glucose levels. Carbohydrate 10 g (see Complications of insulin therapy, above) should be taken every hour or sips every 20 min if nauseated. It is also important to allow for the glucose content in rehydration solutions, for example, Dioralyte powder contains 3.56 g of glucose per sachet.

Table 33.1   Examples of the effects of some important drugs on glucose control and insulin activity

Drug	Effects on diabetes	Comments
Alcohol	May mask the signs of hypoglycaemia	Alcohol should not be consumed in excess and should be taken with food. The carbohydrate content of the drink should also be taken into account (see Counselling)
ACE inhibitors	These can sometimes lead to hypoglycaemia	The dose of insulin or antidiabetic drug may need to be reduced
Beta-blockers	These may mask the awareness of hypoglycaemia by reducing the tremor and tachycardia, while sweating is not affected (as this is cholinergic)	This is most marked with propranolol. This is a reason to choose alternative agents or favour the use of beta$_1$-adrenoceptor antagonists
Corticosteroids	These oppose the actions of insulin and cause hyperglycaemia	The dose of insulin may need to be increased
Isoniazid	Variable effects	Monitoring is appropriate
Lithium	May reduce glucose tolerance	May induce diabetes. Monitoring is appropriate
MAOIs	These may enhance the hypoglycaemic actions of insulin	Monitoring is appropriate
Oral contraceptives	Insulin requirements may be altered	
Thiazides	May increase blood glucose	This is a reason to avoid using thiazides in diabetes
Tobacco smoking	This increases the insulin requirements	Smoking substantially enhances the cardiovascular damage in diabetes

ACE, angiotensin-converting enzyme; MAOIs, monoamine oxidase inhibitors.

Pregnancy is a major issue in patients with diabetes and requires specialist supervision.

Type 2 diabetes mellitus

This is generally associated with increased insulin resistance, in which the body's tissues become less responsive to insulin, leading to increased blood glucose levels. There is also a strong family association. The beta-cells of the islets of Langerhans still produce insulin but there is sometimes a loss of cells or reduced glucose sensitivity. The patient may also have other associated diseases such as obesity, hypertension and hyperlipidaemia. Type 2 diabetes generally presents after the age of 40 years and may have a gradual onset, such that the patient may have the condition for several years (the prediabetic phase) before recognition. This is a persuasive reason for routine blood glucose testing.

Pharmacological basis of management

In mild or initial disease, all that may be required is dietary modification to reduce the amount of simple carbohydrates in the diet, weight loss in obesity and increased exercise to achieve control of blood glucose. The alteration of diet should limit the intake of mono- and disaccharides, increase non-starch polysaccharides and reduce the intake of saturated fat to minimise the risk of atherosclerosis, such that fat is 30–35% calorific intake and carbohydrate is 50–55%. If dietary changes alone are insufficient after 3 months then antidiabetic drugs are used. If these fail to achieve control at maximum doses and optimal combinations then insulin injections may be required. Indeed, type 2 diabetes should be viewed as a progressive disease.

Sulphonylureas

e.g. Chlorpropamide, glibenclamide, gliclazide, glimepiride, glipizide, tolbutamide
The sulphonylureas rely on the fact that the beta-cells can still produce insulin. These drugs act to increase insulin secretion. Pharmacologically,

they are inhibitors of adenosine triphosphate (ATP)-sensitive potassium (K_{ATP}) channels. Subtypes of K_{ATP}-channels are present on many cell types such as beta-cells, smooth-muscle cells, cardiac muscle cells and neuronal cells. In beta-cells, they regulate insulin release. When glucose is present, the production of ATP and the reduction in adenosine diphosphate (ADP) inactivate these channels, leading to cellular depolarisation, which results in calcium influx and insulin secretion. When glucose is low, ATP levels fall and ADP rises, channels open, with membrane hyperpolarization, and this decreases insulin release. Sulphonylureas bind to a receptor associated with these channels, resulting in channel closure, which leads to insulin release.

Meglitinide analogues

Nateglinide, repaglinide
These also act on beta-cells but at a site distinct from the sulphonylurea receptor, causing closure of the K_{ATP}-channels, leading to depolarisation and insulin release. They have a rapid rate of onset and are given at mealtimes to stimulate postprandial insulin secretion, which is relatively short-lived. Their effects may be enhanced by patients having a meal and they are referred to as prandial glucose regulators (PGRs), which may be regarded as producing a more physiological rise in insulin than that produced by sulphonylureas.

Biguanides

Metformin
The action of metformin is less clear. There are several proposed mechanisms of action, including: (1) increased glucose uptake into muscle; (2) reduced uptake of glucose from the gastrointestinal tract; and (3) reduced output of glucose from the liver. Obviously these proposed mechanisms will lead to either reduced entry of glucose in the blood or increased utilisation.

Thiazolidinediones (glitazones)

Pioglitazone, rosiglitazone
These new agents are 'insulin sensitisers' which work by enhancing glucose utilisation in tissues, and so reduce insulin resistance. They activate

the gamma nuclear peroxisome proliferator-activated receptors (PPAR-γ), which alter gene expression and result in insulin-like effects. These include reduced hepatic glucose output, increased glucose transporters (GLUT) in skeletal muscle with increased peripheral glucose utilisation, and the promotion of fatty acid uptake into adipose cells.

Glucosidase inhibitors

Acarbose

Acarbose competitively inhibits the alpha-glucosidases which metabolise oligosaccharides to monosaccharides in the small intestines. This reduces the production of glucose in the gastrointestinal tract, thereby preventing sharp rises in blood glucose after a meal. The subsequent increased presence of carbohydrates in the gastrointestinal tract may lead to flatulence and osmotic diarrhoea as side-effects.

Drug choice

The initial choice is generally between a sulphonylurea and metformin, with the latter being favoured in overweight and obese patients, as it causes weight loss. In choosing a sulphonylurea, age is a consideration. Specifically, elderly patients are more susceptible to the hypoglycaemic effects

of sulphonylureas and this may be reduced by using a short-acting agent such as gliclazide or tolbutamide. Chlorpropamide is not widely used as it is long-acting and may enhance antidiuretic hormone release, leading to hyponatraemia. If monotherapy is inadequate, then a sulphonylurea and metformin are used in combination.

The glitazones are currently licensed as 'add-on' therapies to either a sulphonylurea or metformin but they should not be used in triple combinations. The National Institute of Clinical Excellence (NICE) guidelines (NICE, 2001) indicate that rosiglitazone or pioglitazone should only be added once the combination of a sulphonylurea plus metformin has been proven to be inadequate (or not tolerated). In adding a glitazone, the combination of the glitazone and metformin is preferred, especially in obese patients. This use of a glitazone would be an alternative to adding insulin therapy. Nateglinide is currently licensed as add-on therapy with metformin, and repaglinide is licensed for both monotherapy and in combination with metformin.

Other considerations are detailed in Table 33.2.

Drug interactions

In addition to the effects of drugs on glucose control described above, Table 33.3 gives some important interactions with antidiabetic agents.

Table 33.2   The effects of concurrent conditions on drug choice in type 2 diabetes mellitus

Condition	Effect on drug choice	Comments
Renal impairment	Avoid metformin. Tolbutamide or gliclazide is preferred	The shorter-acting sulphonylureas should be used at a reduced dose
Heart failure	Avoid metformin in severe heart failure. Avoid glitazones in heart failure	
Liver disease	Avoid metformin Avoid glitazones	Risk of lactic acidosis
Hyperlipidaemia	Glitazones may cause modest reductions in triglycerides and increases in HDL	Fibrates may also be chosen to manage hyperlipidaemia (Chapter 12)
Porphyria	Sulphonylureas should be avoided	
Pregnancy	Insulin therapy is generally used in place of oral antidiabetic drugs	

HDL, high-density lipoprotein.

Table 33.3 Examples of some important interactions with antidiabetic drugs

Drugs	Consequences	Comments
Insulin with glitazones	Enhanced actions	This combination is contraindicated but would be a logical insulin-sparing combination
Acarbose with insulin/sulphonylureas	Acarbose may enhance the hypoglycaemic effects of these drugs	Dose reduction of insulin or sulphonylurea may be needed
Chlorpropamide with alcohol	Facial flushing	This does not occur with other sulphonylureas
Glipizide with colestryramine	The absorption of glipizide may be delayed	Glipizide should be taken 1–2 h before colestyramine
Sulphonylureas with fibrates	Enhanced effects of the sulphonylureas	This may be an advantage in poor glucose control or dose reduction of the sulphonylurea may be needed
Tolbutamide/glibenclamide with rifampicin	Rifampicin may increase the metabolism of these agents	The dose of the sulphonylurea may need to be increased
Sulphonylureas with sulphonamides	Enhanced hypoglycaemic effects	This applies to some but not all sulphonamides
Repaglinide with erythromycin, fluconazole, itraconazole, ketoconazole, phenytoin, or rifampicin	These drugs may alter the actions of repaglinide	The manufacturer contraindicates these combinations
Metformin/sulphonylureas with cimetidine	Cimetidine has been reported to increase the activity of sulphonylureas (especially glipizide). Cimetidine may inhibit the renal excretion of metformin	Patients may be advised of the possibility of hypoglycaemia while taking cimetidine and a sulphonylurea. A dose reduction with metformin may be appropriate. Ranitidine does not appear to interact with these antidiabetic drugs

Complications of antidiabetic drug therapy

The main complication of treatment with the sulphonylureas and, to a lesser extent, meglitinide analogues, is hypoglycaemia as they stimulate insulin release. This is most problematic at high doses or in the case of sulphonylureas with long half-lives. Incidences of hypoglycaemia may be managed by sugary drinks (see above) and may require a change in the drug used. The glitazones and metformin are far less likely to cause hypoglycaemia.

The insulin-stimulating effects of sulphonylureas and insulin-sensitising effects of glitazones may lead to weight gain, whilst metformin leads to weight loss.

Monitoring

In view of hepatotoxicity to the prototypic glitazone troglitazone (which has been withdrawn), NICE (2001) recommends that liver function tests are carried out in patients receiving rosiglitazone or pioglitazone before treatment, then every 2 months for the first year and periodically thereafter.

Diabetic complications and their prevention

Diabetic complications have serious consequences for both morbidity and mortality. The complications are macrovascular, microvascular and neuropathy.

Macrovascular complications

Diabetes is associated with a substantial increase in the risk of cardiovascular mortality through ischaemic heart disease and stroke. Furthermore, the risk is substantially enhanced by other cardiovascular risks such as hypertension, hyperlipidaemia, obesity and smoking. Cardiovascular disease occurs prematurely in patients with diabetes, even if they have had good control, and accounts for 70% of deaths in these patients. Strict regulation of blood pressure is essential in diabetes: the British Hypertension Society recommends a target of less than 140/80 mmHg. Evidence from trials indicates that lowering blood pressure *per se* is important and reduces both macrovascular and microvascular complications. Trials with antihypertensive drugs have also focused on specific agents in patients with diabetes. In this respect, the Losartan Intervention for Endpoint Reduction in Hypertension (LIFE) trial (2002) has reported that the angiotensin receptor antagonist losartan is more effective than atenolol at reducing morbidity and mortality in hypertensive patients who have diabetes and/or left ventricular hypertrophy. The Heart Outcomes Prevention Evaluation (HOPE) trial (2000) found that treatment of patients with a high risk for cardiovascular disease with the angiotensin-converting enzyme (ACE) inhibitor ramipril reduced the complications associated with diabetes and also the development of diabetes. Accordingly, ACE inhibitors are often first choice antihypertensives in patients with diabetes. The Heart Protection Study Collaborative Group (2002) has demonstrated in patients with diabetes that simvastatin protects against cardiovascular events, irrespective of their cholesterol levels.

Microvascular complications

Pathological changes in the microcirculation lead to nephropathy and retinopathy. The mechanism of damage is thought to be due to hyperglycaemia leading to glycation of structural proteins and the toxic effects of free radicals and glycation end-products. Accordingly, there is good evidence that good glycaemic control may limit these complications.

Diabetic nephropathy is a long-term consequence of diabetes and may result in end-stage renal failure. In the early stages of diabetes, there is hyperfiltration in the glomeruli. There are subsequent changes in the basement membranes, including glycation, and these lead to microalbuminuria, a marker of renal deterioration. This may be followed by hypertension and proteinuria. Microvascular damage in the retinal circulation may lead to retinopathy which is associated with angiogenesis, haemorrhages and detachment of the retina. Retinopathy is a major cause of blindness.

All patients with type 1 diabetes who have microalbuminuria should receive an ACE inhibitor, regardless of whether they have hypertension. NICE guidance (2002) on renal disease in type 2 diabetes indicated that diabetic nephropathy is likely in patients who have albumin in the urine and/or increased plasma creatinine levels, which is accompanied by retinopathy. In these patients, glycaemic control should aim to achieve levels of glycated haemoglobin (HbA_{1c}) below 6.5–7.5%, blood pressure should be below 135/75 mmHg and an ACE inhibitor should be given for renal and cardiovascular protection. The CALM study group (2000) demonstrated in type 2 diabetes that the angiotensin II receptor antagonist candesartan was equally effective as lisinopril at controlling both blood pressure and microalbuminuria. Furthermore, the combination of candesartan and lisinopril was even more effective. The sartan irbesartan has also been shown to be effective at reducing the incidence of diabetic nephropathy and is licensed for use in type 2 diabetes. This may be an alternative to ACE inhibitors when they are not tolerated, for example due to their associated cough.

The Diabetes Control and Complications Trial (DCCT) (1993) reported that, in type 1 diabetes, intensive insulin therapy to maintain blood glucose as close to normal as possible delayed the onset of and progression of nephropathy, retinopathy and neuropathy. Evidence from the UK Prospective Diabetes Study (UKPDS) (1998a, b) indicated that intensive glycaemic control in type 2 diabetes lowers the risk of microvascular but not macrovascular complications. Furthermore, in overweight subjects metformin was more effective than sulphonylureas in reducing diabetic complications.

Peripheral vascular disease

The vascular damage associated with diabetes is a major risk factor for the development of peripheral vascular disease, leading to ischaemia, and is a major reason for limb amputation.

Neuropathy

Damage to nerves occurs through glycation and the production of polyols. This may lead to impaired nervous conduction and is referred to as neuropathy. The neuropathy may be peripheral, leading to loss of peripheral sensation and ulceration, or autonomic, which may lead to postural hypotension and impotence.

Monitoring

Monitoring of glycaemic control is important in the management of diabetes but is especially important in patients who use insulin and alter their dose according to the level of control. Monitoring is best achieved by measuring blood glucose levels using a reagent stick and simple meter, so that the levels of control may be assessed and the dose of insulin or antidiabetic drugs adjusted accordingly. Long-term monitoring of control is by measuring the levels of HbA_{1c} in the blood. This gives a measure of the long-term control (previous 2 months): a value of 7% or less is associated with reduced diabetic complications. In addition, blood pressure, cholesterol, renal and visual function are routinely monitored.

Over-the-counter considerations

Many medicines, including many over-the-counter (OTC) preparations for coughs and colds, contain sugar and patients should be made aware of this in relation to their daily intake. Sugar-free alternatives are available but may be more expensive and often contain sorbitol, which may cause diarrhoea.

Cornplasters which contain salicylic acid should not be used in patients with diabetes. This is because patients with diabetic neuropathy may have less sensation in the feet and the corrosive effects of cornplasters may go unnoticed, leading to ulceration. All foot problems affecting diabetic patients warrant prompt referral.

Decongestants should be used with caution in patients with diabetes as the beta-adrenoceptor agonist activity may alter glucose control via anti-insulin affects.

Dietary supplements

Insulin therapy or antidiabetic drugs are the only appropriate treatments for diabetes. However, a number of dietary supplements, in addition to a balanced diet, may play some role in the management of diabetes. Examples of these include aloe vera, which has been shown to exert hypoglycaemic actions and may have a potential role as an adjunct to conventional treatment; carnitine may increase glucose utilisation. Other herbal preparations with potential hypoglycaemic activity include burdock, celery, dandelion, eucalyptus, garlic, ginger, ispaghula, juniper, marshmallow, nettle and sage. Studies on animal models of diabetes suggest that evening primrose oil may be of benefit in neuropathy. Hyperglycaemic effects are associated with hydrocotyle, liquorice and rosemary. For a more detailed discussion of this topic, the reader is referred to *Dietary Supplements* by Mason (2001).

Counselling

Diabetes mellitus is a lifelong condition and patients will receive a range of counselling from doctors, specialist nurses and dieticians. Patients may also be directed to organisations such as Diabetes UK for further information and advice. The key to counselling is to ensure good glycaemic control, which is associated with the prevention of diabetic complications. In addition, practical advice which may be given includes the following.

Diabetes

- Give advice regarding the regimen.
- The patient should be made aware of the signs of hypoglycaemia and hyperglycaemia and how to respond to them.

- Patients with diabetes should inform the driving licensing authorities of their condition.
- Patients should be warned to avoid hypoglycaemia whilst driving.
- Patients prescribed insulin and those at risk of hypoglycaemia should carry glucose tablets or similar at all times.
- In addition to dietary advice, special diabetic foods are expensive and of little value.
- It is a misconception that natural fruit juice, honey and reduced-sugar products are low in sugar.
- Patients with diabetes represent a risk group (see Chapter 1) and the importance of consulting their GP should be emphasised.
- Patients with diabetes should consult their GP if they experience problems with their feet, including fungal infections.
- Patients with type 1 and type 2 diabetes (treated with drugs) are exempt from prescription charges.
- Lifestyle advice to reduce cardiovascular risk, including cessation of smoking, should be emphasised.
- Alcohol should only be consumed in moderation and it may mask the signs of hypoglycaemia.
- Alcoholic drinks will also contribute toward the carbohydrate load.
- Low-dose aspirin should be considered for patients with a significant risk of cardiovascular disease.
- Exercise improves insulin sensitivity and reduces cardiovascular risk.
- Advice should be sought before becoming pregnant.
- A medic alert chain or card should be carried if possible to alert doctors that the patient is prescribed insulin. A service is available whereby patients register their insulin regimen and a number is available for emergency doctors to contact if needed.

Type 1 diabetes

- Patients should be advised to maintain adequate supplies of insulin.

- Patients should not stop taking insulin.
- Give advice regarding injection technique.
- Insulins should be stored in a refrigerator but not frozen.
- Different injection sites should be used, although the rate of absorption may differ between sites.
- The dispensed container of insulin should be shown to the patient for confirmation that it is expected by the patient.
- The size of the pen needle should be checked carefully when prescribing and dispensing due to the increasing variety of sizes which reflect different injection techniques.
- Sugary food may be eaten but preferably as part of a meal.
- Needles should be disposed of correctly.

Type 2 diabetes

- Metformin should be taken with or after food.
- Diarrhoea is a common side-effect with metformin and acarbose.
- Nateglinide and repaglinide should be taken just before meals.
- Alcohol should be avoided with chlorpropamide.

Practice points

- Diabetes is a major risk factor for cardiovascular disease and so a healthy lifestyle (including avoidance of obesity and cessation of smoking) is essential.
- Blood pressure should be adequately controlled and ACE inhibitors are effective at reducing diabetic nephropathy.
- The risk of developing type 2 diabetes may be reduced by a lifelong healthy diet, weight control and exercise.
- Type 2 diabetes continues to be underdiagnosed.
- Good glycaemic control may prevent future complications.

CASE STUDY

A 65-year-old woman visits her pharmacist for her third tube of clotrimazole for vaginal thrush in as many weeks and also complains that she is always thirsty. This time her pharmacist refers her to her GP.

Why was a referral made?

- Both recurrent genital thrush and thirst are symptoms of diabetes and should raise suspicion for referral.

On visiting her GP an examination reveals a blood pressure of 160/100 mmHg and biochemistry reveals:

Random glucose   14.0 mmol/L (<11.1 mmol/L)
Creatinine   100 µmol/L (60–120 µmol/L)
Cholesterol   6 mmol/L (ideal <5.2 mmol/L)
Haematology   Normal

She was referred for further glucose tests and then to a dietician. Why was she referred for dietary advice?

- The random glucose level is consistent with diabetes and in type 2 diabetes dietary control should be tried for 3 months to determine whether this alone controls the condition.

Three months later she presents you with a prescription:

Atenolol 50 mg o.d.
Glibenclamide 5 mg daily

Comment on this prescription.

- The atenolol is for blood pressure control, which is essential in diabetes. Although atenolol is effective, it may impair warning signs of hypoglycaemia. Glibenclamide is relatively long-acting and is associated with hypoglycaemia. A shorter-acting agent such as gliclazide or tolbutamide might have been more appropriate, especially in older patients. If the woman was obese then metformin would be more appropriate.

How does glibenclamide act?

- It inhibits K_{ATP}-channels on the beta-cells of the islets of Langerhans, leading to cellular depolarisation and insulin release.

After several weeks she complains to her pharmacist of feeling weak and confused and once again is referred to her GP. This time her random glucose was measured as 3 mmol/L and her blood pressure was 140/90 mmHg. Her GP advised her to drink a sugary cup of tea immediately and her prescription was changed to:

Atenolol 50 mg o.d.
Tolbutamide 1 g daily in divided doses

Why was this change made?

continued

CASE STUDY (continued)

- The confusion and low glucose levels are indicative of hypoglycaemia, which is probably due to glibenclamide. She was changed to tolbutamide, which is less likely to cause hypoglycaemia.

A year later she is under the care of a consultant diabetologist and her prescription was changed to:

Ramipril 2.5 mg daily (with a view to increments over several weeks up to 10 mg)
Tolbutamide 1 g daily in divided doses
Simvastatin 10 mg o.n.

What was the rationale behind these changes?

- The ACE inhibitor is a more logical antihypertensive in patients with diabetes. The HOPE trial indicates that ramipril is protective against diabetic nephropathy and reduces complications of diabetes. The simvastatin has been used to reduce plasma cholesterol and so reduce her overall cardiovascular risk.

How would you counsel the patient with respect to these changes?

- She should initially take the ramipril on retiring to bed at night in case of profound first-dose hypotension.
- Simvastatin should be taken at night when endogenous cholesterol synthesis is greatest.

On changing her medication, she complained of a racing heart. What is the possible explanation for this?

- Abrupt withdrawal of atenolol is associated with tachyarrhythmias due to up-regulation of beta-adrenoceptors on the heart. Withdrawal should be gradual or under close supervision.

References

CALM study group (2000). Randomised controlled trial of dual blockade of the renin–angiotensin system in patients with hypertension, microalbuminuria, and non-insulin dependent diabetes: the candesartan and lisinopril microalbuminuria (CALM) study. *BMJ* 321: 1440–1444.

DCCT (The Diabetes Control and Complications Trial Research Group) (1993). The effect of intensive treatment of diabetes on the development and progression of long-term complications in insulin-dependent diabetes mellitus. *N Engl J Med* 329: 977–986.

Heart Protection Study Collaborative Group (2002). MRC/BHF Heart Protection Study of cholesterol lowering with simvastatin in 20 536 high-risk individuals: randomised placebo-controlled trial. *Lancet* 360: 7–22.

HOPE (Heart Outcomes Prevention Evaluation) study investigators (2000). Effects of an angiotensin-converting-enzyme inhibitor, ramipril, on cardiovascular events in high-risk patients. *N Engl J Med* 342: 145–153.

LIFE (Losartan Intervention for Endpoint Reduction in Hypertension) study investigators (2002). Cardiovascular morbidity and mortality in patients with diabetes in the Losartan Intervention for Endpoint Reduction in Hypertension study (LIFE): a randomised trial against atenolol. *Lancet* 359: 1004–1010.

NICE (2001). Guidance on the use of pioglitazone for type 2 diabetes mellitus. Technology Appraisal Guidance no. 21. London: National Institute of Clinical Excellence (via www.nice.org.uk).

NICE (2002). Management of type 2 diabetes: renal disease – prevention and early management. London: National Institute of Clinical Excellence (via www.nice.org.uk).

UK Prospective Diabetes Study (UKPDS) Group (1998a). Intensive blood-glucose control with sulphonylurea or insulin compared with conventional treatment and the risk of complications in patients with type 2 diabetes (UKPDS 33). *Lancet* 352: 837–853.

UK Prospective Diabetes Study (UKPDS) Group (1998b). Effects of intensive blood-glucose control with metformin on the complications in overweight patients with type 2 diabetes (UKPDS 34). *Lancet* 352: 854–865.

Further reading

Berger J, Moller D E (2002). The mechanisms of action of PPARs. *Annu Rev Med* 53: 409–435.

Mason P (2001). *Dietary Supplements*, 2nd edn. London: Pharmaceutical Press.

NICE (2000). Guidance on rosiglitazone for type 2 diabetes mellitus. Technology Appraisal Guidance no. 9. London: National Institute of Clinical Excellence (via www.nice.org.uk).

Simpson H (2001). Insulin regimens in type 1 diabetes management. *Prescriber* 12: 43–57.

Online resource

www.diabetes.org.uk is the website of Diabetes UK, the operating name of the British Diabetic Association, which provides both patient and professional information (accessed 4 December 2002).

34

Thyroid disorders

The thyroid gland releases predominantly thyroxine (T_4), but also triiodothyronine (T_3), which is the more active hormone; indeed, T_4 may undergo peripheral conversion to T_3. Both of these hormones play important roles in the regulation of cellular metabolism and growth, whilst also influencing activity of the sympathetic nervous system. Clinically there may be excessive activity (hyperthyroidism) or underactivity (hypothyroidism), both of which have widespread pathophysiological effects. Detailed guidance on thyroid disorders and their treatment may be found in Vanderpump *et al.* (1996), which is published on behalf of the Royal College of Physicians (London) and the Society for Endocrinology.

Hyperthyroidism

This is also known as thyrotoxicosis and is generally characterised by elevated levels of T_3 and T_4.

The most common form is Graves disease, which is due to antibodies against the thyroid-stimulating hormone (TSH) receptor, which is responsible for stimulating the release of T_3 and T_4. The antibodies activate the receptor and lead to the increased production of thyroid hormone and there is usually an increase in the size of the thyroid gland (goitre). Other less common causes include toxic multinodular goitre, toxic adenoma and iatrogenic causes. In the latter case, drugs which have a high iodine content such as amiodarone and radiological contrast agents may lead to increased thyroid activity; lithium may rarely cause hyperthyroidism.

Clinical features

Hyperthyroidism is especially common in women and occurs most often between the ages of 20 and 40 years. There may be widespread changes, which include:

- weight loss
- increased appetite
- diarrhoea
- nervousness and irritability
- fatigue
- tremor
- increased sweating
- heat intolerance
- pruritus
- exophthalmos (bulging eyes, seen in Graves disease only)
- eyelid retraction
- goitre
- cardiac arrhythmias, including palpitations and atrial fibrillation
- angina
- precipitation of heart failure
- shortness of breath on exertion
- nausea and vomiting in pregnancy
- palmar erythema

Many of these symptoms may be attributable to the increased action of catecholamines.

Diagnosis

In addition to the above symptoms, biochemistry will reveal increased levels of thyroid hormones but undetectable levels of TSH. This latter finding is due to increased levels of thyroid hormone causing negative-feedback inhibition of TSH release from the pituitary gland. Thyroid function tests may be complicated by concurrent drug treatment, including the use of amiodarone, aspirin, beta-blockers, carbamazepine, corticosteroids, heparin, oestrogens, phenytoin, rifampicin and radiological contrast agents. In this respect, the enzyme inducers carbamazepine, phenytoin and rifampicin may accelerate the metabolism of T_4 and T_3, leading to reduced levels. Corticosteroids may inhibit TSH release, lowering T_4 and T_3. By contrast, heparin may give a rapid but short-lived increase in T_4 and radiological contrast agents may elevate T_4 due to their high iodine content.

Given the non-specific nature of some of the symptoms, thyroid function is often routinely measured in patients presenting with a range of symptoms, for example, palpitations in young adults.

Goals of treatment

These are to achieve a euthyroid state (normal levels of thyroid hormones), and to provide symptomatic relief from the increased sympathetic activity.

Management

To achieve euthyroidism the choice is between the use of antithyroid drugs (thionamides), radioactive iodine to irradiate and destroy part of the thyroid gland and a partial or subtotal thyroidectomy.

Pharmacological basis of management

Thionamides

Carbimazole and propylthiouracil
These decrease the production of thyroid hormones by inhibiting the iodination of thyroglobulin, which occurs via inhibition of thyroperoxidase. The thyroid hormones have long plasma half-lives, so inhibiting their synthesis will take several weeks for an effect to occur. Thionamides may also suppress the immune response, but whether this contributes to their action in hyperthyroidism is unclear.

Beta-blockers

Atenolol, nadolol, propranolol
These are dealt with extensively in Chapter 11. In the context of hyperthyroidism, they will reduce the actions of catecholamines at beta-adrenoceptors, which are augmented in this condition, and will provide relief from symptoms such as tremor, anxiety and palpitations. Non-selective beta-blockers (e.g. propranolol) are required to relieve the tremor. It should also be noted that hyperthyroidism accelerates the metabolism of propranolol.

Treatment

Thionamides are indicated for the first episode of Graves disease with a view to achieving a remission. It is also used in subsequent episodes of Graves disease, in more elderly patients and those with toxic nodular hyperthyroidism to achieve euthyroidism prior to surgery or radio-active iodine for a definitive cure. In the case of drug-induced hyperthyroidism, the causative drug should be stopped and a beta-blocker used to control the symptoms.

Carbimazole is the thionamide of choice, with once-daily administration. It is initially given at higher doses, known as reducing doses, to achieve a euthyroid state, which takes about 1–2 months to achieve. During this time, unless con-traindicated (asthma, chronic obstructive pul-monary disease, uncontrolled heart failure), a beta-blocker is given to control symptoms. Once the euthyroid state is achieved, maintenance therapy with the thionamide at a lower dose may be used, typically for 18 months, and the beta-blocker withdrawn gradually. Alternatively, a high dose of carbimazole may be maintained to suppress thyroid activity completely and com-bined with replacement thyroxine, and this is known as the blocking-replacement regimen. This has the advantage of avoiding hypothy-roidism, which may be induced by antithyroid drugs, and a reduced requirement for monitoring of thyroid function. Despite the use of antithy-roid drugs, the relapse rate is around 50% on dis-continuation of treatment, although it is unclear whether blocking-replacement regimens have a higher success rate.

Other considerations

Pregnancy and breast-feeding
Carbimazole may cause hypothyroidism in the fetus but is generally considered safe in preg-nancy under specialist care, with the lowest effec-tive dose used, and this may be stopped before birth. Propylthiouracil is sometimes preferred as carbimazole may induce fetal aplasia cutis (a localised absence of skin at birth). A blocking-replacement regimen is contraindicated in preg-nancy, as the antithyroid drugs more readily cross the placenta than thyroxine and this may lead to fetal hypothyroidism.

Carbimazole at doses of less than 20 mg is con-sidered safe during lactation, as the amounts in the milk are low. Once again, propylthiouracil is

sometimes preferred as it enters the breast milk to a smaller extent.

Asthma
Hyperthyroidism may sometimes lead to a worsening of asthma. Beta$_2$-agonists should be used with caution as bronchodilators as they may be expected to have enhanced systemic actions in uncontrolled hyperthyroidism. Indeed, the symptoms of toxicity with beta$_2$-agonists may also be confused with those of hyperthyroidism. As commented above, asthma is a contraindica-tion to using beta-blockers in the management of hyperthyroidism. In patients who cannot receive a beta-blocker, calcium channel antagon-ists such as diltiazem may be useful in controlling tachycardia.

Monitoring

No specific monitoring, except thyroid function, is required for treatment with thionamides. However, carbimazole and propylthiouracil may both cause agranulocytosis leading to leuco-penia. If patients report with sore throats, mouth ulcers, bruising or non-specific illness, a full blood count should be carried out and the drug withdrawn if there is leucopenia. Although an alternative thionamide may be used as a replace-ment, there is a high degree of cross-reactivity between agents.

Drug interactions

Drug interactions with antithyroid drugs are limited and detailed in Table 34.1.

Counselling

Lifestyle advice may be helpful in relieving symptoms such as heat intolerance. Caffeine consumption should be reduced, as this may exacerbate symptoms. Ophthalmopathy in Graves disease, presenting as photophobia and grittiness, may be relieved by sunglasses and artificial tears. Drug-specific counselling points are detailed:

Table 34.1 Some important drug interactions with antithyroid drugs

Drugs	Consequences	Comments
Corticosteroids with carbimazole	Increased elimination of prednisolone	The dose of prednisolone may need to be increased
Digoxin with carbimazole	Carbimazole may reduce the plasma levels of digoxin. Patients with hyperthyroidism may be resistant to the actions of digoxin, such that digoxin may be less effective in atrial fibrillation in patients with hyperthyroidism	Higher doses of digoxin may be required initially and then reduced as thyroid levels fall
Theophylline with thionamides	Theophylline levels may rise in patients treated with thionamides for hyperthyroidism	Monitoring may be required and the dose of theophylline may need to be reduced
Warfarin with thionamides	The actions of warfarin may be decreased	The dose of warfarin may need to be increased

- If carbimazole or propylthiouracil is taken without a beta-blocker, it will take several weeks for an improvement in symptoms to be noticed.
- If a beta-blocker is used, it is worth explaining its role to the patient, and that it is not being used for hypertension or angina, which may be indicated on the patient information leaflets. General counselling for beta-blockers is found in Chapter 11.
- Both carbimazole and propylthiouracil may cause agranulocytosis, leading to leucopenia. Patients should report urgently to their general practitioner (GP) with sore throats, mouth ulcers, bruising or non-specific illness.
- Both carbimazole and propylthiouracil may cause mild gastrointestinal disturbances and urticarial rashes. Pruritus may be managed with antihistamines and treatment continued. If this fails, an alternative agent may be tried as cross-sensitivity may not occur.
- Patients should be advised to report symptoms of hypothyroidism, which may indicate over-treatment.

Hypothyroidism

This is simply failure of the thyroid gland to produce sufficient thyroid hormone, leading to reduced circulating levels. The most common form (90%) is Hashimoto's thyroiditis, which is an autoimmune destruction of the thyroid gland. Hypothyroidism may also be induced by antithyroid drug treatment with thionamides, lithium, amiodarone and also radioactive iodine.

Clinical features

As with hyperthyroidism, there is an increased incidence of hypothyroidism in women and this increases with age. There are widespread changes in hypothyroidism which include:

- tiredness
- weight gain
- hypothermia
- cold intolerance
- hoarseness
- bradycardia (rarely angina and heart failure)
- mental slowness
- delayed reflexes
- depression
- anaemia
- dry skin and hair
- goitre
- oedema, leading to puffiness around the eyes
- constipation

Diagnosis

Hypothyroidism is identified on a thyroid function test, which reveals elevated TSH and reduced T_4 levels. In addition there may be macrocytosis and hypercholesterolaemia. In secondary failure due to pituitary or hypothalamic disease, TSH levels will be reduced. Other causes should be considered before starting treatment.

Goals of treatment

These are to achieve a euthyroid state.

Management

Restoring thyroid hormone levels is achieved by administration of levothyroxine (T_4). In young patients the starting dose is usually 50–100 µg/day, which may be increased after 6 weeks by 25–50 µg and thereafter until maintenance levels are achieved. The dose required is the one that leads to correct TSH levels. In elderly patients, and those with ischaemic heart disease, the starting dose used is 25 µg, which is increased every 3–4 weeks by 25 µg, until TSH levels are normalised. The reason to exercise caution in patients with ischaemic heart disease is that T_4 may lead to worsening or uncovering of angina (there is also an increased risk of myocardial infarction and death) by increasing the metabolic rate and sympathetic activity. In patients who experience angina, a beta-blocker may be prescribed. If the TSH levels are suppressed by overtreatment there is a significant risk of atrial fibrillation. Once established, T_4 therapy will need to be used lifelong.

Diabetes mellitus

An increased dose of antidiabetic agents, including insulin, may be required.

Pregnancy

T_4 treatment is continued during pregnancy but the dose may need to be increased to normalise TSH levels.

Drug interactions

Some important interactions with T_4 are detailed in Table 34.2. The interactions relate to altering the effects of T_4 or interacting drugs.

Counselling

Aside from guidance on the regimen, a key counselling point should be to advise patients to consult their GP if they start to suffer from angina or pre-existing angina deteriorates. Additional points:

- It is difficult to distinguish between the strengths of T_4 tablets, as they are all small and white. Patients should make sure that they take tablets of the correct strength.
- If a dose is missed, the missed dose may be taken the next day with the next dose (as T_4 has a long half-life of 7 days).
- Patients should be encouraged to report symptoms of overtreatment, particularly when treatment is initiated. These include diarrhoea, nervousness, rapid pulse, insomnia, tremors or anginal pain. These symptoms may necessitate a reduced dose or the omission of a dose for 1–2 days before restarting at a lower dose.

Over-the-counter medicines in patients with thyroid disorders

Topical or oral sympathomimetic drugs should be avoided in patients with hyperthyroidism, due to the enhancement of catecholamines. Pharmacists can help to remind patients of the need for prompt referral when presenting with signs of infection when prescribed antithyroid medication. Pharmacists may also help to identify patients presenting with symptoms suggestive of thyroid disorder and encourage referral for further investigation. For example, the common request for over-the-counter (OTC) products for fatigue and/or slimming advice may prompt further questioning to identify the possibility of an underlying thyroid disorder.

Table 34.2   Drugs interacting with levothyroxine

Drug	Consequences	Comments
Amiodarone	Reduced effects of thyroxine	Contraindicated by manufacturers. The *British National Formulary* indicates that if amiodarone causes hyperthyroidism, amiodarone should be withdrawn and antithyroid drugs may be required. If hypothyroidism is induced then replacement therapy may be needed
Antiepileptic drugs (carbamazepine and phenytoin)	These enzyme inducers have been reported to lower thyroid hormone levels occasionally	Monitoring may be appropriate
Colestyramine	This may reduce the absorption of levothyroxine	Their use should be separated by 4–6 h
Ferrous sulfate	This may reduce the absorption of thyroxine	Their doses should be separated by 2 h
Digoxin	Hypothyroid patients are relatively more sensitive to digoxin	The dose of digoxin may need to be reduced as thyroxine treatment is established
Sertraline	The effects of thyroxine have been reported to be reduced	The dose of thyroxine may need to be increased
Lofepramine		Its use with levothyroxine is contraindicated by the manufacturers
Theophylline	Reduced effects of theophylline	The dose of theophylline may need to be increased
Tricyclic antidepressants	Thyroxine may accelerate the responses to imipramine and amitriptyline	The manufacturers of lofepramine contraindicate its use with thyroxine
Warfarin	Increased anticoagulant effects of warfarin	The dose of warfarin may need to be reduced

Herbal medicines in patients with thyroid disorders

Kelp is used as herbal treatment for thyroid disorders. However, it has a high iodine content which may lead to hyperthyroidism or hypothyroidism and it should be avoided. Preparations of ephadra should be avoided due to the ephedrine content. Shepherd's purse also has the potential to cause hypothyroidism and should therefore be avoided by patients prescribed thyroid treatment.

Other supplements

Many multivitamin and mineral preparation contain approximately 50–100% of the recommended daily intake of iodine. This is generally provided in the diet, with the possible exception of the vegan diet. Toxicity is rare at these doses but patients prescribed thyroid treatment should be careful to avoid excess doses which may interfere with their treatment.

Practice points

- Both hyperthyroidism and hypothyroidism may present with relatively non-specific symptoms.
- Both may be readily diagnosed by thyroid function tests.
- Both may be managed by drugs; beta-blockers provide symptomatic relief in hyperthyroidism.
- Be alert for leucopenia in patients taking carbimazole and propylthiouracil.

 CASE STUDY

A 35-year-old female with a history of mild asthma developed anxiety, palpitations, rapid pulse and feelings of panic not long after a fall down a full flight of stairs. She put the symptoms down to the fall. Her symptoms worsened until she lost 10 kg (1.5 stone) in a week, developed a tremor, had broken vessels in the eye and the back of the knee and a pulse of 150 beats/min, at which time she visited her GP. She was hyperthyroid and prescribed propranolol and carbimazole. The pharmacist picked up a history of asthma and she was changed to atenolol. She developed a rash on her hands and feet but continued treatment for 2 years, at which point treatment was withdrawn.

- In this case it is possible that the initial palpitations and tachycardia may, in part, have been due to overuse of a beta$_2$-adrenoceptor agonist or its increased sensitivity in hyperthyroidism. The pharmacist was correct to question the use of propranolol and atenolol was only appropriate if symptomatic control was considered absolutely essential as beta$_1$-adrenoceptor antagonists may still lead to bronchospasm in patients with asthma. The rash would have been viewed as an acceptable side-effect of carbimazole.

References

Mehta D K (ed.) *British National Formulary*, latest edition. London: British Medical Association and Royal Pharmaceutical Society of Great Britain.

Vanderpump M P J, Ahlquist J A O, Franklyn J A *et al.* (1996). Consensus statement for good practice and audit measures in the management of hypothyroidism and hyperthyroidism. *BMJ* 313: 539–544.

Further reading

Dale J, Franklyn J (2002). The drug treatment of thyroid disorders. *Prescriber* 13: 50–71.

Online resource

www.british-thyroid-association.org is the website of the British Thyroid Association providing professional and patient advice (accessed 4 December 2002).

Appendix

Formulary of some important classes of drugs, commonly used examples, mechanisms of action and uses

Class	Examples	Actions	Common uses
Gastrointestinal			
Proton pump inhibitors (PPIs)	Omeprazole, lansoprazole, rabeprazole	Irreversible proton pump inhibition	Acid suppression – peptic ulceration, GORD, prophylaxis against NSAID-induced damage
Histamine H_2-receptor antagonists	Ranitidine[a], cimetidine[a]	Antagonism of histamine H_2-receptor	Acid suppression – peptic ulceration, GORD, dyspepsia
Cytoprotective prostaglandin analogue	Misoprostol	Analogue of PGE_1, reduces H^+ secretion and stimulates bicarbonate and mucus secretion	Prophylaxis against NSAID-induced damage
Triple therapy for *Helicobacter pylori* eradication	PPI plus two from amoxicillin, clarithromycin and metronidazole	Acid suppression and *H. pylori* eradication	*H. pylori* eradication in peptic ulceration
Prokinetic drugs	Domperidone[a], metoclopramide	Increase gastric emptying	Bloating and nausea
Laxative	Lactulose[a], senna[a], ispaghula[a]	Lactulose: osmotic. Senna: stimulant. Ispaghula: bulk	Constipation, constipation due to drugs, IBS. Lactulose: also in liver failure to prevent encephalopathy
Antidiarrhoeal agents	Loperamide[a]	Opioid: reduces colonic motility via presynaptic inhibition	Diarrhoea
Antispasmodic agents	Mebeverine[a]	Phosphodiesterase inhibitor?	IBS
Cardiovascular			
Cardiac glycosides	Digoxin	Inhibition of Na/K ATPase	AF, positive inotrope in CHF
Class I antiarrhythmics	Lidocaine (lignocaine)	Inhibition of Na-channels	Ventricular tachycardia
Class II antiarrhythmics	Beta-blockers (including sotalol)	Antagonism of beta-adrenoceptors	Paroxysmal AF
Class III antiarrhythmics	Amiodarone, sotalol	Blockade of K-channels leading to action potential prolongation	AF

Class	Examples	Actions	Common uses
Class IV antiarrhythmics	Verapamil	Blockade of Ca-channels	Supraventricular tachycardia
Thiazide diuretics	Bendroflumethiazide	Inhibition of Na/Cl transporter in DCT	Hypertension, mild CHF (especially elderly)
Loop diuretics	Furosemide (frusemide), bumetanide	Inhibition of Na/K/Cl triporter in loop of Henle; vasodilatation	CHF and LVF, renal failure
Potassium-sparing diuretics	Amiloride	Inhibition of aldosterone-sensitive Na-channels in DCT	Weak diuresis, especially in combination with K-losing diuretics (thiazides and loops)
Potassium-sparing diuretic, aldosterone antagonist	Spironolactone	Aldosterone receptor antagonist	Weak diuresis, especially in combination with K-losing diuretics (thiazides and loops), CHF and liver failure (ascites); Conn's syndrome
Beta-blockers (non-selective)	Propranolol	Antagonism of beta-adrenoceptors	Hypertension, angina, post-MI, anxiety, migraine prophylaxis, hyperthyroidism.
Beta$_1$-blockers	Atenolol, metoprolol, bisoprolol	Antagonism of beta$_1$-adrenoceptors	Hypertension, angina, post-MI; stable CHF (with caution)
ACE inhibitors	Captopril, enalapril, ramipril, lisinopril, perindopril	Inhibition of ACE, reducing synthesis of angiotensin II	Hypertension, post-MI, CHF, diabetic nephropathy
Angiotensin (AT$_1$) receptor antagonist (sartans)	Losartan, candesartan, valsartan	Antagonism of AT$_1$ receptors	Hypertension, CHF? diabetic nephropathy?
Calcium channel antagonists	Verapamil, amlodipine, nifedipine, diltiazem	Inhibition of VSM Ca-channels and cardiac Ca channels (diltiazem, verapamil)	Hypertension, angina. Diltiazem and verapamil: antiarrhythmic
Nitrates	Glyceryl trinitrate[a], isosorbide mononitrate[a]	Act via nitric oxide to increase cGMP	Angina, CHF
Potassium channel activators	Nicorandil	Activation of ATP-sensitive K-channels and release of nitric oxide	Angina
Alpha-blockers	Prazosin, doxazosin, indoramin	Antagonism of alpha-adrenoceptors	Resistant hypertension, prostatic hypertrophy
Centrally acting antihypertensives	Clonidine, moxonidine, α-methyl dopa	Clonidine: central alpha$_2$-adrenoceptors. Moxonidine: central imidazoline receptors	Resistant hypertension
HMG-CoA reductase inhibitors (Statins)	Simvastatin, pravastatin, atorvastatin, fluvastatin	HMG-CoA reductase inhibition in cholesterol synthesis	Reduction of cholesterol in hypercholesterolaemia and in patients with a high CV risk

Class	Examples	Actions	Common uses
Fibrates	Bezafibrate, gemifibrozil	Activates alpha-peroxisome proliferator-activated receptors (PPAR-a)	Hypercholesterolaemia and hypertriglyceridaemia
Bile binding agents	Colestyramine	Binds bile in gastrointestinal tract	Hypercholesterolaemia
Fibrinolytics	Streptokinase	Activates plasminogen to form plasmin	Clot busting in MI, PE
Antiplatelet drugs	Low-dose aspirin[a], clopidogrel	Aspirin: inhibition of platelet COX. Clopidogrel: ADP ($P2Y_{12}$) receptor antagonist	Prevention of MI and CVA. Prophylaxis for CVA in low-risk patients with AF
Injectable anticoagulants	Low-molecular-weight heparins (dalteparin, enoxaparin, tinzaparin), unfractionated heparin	Activates antithrombin III	Immediate anticoagulation
Oral anticoagulants	Warfarin	Vitamin K antagonist	Prophylaxis against thrombosis e.g. DVT, PE, CVA in AF, thrombosis on mechanical heart valves

Respiratory

Class	Examples	Actions	Common uses
Beta$_2$-agonists	Salbutamol, terbutaline	Activation of beta$_2$-adrenoceptors	Relief in asthma, COPD
Beta$_2$-agonists, long-acting	Salmeterol, formoterol	Long-lasting activation of beta$_2$-adrenoceptors	Long-term control in asthma, COPD
Corticosteroids	Beclometasone, budesonide	Anti-inflammatory	Prevention in asthma; 15% of COPD patients also benefit. Nasal use in hayfever[a]
Muscarinic antagonists	Ipratropium	Blockade of vagal bronchoconstriction	Relief in asthma, COPD
Cromones	Sodium cromoglicate	Unclear – may stabilise mast cells/sensory nerves	Prevention in asthma. Nasal and ocular use in hayfever[a]
Xanthines	Theophylline[a]	Phosphodiesterase inhibition, adenosine receptor antagonist	Relief in asthma
Leukotriene receptor antagonist	Montelukast, zafirlukast	Leukotriene receptor antagonist	Prevention in asthma; NSAID-induced bronchospasm
Antihistamines	Loratadine[a], chlorphenamine[a], cetirizine[a]	Antagonism of H$_1$-receptors	Allergy, older sedating agents (diphenhydramine, chlorphenamine, promethazine) for insomnia

Central nervous system

Class	Examples	Actions	Common uses
Benzodiazepines	Diazepam, temazepam	Enhancement of GABA at GABA-A receptors	Anxiety, insomnia. Short-term only

Class	Examples	Actions	Common uses
Z-drugs	Zopiclone, zolpidem	Enhancement of GABA at GABA-A receptors	Insomnia
Antipsychotics	Haloperidol, chlorpromazine, fluphenazine	Dopamine (D_2) receptor antagonists	Schizophrenia
Atypical antipsychotics	Clozapine, olanzapine, risperidone	Dopamine and 5-HT receptor antagonists	Schizophrenia
Antimanic drugs	Lithium	Uncertain	Bipolar affective disorder
Tricyclic antidepressants (TCAs)	Amitriptyline, lofepramine, dosulepin	Inhibition of noradrenaline (norepinephrine) and 5-HT reuptake	Depression. Amitriptyline: neuropathic pain; prophylaxis in migraine, IBS
Serotonin selective reuptake inhibitors (SSRIs)	Fluoxetine, paroxetine, citalopram, sertraline	Inhibition of 5-HT reuptake	Depression, anxiety, panic disorder
Monoamine oxidase inhibitors (MAOIs)	Phenelzine, moclobemide	Inhibition of MAO enzymes (moclobemide is reversible) and catecholamine metabolism	Resistant depression
Other antidepressants	Venlafaxine, reboxetine, mirtazapine	Reboxetine: noradrenaline reuptake inhibitor. Venlafaxine: Serotonin-noradrenaline reuptake inhibitor. Mirtazapine: alpha$_2$-antagonist and 5-HT$_2$ and 5-HT$_3$ antagonist	Depression. Venlafaxine also for anxiety
Antiobesity	Sibutramine, orlistat	Sibutramine: amine reuptake inhibitor. Orlistat: pancreatic lipase inhibitor	Obesity
Antiemetics	Promethazine[a], cyclizine[a], hyoscine[a], metoclopramide, ondansetron	Promethazine and cyclizine: H$_1$-receptor antagonists. Hyoscine: M-receptor antagonist. Metoclopramide: dopamine D$_2$ receptor antagonist. Ondansetron: 5-HT$_3$ receptor antagonist	Promethazine, hyoscine and cyclizine: motion sickness. Metoclopramide: emesis due to anticancer drugs. Ondansetron: emesis due to anticancer drugs; postoperative nausea and vomiting
Non-opioid analgesics	Paracetamol[a], NSAIDs (ibuprofen[a], diclofenac, naproxen, mefenamic acid)	COX inhibition. Paracetamol may inhibit the putative COX-3?	Pain, antipyretic and NSAIDs in inflammation
COX-2 inhibitors	'Coxibs' (celecoxib, rofecoxib). Etodolac and meloxicam	Inhibition of COX-2	Inflammation

Class	Examples	Actions	Common uses
Opioid analgesics	Morphine, tramadol, codeine[a], dihydrocodeine[a]	Opioid receptors	Pain
Opioid antagonist	Naloxone	Opioid receptor antagonist	Reversal of opioids
Antimigraine (triptans)	Sumatriptan, naratriptan	$5-HT_{1D}$-agonists	Treatment of a migraine attack
Antimigraine, prophylaxis	Pizotifen	$5-HT_2$ antagonist	Prevention of migraine
Antiepileptic drugs	Sodium valproate, carbamazepine, phenytoin	Valproate: potentiation of GABA. Carbamazepine and phenytoin: use-dependent inhibition of Na-channels, inhibiting propagation of excitation	Forms of epilepsy: all for tonic-clonic and partial seizures; valproate for absences and myoclonic seizures. Carbamazepine is also used in neuropathic pain and for bipolar affective disorder
Newer antiepileptic drugs	Lamotrigine, gabapentin	Lamotrigine: blockade of Na^+-channels and decreased release of glutamate. Gabapentin: unknown	Certain forms of epilepsy (gabapentin in combination), neuropathic pain
Antiparkinson drugs	L-dopa in carbidopa, ropinirole, benzatropine, selegiline	L-dopa: conversion to dopamine. Ropinirole: dopamine D_2 agonist. Benzatropine: muscarinic antagonist. Selegiline: MAO-B inhibitor	Parkinson's disease
Alzheimer's disease	Donepezil, galantamine, rivastigmine	Acetylcholine esterase inhibitors	Alzheimer's disease
Antimicrobial agents			
Penicillin	Amoxicillin, phenoxymethyl penicillin, flucloxacillin	Inhibition of cross-linking of peptide side chains	Phenoxymethyl penicillin: tonsillitis. Flucloxacillin: impetigo, cellulitis. Amoxicillin: chest infections, otitis media, UTIs
Cephalosporins	Cefalexin, cefotaxime, cefaclor	Binding to beta-lactam-binding sites and inhibiting cell wall synthesis	Septicaemia, pneumonia, meningitis, biliary tract infections, peritonitis, and UTIs
Tetracylines	Tetracycline, doxycycline.	Inhibition of protein synthesis, through interfering with tRNA binding	*Chlamydia*, exacerbation of chronic bronchitis (*Haemophilus influenzae*), periodontal disease, acne, respiratory and genital *Mycoplasma* infections. Doxycycline in malaria prophylaxis

Class	Examples	Actions	Common uses
Macrolides	Erythromycin, clarithromycin	Prevent the translocation movement of the bacterial ribosome along the mRNA and prevent protein synthesis	Suitable alternative in patients who are allergic to penicillin. Respiratory infections, whooping cough, legionnaires' disease, *Campylobacter* enteritis
Aminoglycosides	Gentamicin	Irreversibly bind to the bacterial ribosomes leading to an inhibition of protein synthesis	Gentamicin is used in various infections such as septicaemia, meningitis, acute pyelonephritis and endocarditis
Sulphonamides and trimethoprim	Trimethoprim	Inhibition of folate synthesis and reduces the precursors of DNA and RNA	Pneumonia in AIDS patients, toxoplasmosis and nocardosis. Acute exacerbation of chronic bronchitis, otitis media and UTIs
Antituberculous	Rifampicin, isoniazid, prazinamide, ethambutol	Isoniazid and rifampicin most effective versus continually growing bacteria. Rifampicin versus intermittently dividing bacteria. Pyrazinamide versus rapidly dividing intracellular organisms hence most effective in first 2 months	Tuberculosis
Quinolones	Ciprofloxacin, ofloxacin	Inhibition of bacterial DNA gyrase	*Pseudomonas aeruginosa, Haemophilus influenzae, Campylobacter*
Others	Metronidazole	DNA damage due to toxic oxygen products	Trichomonal vaginosis, giardiasis, pseudomembranous colitis, tumours and rosacea
Antiviral	Aciclovir[a], famciclovir, zanamivir.	Aciclovir: inhibition of herpesvirus DNA polymerase. Zanamivir: a neuramidase inhibitor which prevents the entry and release of the viral particles from the host cells	Aciclovir: herpes simplex and herpes varicella. Zanamivir: influenza
Imidazoles	Clotrimazole[a]	Inhibition of P450-dependent demethylase which converts lanosterol to ergosterol; the accumulation of lanosterol disrupts fungal membrane	Fungal infections
Triazoles	Itraconazole, fluconazole[a]	As for imidazoles	Fungal infections

Class	Examples	Actions	Common uses
Other antifungal agents	Griseofulvin, terbinafine[a], amphotericin	Terbinafine inhibits the conversion of squalene to lanosterol, with the accumulation of squalene causing cell death. Griseofulvin: interferes with fungal microtubules and nucleic acid synthesis	Griseofulvin: suitable for tinea infections but not candidiasis
Endocrine			
Sulphonylureas	Glibenclamide, tolbutamide, gliclazide, glipizide, glimepiride	Inhibition of ATP-sensitive K-channels, leading to insulin release	Type 2 diabetes
Biguanides	Metformin	Activation of AMP kinase? This may increase glucose uptake and reduce glucose production by the liver. It may also suppress lipid synthesis and promote fatty acid oxidation	Type 2 diabetes with obesity
Thiazolidinediones	Rosiglitazone, pioglitazone	'Insulin sensitisers' which work by enhancing glucose utilization in tissues, and so reduce insulin resistance. They activate the gamma nuclear peroxisome proliferator-activated receptors (PPAR-γ)	Type 2 diabetes in combination with sulphonylurea or metformin
Antithyroid	Carbimazole	Decreases the production of thyroid hormones by inhibiting the iodination of thyroglobulin	Hyperthyroidism
Corticosteroids	Prednisolone, hydrocortisone[a], dexamethasone	A range of immunosuppressant actions, including production of lipocortin, which inhibits phospholipase A_2	Anti-inflammatory. Topical hydrocortisone for eczema. Dexamethasone for nerve compression in palliative care
Others			
Topical vitamin D_3 analogues	Calcipotriol	Acts on keratinocyte vitamin D receptors, and has antiproliferative actions and reduces epidermal proliferation	Psoriasis

Class	Examples	Actions	Common uses
Oral retinoids	Acitretin, tretinoin and isotretinoin	Binds to nuclear retinoic acid receptors and affects gene transcription, resulting in antiproliferative actions and normal keratinocyte maturation	Acitretin: psoriasis. Tretinoin and isotretinoin: acne
Folate antagonist	Methotrexate	Inhibits dihydrofolate reductase	Anticancer chemotherapy; immunosuppressant for psoriasis, asthma, Crohn's disease
Immunosuppressants	Aziothioprine, ciclosporin	Aziothioprine: inhibits nucleic acid synthesis and prevents lymphocyte production. Ciclosporin: prevents activation of T-lymphocytes	Immunosuppression including prevention of transplant rejection
5-aminosalicylates	Mesalazine, sulfasalazine	Yield 5-aminosalicylic acid, leading to inhibition of leukotriene and prostanoid formation, scavenging free radicals, and decreasing neutrophil chemotaxis	Ulcerative colitis, Crohn's disease

^{a}Certain preparations of these drugs are available OTC for certain indications.

GORD, gastro-oesophageal reflux disease; NSAID, non-steroidal anti-inflammatory drug; PGE_1, prostaglandin E_1; IBS, irritable bowel syndrome; AF, atrial fibrillation; CHF, chronic heart failure; DCT, distal convoluted tubule; VSM, vascular smooth muscle; LVF, left ventricular failure; MI, myocardial infarction; cGMP, cyclic guanosine monophosphate; ATP, adenosine triphosphate; HMG, hydroxymethylglutaryl; CoA, coenzyme A; CV, cerebrovascular; PE, pulmonary embolism; CVA, cerebrovascular accident; COX, cyclooxygenase; DVT, deep venous thrombosis; COPD, chronic obstructive pulmonary disease; GABA, gamma-aminobutyric acid; 5-HT, 5-hydroxytryptamine; UTIs, urinary tract infections; AIDS, acquired immune deficiency syndrome; AMP, adenosine monophosphate.

Index

Page numbers in **bold** indicate main discussions. Page numbers in *italics* refer to figures and tables.

anion-exchange resins *see* colestyramine
anogenital pruritis 425
antacids 113, 118
  and enteral feeds 27
  GORD 115
  interactions
    antihypertensives *156*
    antimalarials *410*
    quinolones 400
  and renal impairment 220
anthelminthics **408**, 409
  drug interactions *410*
anti-arrhythmics 178, *179*
anti-epileptic drugs *see* anticonvulsants
anti-inflammatory effects, NSAIDs 338, *339*, 340
antibiotics
  acne 420–421
  ADRs *65*, 131, 133, 402
  and alcohol *35*
  case studies 402–403
  concurrent disease and prescribing *396*, 397
  diarrhoea 133
  drug interactions *35*, **397**, *398–399*, 402
  gastrointestinal infections 132
  general counselling **397**, **399–401**
  inflammatory bowel disease 137
  monitoring **401**
  and oral contraceptives 96, 421
  practice points 402
  pregnancy and breast-feeding 397
  prophylaxis 390–391
  resistance **395**
    measures to limit 396–397
  sensitivities *392–393*
  targetting bacterial protein synthesis **391**, **394**
anticancer chemotherapy 372
  ADRs *65*, 75
  emesis 124
anticholinergics
  ADRs *68*, 82
  interactions with cannabis *37*
  psychiatric ADRs 77
  see also antimuscarinic activity, drugs with
anticoagulants 201, **202**
  ADRs *64*
  clinical use 202–203
  drug interactions **205–206**
  and enteral feeds 27
  MI *179*
    secondary prevention 178
  see also thromboembolic prophylaxis; warfarin
anticonvulsants
  ADRs *269*, 270, 271–272, 272–273
  bipolar disorder 287, 288
  drug interactions 271
  food–drug interactions *28*, *29*, *30*
  neuropathic pain **342–343**, 346
  withdrawal **272**

  see also phenytoin
antidepressants
  anxiety disorders 305, *306*, 307
  case studies 297–298
  combinations 289, *290*, 298
  counselling **294–296**
  drug choice *283–284*
    and concurrent illness **288–289**
  drug interactions **289**, *291–292*
  future developments 296
  monitoring **289**, **290**, **292**
  OTC considerations **292–294**
  seizure threshold, lowering 270
  treatment failure 286
  withdrawal 62, 292
  see also monoamine oxidase inhibitors (MAOIs);
    selective serotonin reuptake inhibitors (SSRIs);
    tricyclic antidepressants
antidiabetic agents and alcohol *35*
antiemetics **124**, **125**
  drug interactions 127
antifungals **422**, **423**
  food–drug interactions *29*
antihistamines
  ADRs *64*
  allergic reaction 238
  allergic rhinitis **234**, 235, 236
  and anaphylaxis 238
  counselling 128
  drug interactions *237*
  intravenous, anaphylaxis 238
  misuse 36, 37
  non-sedating 234, 236
  pruritis 143
  side-effects 125
antihypertensives
  and alcohol *35*
  drug interactions 153, *154*
  indications and contraindications *152*
  renal failure 217, 219
  resistance 153
  see also angiotensin converting enzyme (ACE)
    inhibitors; hypertension
antimalarials 359, **405–406**
  counselling 367, **406**, **407**
  drug interactions *410*
  monitoring 364
  pregnancy 409
  renal impairment 364
antimicrobial agents *see* antibiotics
antimotility agents, diarrhoea 132–133
antimuscarinic activity, drugs with
  allergic rhinitis **235**
  antipsychotics 322–323, 330
  asthma 244
  gastrointestinal effects 124, 133, 134
  side effects **65**, **68**, 125
  see also anticholinergics